Immunological Aspects of
Infectious Diseases

Immunological Aspects of Infectious Diseases

EDITED BY

GEORGE DICK

Professor of Pathology, London University
Honorary Consultant, Institute of Child Health
Assistant Director, British Postgraduate Medical Federation
Postgraduate Dean, S.W. Thames Regional Health Authority,
London, England

ISBN-13: 978-94-011-6193-0   e-ISBN-13: 978-94-011-6191-6
DOI: 10.1007/978-94-011-6191-6

Published by
MTP Press Limited
Falcon House
Lancaster, England

British Library Cataloguing in Publication Data
Immunological aspects of infectious diseases.

    1. Communicable diseases—Immunological aspects.
I. Dick, George
616.9   RC112

Contents

List of Contributors   vii

Preface   ix

1   Non-specific resistance to infection: *R. J. Elin*   1

2   Immune responses to fungal infections: *D. W. R. Mackenzie*   21

3   Normal immune responses to protozoal infections: *J. P. Ackers*   77

4   Defects in host-defence mechanisms: *J. L. Meakins and N. V. Christou*   117

5   Immunodeficiency: *A. R. Hayward*   151

6   Immune status of the malnourished host: *R. M. Suskind*   201

7   Allergy: *J. Pepys*   215

8   Mechanisms of anergy in infectious diseases: *W. E. Bullock*   269

9   Immune complexes and tissue injury: *P. Casali, L. H. Perrin and P.-H. Lambert*   295

10   Infection in the compromised host: *E. H. Nauta*   343

11   Autoimmunity in infectious disease: *L. E. Glynn*   389

12   Immunology of chronic infections: *J. L. Turk*   421

13   Immunology of persistent and recurrent viral infections: *C. J. Gibbs, Jr., G. J. Nemo and A. R. Diwan*   453

14   Immunology of slow infections: *J. M. Adams*   497

Index   513

List of Contributors

J. P. Ackers
Department of Medical Protozoology,
London School of Hygiene and Tropical
    Medicine,
London WC1E 7HT, UK

J. M. Adams
Professor Emeritus of Pediatrics,
School of Medicine,
The Center for Health Sciences,
Los Angeles, CA 90024, USA

W. E. Bullock
Professor and Director,
Division of Infectious Diseases,
University of Kentucky,
Lexington, KY 40506, USA

P. Casali
WHO Immunology Research and Training
    Centre,
Department of Medicine,
University of Geneva,
Hôpital Cantonal,
1211 Geneva 4, Switzerland

N. V. Christou
Department of Surgery and Microbiology,
McGill University,
Montreal, Quebec, Canada

G. Dick
Professor of Pathology,
University of London,
British Postgraduate Medical Federation,
London WC1N 3EJ, UK

A. R. Diwan
Laboratory of Central Nervous System
    Studies,
National Institute of Neurological and
    Communicative Disorders and Stroke,
National Institutes of Health,
Bethesda, MD 20014, USA

R. J. Elin
Chief,
Clinical Pathology Department,
National Institutes of Health,
Bethesda, MD 20014, USA

C. J. Gibbs, Jr.
Laboratory of Central Nervous System
    Studies,
National Institute of Neurological and
    Communicative Disorders and Stroke,
National Institutes of Health,
Bethesda, MD 20014, USA

L. E. Glynn
Former Director,
Kennedy Institute of Rheumatology,
London W6 7DW, UK

A. R. Hayward
Associate Professor of Pediatrics and
    Microbiology,
University of Colorado Medical School,
Denver, Colorado, USA

P.-H. Lambert
Centre de Transfusion,
Hôpital Cantonal,
CH-1211 Geneve 4, Switzerland

D. W. R. Mackenzie
Professor of Medical Mycology,
University of London,
London School of Hygiene and Tropical
    Medicine,
London WC1E 7HT, UK

J. L. Meakins
Assistant Professor of Surgery and
    Microbiology,
McGill University,
Montreal, Quebec, Canada

LIST OF CONTRIBUTORS

E. H. Nauta
Andreas Ziekenhuis,
Amsterdam, The Netherlands

G. J. Nemo
Laboratory of Central Nervous System
  Studies,
  National Institute of Neurological and
  Communicative Disorders and Stroke,
National Institutes of Health,
Bethesda, MD 20014, USA

J Pepys
Professor of Clinical Immunology,
University of London,
Cardiothoracic Institute,
Fulham Road,
London SW3, UK

L. H. Perrin
WHO Immunology Research and Training
  Centre,
Department of Medicine,
University of Geneva,
Hôpital Cantonal,
1211 Geneva 4, Switzerland

R. M. Suskind
Associate Professor of Pediatrics and
  Clinical Nutrition,
Clinical Research Center,
Massachusetts Institute of Technology,
Cambridge, MA 02142, USA

J. L. Turk
Professor of Pathology,
The Royal College of Surgeons,
University of London,
London WC2A 3PN, UK

Preface

In the first place may I say how grateful I and others are to those who have contributed chapters for this book; all of them are well known for their research on the subject on which they have written and each has indicated the background to his own specialist field by providing an extensive bibliography giving this book a total reference list of over 2,500.

Although there have been enormous advances in immunology over recent years, much of the new knowledge in relation to infectious diseases was scattered over the world's literature and is now brought together in a single volume. Furthermore, while a number of previously unknown infectious diseases have recently been discovered (e.g. Marburg and Lassa virus infections and Legionnaires' disease) to which many new techniques have been applied, there seemed to be no clear statement of the rationale for their use, or for their further exploitation in some of the more common infectious diseases which are discussed in this book.

The host–parasite interaction, as pointed out by R. J. Elin, may be of no consequence, or it may result in colonization, subclinical infection, symptomatic disease, or death, and the first chapter of this book focuses on some of the *non-specific* factors which may affect the response of the host to invading micro-organisms. The normal responses to infections with viruses and bacteria which are the stock-in-trade of those interested in infectious disease have not been separately treated but are summarized in the introduction to Chapter 10. On the other hand, while the host reactions to fungal infections mirrors that to other micro-organisms, the nature of these reactions are largely determined by the *type* of infection, which is discussed by D. W. R. Mackenzie, as well as individual immune responses in some of the commoner mycoses and the application of immunodiagnostic tests to the recognition of the diseases which they produce and their epidemiology.

To most of us, the objective of understanding the immunological response to a parasite is to increase our knowledge of the pathogenesis of the disease in question, so that it may be controlled or prevented by treatment or by vaccines. As far as protozoal infections are concerned, J. P. Ackers, in critically reviewing the immune responses to the major protozoal infections of man, reminds us that when the immunological techniques which had been so successful in the control of microbial infections were applied to the parasitic infections it was soon realized that there was something special about the immune response to protozoa. He discusses these responses in detail with particular reference to antigenic variations and persistence of the parasite in the host. This important contribution leads to many questions on the methods of controlling parasitic infections of man and animals which are such enormous problems in developing countries.

It is only in the last few years that various defects in host response have been identified and their importance defined, particularly in relation to recurrent infections. The *primary* immunodeficiencies are summarized by J. L. Meakins and N. V. Christou and are discussed in greater detail by A. R. Hayward, who has presented a comprehensive study of the clinical picture, cause, and where possible treatment of the known immunodeficient diseases of man. The recognition of these conditions must obviously increase as more and more becomes known of the minutiae of immune responses. Most of the immuno-deficiencies which are usually recognized are very often severe and have a fatal outcome from infection unless identified and treated. Some of them are extremely rare and have either a single gene inheritance or sometimes some other characteristic phenotypic manifestation. The importance of less serious immunodeficiencies in allergy and autoimmunity are now becoming apparent.

It is only recently that the importance of *acquired* defects of host defence. such as advanced age, major surgery, trauma, shock and diabetes and uraemia, etc. have been recognized and the part which they play in producing alterations in host resistance in some individuals has been appreciated. The investigations of persons likely to develop sepsis (with its related mortality) is a problem not only for physicians and surgeons, but is of importance to immunologists who may be able to identify the basic alterations in the host defences of these individuals by suitable immunological tests.

The individual family with a primary immunodeficiency is a fascinating but trivial problem compared with that of millions of children in the world who may be suffering from an immunological defect due to malnutrition. A number of immune parameters which are depressed in protein-calorie malnutrition are discussed by R. M. Suskind who points the way for further investigations of this most important problem with particular reference to the effect of protein-calorie malnutrition on polymorphonuclear leukocyte activity.

The recent research work of J. Pepys has provided a much more complete understanding of skin tests in allergy and of their clinical value and interpretation. While IgE is well recognized as the main mast cell sensitizing antibody, evidence is now accumulating of the facilitating effect of IgA in IgE-antigen reactions and also of a heat stable, short-term sensitizing (STS) antibody in the IgG complex which is capable of passive sensitization of mast cells for only a few hours: this observation throws new light on the interpretation of skin-prick tests which are discussed in detail. Further studies of type III reactions are now leading to much greater understanding of delayed hypersensitivity reactions and the significance of this type of reaction in bacterial, viral, fungal and protozoal disease. To all this has been added the newer techniques which are now available for antibody assays.

At the opposite pole to *allergy* is *anergy*, which was the term which Von Pirquet applied 'quite generally to the absence of clinical manifestation of reaction'. Anergy must be one of the most poorly understood subjects in immunology, however as W. E. Bullock points out, the recent demonstration of an immunoregulatory control system in mammals which exerts suppressor effects on the immune response has provided some insights into its mechanism. This is discussed in detail with reference to infectious diseases, paying particular attention to the clinical phenomenon of delayed-type hypersensitivity and cell-mediated immunity: Bullock concludes that continued investigations along these lines may lead to the concept of 'positive anergy'.

In addition to the tissue injury produced by an infectious agent *per se* or which results from cellular responses to it, there are now many examples of injury associated with humoral antibody which are largely elicited by immune complexes. The nature and detection of these immune complexes and the literature on this subject are discussed and reviewed by P. Casali, L. H. Perrin and P.-H. Lambert.

Infection in the compromised host has been reviewed by E. H. Nauta who after summarizing the normal defence mechanisms of the body describes disturbances of these mechanisms and their clinical manifestations, prevention and treatment with particular reference to bacterial, viral, fungal and protozoal infections in acute leukaemia, in Hodgkin's disease and other myeloproliferative diseases and in organ transplant patients, etc. To all this he brings his personal experience of the diagnosis and prognosis of infections in the compromised host.

Autoimmunity implies loss of tolerance and L. E. Glynn discusses the ways in which infectious diseases may interfere with immunological tolerance and overcome it. T cells are more easily rendered tolerant than B cells and natural tolerance to most autochthonous antigens is of the T-cell variety; for an infection to induce an autoimmune reaction it would only be necessary for T cells to be activated. Probably the most important cause of autoimmunization is due to cross-reactions of antigens of the parasite and the host: the chemical characteristics of these antigens and the enhancement of the immune response by micro-organisms and other substances is discussed in detail. The whole story is exemplified with a discussion of autoimmune phenomena associated with infectious diseases such as those due to *T. pallidum*, and to streptococci in relation to rheumatic fever and to glomerulonephritis. Although infections with viruses (because of the nature of these agents) might be expected to be the most likely micro-organism to be associated with autoimmune disease, so far there is no direct evidence of their role in this respect in many of the virus diseases where they are strongly suspected.

The chapter on chronic infections by J. L. Turk brings together many of the facets of the immunological aspects of infectious disease which are discussed in earlier chapters. Attention is focused on the role of bacteria in chronic diseases, and particular attention is paid to the clinical spectrum of leprosy, tuberculosis, syphilis and also to some parasitic and fungal infections.

In the final chapters C. J. Gibbs and his colleagues and J. M. Adams discuss the role of viruses in chronic, persistent and recurrent viral infections and in slow infections. The pre-requisites for chronic infections are the ability of the infecting agent to avoid host-defence mechanisms and second to be of such low toxicity or invasiveness that the host can survive a prolonged state of parasitism. The recent *in vivo* and *in vitro* studies which have led to a better understanding of persistent viral infections and the role of the immune response in these infections in man are discussed.

J. M. Adams takes us beyond both conventional and unconventional 'viruses' towards the immunology of diseases not yet known to be caused by classical infective agents. The understanding of these conditions has made enormous strides in recent years based on the appreciation that scrapie was caused by an agent which produced a similar histopathology to that of Kuru. Further study of these slow infections may lead to an understanding of diseases such as multiple sclerosis and of the disease which finally affects most of us – old age – if not cerebral dementia.

G.D.

1
Non-specific Resistance to Infection

R. J. ELIN

1.1 INTRODUCTION   1

1.2 VITAMINS   2
   1.2.1 *Vitamin A*   2
   1.2.2 *Vitamin C*   3
   1.2.3 *Vitamin E*   5

1.3 MINERALS   5
   1.3.1 *Iron*   6
   1.3.2 *Zinc and copper*   8

1.4 MICROBIAL PRODUCTS   9
   1.4.1 *Bacterial endotoxins*   9
   1.4.2 *Adjuvants*   12

1.5 THE SPLEEN   12

1.6 SUMMARY   13

1.1 INTRODUCTION

The ability of vertebrates to combat invasion by micro-organisms can be divided into two different mechanisms: a specific immunity based upon the development of humoral (antibodies) or cellular factors and a so-called natural or non-specific resistance that is not unique to the invading micro-organism. The remaining chapters in this book focus on several aspects of the first mechanism, i.e. the influence of the immune system in host resistance to infectious diseases.

The defence mechanisms of the body against pathogenic micro-organisms that are not mediated by the specific action of the immune system comprise the host's non-specific resistance to infection. These mechanisms include both humoral and cellular components. The inhibition of infection by non-specific mechanisms is affected by substances that alter humoral or cellular factors of the host to induce the non-specific resistance. Usually, these substances do not directly affect the infecting micro-organism. These substances are termed non-specific since they induce protection against a spectrum of micro-organisms. A large number of humoral and cellular factors may enhance the resistance of the host to infection, but only a few of these factors have been studied in sufficient detail to establish a relationship to non-specific resistance to infection. The remainder of this chapter will focus on three groups of compounds—vitamins, minerals and microbial products—and an organ, the spleen, which have clearly been shown to be related to non-specific resistance to infection.

1.2 VITAMINS

The experimental evidence that vitamins A, C and E are required to maintain normal host defence mechanisms against infection or induce non-specific resistance to infection is reviewed below.

1.2.1 Vitamin A

An excess of vitamin A induces non-specific resistance to infection, and a deficiency of vitamin A causes an enhanced infection with a challenge organism in experimental animals. The injection of vitamin A into mice produced significant protection compared with the control group when these animals were challenged with either *Pseudomonas aeruginosa*, *Listeria monocytogenes* or *Candida albicans*[1]. Those animals treated with vitamin A and infected with *P. aeruginosa* cleared the bacteria from the blood more rapidly than the control group. The vitamin A had no effect on the growth of these organisms *in vitro* at concentrations greater than that achieved in the experimental animal. Thus parenteral administration of vitamin A enhances the resistance of mice to challenge with these bacteria and fungal micro-organisms.

In deficiency states of vitamin A, bacterial, viral and parasitic infections are more pronounced. A deficiency of vitamin A appears to enhance the virulence of *Mycobacterium tuberculosis* and other bacteria in man and the chick[2-4]. The response of the chick to challenge with Newcastle disease virus is impaired with dietary vitamin A deficiency[5]. The rate of parasitaemia is significantly increased in vitamin A-deficient rodents challenged with either *Plasmodium berghei* or *Trypanosoma musculi*[6,7]. Thus a deficiency of vitamin A impairs host defence mechanisms for a variety of micro-organisms.

The mechanisms by which vitamin A increases host resistance to infection have not been defined, although vitamin A is an effective adjuvant[8,9] and has been shown to labilize lysosomal membranes[10], both of which may affect the response of a host to an infectious agent. It is well established that a deficiency of vitamin A induces squamous metaplasia of respiratory epithelia which may alter host defence mechanisms for respiratory infections[11]. However, studies of the relationship between vitamin A and infection have been limited almost entirely to experimental animals, and the clinical importance of these experimental findings is unknown. Since a chronic intake of vitamin A greatly in excess of the requirement clearly results in a toxic syndrome in man known as hypervitaminosis A, further investigation will be needed to determine the possible clinical relevance, the spectrum of micro-organisms, and the mechanism of non-specific resistance before this vitamin can be recommended therapeutically[12].

1.2.2 Vitamin C

The medical literature for the past 35 years has reflected the controversy over the efficacy of vitamin C at preventing or altering the symptoms of the common cold and enhancing resistance to infectious diseases. The early clinical trials assessing the value of vitamin C as a prophylactic agent against the common cold and other infectious diseases were more positive than negative[13-18]. Some of these studies would have been considered poorly controlled because they did not employ the techniques of randomization and double blinding[13-15].

In 1970, Professor Linus Pauling published his now famous book entitled, *Vitamin C and the Common Cold*[19]. In the book, Pauling emphasized that vitamin C is indeed a 'vitamin' for only a few species; an exogenous source of vitamin C is required only by man, other primates, guinea-pigs, flying mammals, and certain highly evolved birds[20]. These animals must obtain vitamin C in the food they eat because they lack the enzyme L-gulonolactone oxidase which catalyses the final step in the microsomal conversion of D-glucuronic acid to L-ascorbic acid[21]. It was noted that man has a relatively low concentration of vitamin C compared with animals that can synthesize the vitamin, and these animals with an endogenous source of vitamin C seem to be free from the common cold[22]. Thus the implication is that dietary supplements of vitamin C might alter the response or prevent the common cold.

During the past 7 years, the intense public interest in this area has mandated several clinical trials which have employed techniques of randomization and double blind[23-30]. These trials were conducted by four different groups of investigators. Three studies have now been published by the group in Toronto, Canada[23-25]. The first study was conducted specifically to evaluate Professor Pauling's claim that the intake of 1 g of vitamin C per day would substantially reduce the frequency and duration of colds[23]. The results of this study showed that the average number of colds per subject was not statistically different between the two groups; however, those on vitamin C experienced 30% fewer days' disability and this difference was significant ($p < 0.001$) compared with the placebo group. The second trial was designed to examine the effect of prophylactic and therapeutic dosages of vitamin C, but the results were less than clear-cut, in part due to the complexity of the experimental design[24]. The third trial assessed dosage. Subjects were randomly allocated to one of three treatment groups: placebo, 500 mg of vitamin C weekly and 1500 mg of vitamin C daily. Subjects in both vitamin groups experienced less severe illness than subjects in the placebo group ($p < 0.05$). The authors concluded that supplementary vitamin C can reduce the burden of winter illness, but dietary supplementation could be done weekly with an amount less than 1 g[25].

A group in England assessed the prophylactic value of placebo and 200 mg or 500 mg of vitamin C in school children over a 9-month period. They found that catarrhal cold symptoms were reduced by over 50% in girls taking 500 mg of vitamin C daily, but there was no consistent effect in boys[26,27].

A third group studied Navajo school children in Arizona[28,29]. The first trial showed no difference between treatment groups in the number of respiratory illnesses, but those children receiving vitamin C had fewer days of morbidity[28]. A second trial to corroborate the first trial showed no differences in the number of children becoming ill, the number of episodes or the mean illness duration between the placebo and vitamin C groups[29].

The fourth group conducted a trial among employees at the National Institutes of Health[30]. In this trial, the incidence of colds was not statistically different between the two groups, but the group receiving vitamin C had a significant reduction in morbidity. The validity of this study is questionable since many of the subjects were aware of their treatment group.

The results of these several clinical trials fail to give a clear mandate for the prophylactic use of vitamin C. The data somewhat suggest that vitamin C does not alter the incidence of upper respiratory infections, but that it may reduce the severity of symptoms and the duration of illness.

Studies in experimental animals support the theory that vitamin C induces non-specific resistance to infection. Vitamin C deficiency in guinea-pigs creates a higher incidence of bacterial pneumonia and septicaemia[31]. Mortality in these animals is increased following challenge with *Staphylococcus aureus*, *Streptococcus pneumoniae* or *Streptococcus pyogenes*. In addition, increased dietary vitamin C markedly reduces mortality in guinea-pigs infected with *Mycobacterium tuberculosis* and increases resistance in these animals to re-infection[32]. Thus in the guinea-pig vitamin C appears to afford a degree of protection to a variety of bacteria.

What are the possible mechanisms by which vitamin C enhances resistance to infection? Vitamin C potentiates chemotaxis of normal polymorphonuclear leukocytes[33]. Vitamin C has been shown to stimulate hexose monophosphate shunt activity in resting polymorphonuclear leukocytes and macrophages *in vitro* to a similar activity to that seen following phagocytosis[34]. These enhancements of leukocyte function by vitamin C may correct the defect in Chediak-Higashi syndrome[35], in which patients suffer frequent and severe pyogenic infections that are secondary to abnormal function of polymorphonuclear leukocytes. The impaired bacterial activity of the leukocytes appears to be related to delayed delivery of lysosomal contents into phagosomes[36], a functional defect which may be related to abnormal microtubular assembly in polymorphonuclear leukocytes in this syndrome[37]. The treatment of leukocytes from patients with Chediak–Higashi syndrome with agents that increase cyclic 3',5'-guanosine monophosphate (cyclic GMP) concentration will improve microtubular function[37]. Studies *in vitro* have demonstrated that vitamin C will increase cyclic GMP concentrations in monocytes[33]. In a case report, a patient with Chediak–Higashi syndrome was treated with vitamin C, and the defect in chemotactic migration and bactericidal activity of leukocytes was corrected to normal[35]. Thus there is evidence that vitamin C affects leukocyte function, which is a prime element in host-defence mechanisms against infectious diseases.

1.2.3 Vitamin E

A relationship of vitamin E to resistance to infection has been documented. Supplementing a standard chick ration with either vitamin E or vitamin A increased the protection of 6-week-old immunized chickens against *E. coli* infection by decreasing mortality from about 40% to 5%[38]. Interestingly, the combination of the two vitamins did not give as much protection as either vitamin alone. Further studies will be needed to define the significance of vitamin E in non-specific resistance to infection.

1.3 MINERALS

Serum concentrations and metabolic homeostasis for several minerals (iron, zinc, copper, chromium, cobalt, gallium, iodine and manganese) are altered in infectious processes[39,40]. For several of these minerals additional research is needed to establish a possible link to host-defence mechanisms. However, studies concerning infection-induced alterations in iron, zinc, and copper metabolism have now advanced beyond the purely descriptive stages and suggest that these elements have a role in host-defence mechanisms.

1.3.1 Iron

There is a growing body of experimental and clinical evidence to suggest that the iron status of an individual may affect his resistance to infection. I will discuss initially some of the studies *in vitro* which indicate the importance of iron in infection and then evaluate hyperferraemia, hypoferraemia and resistance to infection.

Iron is essential for bacterial growth. Iron-chelating agents cause a selective inhibition of DNA synthesis in living cells *in vitro* which suggests that iron plays a crucial role in mitosis[41]. Since iron is needed for cell division, it is not surprising that comparable quantities of iron are required for the growth of plant, animal and microbial cells[42]. Thus, if micro-organisms are going to invade a host successfully, they must acquire iron from the host for continued normal growth.

Although the quantity of iron in some host fluids, such as milk and plasma, is more than adequate for microbial growth, the amount of free ionic iron in these body fluids available to micro-organisms for normal growth is too low by a factor of several thousand, because iron-binding proteins present in healthy human hosts (such as lactoferrin and transferrin) are present in sufficient quantity to bind all iron. This is due to the very high association constant (10^{30}) for iron which is characteristic of these iron-binding proteins[42]. Over three decades ago, Schade and Caroline were first to describe the prevention of bacterial growth by iron-binding proteins in egg white and plasma which was reversed by the addition of iron in excess of the binding capacity of these proteins[43,44]. Several investigators have confirmed that the inhibition of growth of a variety of bacteria and fungi by normal serum can be reversed by the addition of iron[45,46]. Thus the availability of free iron in body fluids determines the growth potential for most micro-organisms in these fluids.

Many pathogenic bacteria synthesize iron-chelating agents (siderophores) which can remove iron from the iron-binding proteins. These microbial siderophores have association constants for iron of 10^{30} or more, and at least some of them are capable of withdrawing iron from 30% saturated transferrin[42]. Some of the siderophores have been chemically characterized as phenolates, hydroxamates, or lipopolysaccharides[47]. Thus the resolution of the contest between the invading micro-organism and the defence mechanisms of the host depends upon the iron concentration and iron metabolism of the host.

From the above *in vitro* observations it could be postulated that states of increased iron availability might predispose to infection. Conversely, iron deficiency might protect the individual against infection. The actual clinical situation is considerably more complex and not yet clear.

In a variety of clinical conditions marked by iron overload, the incidence of infection appears to be increased. Hyperferraemic states occur in individuals who have the following: (1) occult or overt haemolytic anaemia, (2) destruction of liver cells containing ferritin, and (3) an overload of iron from exogenous sources. One of the best examples of haemolytic anaemia is sickle cell disease. Bacterial infection is still the single most common cause of death in sickle cell disease, and the incidence of bacterial meningitis is 300 times greater than in normal siblings[48]. Increased susceptibility to salmonella infections, bartonellosis and malaria is known to be associated with the haemolysis present in sickle cell disease[49]. Systemic salmonellosis is common in persons with viral hepatitis[42]. Following a single injection of iron sorbitol citrate, patients with chronic pyelonephritis had an exacerbation of their infection as documented by increased numbers of white blood cells in urine[50]. A similar increase in white blood cells did not occur in non-infected controls or in patients with non-infectious renal disease[50]. On the other hand, patients with an iron overload due to haemochromatosis or multiple blood transfusions are not notably prone to infection[51].

Hypotransferrinaemic states with an increased percentage saturation may predispose to infection. The incidence of bacterial infection is far higher in children with kwashiorkor (reduced transferrin concentration) than in normal children[52]. There is evidence that the administration of iron to patients with abnormally low transferrin concentrations may result in overwhelming infection and death[52]. Thus in several diseases an increase in the percentage iron saturation of transferrin predisposes the host to infection.

The incidence of infection in iron-deficient human populations is increased rather than decreased. The *in vitro* data suggest that hypoferraemia should be advantageous to the host and disadvantageous to the microbial invader. However, there is widespread belief with some supporting data that iron deficiency predisposes to infection[53].

Several clinical surveys have attempted to correlate the iron status of an individual with the risk of infection. Infection has been reported as the most common symptom for which iron-deficient children seek medical advice[54]. The World Health Organization has reported that individuals with nutritional anaemia tend to have a higher incidence of infections[55]. Several studies have been made of iron supplementation; the first longitudinal study of the effects of iron supplementation in the first year of life was reported in 1928 among infants from low-income families in London[56]. A modest decrease in the number of episodes of bronchitis and gastroenteritis in iron-supplemented children was reported, but, as might be expected, the study was not double blind and defects in the design of the study permit alternative interpretations[56]. The frequency of respiratory infections was reported to be significantly less during the first year of life in infants from Chicago's inner city who were given an iron-fortified formula[57]. However, criteria for the diagnosis of respiratory tract infection were not defined, and precautions to minimize bias on the part of the observers were not taken. Other studies have failed to show a relationship between iron deficiency and the incidence of infection[58,59]. The third possibility, that iron deficiency may protect against infection, has also been reported[60]. Sixty-seven older children and adults with severe iron deficiency anaemia had a lower frequency of bacterial infections than did 43 patients with other types of severe anaemia. However, the study did not include an evaluation of any control group of healthy subjects, which compromises the interpretation of the results. The differences in results among these clinical surveys may be related to different degrees of iron deficiency in the study populations and an effect of iron deficiency on other host-defence mechanisms.

The immune response and leukocyte function are altered by iron deficiency. Lymphocyte transformation was decreased in 12 iron-deficient patients when purified protein derivative (PPD) was used as the antigen[61]. In addition, the production of macrophage migration inhibition factor was reduced when lymphocytes were stimulated with *Candida* but not when PPD was employed. An important control for the study, i.e. characterization of lymphocyte function after correction of iron deficiency, was not done. Thus it is possible that differences in lymphocyte response reflect differences in the exposure of tested subjects to environmental antigens rather than differences in functional capacity. Lymphopaenia and depressed lymphocyte transformation response in iron-deficient subjects have been reported, which returned to normal after correction of their iron status[62]. Other groups have also reported deficient cellular immunity in iron-deficient subjects that was corrected after the administration of oral or parenteral iron[63,64]. There is a report that granulocyte function is impaired in iron deficiency[65]. In that report. the rate of killing of *Staphylococcus albus* by granulocytes was decreased in eight of nine iron-deficient patients, with a return of bacteriocidal rates in six subjects to the normal range following the administration of iron. However, iron deficiency was not the sole determinant of compromised granulocyte function, since four patients without evidence of iron deficiency had subnormal bacteriocidal rates. Thus secondary effects of iron deficiency on the immune system and leukocyte function will alter host-defence mechanisms to invading micro-organisms.

Much work has been done in an attempt to define the relationship between iron metabolism and resistance to infection. The literature tends to support two apparently contradictory positions: that both an increase and a decrease in iron concentration may predispose the host to infectious diseases. It is clear that a great deal of work will be needed to define the role of iron in the conflict between micro-organism and host.

1.3.2 Zinc and copper

A definite alteration in serum zinc and copper concentrations occurs during infection, which may or may not be related to resistance to infection. Serum zinc concentrations closely parallel those of iron, i.e. the serum zinc concentration declines rapidly and appreciably during both generalized and inflammatory reactions. Patients with bacterial, viral, parasitic, and rickettsial infections have been confirmed to have reduced serum zinc concentrations[39,66]. Although serum zinc concentrations decline as rapidly as those of serum iron, the magnitude of the depression in serum zinc is not generally as great; zinc concentrations decline approximately 70% and iron concentrations 50% of normal. Hepatitis is an exception in that serum iron increases due to the liberation of ferritin, but serum zinc concentrations decline to values comparable to those observed in other types of acute infection[67].

Serum copper concentrations increase during infections and inflammatory reactions with a concomitant increase of the copper-binding protein ceruloplasmin[68]. The increase in serum copper concentration is believed to be secondary to an increased hepatic synthesis and release of ceruloplasmin[69]. The mechanism and significance of the accelerated production of ceruloplasmin are not known, but the phenomenon is similar to the accelerated production of many other specific serum proteins during infection or other inflammatory states. The term 'acute phase reactant proteins' has been applied to this group of proteins which includes haptoglobin, α_1-antitrypsin, fibrinogen, C-reactive protein and others. The increase of these proteins in serum appears to be mediated by a protein molecule termed 'leukocytic endogenous mediator' which appears to arise from phagocytizing cells[69]. The relationship, if any, between zinc, copper, and acute phase reactant proteins and resistance to infection has yet to be determined.

1.4 MICROBIAL PRODUCTS

Two classes of microbial products, namely bacterial endotoxins and adjuvants derived from mycobacteria, have been shown to enhance non-specific resistance to infection in experimental animals. In addition, low molecular weight synthetic adjuvants which have a chemical structure similar to portions of the mycobacteria cell wall will be discussed.

1.4.1 Bacterial endotoxins

The concept of non-specific resistance to infection arose more than 80 years ago. In 1893 Klein noted that 'six different species of bacteria contain in their protoplasm a poisonous principle, which appears to be the same for all species'[70]. He recognized the non-specific nature of this phenomenon when stating that 'the refractory condition produced by intraperitoneal injection of a non-fatal dose of one of the above six species holds good against all the other five'. Two years later Sobernheimm showed that a temporary immunity to cholera infection could be produced in guinea-pigs by injections of *Escherichia coli*[71]. In 1955, Rowley made the observation that mice had a greatly reduced susceptibility to several different strains of *E. coli* if the mice had been injected with *E. coli* cell walls 24 hours before challenge with the bacteria[72]. The active component in the *E. coli* cell wall which induced the non-specific resistance to infection was subsequently shown to be endotoxin[73,74]. Since that time, several investigators have shown that a variety of bacterial endotoxins will induce resistance to infection with the following challenge organisms: bacteria (*E. coli, Klebsiella, Streptococcus pneumoniae, Pseudomonas, Salmonellae*, and *Staphylococci*)[72,75–77], fungi (*Candida* and *Cryptococcus*)[78–80], parasites (*Plasmodia* and *Prypanosoma*)[81,82] and viruses (*Ectromelia* and Newcastle disease virus)[83–85].

Bacterial endotoxins are biologically active compounds present in the cell wall of Gram-negative bacteria. Using chemical methods of extraction and purification, bacterial endotoxins can be obtained as relatively pure chemical complexes that consist mainly of lipids, polysaccharides and small quantities of amino acids[86]. The chemical name, lipopolysaccharide (LPS), has been used synonymously with bacterial endotoxin. The lipid part of the LPS molecule is primarily responsible for the biological activity of this compound, including the induction of non-specific resistance to infection[86].

The mechanism of non-specific resistance to infection secondary to endotoxin administration is unclear. Bacterial endotoxins have myriad biological activities that affect all systems of the body. The administration of endotoxin induces changes in granulocytes, body temperature, mineral metabolism, vascular reactivity, coagulation and other systems, as well as changes in resistance to infection. Thus the resistance to infection has been attributed to several different cellular and non-cellular mechanisms.

The changes in host susceptibility to infection following the administration of endotoxin have been shown to follow a consistent pattern. During the first few hours following the administration of endotoxin, there is an increase in host susceptibility to infection, the so-called 'negative phase'. This is followed by a prolonged increase in non-specific resistance to infection that reaches a maximum approximately 24 hours after the administration of endotoxin in experimental animals[87,88]. This is followed by a return to approximately the same immunity to infection as in control animals, but a second period of enhanced resistance to infection occurs at approximately the sixth day after endotoxin administration[87,88]. In addition, repeated administration of endotoxin results in the development of tolerance to several systemic responses such as fever, lethality and granulocytopenic effect, but tolerance does not occur for non-specific resistance to infection[76]. In other studies, the rate of growth of the challenge organism is reduced in several tissues when animals are treated with endotoxin[89].

The effect of endotoxin on cellular components, i.e. granulocytes and the reticuloendothelial system (RES), has been implicated in non-specific resistance to infection. Endotoxin induces a transient leukopenia followed by marked granulocytosis. The granulocytosis is dependent on an adequate bone marrow reserve of granulocytes and on a normal granulocyte-releasing mechanism[90]. Studies *in vitro* have shown that LPS can induce a series of metabolic changes in granulocytes resembling those associated with phagocytosis[91]. Since granulocytes are a prime factor in the control of invading micro-organisms, the granulocytosis and increased metabolic activity of these cells induced by LPS may significantly alter the infectious process. On the other hand, LPS is a potent stimulator of RES activity, as shown by enhanced blood clearance of colloidal carbon[92]. This alteration in the activity of the RES has been related to the enhancement of non-specific resistance[92].

Two humoral factors, C-reactive protein (CRP) and serum iron, have been linked to non-specific resistance induced by endotoxin. The concentration of CRP is significantly increased in experimental animals 24 hours after the administration of endotoxin[93]. Studies *in vitro* show that CRP can agglutinate and reduce the growth rate of bacteria[94]. These observations suggest a possible role of CRP for endotoxin-induced non-specific resistance.

The effect of iron on non-specific resistance to infection has already been discussed. A relationship between serum iron concentration and endotoxin in non-specific resistance has been shown *in vitro* and *in vivo*. Studies *in vitro* have shown a positive correlation between the growth of micro-organisms and the percentage iron saturation of the serum obtained daily from mice for 10 days after endotoxin or saline injection[88]. Studies *in vivo* in which iron was injected into control and endotoxin-treated mice at the time of challenge showed that the rate of mortality of the mice was directly related to the concentration of iron injected[88]. The endotoxin-induced non-specific resistance was negated and reversed by iron administration. Thus the above studies suggest that endotoxin-induced changes in iron metabolism influence the mechanism of non-specific resistance to infection.

The induction of non-specific resistance by endotoxins is not related to some of the other biological activities of these molecules. Endotoxins can be detoxified by alkylation (succinylation or phthalylation). Sodium phthalate derivatives of several endotoxin preparations have been shown to be at least 10 000 times less toxic than the parent endotoxin when assayed by pyrogenicity in rabbits and by lethality in mice rendered susceptible to endotoxins by actinomycin D[95]. These detoxified endotoxins retain their adjuvant activity, capacity to protect mice against lethal radiation and blast transformation of murine B-lymphocytes. However, these alkylated preparations do not induce non-specific resistance to infection in mice[95]. Since endotoxins are potent mitogens of murine B-lymphocytes, several non-toxic B-cell mitogens were assayed for the induction of non-specific resistance, but these non-toxic mitogens did not protect mice[96]. Thus the various biological functions of endotoxins can be separated and are not uniformly related to their toxicity.

1.4.2   Adjuvants

A non-toxic, water-soluble adjuvant has been prepared by lysozyme digestion of delipidated cells from *Mycobacterium smegmatis*[97]. The intravenous administration of this adjuvant to mice induced resistance to infection with a fungus, a Gram-negative bacterium and a Gram-positive bacterium[98]. This adjuvant did not afford protection when the animals were challenged with a malarial parasite. It induced non-specific resistance when administered just prior to challenge and did not significantly change the serum iron concentration. These differences clearly separate the type of resistance induced by this compound from that induced by bacterial endotoxins.

The minimal structure (N-acetyl-muramyl-L-alanyl-D-isoglutamin) capable of duplicating the activity of mycobacteria in Freund's complete adjuvant has been synthesized[99,100]. In contrast to mycobacterial adjuvant preparations which function only in the form of water-in-oil emulsions, this compound and synthetic analogues in aqueous solutions augment the humoral immune responses of mice[100]. Recently, some of these synthetic adjuvants and analogues have induced non-specific resistance to infection in mice when given orally, intravenously or interperitoneally[101]. Many of these synthetic compounds do not produce the toxic effects associated with bacterial endotoxins. It is hoped that further investigations with these synthetic compounds may eventually lead to clinical trials of their efficacy for producing non-specific resistance in humans.

1.5   THE SPLEEN

An innate form of non-specific resistance to infection is present in the spleen. The spleen has been a rather mysterious organ ever since the time of Galen who thought it was a source of black bile and melancholy. Although its function in humans is still poorly understood, studies during the last decade have clearly defined the importance of the spleen in resistance to infection. A series of clinical studies have documented the fact that splenectomy or functional asplenia predisposes an individual to infection with bacteria, parasites, viruses or fungi[102-107]. In an analysis of 2796 asplenic patients from 23 reports, Singer noted that sepsis occurred in 119 (4.25%) patients, and 71 (2.52%) of them died because of the septic disease[108]. Death from post-splenectomy sepsis was found to be 200 times as prevalent as death due to sepsis in the population at large[108]. If the spleen was surgically removed, the interval between surgery and infection was shorter (weeks to months) in infants than in older children and adults (as long as 14 years). However, there does not seem to be a time limit beyond which an asplenic person may be considered safe from infection.

Bacterial infection after splenectomy can be fulminant with large numbers of bacteria invading the blood and cerebrospinal fluid, sometimes leading to septic shock and disseminated intravascular coagulation[104]. In approximately 50% of the cases, the offending organism is *Streptococcus pneumoniae*, whereas the remaining 50% of the infections are primarily caused by *Haemophilus influenzae, Neisseria meningitidis, Staphylocuccus aureus, Escherichia coli,* and group A *Streptococci*[103, 108–110].

The detrimental effects of surgical or functional asplenia are probably related to the role of the spleen in the clearance of particulate antigens and impaired production of specific antibodies and other substances that activate phagocytosis. The spleen may act partly as a mechanical filter since it is efficient at clearing particles of approximately 1 micron in size. Although the mechanisms associated with these events are unclear, studies in experimental animals verify the primary importance of the spleen in the clearing and trapping of cellular antigens[111]. Thus, without a functioning spleen, a major mechanism for clearing bacteria from the blood is absent.

Removal of the spleen has little effect on the net functional potential of antibody synthesis, although it has been established that certain antibody concentrations are decreased. Splenectomized animals have deficient and delayed production of opsonizing 19S antibodies during a primary response, and during a secondary response production of 7S antibodies is also deficient[112, 113]. Children who have been splenectomized have decreased serum concentrations of IgM compared with controls, and a fall has been observed in the post-splenectomy period[113, 114]. In addition, the spleen is the site of production of a non-specific serum immunoglobulin that coats neutrophils and enhances their bacterial phagocytic activity[115]. This immunoglobulin is an IgG that on tryptic digestion releases a bioactive tetrapeptide named Tuftsin after Tufts University[116]. Tuftsin is capable of stimulating phagocytosis and seems to be lacking in the sera of splenectomized subjects. Thus the spleen has important cellular and humoral factors that provide the host with non-specific resistance to infection.

1.6 SUMMARY

Host–parasite interaction may be of no consequence or may result in colonization, subclinical infection, symptomatic disease or death. The factors that determine who among us is chosen to follow one path rather than the other remain poorly defined. The first chapter of this book has focused on four areas (vitamins, minerals, microbiological products and the spleen) that may significantly affect the response of a host to an invading microorganism. The spleen provides innate non-specific resistance to infection. Nutrition and disease processes determine the concentrations of certain vitamins and minerals which are important for the normal resistance of a host to infection. Certain microbiological products can enhance the resistance of an animal to an infectious agent. It is this area that holds the most promise for the future, since agents may be discovered that can be given to a host to enhance his resistance to infection. Future research will undoubtedly define other important areas that induce or influence non-specific resistance to infection in the host.

ACKNOWLEDGEMENTS

I am most grateful to Dr Sheldon M. Wolff for his guidance and support of our research efforts about factors affecting resistance to infection. Sincere thanks are due to Mrs Elsa Elkin for her excellent assistance in preparing this manuscript.

References

1. Cohen, B. E. and Elin, R. J. (1974). Vitamin A-induced non-specific resistance to infection. *J. Infect. Dis.*, **129**, 597
2. Getz, H. R., Long, E. R. and Henderson, H. J. (1951). A study of the relation of nutrition to the development of tuberculosis – Influence of ascorbic acid and vitamin A. *Am. Rev. Tuberc.*, **64**, 381
3. Solotorovsky, M., Squibb, R. L., Wogan, G. N., Siegel, H. and Gala, R. (1961). The effect of dietary fat and vitamin A on avian tuberculosis in chicks. *Am. Rev. Respir. Dis.*, **84**, 226
4. Valenton, M. J. and Tan, R. V. (1975). Secondary ocular bacterial infection in hypovitaminosis A xerophthalmia. *Am. J. Ophthalmol.*, **80**, 673
5. Bang, F. B., Bang, B. G. and Foard, M. (1975). Acute Newcastle viral infection of the upper respiratory tract of the chicken. II. The effect of diets deficient in vitamin A on the pathogenesis of the infection. *Am. J. Pathol.*, **78**, 417
6. Krishnan, S., Krishnan, A. D., Mustafa, A. S., Talwar, G. P. and Ramalingaswami, V. (1976). Effect of vitamin A and undernutrition on the susceptibility of rodents to a malarial parasite *Plasmodium berghei*. *J. Nutr.*, **106**, 784
7. Lee, C. M., Aboko-Cole, G. F. and Fletcher, J. (1976). Effect of malnutrition on susceptibility of mice to *Trypanosoma musculi*: vitamin A deficiency. *Z. Parasitenkd.*, **49**, 1
8. Dresser, D. W. (1968). Adjuvanticity of vitamin A. *Nature*, **217**, 527
9. Jurin, M. and Tannock, I. F. (1972). Influence of vitamin A on the immunological response. *Immunology*, **23**, 283
10. Dingle, J. T. (1963). Action of vitamin A on the stability of lysosomes *in vivo* and *in vitro*. In: *CIBA Foundation Symposium on Lysosomes* (A. V. S. DeReuck and M. D. Cameron, eds.), p. 384 (Boston: Little, Brown & Co.)
11. Hayes, K. C. (1971). On the pathophysiology of vitamin A deficiency. *Nutr. Rev.*, **29**, 3
12. Mandel, H. G., Weiss, W. P. (1965). Fat-soluble vitamins. In: *The Pharmalogical Basis of Therapeutics*, 3rd edition (L. S. Goodman and A. Gilman, eds.), p. 1681 (New York: Macmillan)
13. Glazebrook, A. J. and Thomson, S. (1942). The administration of vitamin C in a large institution and its effect on general health and resistance to infection. *J. Hyg.*, **42**, 1
14. Dahlberg, G., Engel, A. and Rydin, H. (1944). The value of ascorbic acid as a prophylactic against 'common colds'. *Acta Med. Scand.*, **119**, 540
15. Barnes, F. E. (1961). Vitamin supplements and the incidence of colds in high school basketball players. A preliminary report. *N. C. Med. J.*, **22**, 22

16. Cowan, D. W., Diehl, H. S. and Baker, A. B. (1942). Vitamins for the prevention of colds. *J. Am. Med. Assoc.*, **120**, 1268
17. Franz, W. L., Heyl, H. L. and Sands, W. (1956). Blood ascorbic acid level in bioflavonoid and ascorbic acid therapy of common cold. *J. Am. Med. Assoc.*, **162**, 1224
18. Ritzel, G. (1961). Kritische Beurteilung des Vitamins C als Prophylacticum und Therapeuticum des *Erkältungskrankheiten*. *Helv. Med. Acta*, **28**, 63
19. Pauling, L. (1970). *Vitamin C and the Common Cold* (San Francisco: W. H. Freeman and Co.)
20. Chatterjee, I. B. (1973). Evolution and the biosynthesis of ascorbic acid. *Science*, **182**, 1271
21. Chatterjee, I. B., Chatterjee, G. C., Gosh, N. C., Gosh, J. J. and Guha, B. C. (1960). Biological synthesis of L-ascorbic acid in conversion of L-gulonolactone into L-ascorbic acid. *Biochem. J.*, **74**, 193
22. Pauling, L. (1970). Evolution and the need for ascorbic acid. *Proc. Nat. Acad. Sci.*, **67**, 1643
23. Anderson, T. W., Reid, D. B. and Beaton, G. H. (1972). Vitamin C and the common cold: a double-blind trial. *Can. Med. Assoc. J.*, **107**, 503
24. Anderson, T. W., Suranyl, G. and Beaton, G. H. (1974). The effect on winter illness of large doses of vitamin C. *Can. Med. Assoc. J.*, **111**, 31
25. Anderson, T. W., Beaton, G. H., Corey, P. N. and Spero, L. (1975). Winter illness and vitamin C: the effect of relatively low doses. *Can. Med. Assoc. J.*, **112**, 823
26. Wilson, C. W. M. and Loh, H. S. (1973). Common cold and vitamin C. *Lancet*, **i**, 638
27. Wilson, C. W. M., Loh, H. S. and Foster, F. G. (1973). The beneficial effect of vitamin C on the common cold. *Europ. J. Clin. Pharmacol.*, **6**, 26
28. Coulehan, J. L., Reisinger, K. S., Rogers, K. D. and Bradley, D. W. (1974). Vitamin C prophylaxis in a boarding school. *N. Engl. J. Med.*, **290**, 6
29. Coulehan, J. L., Eberhard, S., Kapner, L., Taylor, F., Rogers, K. and Garry, P. (1976). Vitamin C and acute illness in Navajo school-children. *N. Engl. J. Med.*, **295**, 973
30. Karlowski, T. R., Chalmers, T. C., Frenkel, L. D., Kapikian, A. Z., Lewis, T. L. and Lynch, J. M. (1975). Ascorbic acid for the common cold: a prophylactic and therapeutic trial. *J. Am. Med. Assoc.*, **231**, 1038
31. Perla, D. and Marmorston, J. (1937). Role of vitamin C in resistance. *Arch. Pathol.*, **23**, 543
32. Steinbach, M. M. and Klein, S. J. (1941). Vitamin C in experimental tuberculosis. *Annu. Rev. Tuberc.*, **43**, 403
33. Sandler, J. A., Gallin, J. I. and Vaughan, M. (1975). Effects of serotonin, carbamylcholine, and ascorbic acid on leukocyte cyclic GMP and chemotaxis. *J. Cell. Biol.*, **67**, 480
34. McCall, C. E., DeChatelet, L. R., Cooper, M. R. and Ashburn, P. (1971). The effects of ascorbic acid on bactericidal mechanisms of neutrophils. *J. Infect. Dis.*, **124**, 194
35. Boxer, L. A., Watanabe, A. M., Rister, M., Besch, H. R. Jr., Allen, J. and Baehner, R. L. (1976). Correction of leukocyte function in Chediak–Higashi syndrome by ascorbate. *N. Engl. J. Med.*, **295**, 1041
36. Stossel, T. P., Root, R. K. and Vaughan, M. (1972). Phagocytosis in chronic granulomatous disease and the Chediak–Higashi syndrome. *N. Engl. J. Med.*, **286**, 120
37. Oliver, J. M. (1976). Impaired microtubule assembly in Chediak–Higashi syndrome neutrophils correctable by cyclic GMP and cholinergic agents. *Am. J. Pathol.*, **85**, 395
38. Tengerdy, R. P. and Nockels, C. F. (1975). Vitamin E or vitamin A protects chickens against *E. coli* infection. *Poult. Sci.*, **54**, 1292
39. Beisel, W. R. (1976). Trace elements in infectious processes. *Med. Clin. North Am.*, **60**, 831
40. Beisel, W. R., Pekarek, R. S. and Wannemacher, R. W. Jr. (1974). The impact of infectious disease on trace-element metabolism of the host. In: *Trace Element Metabolism in Animals* (W. G. Hoekstra et al., eds.), p. 217 (Baltimore: University Park Press)
41. Robbins, E. and Pederson, T. (1970). Iron: its intracellular localization and possible role in cell division. *Proc. Nat. Acad. Sci. USA*, **66**, 1244
42. Weinberg, E. D. (1974). Iron and susceptibility to infectious disease. *Science*, **184**, 952

43. Schade, A. L. and Caroline, L. (1944). Raw hen egg white and the role of iron in growth inhibition of *Shigella dysenteriae, Staphylococcus aureus, Escherichia coli* and *Saccharomyces cerevisiae. Science,* **100**, 14

44. Schade, A. L. and Caroline, L. (1946). An iron-binding component in human blood plasma. *Science,* **104**, 340

45. Kochan, I. (1973). The role of iron in bacterial infections, with special consideration of host-tubercle bacillus interaction. *Curr. Top. Microbiol. Immunol.,* **60**, 1

46. Elin, R. J. and Wolff, S. M. (1973). Effect of pH and iron concentration on growth of *Candida albicans* in human serum. *J. Infect. Dis.,* **127**, 705

47. Kochan, I., Kvach, J. T. and Wiles, T. I. (1977). Virulence-associated acquisition of iron in mammalian serum by *Escherichia coli. J. Infect. Dis.,* **135**, 623

48. Barrett-Connor, E. (1971). Bacterial infection and sickle cell anemia. An analysis of 250 infections in 166 patients and a review of the literature. *Medicine (Baltimore),* **50**, 97

49. Weinberg, E. D. (1972). Systemic salmonellosis: A sequela of sideremia. *Tex. Rep. Biol. Med.,* **30**, 277

50. Briggs, J. D., Kennedy, A. C. and Goldberg, A. (1963). Urinary white-cell excretion after iron-sorbitol-citric-acid. *Br. Med. J.,* **2**, 352

51. The relationship between infection and the iron status of an individual (1975). *Nutr. Rev.,* **33**, 103

52. McFarlane, H., Reddy, S., Adcock, K. J., Adeshina, H., Cooke, A. R. and Akene, J. (1970). Immunity, transferrin, and survival in kwashiorkor. *Br. Med. J.,* **4**, 268

53. Chandra, R. K. (1976). Iron and immunocompetence. *Nutr. Rev.,* **34**, 129

54. Shaw, R. and Robertson, W. O. (1964). Anemia among hospitalized infants. *Ohio Med. J.,* **60**, 45

55. *Nutritional Anaemias* (1968). World Health Organization Technical Report Series No. 405

56. MacKay, H. M. M. (1928). Anaemia in infancy: prevalence and prevention. *Arch. Dis. Child.,* **3**, 117

57. Andelman, M. B. and Sered, B. R. (1966). Utilization of dietary iron by term infants. A study of 1048 infants from a low socioeconomic population. *Am. J. Dis. Child.,* **111**, 45

58. James, J. A. and Combes, M. (1960). Iron deficiency in the premature infant. Significance, and prevention by the intramuscular administration of iron-dextran. *Pediatrics,* **26**, 368

59. Burman, D. (1972). Haemoglobin levels in normal infants aged 3 to 24 months, and the effect of iron. *Arch. Dis. Child.,* **47**, 261

60. Masawe, A. E., Muindi, J. M. and Swai, G. B. (1974). Infections in iron-deficiency and other types of anaemia in the tropics. *Lancet,* **ii**, 314

61. Joynson, D. H., Walker, D. M., Jacobs, A. and Dolby, A. E. (1972). Defect of cell-mediated immunity in patients with iron-deficiency anaemia. *Lancet,* **ii**, 1058

62. Fletcher, J., Mather, J., Lewis, M. J. and Whiting, G. (1975). Mouth lesions in iron-deficient anemia: relationship to *Candida albicans* in saliva and to impairment of lymphocyte transformation. *J. Infect. Dis.,* **131**, 44

63. Bhaskaram, C. and Reddy, V. (1975). Cell-mediated immunity in iron- and vitamin-deficient children. *Br. Med. J.,* **3**, 522

64. Chandra, R. K. and Saraya, A. K. (1975). Impaired immunocompetence associated with iron deficiency. *J. Pediatr.,* **86**, 899

65. Arbeter, A., Echeverri, L., Franco, D., Munson, D., Vales, H. and Vitale, J. J. (1971). Nutrition and infection. *Fed. Proc.,* **30**, 1421

66. Halsted, J. A. and Smith, J. C. Jr. (1970). Plasma-zinc in health and disease. *Lancet,* **i**, 322

67. Henkin, R. I. and Smith, F. R. (1972). Zinc and copper metabolism in acute viral hepatitis. *Am. J. Med. Sci.,* **264**, 401

68. Markowitz, H., Gubler, C. J., Mahoney, J. P., Cartwright, G. E. and Wintrobe, M. M. (1955). Studies on copper metabolism. XIV. Copper, ceruloplasmin and oxidase activity

in sera of normal subjects, pregnant women, and patients with infection, hepatolenticular degeneration and the nephrotic syndrome. *J. Clin. Invest.*, **34**, 1498

69. Pekarek, R. S., Powanda, M. C. and Wannemacher, R. W. Jr. (1972). The effect of leukocytic endogenous mediator (LEM) on serum copper and ceruloplasmin concentrations in the rat. *Proc. Soc. Exp. Biol. Med.*, **141**, 1029

70. Klein, E. (1893). The anti-cholera vaccination: an experimental critique. *Br. Med. J.*, **1**, 632

71. Sobernheimm, G. (1895). Untursuchungen über die specifische bedeutung der choleraimmunität. *Z. Hyg. Infektionskr.*, **20**, 438

72. Rowley, D. (1955). Stimulation of natural immunity to *Escherichia coli* infections. Observations on mice. *Lancet*, **268**, 232

73. Landy, M. (1956). Increase in resistance following administration of bacterial lipopolysaccharides. *Ann. N.Y. Acad. Sci.*, **66**, 292

74. Rowley, D. (1956). Rapidly induced changes in the level of non-specific immunity in laboratory animals. *Br. J. Exp. Pathol.*, **37**, 223

75. Margherita, S. S. and Friedman, H. (1965). Induction of non-specific resistance by endotoxin in unresponsive mice. *J. Bacteriol.*, **89**, 277

76. Berger, F. M. and Fukui, G. M. (1963). Endotoxin induced resistance to infections and tolerance. *Proc. Soc. Exp. Biol. Med.*, **114**, 780

77. Sultzer, B. M. (1968). Endotoxin-induced resistance to staphylococcal infection: cellular and humoral responses compared in two mouse strains. *J. Infect. Dis.*, **118**, 340

78. Kimball, H. R., Williams, T. W. and Wolff, S. M. (1968). Effect of bacterial endotoxin on experimental fungal infections. *J. Immunol.*, **100**, 24

79. Wright, L. J., Kimball, H. R. and Wolff, S. M. (1969). Alterations in host responses to experimental *Candida albicans* infections by bacterial endotoxin. *J. Immuno.*, **103**, 1276

80. Kobayashi, H., Yasuhira, K. and Uesaka, I. (1969). Effect of *Escherichia coli* and its endotoxin on the resistance of mice to experimental cryptococcal infection. *Jpn. J. Microbiol.*, **13**, 223

81. McGregor, R. R., Sheagren, J. N. and Wolff, S. M. (1969). Endotoxin-induced modification of *Plasmodium berghei* infection in mice. *J. Immunol.*, **102**, 131

82. Singer, I., Kimble, E. T. III and Ritts, R. E. Jr. (1964). Alterations of the host-parasite relationship by administration of endotoxin to mice with infections of trypanosomes. *J. Infect. Dis.*, **114**, 243

83. Gledhill, A. W. (1959). Sparing effect of serum from mice treated with endotoxin upon certain murine virus diseases. *Nature*, **183**, 185

84. Wagner, R. R., Snyder, R. M., Hook, E. W. and Luttrell, C. N. (1959). Effect of bacterial endotoxin on resistance of mice to viral encephalitides. *J. Immunol.*, **83**, 87

85. Finkelstein, R. A. (1961). Alteration of susceptibility of embryonated eggs to Newcastle disease virus by *Escherichia coli* and endotoxin. *Proc. Soc. Exp. Biol. Med.*, **106**, 481

86. Elin, R. J. and Wolff, S. M. (1973). Bacterial endotoxins. In: *Handbook of Microbiology*, Vol. II, *Microbial Composition* (A. I. Laskin and H. A. Lechevalier, eds.), p. 215 (Cleveland: CRC Press)

87. Hasenclever, H. F. and Mitchell, W. O. (1963). Endotoxin-induced tolerance to toxic manifestations of *Candida albicans*. *J. Bacteriol.*, **85**, 1088

88. Elin, R. J. and Wolff, S. M. (1974). The role of iron in non-specific resistance to infection induced by endotoxin. *J. Immunol.*, **112**, 737

89. Hill, A. W., Hibbitt, K. G. and Shears, A. L. (1974). Short-term effects of non-specific resistance induced by endotoxin on the distribution and viability of bacteria injected into mice. *Br. J. Exp. Pathol.*, **55**, 448

90. Marsh, J. C. and Perry, S. (1964). The granulocyte response to endotoxin in patients with hematologic disorders. *Blood*, **23**, 581

91. Cline, M. J., Melmon, K. L., Davis, W. C. and Williams, H. E. (1968). Mechanism of endotoxin interaction with human leucocytes. *Br. J. Haematol.*, **15**, 539

92. Golub, S., Groschel, D. H. M. and Nowotny, A. (1968). Factors which affect the reticuloendothelial system uptake of bacterial endotoxins. *J. Reticuloendothel. Soc.*, **5**, 324

93. Patterson, L. T., Harper, J. M. and Higginbotham, R. D. (1968). Association of C-reactive protein and circulating leukocytes with resistance to *Staphylococcus aureus* infection in endotoxin-treated mice and rabbits. *J. Bacteriol.*, **95**, 1375

94. Patterson, L. T. and Higginbotham, R. D. (1965). Mouse C-reactive protein and endotoxin-induced resistance. *J. Bacteriol.*, **90**, 1520

95. Chedid, L., Audibert, F., Bona, C., Damais, C., Parant, F. and Parant, M. (1975). Biological activities of endotoxins detoxified by alkylation. *Infect. Immun.*, **12**, 714

96. Parant, M., Galelli, A., Parant, F. and Chedid, L. (1976). Role of β-lymphocytes in nonspecific resistance to *Klebsiella pneumoniae* infection of endotoxin-treated mice. *J. Infect. Dis.*, **134**, 531

97. Adam, A., Ciorbaru, R., Petit, J. F., Lederer, E., Chedid, L., Lamensans, A., Parant, F., Parant, M., Rosselet, J. P. and Berger, F. M. (1973). Preparation and biological properties of water-soluble adjuvant fractions from delipidated cells of *Mycobacterium smegmatis* and *Nocardia opaca*. *Infect. Immun.*, **7**, 855

98. Elin, R. J., Wolff, S. M. and Chedid, L. (1976). Non-specific resistance to infection induced in mice by a water-soluble adjuvant derived from *Mycobacterium smegmatis*. *J. Infect. Dis.*, **133**, 500

99. Chedid, L., Audibert, F., Lefrancieer, P., Choay, J. and Lederer, E. (1976). Modulation of the immune response by a synthetic adjuvant and analogs. *Proc. Nat. Acad. Sci. USA*, **73**, 2472

100. Audibert, F., Chedid, L., Lefrancier, P. and Choay, J. (1976). Distinctive adjuvanticity of synthetic analogs of mycobacterial water-soluble components. *Cell. Immunol.*, **21**, 243

101. Personal communications from Dr Louis Chedid, Institut Pasteur, Paris, France

102. Smith, C. H., Erlandson, M. E., Stern, G. and Hilgartner, M. W. (1962). Post-splenectomy infection in Cooley's anemia. *N. Engl. J. Med.*, **266**, 737

103. Eraklis, A. J., Kevy, S. V., Diamond, L. K. and Gross, R. E. (1967). Hazard of overwhelming infection after splenectomy in childhood. *N. Engl. J. Med.*, **276**, 1225

104. Bisno, A. L. and Füeeman, J. C. (1970). The syndrome of asplenia, pneumococcal sepsis, and disseminated intravascular coagulation. *Ann. Intern. Med.*, **72**, 389

105. Jones, J. F., Stutz, F. H., Manuele, V. J. and Allen, R. G. (1975). Atypical rubeola infection after splenectomy. *N. Engl. J. Med.*, **292**, 111

106. Schimpff, S. C., O'Connell, M. J., Greene, W. H. and Wiernik, P. H. (1975). Infections in 92 splectomized patients with Hodgkin's disease. A clinical review. *Am. J. Med.*, **59**, 695

107. Chilcote, R. R., Baehner, R. L., Hammond, D. and the Investigators and Special Studies Committee of the Children's Cancer Study Group. (1976). Septicemia and meningitis in children splenectomized for Hodgkin's disease. *N. Engl. J. Med.*, **295**, 798

108. Singer, D. B. (1973). Post-splenectomy sepsis. *Perspect. Pediatr. Pathol.*, **1**, 285

109. Diamond, L. K. (1969). Splenectomy in childhood and the hazard of overwhelming infection. *Pediatrics*, **43**, 886

110. Donaldson, S. S., Moore, M. R. and Rosenberg, S. A. (1972). Characterization of postsplenectomy bacteremia among patients with and without lymphoma. *N. Engl. J. Med.*, **287**, 69

111. Likhite, V. V. (1976). Immunological impairment and susceptibility to infection after splenectomy. *J. Am. Med. Assoc.*, **236**, 1376

112. Lozzio, B. B. and Wargon, L. B. (1974). Immune competence of hereditarily asplenic mice. *Immunology*, **27**, 167

113. Schumacher, M. J. (1970). Serum immunoglobulin and transferrin levels after childhood splenectomy. *Arch. Dis. Child.*, **45**, 114

114. Claret, I., Morales, L. and Montaner, A. (1975). Immunological studies in the post-splenectomy syndrome. *J. Pediatr. Surg.*, **10**, 59
115. Constantopoulos, A. and Najjar, V. A. (1972). Tuftsin, a natural and general phago-cytosis-stimulating peptide affecting macrophages and polymorphonuclear leukocytes. *Cytobios*, **6**, 97
116. Constantopoulos, A., Najjar, A. V. and Smith, J. W. (1972). Tuftsin deficiency: a new syndrome with defective phagocytosis. *J. Pediatr.*, **80**, 564

2
Immune Responses to Fungal Infections

D. W. R. MACKENZIE

2.1	INTRODUCTION	22
2.2	THE FUNGAL CELL	23
	2.2.1 *Fungal spores*	24
.2.3	TYPES OF INFECTION WITH FUNGI	25
	2.3.1 *Superficial infections*	25
	2.3.2 *Diseases of implantation (subcutaneous mycoses)*	25
	2.3.3 *Respiratory (systemic) mycoses*	25
	2.3.4 *Opportunist mycoses*	26
	2.3.5 *Fungal diseases caused by respiratory hypersensitivity*	26
2.4	NON-SPECIFIC TISSUE REACTIONS IN FUNGAL DISEASES	26
2.5	TYPES OF IMMUNE RESPONSE	27
	2.5.1 *Cellular responses*	27
	2.5.2 *Humoral responses*	28
	2.5.3 *Standardization of immunodiagnostic reagents*	29
2.6	THE IMMUNE RESPONSE AND DIAGNOSIS	30
	2.6.1 *Cell-mediated studies*	30
	2.6.2 *Serological studies*	31
	2.6.2.1 *Detection of antibody*	31
	2.6.2.2 *Detection of antigen*	33
2.7	THE IMMUNE RESPONSE AND PATHOGENESIS	34
2.8	MODIFICATIONS OF THE IMMUNE RESPONSE	35

2.9   IMMUNE RESPONSES IN INDIVIDUAL MYCOSES   36
    2.9.1   *Dermatophytoses (ringworm)*   37
    2.9.2   *Chromomycosis, mycetoma and sporotrichosis*   39
        2.9.2.1   *Chromomycosis*   39
        2.9.2.2   *Mycetoma*   39
        2.9.2.3   *Sporotrichosis*   40
    2.9.3   *Histoplasmosis*   41
        2.9.3.1   *Skin tests*   41
        2.9.3.2   *Antibody formation*   43
        2.9.3.3   *Protective immunity*   44
    2.9.4   *Coccidioidomycosis*   45
        2.9.4.1   *Serology*   47
        2.9.4.2   *Immunity*   48
    2.9.5   *Blastomycosis*   48
    2.9.6   *South American blastomycosis (paracoccidioidomycosis)* 50
        2.9.6.1   *Skin reactivity*   51
        2.9.6.2   *Serological tests*   51
    2.9.7   *Cryptococcosis*   52
    2.9.8   *Opportunist mycoses*   54
        2.9.8.1   *Candidiasis*   55
        2.9.8.2   *Aspergilloma*   60
        2.9.8.3   *Invasive aspergillosis*   60

2.10   DISEASES CAUSED BY RESPIRATORY HYPER-
    SENSITIVITY   60
    2.10.1 *Allergic bronchopulmonary aspergillosis*   61
    2.10.2 *Farmer's lung (extrinsinc allergic alveolitis)*   62

2.1   INTRODUCTION

Fungi do not rank with bacteria, viruses or protozoa as causes of human disease. Mycoses are generally associated with morbidity rather than mortality and, since they are not notifiable, accurate data on their prevalence are almost unobtainable. In addition, countries where mycoses are believed to be of major public health significance are not necessarily those where expertise in mycological diagnosis, management and reporting are available.

Fungi can nevertheless cause much suffering, and ringworm infections involving skin are amongst the commonest infectious diseases occurring in some parts of the world. Hammerman *et al.*[1] have estimated that in the United States mycoses are annually responsible for 300–400 deaths, for over 8 700 hospital admissions and for the outlay of over $9 000 000 in costs.

Establishment of infection by a pathogenic fungus is almost always accompanied by measurable responses in the immune state of the patient. In some instances deviation from the 'normal' immune state appears to be the principal cause of susceptibility to infection. In common with all other micro-organisms fungi are immunogenic, the type, extent and duration of response depending to a large extent on the degree of colonization or invasion. When the fungus grows only on hairs, for example, no inflammatory or immune responses can be detected. When living tissues are invaded or affected, however, T- and B-cell responses are almost always elicited. These can be of great value in diagnosis of individual cases and in population studies involving the measurement of acquired skin-test sensitization. In this chapter, consideration is given to specific immune responses in fungal diseases caused by infection or hypersensitization.

2.2 THE FUNGAL CELL

Fungi are highly successful life forms, abundant in most environments inhabited by man and enormously varied in their morphology, metabolism and reproductive capacities. Many are unicellular and microscopic. Others may aggregate into large and complex specialized structures associated with reproduction. The most common vegetative form assumed by fungi is the hypha, a branching microscopic filament which can colonize suitable substrates very rapidly. Diagrammatic representations of a fungal hypha and a unicellular yeast cell are shown in Figure 2.1.

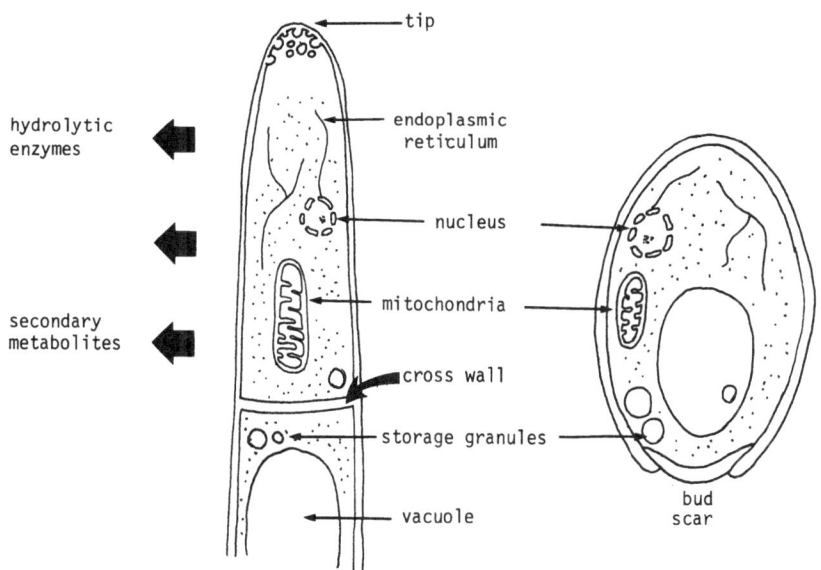

Figure 2.1 Diagrammatic representations of a fungal hypha (left) and a yeast cell (right)

Extensive growth takes place only in the tip region. Behind this is an area of active metabolism. Enzymes secreted into the substrate break down large molecules and allow their transport through the cell wall and cytoplasmic membrane. The cytoplasm is rich in membranes, ribosomes and enzymes. Fungi are eukaryotic, their nuclei being bounded by nuclear membranes which are interrupted by pores. Gradients of age and metabolic activity exist behind the growing tip. As the hypha ages, i.e. in portions increasingly close to the point of origin of the hypha, various changes occur in physiology and vegetative organization. These include progressive senescence and finally death of the hypha. Cytoplasm becomes scarcer due to the formation of prominent vacuoles. Products of secondary metabolism appear increasingly in the substrate as the hypha ages, and integrity of the cell wall diminishes. Eventually, through a form of autolysis, the remaining cytoplasmic contents are discharged into the environment.

Several fungi, notably the yeasts, are basically unicellular. Although filamentous growth is reduced or absent, their organizational differences compared with hyphal fungi (moulds) are more apparent than real. Life processes are to a large extent common to the two forms and their distinctive qualities relate more to mechanisms of cellular division than to fundamental differences in their biosynthetic patterns. Several pathogenic fungi can be hyphal or yeastlike, depending on the conditions under which growth is taking place. This phenomenon is known as dimorphism, and in some instances may represent an adaptation towards a parasitic mode of life. It should be realized that not all dimorphic fungi are pathogenic and that not all pathogenic fungi are dimorphic. The biochemical basis of pathogenicity is imperfectly understood in fungi, but it is generally accepted that infectivity and virulence are controlled by a variety of factors, both of the host and of the parasite. It should also be realized that chemical as well as morphological differences exist between yeast and filamentous forms of a dimorphic fungus. Such considerations may be of relevance in explaining specific immune responses in a subject where infection may be initiated by one form and maintained or extended by the other.

2.2.1 Fungal spores

Fungi produce enormous numbers and varieties of spores. These are formed during and after establishment of the vegetative phase of growth. Many species produce spores (conidia) on specialized aerial hyphae, which are released into the air and are responsible for dispersion of the mould from its original habitat. These conidia are often minute and many are of a size (5 μm in diameter) which assures deep penetration and retention in the terminal portions of the respiratory tract. Airborne spores can be inhaled in large numbers and they are recognized as important mediators of respiratory allergy.

In terms of the immune response to infection, the major eliciting elements associated with the vegetative fungal cell are cell walls and cytoplasm, together with the extracellular products released through normal metabolic or autolytic mechanisms. Both chemical and physical natures of the individual components are of importance in determining the type of response, or indeed whether a specific reaction occurs at all. Airborne spores constitute a separate category of immunogen, the associated diseases having an allergic rather than an infective basis.

2.3 TYPES OF INFECTION WITH FUNGI

Infections caused by fungi fall into several distinct categories. Features of the diseases and their causal agents can be summarized as follows:

2.3.1 Superficial infections

(1) *Principal types* – Ringworm (dermatophytosis; tinea); Pityriasis versicolor; Piedra.

(2) *Features of the disease* – Acquired by contagion; primary site of multiplication is skin and appendages; lesions restricted, often self-limiting, mild and asymptomatic; acute and chronic forms occur; living tissues not invaded; prognosis in untreated cases not grave; immune response usually absent, but infections with ringworm result in acquired hypersensitivity.

(3) *Features of the pathogen* – Normally parasitic, occasionally saprophytic; transmitted from active lesion; not dimorphic.

2.3.2 Diseases of implantation (subcutaneous mycoses)

(1) *Principal types* – Chromomycosis; Mycetoma; Sporotrichosis.

(2) *Features of the disease* – Acquired by traumatic implantation; primary site of multiplication is subcutaneous tissues; lesions chronic; self-limiting forms unknown or uncommon; formation of nodules, tumefactions, or ulcers; deeper tissues may become involved; serological tests may aid diagnosis; some geographical localization.

(3) *Features of the pathogen* – Saprophytic; characteristic morphology *in vivo*; apart from sporotrichosis, multiple aetiology.

2.3.3 Respiratory (systemic) mycoses

(1) *Principal types* – Histoplasmosis; Paracoccidioidomycosis; Coccidioidomycosis; Cryptococcosis; Blastomycosis.

(2) *Features of the disease* – Acquired by inhalation of airborne spores; primary site of multiplication is lungs; acute and chronic forms found; usually mild and self-limiting; disseminated forms rare; affects any part of

the body; prognosis in untreated disseminated cases grave; infected individual becomes sensitized (skin-test positive); antibody formation prognostically and diagnostically helpful; apart from cryptococcosis, diseases have geographical localizations.

(3) *Features of the pathogen* – Soil saprophytes; apart from cryptococcosis, causal agent is dimorphic; causal agents share antigens (i.e. cross-reactions occur in immunodiagnostic tests).

2.3.4 Opportunist mycoses

(1) *Principal types* – Candidiasis; Phycomycoses; Invasive aspergillosis; Aspergilloma.

(2) *Features of the disease* – Acquired by introduction of agent to areas of impaired host response, i.e. recognizable predisposition of host; immune responses may or may not be suppressed; duration may or may not depend on duration of patient's susceptibility; localized and disseminated forms; acute, subacute or chronic.

(3) *Features of the pathogen* – Saprophytic, acquired from the environment (e.g. *Aspergillus*, *Mucor*) or commensal, acquired endogenously (e.g. *Candida*); limited innate pathogenicity.

2.3.5 Fungal diseases caused by respiratory hypersensitivity

(1) *Principal types* – Extrinsic mould asthma; allergic aspergillosis; extrinsic allergic alveolitis (Farmer's Lung, Bird Fancier's Disease, etc.).

(2) *Features of the disease* – Acquired by exposure of sensitized subjects to fungal allergens; immunopathogenic basis; Type 1 and/or Type 3 predominating; no tissue invasion by agent(s); antibody production common, IgG or IgE.

(3) *Features of allergenic agents* – Common saprophytes in man's environment; spores usually minute; spores abundant according to season and/or environment.

2.4 NON-SPECIFIC TISSUE REACTIONS IN FUNGAL DISEASES

Tissue responses to the presence of fungi vary according to their specific identity and site of proliferation, and the duration of infection. There is sometimes a tendency[2] for the inflammatory reaction to be low-grade, viable cells being present and persisting within macrophages or giant cells.

In general, however, inflammatory responses are comparable to those occurring in infections caused by bacteria, parasites and other infectious agents. No one tissue change is completely pathognomonic for any one mycosis, and in most instances a mixture of responses is present. The precise extent to which natural or acquired resistance determines or influences histopathological characteristics of infection is still largely unknown. *Histoplasma* cells may develop abundantly in the cytoplasm of macrophages in some subjects, and may spread unchecked to produce disseminated disease. In most individuals, however, an epithelioid granulomatous reaction is developed, which, together with fibrosis, has the effect of localizing the fungus and minimizing its spread[3].

The first line of inflammatory defence is represented by the neutrophil, and indeed phagocytosis is the earliest and most efficient mechanism for preventing establishment of infection. Chronic inflammatory reactions, including lymphocytes, plasma cells, macrophages and smaller numbers of neutrophils, are common in established lesions. Chronic suppuration and fibrosis are present in most mycoses, but in some (e.g. phycomycoses) inflammation is minimal, tissue damage resulting primarily from invasion and thrombosis of blood vessels.

To a large extent, immune responses to fungal disease are linked to both qualitative and quantitative aspects of the associated inflammatory response. Any modification of these responses whether determined by genetic, pathological or therapeutic factors will be accompanied by a shift from the anticipated pattern of immune response. These changes have a profound effect in modifying the establishment, progress and outcome of infection.

Non-specific defence mechanisms have an important primary role in denying fungal pathogens access to otherwise susceptible tissues, but they also have a regulatory role in determining chronicity and histopathological characteristics of the disease, and the nature, extent and duration of the immune reactions.

2.5   TYPES OF IMMUNE RESPONSE

Fungal cells and their extracellular products are rich sources of antigens. Their recognition by the immune system is manifested by the development of both cellular and humoral responses. Quantitative and qualitative variations occur in the immune responsiveness, depending on the chemical nature of the immunogens and their mode of presentation. Another major modifying influence is the integrity of the body's defence mechanisms, both non-specific and specific. Individuals with immune deficiencies, whether inherent or induced by immunosuppressive treatment, are particularly prone to fungal infections, their susceptibility being unequivocally linked to the ineffectiveness of their immune responses.

2.5.1   Cellular responses

Apart from the most superficial of fungal infections, where no direct contact exists between fungal material and the immune system, infected individuals acquire Type IV (delayed) hypersensitivity which is generally demonstrable 10–14 days after infection. Skin tests with fungal extracts or culture filtrates result in a tuberculin-like reaction 24–48 hours later.

The acquisition of cellular hypersensitivity may also be demonstrated by tests *in vitro* such as macrophage migration inhibition or blast formation of sensitized lymphocytes in the presence of antigen.

Cellular responses are believed to be of fundamental importance in acquired resistance to infection with pathogenic fungi. A link between cell-mediated immunity and resistance is probably present in all mycoses where the causal fungi are capable of tissue invasion, but proof is often lacking.

2.5.2   Humoral responses

Antibodies to fungi are produced in most mycotic infections. Their production depends in part on contact being established between fungus or fungal metabolite and the antibody producing mechanism, and partly on the ability of the infected host to mount an active antibody response.

In the course of an acute respiratory infection such as histoplasmosis, establishment of the pathogen and its subsequent proliferation give rise to antibody production which is first detectable 10–14 days later. To some extent, the type of antibody and its titre reflect the status and progress of infection. Serological tests have therefore an important role in the diagnosis of deep-seated infections and in evaluating the response of the patient to treatment. Evidence that antibodies *per se* have a protective effect against fungal disease is fragmentary and largely inconclusive. Protection can sometimes be demonstrated in experimentally infected animals, by passive transfer of serum[4], but tends to be relative rather than absolute, and is unlikely to be the sole mechanism of acquired resistance. Fungi produce many different antigens. The majority of these are protein, and are often associated with cytoplasmic contents. Cell-wall antigens are usually predominantly polysaccharide or glycopeptide, and may be produced in abundance. In view of the number and range of antibodies produced, it is hardly surprising to find that the antibody response can vary qualitatively as well as quantitatively. Using two-dimensional gel electrophoresis Axelsen[5] demonstrated the existence of 78 distinct water-soluble antigens in *Candida albicans*.

For more than three decades, attention has been focussed on the application of serological tests to the diagnosis of fungal infections. Different techniques have been applied to the detection and quantitation of different antibodies. Many of these tests are accurate and reliable, and serodiagnosis is rightly valued for its ability to obtain information of direct relevance to the recognition and management of diseases caused by fungi. These tests are considered more fully below.

In common with most other pathogenic micro-organisms, the biochemical basis for fungal pathogenicity is not understood. It is therefore not yet possible to distinguish between antigens which are implicated in the disease process from those which are pathogenically irrelevant. Perhaps surprisingly, only Biguet and his colleagues in Lille[6] have combined cytochemical and immunological techniques and shown the enzymatic nature and substrate specificity for single antigens present in extracts of fungi pathogenic for humans. Such studies are likely to lead to a better understanding of mechanisms of pathogenicity and to provide a basis for discriminating between relevant and irrelevant antigens.

Immunoglobulins occurring in mycotic infections may be IgG, IgA or IgM, the predominant class depending on the host, the pathogen and the type of infection. Where respiratory allergy is involved, raised IgE titres may be present. Their detection is generally by well-established procedures, including whole cell or inert particle agglutination, complement fixation, double diffusion or electrophoresis in agar or agarose gel, and immuno-fluorescence. Some tests are better developed than others, and are described in some detail in the section dealing with serological testing.

Fungi[7] and actinomycetes[8] are known to be capable of activating complement by the alternative pathway. It is not yet known how common activation of complement by the alternative pathway is in the mycoses, and how significant a role this might play in pathogenesis. Such a mechanism could account for some of the pathological responses seen in conditions such as extrinsic allergic alveolitis, where prior hypersensitivity was thought to be prerequisite to the production of disease but where some affected subjects have no history of exposure.

Antibody-mediated killing of fungi has not received much attention, and there is little evidence to suggest that complement is involved directly in causing the death of parasitic fungal cells. Diamond[9] has shown that mono-nuclear cells can kill *Cryptococcus neoformans* by a non-phagocytic mechanism in the presence of anti-cryptococcal antibody. The C-3 component of complement activated by cells of *C. albicans* by the alternative pathway has been shown by Yamamura and Valdimarsson[10] to be directly implicated in their intraphagocytic killing. It is not yet known how widespread and significant this defence mechanism may be in combating fungal infections.

2.5.3 Standardization of immunodiagnostic reagents

For some serological tests, commercially produced diagnostic kits are available. For others, tests are still under development and are undertaken only by specialist laboratories. It is difficult to compare results obtained at different centres because of the lack of reference reagents and procedures. Standardization of fungal antigens – whether used for skin or serological testing – has only recently been given consideration at an international level.

In common with other substances used for detection of hypersensitivity or antibody, fungal extracts are best characterized by their biological reactivity. Physicochemical measurements do not correlate well with the activities of fungal extracts in skin or serological tests. Huppert et al.[11] showed that different batches of coccidioidin could have similar carbohydrate and protein contents, but could differ in optimum reactivities for the complement fixation test. Two principal problems face those engaged in serodiagnostic work, viz. minimizing batch-to-batch variation of their reagents, and equating their results with those obtained by others. In the case of skin-test materials, e.g. histoplasmin, variation is minimized by the production of large amounts of the test material. There are obvious advantages in having internationally accepted reference reagents including the ability to co-ordinate results obtained at different centres. The need for such references has recently been recognized by the World Health Organization, and the first WHO reference antigen for a fungus may soon be designated.

2.6   THE IMMUNE RESPONSE AND DIAGNOSIS

2.6.1   Cell-mediated studies

Individuals recovering spontaneously from respiratory mycoses such as histoplasmosis and coccidioidomycosis retain positive skin-reactivity for several years. Skin tests with histoplasmin and coccidioidin can therefore be of value in estimating the proportion of a population exposed to (and previously infected with) these agents. In most cases, a positive skin test is of epidemiological rather than of diagnostic value. In endemic areas, where a high proportion of subjects have been affected, the majority of individuals will be reactive. For histoplasmosis, 85% of the population in an endemic area may react to intradermal testing with histoplasmin. The situation is different, however, when a subject living outside the endemic areas pays a brief visit to a region where the pathogen is known to exist, and acquires a respiratory infection during or shortly after the visit. In such a case a positive skin test may be helpful in establishing the true nature of the infection.

Skin tests may be negative in the early stages of infection, in elderly subjects, and in patients with severe or disseminated disease. A constantly recurring problem in interpreting immunodiagnostic tests for the mycoses is the widespread existence of cross-reacting antigens amongst the causal agents. Specificity of reaction is relative rather than absolute, and this has always to be borne in mind. Goodman et al.[12] have demonstrated marked cross-reactivity in the cutaneous responses of guinea-pigs sensitized to Histoplasma capsulatum and a range of other fungi. Thus, histoplasmin-positive skin tests were obtained in the majority of animals sensitized with Aspergillus fumigatus, Penicillium spp. and Coccidioides immitis. Reduced but possibly significant cross-reactions were also obtained with Blastomyces,

Geotrichum, *Sporothrix* and other pathogenic and non-pathogenic representatives.

A positive skin test implies previous exposure to the agent rather than active infection. More correctly, a positive skin test merely indicates sensitization. This may or may not be associated with active infection.

Many of the earlier studies on skin hypersensitivity to fungal infections were made on human or experimental dermatophytoses (ringworm). Some 7–10 days after infection, Type IV responses can be demonstrated following the intradermal injection of trichophytin. Accompanying this sensitization is an increased resistance to re-infection. The hypersensitive state is demonstrable for some years after the lesions have healed. Trichophytin sensitivity is specific for dermatophytes but is not species-specific. Of considerable interest is the tendency for patients infected with *Trichophyton rubrum*, but not other species, to be anergic when tested with trichophytin. In one series reported by Hanifin et al.[13] 12 of 14 patients with *T. mentagrophytes* responded to trichophytin, in contrast to only 12 of 49 patients infected with *T. rubrum*. This phenomenon, described independently by Jones et al.[14] can also be revealed by lymphocyte stimulation studies[13]. Similar findings have been reported by Abraham et al.[15].

Type I immune (immediate) responses are also detected by the skin testing of a proportion of subjects with dermatophytosis. They may be common, occurring in as many as 85% of infected adults, but the correlation with an accelerated response to re-infection is poor, and reactions are frequently noted amongst non-infected subjects.

Tests *in vitro* for cell-mediated immunity have been used increasingly in the study of peripheral macrophages and lymphocytes from patients or experimental animals infected with superficial, subcutaneous or systemic mycoses. Specific sensitization has been demonstrated for a wide range of mycotic diseases including aspergillosis, candidiasis, coccidioidomycosis, cryptococcosis, dermatophytosis, histoplasmosis, sporotrichosis and paracoccidioidomycosis.

Walters et al.[16] have described a leukocyte adherence inhibition test, where homologous, but not heterologous, antigens will prevent peripheral leukocytes from patients with dermatophytosis from settling on to a glass slide. In view of the common occurrence of cross-reacting antigens amongst the dermatophytes, this is a surprising and, as yet, unconfirmed finding.

2.6.2 Serological studies

2.6.2.1 *Detection of antibody*

The basic approach to serodiagnostic testing in the mycoses has been chosen (and justified) on the basis that changes in levels of detectable antibodies bear a direct relationship to changes in the host–parasite relationship.

Bearing in mind the limitations imposed by cross-reactivity of antigens obtained from different fungi on the one hand, and differences in the antigens produced at different stages of infection on the other, traditional methodology and concepts have undoubtedly provided valuable ancillary laboratory diagnostic procedures. Provided antibodies are produced during the course of infection, their detection and quantitation can provide a measure of pathogenic involvement and host response.

Serological tests, particularly those directed towards recognition of precipitating, agglutinating and complement-fixing antibodies, have been of great value in the major respiratory mycoses such as histoplasmosis and coccidioidomycosis. Serological tests are seldom of value when not related to the history and condition of the patient. It may nevertheless be helpful to realize that tests on a single serum may give results which are very uncommon and which might raise the possibility of a fungal infection. Antibodies to *Candida* can be demonstrated in the serum of healthy subjects, but this is not

Table 2.1 Serological tests in common use as diagnostic aids for diseases caused by fungi and actinomycetes

Disease	Tests
Aspergillosis	Double diffusion/counter immunoelectrophoresis*, indirect fluorescent antibody
Blastomycosis	Double diffusion, complement fixation
Candidiasis	Double diffusion/counter immunoelectrophoresis*, whole cell agglutination, haemagglutination*, indirect fluorescent antibody*
Chromomycosis	Double diffusion
Coccidioidomycosis	Double diffusion*, complement fixation*
Cryptococcosis	Whole cell agglutination, latex agglutination*, indirect fluorescent antibody
Farmer's Lung	Double diffusion/counterimmunoelectrophoresis, complement fixation, haemagglutination, indirect fluorescent antibody
Histoplasmosis	Double diffusion*, latex agglutination*, complement fixation*
Mycetoma	Double diffusion
Paracoccidioidomycosis	Double diffusion/counterimmunoelectrophoresis, complement fixation
Sporotrichosis	Double diffusion/counterimmunoelectrophoresis, whole cell agglutination, indirect fluorescent antibody

*Commercially available

true for *Histoplasma* or *Coccidioides*. As serological tests become more widely used and as better links become established between laboratory and clinical findings, an increase can be anticipated in their diagnostic value. Table 2.1 shows the most widely used serological tests for the principal mycoses.

2.6.2.2 *Detection of antigen*

Since the first recognition by Neil *et al.*[17] that free capsular polysaccharide of the pathogenic yeast *Cryptococcus neoformans* can be detected in the tissue fluids of patients with cryptococcosis, the latex agglutination test has been developed into a test of encouraging reliability and specificity. In the past 5 years it has become increasingly obvious that traditional serological tests have a limited value in detecting infections which are at an early stage, or which affect patients whose immune response has been impaired. In such patients, it can be anticipated that *antigen* rather than antibody may be present, and much investigative attention is now being directed towards the detection of antigenaemia. New technical difficulties have to be recognized and overcome. In general, a marked increase in sensitivity is required, and efforts have therefore been made to adopt techniques based on radio-immunoassay or enzyme-linked immunosorbent assays (ELISA). At the time of writing, reports on their successful application to the problem have not yet appeared, but demand for such tests should assure their eventual addition to the diagnostic capabilities of the microbiological laboratory.

Miller *et al.*[18], using gas-liquid chromatography, demonstrated peaks which were present in the sera of six patients with candidaemia and in culture filtrates of *C. albicans*. These components were also shown to be associated with the yeast cells. They were shown to be mannose derivatives, and were not present in normal sera, nor in sera from patients with bacteraemia. Weiner and Yount[19] were also able to demonstrate mannanaemia in patients with candidiasis, using a haemagglutination inhibition technique. The first report on the use of an ELISA procedure was that of Warren *et al.*[20]. Mannan was detected in the serum of experimentally infected animals and in the sera of three patients with evidence of *Candida* infection. Mackenzie and Georgakopoulos[21] later reported the presence of mannan in the sera of patients who had clinical evidence of candidiasis but who were forming no detectable antibodies. Protein antigen was detected in the serum of a patient with chronic mucocutaneous candidiasis by Axelsen and Kirkpatrick[22] using two-dimensional immunoelectrophoresis with the patient's serum in an intermediate gel. The diseases in which the greatest need for antigen detection can be recognized are those which affect severely compromised patients, e.g. those receiving heavy immunosuppression. They would include candidiasis, invasive aspergillosis and phycomycosis. Encouragement for this approach is provided by reports such as that by Young and Bennett[23] which showed that antibody responses were lacking in 15 patients with widespread invasive aspergillosis. Should it prove practicable to introduce tests for detection of antigen rather than antibody on a routine basis, the laboratory would acquire a valuable new diagnostic aid, and the correct treatment for patients developing a serious mycotic infection could be indicated and administered much earlier than can be achieved at present.

2.7   THE IMMUNE RESPONSE AND PATHOGENESIS

Establishment of a fungal infection involves a complex series of interactions between host and parasite. In most instances immune responses accompany the pathogenic process, and on some occasions the host's immune mechanism contributes directly to the disease process. This is exemplified by the role of hypersensitivity in mediating extrinsic mould asthma, allergic aspergillosis and extrinsic allergic alveolitis. There is ample evidence that the immune state and responsiveness of the host play an important role in susceptibility to infection and determination of its outcome. The anticipated progress of an experimental infection can be markedly influenced by alterations in the immune state. Vaccines have had little application in the management of patients with fungal infections, although these have been used in the past[24] particularly in cases of intractable candidiasis. Some recent attention has been paid to the development of protective vaccines for animal mycoses. In the USSR success has been claimed in preventing cattle ringworm by the subcutaneous administration of a vaccine (TF-130) prepared from *T. verrucosum*[25]. Immunity in vaccinated animals was claimed to persist for 7 years. Millions of animals have now been treated, and an overall effectiveness of 95.37% has been reported[26]. Protection is presumably linked to acquired hypersensitivity. Antibodies can be demonstrated in natural or experimental infections of animals[27] and in natural infections of man[28], but there is no indication that they influence the eventual outcome of the disease. Experimental vaccines have also been developed against coccidioidomycosis. Levine and Kong[29] showed that mice immunized with heat-killed spherules were resistant to 200 LD50 of arthrospores administered intranasally. Similar protection has been reported in experimentally infected monkeys[30], and the vaccine was eventually used to a limited extent in human volunteers[31].

Type I (immediate) responses, mediated by IgE immunoglobulin, are elicited in sensitized atopic individuals and are responsible for the marked symptoms which appear following exposure to the airborne allergens. Fungal spores are abundant in the atmosphere, and are common causes of conjunctivitis, rhinitis and asthma. Atopy is also a component of allergic aspergillosis (p. 61).

Immune complexes are implicated in extrinsic allergic alveolitis, lung responses to inhalation being related to the formation of antigen–antibody complexes in the lung (p. 63). It is not known if immune complexes contribute to the pathology of mycotic infections. Modification of the immune response may be accompanied by a marked improvement in the patient's condition. Immunotherapy is not widely used in the management of patients with fungal infections, although desensitization can be helpful in reducing symptoms caused by mould allergy. Treatment with transfer factor has produced clinical improvement in patients with coccidioidomycosis[32] and chronic mucocutaneous candidiasis (p. 58), but in neither instance has this form of treatment become well-established. It is a commonly held belief that cellular immunity is of greater protective value against fungal infections than antibody production. This view is supported by the observation that patients with recognizable immune deficiencies are particularly prone to fungal infections. Candidiasis in experimental animals is more severe when cellular responses are inhibited by immunosuppressive agents such as cyclophospha-mide[33]. Cutler[34] injected thymus-deficient mice with *C. albicans* and found their resistance to infection was not impaired. Similar studies on thymec-tomized mice[35] suggest that, in experimental infections, absence of T cells does not correlate with absolute susceptibility. In these studies it is clear that other mechanisms (including phagocytosis) were functioning and were effectively limiting infection.

Some evidence for an active role of cellular hypersensitivity has been provided by Mahgoub[36]. Mycetoma is a subcutaneous mycosis characterized by its distinctive history and its clinical and histopathological appearance. Mahgoub has shown that a significant number of infected subjects have diminished skin reactivity to tuberculin and to a sensitization course with dinitrochlorobenzene (DNCB). Since the histopathological response tends to be neutrophilic rather than lymphocytic there is some suggestion that patients with mycetoma are immunologically deficient. Candidiasis is another mycosis where immune deficiency is known to be a major cause of host susceptibility. All available evidence to date suggests that the agents causing candidiasis and mycetoma exploit rather than create susceptibility and do not play an active role in regulating the immune mechanism of the host to their advantage.

2.8 MODIFICATIONS OF THE IMMUNE RESPONSE

Immunological responses are important components in the elaborate defence mechanisms of the body. When reduced or absent the integrity of the complicated protective barrier systems can be weakened or broached, and infection may be established or enhanced. Fungi such as *Candida* are common opportunistic pathogens, causing infection by exploiting host susceptibility rather than by their own inherent powers of pathogenicity. Individuals with altered immune responses are particularly prone to fungal infections. In some instances the immune deficiencies are acquired congenitally; in others immune reactivity is diminished by disorders which affect the immune system directly or where the effect is related to treatments which are themselves immunosuppressive.

Disorders of non-specific immunity, e.g. deficient phagocytosis or meta-bolic diseases such as diabetes, are exploited by fungi as well as other micro-organisms, but will not be considered further. Predisposition to fungal infection has been recognized for both thymic-independent and -dependent systems (see Chapter 4). In the former category *Candida* infections have been associated with the Wiskott–Aldrich syndrome and hypogamma-globulinaemia. They are also found in patients with thymic aplasia (DiGeorge's and Nezelof's syndromes), thymic dysplasia with agamma-globulinaemia (Swiss type) or with other defects in cellular immunity which are not obviously associated with abnormalities of the thymus. (See chronic mucocutaneous candidiasis, p. 58.) Infections in subjects with humoral rather than cellular deficiencies tend to be bacterial. Where T-cell deficiencies are present, the pathogenic agents are more commonly viral or fungal. Cell-mediated functions are adversely affected by malignant lymphomas such as Hodgkin's disease, and by immunosuppressive or lympholytic therapy. Increased susceptibility is often exploited by opportunistic pathogens such as *Cryptococcus, Candida, Mucor, Absidia, Rhizopus, Nocardia* and *Aspergillus*. Table 2.2 lists common associations between immune deficiency disorders and opportunistic mycoses.

Table 2.2 Immune deficiency disorders and opportunist mycoses

Disorder	Predominant fungal agents
Leukaemia	*Aspergillus*
Lymphoma	*Cryptococcus*
Dysgammaglobulinaemia	*Candida*
Thymic aplasia	*Candida*
Wiskott–Aldrich syndrome	*Candida*
Ataxia-telengiectasia	*Candida*

Reduction of immune responses may result from a wide range of unrelated causes. These include malnutrition, chronic bacterial disease, arthritis, haemolytic anaemia, chronic enteritis, complement deficiencies, Hodgkin's disease and the use of cytotoxic or immunosuppressive drugs. Providing an opportunity is presented, infection can result. A similar exploitation can result following compromise of non-immune systems.

2.9 IMMUNE RESPONSES IN INDIVIDUAL MYCOSES

In this section, consideration is given to the immune responses which follow infection by different mycoses, to the application of immunodiagnostic tests to the recognition and management of disease, and to epidemiological studies of the prevalence of specific cutaneous hypersensitivity. Individual mycoses considered are those listed in section 2.3.

2.9.1 Dermatophytoses (ringworm)

Dermatophytes grow only in the fully keratinized portions of the skin and are normally confined to the stratum corneum, to the nail plate and to the hair shaft. Species normally affecting animals (zoophilic) or living in soil (geophilic) tend to produce acute, inflammatory and comparatively short-lived infections of man. In contrast, anthropophilic species, which are adapted to a parasitic existence on man, tend to produce lesions which are less inflammatory but longer lasting. About 37 species have been described in the genera: *Microsporum* (14 species), *Trichophyton* (22 species) and *Epidermophyton* (1 species).

Although external to the body in the sense that there is no direct contact between fungal and living host cells, dermatophytes nevertheless evoke specific immune responses in the form of skin sensitization and antibody formation.

It has been known since 1908[37] that a resistance to re-infection develops following spontaneous recovery from a primary infection. This resistance is manifested by acceleration of the disease process and a reduction in its severity.

There is some correlation between the degree of inflammation and the extent of induced resistance, but resistance to re-infection can generally be demonstrated even in subjects with non-inflammatory ringworm. This resistance is associated with acquired hypersensitivity, and intradermal injection of trichophytin, a concentrated culture filtrate, elicits responses which can be either Type IV or Type I.

Trichophytin is prepared from pooled culture filtrates of several species of dermatophytes. Several preparations are available commercially. They are useful in recognizing hypersensitivity, but their basic crudity and lack of standardization limits their diagnostic applications.

Studies on the immunochemical nature of dermatophyte extracts have led to the recognition of several chemically defined groups of antigens. Barker et al.[38] isolated a glycopeptide containing galactose and mannose. Degradation of the carbohydrate part caused a reduction in the immediate response whilst elimination of the peptide caused a reduction in the delayed reaction. Cell-wall polysaccharides of dermatophytes have been studied extensively by Bishop and his colleagues. Two distinct galactomannans which differ in linkage of the D-mannopyranose units in the linear portions of the chains have been described[39]. The same group also studied cell-wall glucan and described three keratinases, one of which is extracellular, the other two being cell-associated[40].

Immunochemical studies suggest that there are marked similarities between the polysaccharides isolated from different dermatophytes. Their chemical similarity[41] is reflected in cross-reactivities in skin tests for Type I and Type IV hypersensitivities and in precipitin tests of patients' sera in agar gel immunodiffusion tests[42]. Noguchi *et al.*[43] studied antibody responses in rabbits immunized with phenol extracts of *T. mentagrophytes*. It was found that precipitating, complement-fixing and haemagglutinating antibodies were produced. IgG was the predominating immunoglobulin but IgM was also present and caused haemagglutination of red cells coated with dermatophyte antigens.

Antigen specificity of dermatophyte galactomannans were shown by Grappel[39] to be associated with different determinants. Removal of D-galactofuranoside units from galactomannan I by acid hydrolysis of parent polysaccharide had no effect on antigenicity. In contrast, mannan derived by hydrolysis of galactomannan II differed from the parent material when compared by immunodiffusion and by complement-fixing tests. Cross-reactions were demonstrated between *Candida* and *M. quinckeanum* (= *T. mentagrophytes* var. *quinckeanum*) when mannan from three species of *Candida* was shown to react to antiserum prepared against the dermatophyte.

Antibodies produced in rabbits injected with mycelium of *T. mentagrophytes* were shown by Grappel *et al.*[44] to inhibit growth of the dermatophyte. Immunoglobulins prevented growth when incorporated into culture media at a concentration of $50\,\mu g/ml$. At lower concentrations morphological changes were produced in the hyphae. Antibodies to extracellular keratinase caused only partial inhibition of growth, but they were able to fix complement and, interestingly, to inhibit their proteolytic activity[45]. These keratinases were shown to inhibit macrophage migration *in vitro*[46] and elicit type IV responses in sensitized guinea-pigs[47].

Immunotherapeutic procedures have been used in attempts to eradicate ringworm infections. The approach has been largely discontinued following the introduction of griseofulvin therapy, but some earlier successes have been claimed. Loughin and Olaru[48], for example, treated 680 infected patients with TCA extracts of *T. mentagrophytes*, and reported that almost 80% recovered without any additional therapy. Huppert and Keeney[49] noted a four-fold reduction in experimental ringworm of the foot by prior local immunization with an extract of the infecting agent. There is a real possibility that the therapeutic value of immunoprophylaxis has been underrated. Intractable ringworm is by no means unknown in this griseofulvin era, and a reappraisal of the benefits to be gained by controlled manipulation of the immune responses of the host may be profitable.

Subjects infected with ringworm may have id reactions. These are produced as a result of interaction between fungal antigens and skin-sensitizing antibodies. The lesions may have a grouped or diffusely scattered follicular distribution on the trunk and limbs, or may appear as papules, vesicles and occasionally bullae on the palms or the sides of the fingers. Fungal elements are lacking, but are always present at a site which is usually some distance removed from the id eruptions, e.g. the toespaces or scalp. The most common eliciting condition is ringworm of the feet. Subjects with id eruptions always have a positive skin test to trichophytin. The lesions disappear following successful treatment of the primary infection or administration of cortico-steroids topically. It should be noted that steroids may radically alter the appearance of dermatophyte lesions and make their recognition difficult.

The association between chronicity of infection with *T. rubrum* and the immune state of the patient was established by Jones *et al.*[50]. Recurrent infections occurred in only 7% of subjects with Type IV responses to trichophytin prepared from *T. mentagrophytes* but in 75% who demonstrated a Type I response, alone or in association with a Type IV reaction. The association related to chronicity rather than to infection as such.

The immunology of dermatophytes and dermatophytic infections has been recently reviewed by Grappel[45].

2.9.2   Chromomycosis, mycetoma and sporotrichosis

2.9.2.1   *Chromomycosis*

Little is known about immune responses in this mycosis. Antibodies to the species causing the condition have been demonstrated in the sera of patients by gel diffusion[51] and complement-fixation[52,53] tests, but studies on cellular immunity are lacking and no suitable animal model has been developed. It is not yet known if infection is associated with diminished immunity, although this possibility is at least suggested by the fact that although the causative agents are abundant in nature, infections are comparatively un-common.

2.9.2.2   *Mycetoma*

Subjects with mycetoma develop antibodies to the infecting agent. Although cross-reactions occur between several of the causal organisms it is generally possible to distinguish between infections caused by fungi (eumycetoma) and actinomycetes (actinomycetoma). The latter usually respond to chemo-therapy, whereas infections caused by fungi do not. There is, therefore, an important need to recognize the type of mycetoma, and serological tests, principally detection of precipitins, are a valuable laboratory aid to diagnosis[54].

As noted, Mahgoub[36] has recently shown that patients with mycetoma tend to be anergic. Of 72 patients with the condition, 56 (78%) were tuberculin-negative, compared to 34 (47%) of controls. Moreover 11 of 13 patients could not be sensitized with DNCB although all five control subjects were readily sensitized. These findings do at least suggest the possibility that individuals with mycetoma have an immune cellular de-ficiency. That the agents exploit rather than create the defect is suggested by the wide range of unrelated fungal and actinomycete species involved, and the fact that anergy exists towards mycobacterial and experimental immunogens.

2.9.2.3 Sporotrichosis

Patients with sporotrichosis usually develop antibodies and since the agent (*Sporothrix schenckii*) is often sparse in infected tissues, and distinctive clinical features may be lacking, serodiagnostic tests are often helpful in establishing a diagnosis.

Several procedures have been recommended. Agglutination of yeast cells or latex particles coated with antigen[55-57] is reliable and sensitive. Precipitin and complement-fixation tests are thought to be less specific[58] although they may be of value as a screening procedure. An indirect immunofluorescent procedure is also useful in detecting antibody, but optimum conditions for the test may not yet have been established. If the predominant immunoglobulin class of antibody in the serum of patients with sporotrichosis is IgG, there may be an advantage in developing the fluorescent antibody test further.

Cutaneous reactivity to sporotrichin is present in most patients with sporotrichosis. Martins de Castro[59] reported positive skin tests in 64 of 65 patients with proven infection. There is evidence to suggest that patients with sporotrichosis will almost always react to sporotrichin and that a negative test may help to exclude the diagnosis. Specificity of the reaction, however, is apparently low, positive reactions being obtained in patients with unrelated conditions. Gonzalez Ochoa[60] has reported that polysaccharide antigen prepared from the filamentous phase elicits positive skin reactions only in patients with active infection. Following elimination of infection, cutaneous reactivity is lost within 3 years. In contrast, reactivity to yeast-phase antigen is maintained more or less indefinitely. Individuals with disseminated infection may be anergic[61]. The role of acquired immunity in resistance to sporotrichosis has been reviewed by Lurie[62]. In this mycosis, yeast-like organisms of *S. schenckii* are often sparse, and may be difficult to detect even in tissues stained specially for fungi. In some patients, however, fungal elements are abundant. Padilha Goncalves[63] and his associates[61] have suggested that, when entry of the pathogen is through the skin and the typical chancre-like lesion is formed, acquired immunity in the form of antibodies and cell-mediated immunity develops and spread of the disease is checked. In these circumstances yeast cells of *Sporothrix* are scarce in the tissues. Dissemination, which occurs infrequently, may be potentiated by lack of immunity and/or entry of the pathogen into the body by inhalation or injection. Characteristically in such patients skin reactivity to sporotrichin is absent and the organisms are abundant in infected tissues. In previous reviews of sporotrichosis[64,65] about 50% of reported cases were in patients with malignant disease. Occupation is another factor increasing the likelihood of infection, as in individuals such as nursery workers exposed to plants and soil who thus come into frequent contact with *S. schenckii*[66]. Ingrish and Schneidau[67] reported that 58% of nursery workers had a positive skin test to sporotrichin compared with 11% of a control population.

Steel *et al.*[68] examined cellular responses to sporotrichin using skin tests and lymphocyte transformation. Cross-reactivity was checked by simultaneous tests with antigens derived from *Candida albicans* and *Coccidioides immitis*. Positive skin responses were obtained in only five of the 143 control subjects tested with sporotrichin, in contrast to the 116 reacting to *C. albicans* and four reacting to *Coccidioides*.

Blastogenic responses of peripheral blood lymphocytes correlated well with the skin-test results. One patient with articular sporotrichosis had positive skin and lymphocyte transformation tests. Since marked cross-reactivity was noted in this study between results with *S. schenckii* and *C. albicans*, the authors suggest that the co-existence of intact cellular immune responses and exposure to *C. albicans* may lead to a state of refractoriness to infection with *S. schenckii*.

Antigenic determinants of the cell-wall polysaccharides of *S. schenckii* and related fungi have been studied by Lloyd and Travassos[69], and shown to be associated with rhamnose-containing mannans. Precipitation and inhibition data showed that the immunodominant structure was α-L-Rha$p$-$(1 \rightarrow 2)$-α-L-Rha$p$-$(1 \rightarrow 3)$-D-Man-$(1 \rightarrow$. Of interest was the finding that of the fungi tested only *S. schenckii* produced polysaccharides with large amounts of α-L-Rha$p$-$(1 \rightarrow 2)$-α-L-Rha$p$-$(1 \rightarrow$ side chains, and that these were formed at 25 °C but not at 37 °C.

2.9.3 Histoplasmosis

2.9.3.1 *Skin tests*

Individuals infected with *Histoplasma capsulatum* acquire skin sensitivity to histoplasmin, and skin tests have provided an invaluable means of defining endemic areas. It was realized a little over three decades ago that histoplasmosis, far from being a rare and uniformly fatal mycosis, was exceedingly common, and moreover, was generally mild and self-limiting. This awareness stems from the finding that many US military recruits during World War II had radiological evidence suggesting pulmonary tuberculosis but were negative in the tuberculin skin test. Only when the histoplasmin skin test was introduced routinely in the early 1940s was it realized that the aetiology of many subjects with non-tuberculous pulmonary calcification was fungal[70]. This discovery heralded the modern era of medical mycology, where the attention of clinicians, pathologists and epidemiologists, was drawn to infections of man caused by inhalation of airborne spores. Histoplasmin is still widely used and skin-test surveys have been of great value in building up information on the world-wide distribution and prevalence of skin-test reactions[71].

Histoplasmin is prepared by ammonium sulphate precipitation of an asparaginate broth culture filtrate in which the mycelial phase of the dimorphic fungus *H. capsulatum* has been growing for several months. Batches of histoplasmin are tested against a battery of skin-sensitive individuals. Selection of a reference reagent is made on the basis of such factors as sensitivity, specificity and stability. Batch-to-batch variation is minimized by the simple expedient of producing the skin-test material in large quantities. The current histoplasmin used by the US Public Health Service (H42) has now been in use for nearly three decades[72]. Histoplasmin is produced commercially in the United States. Information obtained by reactivity to histoplasmin has greatly increased our knowledge of this disease and its distribution, and there is no denying its eminence as a tried and trusted reagent. It is nevertheless the case that the mode of production of histoplasmin owes more to the precedent set by production of tuberculin and coccidioidin than to any carefully formulated approach based on an understanding of the growth requirements and characteristics of the agent in general and the precise immunochemical nature of the active allergens. The culture filtrate contains a wide range of secondary metabolites and an undetermined number of products released into the culture medium by dissolution of the mycelium. The parasitic phase of *Histoplasma* is yeast-like, not mycelial, and it might have been anticipated that immunologically active yeast-cell components would provide a suitable source of antigens for both skin and serological tests. In view of the amount of research into all aspects of histoplasmosis which has been initiated over the past three decades it is perhaps surprising that so little attention has been paid to the extraction, characterization and application of purified skin-test antigens. The failure of investigators to focus on this area is all the more surprising in view of the known cross-reactivity of histoplasmin with extracts of other pathogenic and non-pathogenic fungi. One of the few series of attempts in recent years to define more precisely the immunochemical nature of the active components of histoplasmin has been the studies by Sprouse and his colleagues in Oklahoma[73-75]. It was shown that crude histoplasmin fractionated on G-25 Sephadex columns yielded active skin-test material which had characteristics of a protein-carbohydrate complex. One fraction, HPDd$_{11}$, was reactive in guinea-pigs infected with *H. capsulatum* but not *Blastomyces dermatitidis*. Similar studies by O'Connell *et al.*[76] with different fractionating procedures led to the recognition of carbohydrate-rich fractions with potent skin activity from *H. capsulatum*. The principal theoretical advantages to be gained by this type of approach are elimination of non-reactive substances, ability to dehydrate and reconstitute to known potency on the basis of dry weight, and an overall improvement in standardization of the preparation and use of the product.

The histoplasmin skin test is read at 48–72 hours. Positive reactions are indicated by induration diameters of 5 mm or greater. Skin sensitivity suggests past or present infection, without distinguishing between them. A negative reaction does not necessarily exclude infection, but may represent anergy, tolerance, an improperly performed test or an impotent antigen[77]. Cross-reactions have been referred to on p. 30 but the principal cross-reacting pathogens are *Blastomyces* and *Coccidioides*. Interpretations of skin tests should take into account the clinical history of the patient and geographical origins or travels. The proportion of subjects reacting to histoplasmin in an endemic area may be 85% or higher[71]. The diagnostic value of a histoplasmin skin test is proportional to the length of time the patient had spent in the endemic area. In the States bordering on the Mississippi valley, where histoplasmin reactivity ranges from 40 to 90%, a positive skin test is likely to be of greater assistance in detecting anergy than in establishing a diagnosis.

2.9.3.2 *Antibody formation*

Antibody formation following infection with *H. capsulatum* has been studied intensively, and serodiagnostic tests have been developed to the point where they can make a positive and reliable contribution to both diagnosis and prognosis of the disease. Two basic types of antigen are used, viz. histoplasmin (mycelial-phase culture filtrate) and killed whole yeast-phase cells. Many different serological procedures have been evaluated, but the most common – and most reliable – tests are complement fixation (CF), double diffusion (DD) and latex agglutination (LA).

(a) *Complement fixation* – The procedure most widely used is the Laboratory Branch Complement Fixation (LBCF) test[78] and the most widely used antigens are histoplasmin and merthiolate-treated whole yeast cells. Antibodies are generally demonstrable 2–4 weeks after exposure, their appearance often coinciding with the onset of symptoms. Titres of 1:8 or greater are regarded as presumptive evidence of active infection. The higher the titre the greater the likelihood of severe disease. Low titres do not necessarily exclude severe infection, and rising or falling titres correlate better with disease, corresponding to progression and improvement respectively. As with all serological tests interpretations on single serum specimens are difficult or impossible to make, and serial examinations should be made wherever possible. The CF test is more frequently positive in patients with chronic active pulmonary histoplasmosis than with primary acute respiratory infection.

(b) *Immunodiffusion* – Double diffusion in agar gel was first used as a routine serodiagnostic procedure for histoplasmosis by Heiner[79]. Using technological methodology characterized equally by simplicity and effectiveness, Heiner distinguished several precipitinogens two of which, the 'H' and 'M' antigens, have proved to be of considerable serodiagnostic value.

Antibodies to the H antigen are produced during active and recent disease. In contrast M precipitins occur in the sera of patients with acute and chronic infections and persist following resolution of the disease. Correlations exist between the type of serum precipitin present and the state of development of the disease process. Thus, M precipitins appear early; in mild, self-limiting histoplasmosis H precipitins may not develop at all. As the disease progresses H antibody becomes apparent along with an increasing CF titre to yeast-phase *H. capsulatum*[80]. In remission, the H-precipitin band disappears and the CF titre declines. The H band is usually found in association with the M band, but the latter is often found alone.

Skin tests with currently available histoplasmin may boost antibody levels, and for this reason serum for antibody studies should always be drawn before skin testing – or at least within 2–3 days following the skin test, before antibodies have developed[81]. The proportion of subjects showing elevated CF titres to histoplasmin following a skin test ranges from 3 to 58%. Maximum antibody levels are noted 2–3 weeks following the test and persist up to 6 months. Elevated CF titres to yeast-phase antigen are encountered less frequently, varying from 0 to 14%. The appearance of M precipitins following a single positive skin test is more common, occurring in 12–90% of subjects. Kaufman *et al.*[82] have attempted to eliminate this problem by the use in skin tests of sensitized subjects with histoplasmin deficient in the M component. In their studies no humoral boosting effect was noted. Repeated skin tests with histoplasmin do not induce Type IV hypersensitivity in infected subjects. The booster effect noted in levels of CF or precipitating antibodies occurs only following a positive skin-test reaction.

Both H and M antigens have been obtained from yeast-phase *H. capsulatum*[83]. Their chemical nature has not yet been fully defined, but from studies made to date, they would appear to contain both protein and polysaccharide components[74]. Deproteinization of histoplasmin renders it ineffective in skin tests[84] and in serological tests[85]. Kobayashi[86], however, isolated from culture filtrate an immunologically active polysaccharide containing glucose and mannose but only 0.39% nitrogen and no detectable amino acids.

(c) *Latex agglutination* – The latex agglutination test, in which polystyrene particles coated with mycelial-phase histoplasmin are agglutinated by serum antibodies, is often used in recognizing early serological responses in acute histoplasmosis[87]. This procedure may be particularly useful when sera are anti-complementary, but it is not a substitute for the CF test and is not by itself diagnostically or prognostically helpful.

2.9.3.3 *Protective immunity*

Protective immunity in histoplasmosis is thought to be cellular[88]. Garcia and Howard[89] showed that mice inoculated intraperitoneally with intact yeast cells or cell walls were protected for 21 days against intravenous challenge with *H. capsulatum*. Restriction of the intracellular growth of *H. capsulatum* within mouse peritoneal cells was noted by Howard *et al.*[90] and thought to be mediated by lymphocytes. Partially purified lymphocytes from the peritoneal cavity of mice immunized by sublethal infection inhibited intracellular growth of *H. capsulatum in vitro* within macrophages obtained from normal mice. Studies by Domer[91] showed that treatment of *H. capsulatum* yeast cells with lipid solvents inhibited transformation of lymphocytes from sensitized guinea-pigs. Variations in lymphocyte reactivity to histoplasmin were noted in patients with chronic pulmonary histoplasmosis and periods of exacerbation were associated with diminished lymphocyte reactivity in two of three patients. In contrast the third patient had marked lymphocyte responsiveness to histoplasmin at the time of active disease. Variation in the lymphocyte responses of these three patients was marked, both general and specific defects being noted in the subjects with diminished cellular immunity, and the third subject showing no reduction in blastogenesis.

Experimental studies on acquired resistance to histoplasmosis have suggested that ribosomes may induce protective immunity in mice[93]. Spleen cells or peritoneal cells from animals sensitized with live cells of *H. capsulatum* provided 90–100% protection to intravenous challenge. This figure was comparable to the protection obtained with ribosomes or live cells[94]. No such protection was seen in animals receiving serum from immunized animals prior to challenge.

Transfer factor was shown by Smith *et al.*[95] to cause transient restoration of skin-test and lymphocyte responsiveness to histoplasmin in a patient with anergic chronic pulmonary histoplasmosis. Acquired immunity is strongly suggested by the finding that experimentally infected dogs subjected to re-infection challenge acquire almost complete protection[96]. It is not yet known if re-infection histoplasmosis is *endogenous*, resulting from suppression of immunity and subsequent proliferation of *H. capsulatum* from formerly quiescent foci in the reticuloendothelial system[96], or *exogenous*, resulting from exposure to aerosol infection which overwhelms the acquired resistance of the host[97]. Presumably both types of pathogenesis may exist, for there is no reason to suppose that a single mechanism must be involved.

2.9.4 Coccidioidomycosis

The immune responses in patients acquiring coccidioidomycosis are comparable to those seen in histoplasmosis. In most instances the infection, acquired by the respiratory route by the inhalation of airborne spores, is benign, mild, usually inapparent and self-limiting. Disseminating disease is rare and has a high fatality rate. Following mild primary acute coccidioido-mycosis, chronic pulmonary disease may become established, or there may be systemic involvement affecting bones, meninges, joints, and both sub-cutaneous and cutaneous tissues. The inflammatory response may be pre-dominantly suppurative in rapidly disseminating disease, or granulomatous in chronic or slowly progressive infection. The agent grows saprophytically in the upper soil layers and man becomes infected following inhalation of airborne spores. The geographical distribution is more restricted than that of histoplasmosis, being confined to the arid south-western United States and northern Mexico. Other endemic areas exist in Central America, Venezuela, Colombia, Argentina and Paraguay.

Most subjects with non-progressive primary coccidioidomycosis develop cutaneous reactivity within the first week of illness, and by the third week virtually all infected individuals have demonstrable Type IV hypersensitivity to coccidioidin[98]. Anergy is common in patients with severe pulmonary cavitation or extensive dissemination, cellular reactivity being impaired to other skin-testing reagents as well as coccidioidin[99]. Cross-reactivity between coccidioidin and other fungal antigens is generally thought to be less pro-nounced than with histoplasmin, but 10–35% of guinea-pigs sensitized to *C. immitis* were found to react to *Aspergillus fumigatus*, *A. terreus* and *Nocardia asteroides*, compared with 75% of animals reacting to homologous antigen[12]. Cross-reactions have been noted with coccidioidin in patients infected with *Histoplasma* and *Blastomyces*[100]. Earlier studies of the development of cutaneous reactivity in natural infections have been followed by investigations of the responsiveness of macrophages or lymphocytes in the presence of coccidioidin[101–104].

Lymphocyte stimulation shows a good correlation with cutaneous reactivity. Cox *et al.*[104] noted that lymphocyte responses were demonstrable *in vitro* when obtained from healthy, coccidioidin skin-test positive subjects and healthy skin-test reactors who had primary asymptomatic coccidioido-mycosis. In contrast no cellular responses were observed *in vivo* or *in vitro* in patients with active pulmonary coccidioidomycosis or with disseminated disease. Responses of five patients who had been in clinical remission for a year or more were intermediate. A similar correlation with macrophage inhibition has not been recorded. Sinski *et al.*[102] reported erythema, oedema and an induration-like reaction to intradermal injection of coccidioidin in sensitized guinea-pigs, but no migration inhibition of peritoneal exudate macrophages was observed. Progressive loss of cutaneous reactivity in guinea-pigs sensitized with coccidioidin and tuberculin was reported by Ibrahim and Pappagiannis[105] following repeated daily injection of coc-cidioidal antigen. The anergy was specific to *Coccidioides*, the skin response to tuberculin being unaffected. The rate at which sensitivity was lost was influenced by the antigen dose. Reactivity to coccidioidal antigen was restored several days after discontinuing injection of antigen.

The active principle of coccidioidin appears to be a glycoprotein com-plex[106] with a molecular weight of 31 700. Anderson *et al.*[107] studied skin-test reactivities of individual fractions isolated from mycelial culture filtrate and autolysates. Their findings suggested that activity was not confined to a single component, and that antigenicity was associated with a range of molecular components rather than a single discrete antigen. Using two-dimensional immunoelectrophoresis, Huppert et al.[108] showed that coccidioidin contained some antigens which were *Coccidioides*-specific and others which cross-reacted with *Histoplasma* and *Blastomyces*.

In nature, *Coccidioides* exists in the form of a mycelium of which individual hyphae disintegrate to produce the infectious arthrospores. In infected tissues, however, *Coccidioides* develops large (30–60 μm diameter) globular spherules, which, when mature, contain endospores. By manipulating cultural conditions, it is possible to grow the parasitic phase of this dimorphic fungus *in vitro*, and attempts have been made to develop spherulin – which is produced by lysing spherules – as a skin-test reagent[109,110]. Initial studies have been promising. Levine et al.[111] reported that 64% of 243 residents of an endemic area in Mexico reacted to spherulin, in contrast to a 41% reactivity obtained with coccidioidin. All coccidioidin reactors were spherulin-positive, but in 35% of the spherulin reactors skin tests with coccidioidin were negative. Moreover, one individual with disseminated disease reacted to spherulin but not to coccidioidin. Later studies[112] tended to confirm that, in contrast to coccidioidin, spherulin elicited cutaneous reactions in patients with disseminated coccidioidomycosis. Its effectiveness in stimulating sensitized lymphocytes was demonstrated by Cox et al.[104].

2.9.4.1 *Serology*

In addition to the development of a positive skin test to coccidioidin most subjects with symptomatic disease develop antibodies which can be detected and measured by appropriate serological procedures. Precipitating antibodies appear in the majority of cases 1–3 weeks after primary infection. They are readily detectable by tube precipitin, double diffusion or counter-immuno-electrophoresis procedures, and are generally short-lived, seldom being detectable after 4–6 months. They can reappear following spread or relapse.

Complement-fixing antibodies also appear early in the disease, but persist longer. The studies made by Smith and his colleagues[113] established the diagnostic and prognostic value of rising and falling titres, which correspond to dissemination and resolution respectively, CF titres rise in proportion to severity of infection and decline as the patient improves. By using both precipitin and CF tests, positive serological tests can be anticipated in over 90% of primary symptomatic cases of coccidioidomycosis[114]. Unlike histo-plasmin, a positive coccidioidin skin test does not elicit an antibody response.

An additional serological screening test is the latex particle agglutination technique where results coincide fairly closely with the tube precipitin test.

As with most systemic mycoses, no single serological method is adequate for detection of all definite or probable cases of infection and better results are always obtained when a combination of tests are used, such as double diffusion and complement fixation.

Counterimmunoelectrophoresis appears to be a reliable substitute for double diffusion[115]. Coccidioidomycosis of the central nervous system may be suggested by the demonstration of complement fixation by cerebrospinal fluid (CSF). Smith *et al.*[113] showed that this occurred in about 75% of patients with coccidioidal meningitis. More recently it has been shown that specific precipitins can be demonstrated in CSF concentrated and tested by double diffusion. A positive double diffusion test with a specimen of CSF is not by itself diagnostic, but is more reliable when there are also increased cells and protein and decreased sugar[116].

2.9.4.2 *Immunity*

Patients who recover from infection, whether or not it is symptomatic, are usually immune to re-infection. When re-infection does occur, it is rarely exogenous[117]. In most instances reactivation of a latent focus of infection takes place by a depression of the acquired immunity of the host. A characteristic feature of a proportion of cases with spontaneously acquired infection is the development of erythema nodosum and erythema multiforme – cutaneous expressions of hypersensitivity relating to the development of cell-mediated immunity. Appearance of these nodules coincides with the development of resistance to infection and containment of the disease. This response is more common in women than in men, and in white rather than dark-skinned individuals.

The basis for resistance to coccidioidomycosis appears to be closely linked with cell-mediated immunity. Attempts have been made to produce a vaccine, and although protection – albeit quantitative rather than qualitative – can be produced in animals immunized with coccidioidin[29], immune responses in inoculated humans have been variable[31]. There is some evidence from experimental studies to suggest that immune responses may include a specifically conditioned augmentation of phagocytic activity. Transfer factor (TF) has been used in attempts to restore cellular immunity to coccidioidomycosis. Graybill *et al.*[32] reported prolonged clinical remissions in two of three patients receiving TF. Temporary remission was also reported in a single patient treated with TF by Valasco-Castrejon *et al.*[118] but Cloninger *et al.*[119] reported a cure with TF in a patient with coccidioidal osteomyelitis who had failed to respond to amphotericin.

2.9.5 Blastomycosis

The fungus causing blastomycosis (= North American Blastomycosis) is *Blastomyces dermatitidis.* In common with *Histoplasma* and *Coccidioides,* it is dimorphic, being yeast-like (Y) in infected tissues and mycelial (M) when grown *in vitro*. Although not closely related to either *Coccidioides* or *Histoplasma*, antigens extracted from Y and M forms cross-react with antigens extracted from *Histoplasma* when tested against heterologous antisera. Cross-reactions with *Aspergillus* have also been reported[120]. *Blastomyces* is known to produce a systemic mycosis in Africa as well as the North American continent. So far as can be determined, the causal agents belong to the same species, although fluorescent antibody studies suggest that antigenic differences exist[121]. The African type appeared to be more closely related antigenically to *Paracoccidioides brasiliensis*, the cause of South American blastomycosis, than to American isolates of *B. dermatitidis*.

Lack of specificity has proved a major problem in studying immune responses in blastomycosis. Galactomannans from *B. dermatitidis* when tested in agar gel double diffusion against rabbit antisera show identical reactions to similar polysaccharides obtained from *Histoplasma* and *Paracoccidioides*[122]. Sera from patients with histoplasmosis and blastomycosis cross-react when tested by skin or serological tests against heterologous antigens. For this reason, no skin-test material is currently available from a commercial source. Complement-fixing tests are of little diagnostic value, and are positive in only about 50% of sera from patients with culturally or histologically proven infection. Moreover, positive reactions may occur in patients with other mycoses such as coccidioidomycosis, histoplasmosis and paracoccidioidomycosis.

The precipitin (double diffusion) test, using antigen from yeast-phase *B. dermatitidis* is more helpful, with a sensitivity of about 80% and a satisfactory specificity[123]. Disappearance of precipitins is a favourable prognostic sign, but they may persist for 30 days after successful treatment of the disease. Kaufman[124] has described two antigens (A and B) associated with Y-phase *B. dermatitidis*. Antibodies to A or A and B are thought to indicate recent or current infection.

Despite the unpredictable response of infected subjects to intradermal tests with blastomycin (concentrated mycelial-phase culture filtrate), acquired resistance to infection is thought to be related to cellular rather than humoral responses. Type IV hypersensitivity has been transferred by spleen cells from mice sensitized with *B. dermatitidis*[125]. Acquisition of hypersensitivity in mice coincided with a significant protection from the lethal effect of subsequent intraperitoneal challenge[126]. Furcolow and Smith[127] postulate that the ineffectiveness of the blastomycin may be more apparent than real. It is suggested that infections may be uncommon, and that a negative skin test may actually mean that there has been no prior infection. Sarosi and King[128] followed 18 subjects involved in a point-source epidemic for 3 years and showed not only that cutaneous reactivity was demonstrable in 16 of the infected individuals (89%) but that it diminished quite rapidly following spontaneous recovery. At present, both the value and reliability of a skin test are unknown. Hints of the existence of specific cell-wall components have been provided by Lancaster and Sprouse[129,130] using acrylamide gel electrophoresis and experimentally infected guinea-pigs.

Similar studies by Deighton et al.[131] showed an encouraging degree of specificity for a cell-wall fraction of B. dermatitidis in tests for skin reactivity, macrophage inhibition and lymphocyte transformation.

Vaccination studies have received little attention in experimental blastomycosis, although Landay et al.[132] showed that mice immunized with the insoluble component of disrupted B. dermatitidis yeast cells were partially protected against lethal challenge with a spore-mycelium suspension but not with yeast cells. The occurrence of blastomycosis in immunosuppressed subjects has been reported[133,134] but is apparently not a commonly recognized association.

2.9.6 South American blastomycosis (paracoccidioidomycosis)

This chronic, progressive, granulomatous disease affects mainly the lungs, oral mucosa and skin, with a tendency to spread and involve lymph nodes, adrenals and other viscera[135]. The prognosis in untreated disseminated infections is poor and the mortality amongst children in one series reported from Brazil by Castro and Negro[136] was 31%. The aetiological agent is *Paracoccidioides brasiliensis*, a dimorphic fungus with characteristic yeast and mycelial phases. The disease is apparently confined to the Latin American countries of the New World. Although different forms of the disease exist the lung is the most likely and most frequent portal of entry of the pathogen from an exogenous source[137,138]. The natural reservoir of *Paracoccidioides* in unknown, although Borelli[139] suggests that an underground habitat is probable.

Several features of the disease are unusual. Clinically defined paracoccidioidomycosis is much more common in males than in females. In one report, 66 of 68 patients studied for patterns of immunoglobulin class responses to infection were male[140]. In this study, IgG levels were consistently high, but IgM and IgA values were within normal limits. The marked susceptibility of males to infections with *Paracoccidioides* has been borne out by other studies, but a clear distinction must be made between infection and disease. On the basis of cutaneous reactivity to *Paracoccidioides* antigen, it would appear that although the infection rates are similar for both sexes, there is a distinct tendency for overt disease to be expressed in males.

Another unusual finding in paracoccidioidomycosis is the latent state which may follow establishment of infection. It is not uncommon for lesions to appear in individuals decades after their last residence in an endemic zone. In view of the variety of clinical expressions and histories associated with this disease it is clear that its course is influenced by a variety of factors.

2.9.6.1 Skin reactivity

It has been known for more than 50 years[141] that infected subjects acquire skin hypersensitivity. Fava Netto et al.[142] skin-tested 100 patients with two types of antigen derived from *Paracoccidioides, viz.* polysaccharide and culture filtrate. Reactions were not always obtained, being negative in 23–33% of infected subjects. Musatti et al.[143] reported that almost half of 19 patients studied showed depressed cell-mediated responses to *Paracoccidioides* antigen, failure to develop sensitization to 2,4-dinitrochlorbenzene (DNCB), and unresponsiveness of lymphocytes to *P. brasiliensis* antigen or phytohaemagglutinin. Of particular interest in this study was the observation of a factor present in the plasma of some patients which reduced the ability of lymphocytes to undergo blastogenesis. This factor inhibited lymphocytes from patients and healthy subjects, and its absence correlated with a demonstrable Type IV skin hypersensitivity. Cross-reactions to histoplasmin were reported by Negroni et al.[144] in 50% of 56 patients with paracoccidioidomycosis. In this same study, the paracoccidioidin skin test was positive in 2–3 of 15 patients with proven histoplasmosis. Cross-reactions also occur in patients with sporotrichosis[145]. The value of the paracoccidioidin skin test in epidemiological studies was demonstrated by Greer et al.[146]. In studying the dermal sensitivity of family contacts of 22 patients with *P. brasiliensis* infection, it was shown that although active disease was not demonstrated in the spouses of the patients, positive skin tests suggested that they were 3–5 times more likely to be infected than other adults.

Patients with paracoccidioidomycosis have been shown to have reduced percentages of T cells; affected lymph nodes showed a depletion of T lymphocytes in the paracortical area and there was a reduction in size of the follicles[147]. Restoration of immune responsiveness with transfer factor was reported by Mendes[148] in two out of five patients with skin-test anergy to microbial antigens and DNCB. In one patient there was a clinical improvement following administration of transfer factor which was described as dramatic.

2.9.6.2 Serological tests

Serological tests have been widely used as a laboratory diagnostic procedure[149]. CF antibodies were demonstrated in sera of patients more than six decades ago. Results with this test correlate well with the evolving condition, titres rising as the disease progresses and falling with successful therapy. Favo Netto[150], using a yeast-phase polysaccharide antigen, obtained positive CF titres in 83 of 100 patients. In a later study[151] it was reported that the first antibodies to appear in paracoccidioidomycosis were precipitins. They were also the first to disappear as the patient improved on therapy. CF antibodies appeared later and persisted longer. Low titres are present in mild, localized forms and high in disseminated forms. Simultaneous testing with CF and gel diffusion procedures gave positive results in over 98% of patients with active disease. Restrepo summarized findings on over 1000 CF and precipitin tests. On 61 patients studied in Colombia[152] positive results were obtained in 95% and 79% of the precipitin and CF tests respectively. In other studies Restrepo and Drouhet[153], using immunoelectrophoresis, showed that paracoccidioidin could be resolved into five bands, designated A–E. Restrepo has also reported that one antigen from *P. brasiliensis* (antigen 3) was identical to the M antigen of *Histoplasma capsulatum*. One specific antigen designated E has been investigated by Yarzabal and his associates[154–158]. This antigen was shown to be a protein with cationic mobility and was further characterized as having alkaline phosphatase activity. One fraction designated E_2, obtained by affinity chromatography, appeared to be the specific antigenic determinant for the immunoelectrophoretic band E. It reacted in gel diffusion tests only against the sera from patients with paracoccidioidomycosis.

2.9.7 Cryptococcosis

Cryptococcosis is acquired by the inhalation of the pathogenic yeast *Cryptococcus neoformans* from an exogenous source, which is commonly soil contaminated with pigeon faeces. Most individuals have an innate resistance, and proliferation of the yeast in the lung following inhalation is usually both minimal and self-limiting. Exceptionally, dissemination from a pulmonary focus may occur, with the formation of lesions in skin, bone and internal organs. Involvement of the central nervous system with subacute or chronic meningitis is the most familiar form of the disease, with a high mortality rate unless diagnosed early and treated vigorously.

Cryptococcosis is commonly associated with co-existing disease, particularly of the reticuloendothelial and lymphatic systems. It is also found in patients receiving immunosuppressive or corticosteroid treatment and renal transplants[159–161]. A common association exists between cryptococcal meningitis and Hodgkin's disease, but a variety of chronic systemic diseases have been recognized as predisposing towards cryptococcosis, including sarcoid, lupus erythematosus, diabetes, malignant diseases of the blood and endocrine disorders.

Cells of *C. neoformans* in infected tissues are usually surrounded by a large polysaccharide capsule. In the spinal fluid of patients with CNS infections, soluble capsular material can be detected by the latex agglutination (LA) test, using polystyrene particles coated with immunoglobulin from hyperimmune rabbit antiserum. Capsular antigen can be detected and quantitated in cerebrospinal fluid and serum, and the titres bear a direct relationship to the severity of infection. High LA titres have a poor prognosis[162]. Improvement on therapy (amphotericin B alone or in combination with 5-fluorocytosine) is accompanied by a falling LA titre and antigen eventually disappears from the serum and is replaced by antibody. False positive LA tests occur in the presence of rheumatoid factor, but can be eliminated by prior treatment of the serum with a reducing agent such as dithiothreitol[163]. Specificity of the cryptococcal LA test is good, and the correlation with active disease is excellent. Not all patients with proven cryptococcosis have a positive test however. In one series of 48 patients whose CSF or sera were examined in the author's laboratory, antigen was detected in 33 of 35 CNS infections and in four of six infections involving the viscera or blood, but in only one of seven patients with localized cryptococcal lesions of skin, bone or lymph node.

Antibody responses are less specific but may be of value in detecting early stages of infection and monitoring the effect of therapy. They are generally detected and measured by agglutination and indirect fluorescent antibody tests. Positive results are obtained with less than 50% of sera from proven cases. Specificities of the indirect fluorescent antibody (IFA) and agglutination tests have been reported as 79% and 95% respectively[164]. Blumer and Kaufman[165] found increased levels of IgM immunoglobulin in the sera of 11 patients with cryptococcosis. By using fluorescein-labelled monospecific anti-human IgG and IgM, they showed that IgG was the immunoglobulin reacting in the IFA test. Antibodies from patients with other mycotic infections which cross-reacted in the IFA test were also shown to be IgG. Their studies failed to establish a correlation between infection with *C. neoformans* and levels of specific IgM antibody.

A contributory role for antibody in the elimination of *C. neoformans* was indicated by Diamond and Bennett[166]. Mononuclear cells from humans were able to kill *C. neoformans* cells by a non-phagocytic mechanism providing antibody was present. This may be an important means of eliminating the comparatively large yeast cells of *C. neoformans* which are not readily phagocytosed, particularly when heavily encapsulated. Only small quantities of antibody were required to mediate the extracellular killing of *C. neoformans*, some effect being noted with rabbit antiserum even at a 1:20 000 dilution. It may be that this finding is directly linked to the general observation that appearance of antibody in patients with cryptococcosis usually correlates with cure.

Phagocytosis and intracellular killing of *C. neoformans* has been demonstrated *in vitro*[167]. Phagocytosis by neutrophils was not markedly altered by specific antibody or by soluble capsular material, but size of the capsule was an important factor. Inhibition of phagocytosis by capsular polysaccharide has nevertheless been reported[168]. Diamond and his associates[169-172] have shown that *C. neoformans* can activate complement by the alternative pathway and have demonstrated in guinea-pigs that the later components (C3–C9) are of importance in clearing cryptococci from extraneural sites. Yeast cells from the spinal fluid of patients with cryptococcal meningitis were found to have no demonstrable absorbed complement on their surfaces. In contrast, cryptococcal cells from such patients readily opsonized cryptococci.

Diamond and Bennett[173] reported a functional abnormality in the T cells of patients with disseminated cryptococcosis. Incorporation of tritiated thymidine by lymphocytes of seven patients was significantly decreased in comparison to that by 12 healthy subjects with a positive skin test to cryptococcin. This study suggested that the cell abnormality was associated with susceptibility to disseminated cryptococcosis. It is not known whether this represents a basic underlying immune deficiency or whether it results from previous infection. The abnormality of T-cell function was found to persist for some months after successful therapy of the disease.

Graybill and Alford[174] studied cell-mediated immunity in cryptococcosis and showed that lymphocytes from two of 13 patients with cryptococcosis failed to transform *in vitro* in the presence of cryptococcal cell extract (cryptococcin). Reactions were obtained with lymphocytes from 50% of the 24 healthy controls and with three of six control subjects who worked in a laboratory where *C. neoformans* was grown. Only one control subject had a positive skin test to cryptococcin.

Skin-test preparations to date have had a low level of specificity, and have not yet been widely used in epidemiological surveys. Muchmore *et al.*[175] reported positive skin tests in 32% of 82 subjects living in a small community in Oklahoma. Atkinson and Bennett[176] using a urea extract antigen found a high proportion of reactions amongst cryptococcal patients, but cross-reactions were observed in patients with other mycoses. Further refinement of the test may be possible, using different fractions, cellular or culture filtrates. Until a reliable reagent becomes available, the numbers of subclinical infections with *C. neoformans* will remain speculative.

2.9.8 Opportunist mycoses

A wide range of fungi normally regarded as non-pathogenic are capable of exploiting diminished resistance of the host. Such organisms exist saprophytically or commensally in the human external or internal environment respectively, sometimes in fairly large numbers. Common representatives include *Aspergillus, Candida, Mucor, Rhizopus, Absidia, Sporothrix* and *Fusarium*. The list is long, and the distinction between opportunistic and innate or primary pathogenicity is often obscure. Thus the agents of mycetoma are normally harmless to man, and can be regarded as opportunist since they appear to become established as pathogens only when implanted in the skin by trauma and perhaps only into individuals with an immune defect.

Similarly *Cryptococcus* is apparently more frequent as an opportunist than as a primary pathogen. In one sense, all mycoses have an element of opportunism, but consideration will be restricted to infections where establishment is promoted primarily by loss of metabolic, physiological or immunological integrity of the host. Among the commonly recognized causes of susceptibility are diseases such as diabetes, leukaemia, lymphoma, aplastic anaemia and cancer. Treatment with drugs (e.g. antibiotic, immunosuppressive, cytotoxic, corticosteroid or contraceptive) or surgery (e.g. cardiac, abdominal, transplantation or the use of indwelling catheters) also predispose to opportunist infections, as do physical factors such as burns, wounds and X-rays.

2.9.8.1 *Candidiasis*

Candidiasis has a wide range of clinical expression, with infections which are cutaneous, mucosal or deep-seated; localized or generalized; acute, subacute or chronic. The most common agent is *Candida albicans*, but several other species may be implicated, notably *C. parapsilosis*, *C. tropicalis*, *C. krusei* and *C. guilliermondii*. Mucosal candidiasis (thrush) is quite common, with localized, superficial vegetations occurring in the oral cavity, vagina, bronchial or alimentary systems. Candidiasis of the skin affects areas with opposing skin surfaces (intertrigo) and the lateral nail tissues (paronychia). Other skin involvement includes chronic mucocutaneous candidiasis and napkin rash of infants. Deep-seated candidiasis includes urinary and pulmonary candidiasis, *Candida* meningitis, *Candida* septicaemia and *Candida* endocarditis. Finally, allergic responses to *Candida* include id eruptions, eczema and asthma.

C. albicans is a normal member of the alimentary tract and may often be recovered in considerable numbers from mouth swabs or stools of healthy individuals. Predisposition is almost always present and many different causes of susceptibility have been recognized. Prominent amongst these are immune deficiencies, defects in phagocytic function and a wide range of physiological and endocrine disorders, malignancies, post-operative states and drug therapies.

(a) *Principal antigens* – Associated with the yeast cells of *C. albicans* are cell-wall polysaccharide (mannan) and cytoplasmic proteins. Using two-dimensional immunoelectrophoresis, Axelsen[177] detected and enumerated 78 water-soluble antigens, and suggested a simple means for standardization. Most antigens used in detection of humoral or cellular responses have not been well characterized and contain variable quantities of cell-wall and cytoplasmic material. Comparison of results from different investigations is made difficult by the absence of standardized products. In an attempt to rectify this situation, a Committee of the International Union of Immunological Societies has recommended the adoption of three reference antigens prepared from *C. albicans*, viz. whole cell extract, purified mannan and purified cytoplasmic protein, where mannan has been removed by complexing with cancanavalin A.

(b) *Antibodies* – Antibodies to mannan are exceedingly common in human sera. Providing a sufficiently sensitive technique is used, they can almost invariably be found. Antibodies to cytoplasmic protein are less common and for this reason they were originally considered to be of greater diagnostic significance. Antibodies to mannan and protein antigens are readily distinguished in gel diffusion tests, but as with most serological procedures, attempts to ascribe significance using the results obtained on single samples of serum are rarely successful. Much confusion exists over the value of serological testing, and much of this has been caused by a failure to realize the dangers of over-simplification. Thus antibodies to protein are *not* always significant, and antibodies to mannan are *not* always meaningless. Used with care and discrimination, however, serological tests can be of great value in recognizing candidiasis and in monitoring responses to therapy. It is essential to distinguish circumstances where serology is helpful from those where it is not. Tests for antibody are of little diagnostic value in patients with superficial lesions such as oral or vaginal thrush or with colonization of the lower urinary tract. They are more reliable in the evaluation of patients with deep-seated infections such as endocarditis, peritonitis, wound sepsis and visceral infection.

Candida endocarditis is an uncommon condition. Serial examinations of sera may provide the first clue to the presence of *Candida* in an infected heart valve. High or rising antibody titres should alert the clinician to the possibility of candidiasis. Patients with subacute bacterial endocarditis often develop rises in *Candida* antibody titres which are not pathognomonic[178]. Similarly patients receiving open-heart surgery commonly show transient antibody rises in the second week after operation[179]. Given realization of these limitations. and the invariable need to view serodiagnostic tests in the light of the condition and history of the patient, antibody studies can nevertheless be a useful measure of immune responses to infection or colonization.

The tests most commonly used are agar or agarose gel diffusion and counterimmunoelectrophoresis for the detection of precipitins and whole cell or inert particle agglutination. Complement fixation tests are rarely used because of the frequency with which antibodies can be detected in healthy subjects or in patients with superficial infection[180]. Lehner[181], using immunofluorescence, measured the antibody responses and immunoglobulin classes in patients with different types of candidiasis. Significant titres of IgG were found in 78% of the sera, IgM in 51% and IgA in 30%. Later studies[182] showed that precipitins belonged to the IgG class; agglutinins were predominantly IgM but IgG and IgA classes were also represented. Muller[183] considered that the predominant immunoglobulin to *Candida* cell-wall polysaccharide in the early stages of infection is IgM, and that this is later replaced by IgG. She has proposed that, in early infections, IgM will best be detected by haemagglutination, using sheep red cells coated with *Candida* polysaccharide. Later stages would be more suitably evaluated by an indirect immunofluorescent procedure, where the response is effected largely by IgG immunoglobulin. Antibodies to *C. albicans* can be detected in patients receiving cytostatic drugs[184]. Intravaginal immunization of women with *C. albicans* produced a marked increase in secretory IgA immunoglobulin[185]. A similar predominance of secretory IgA was reported by Mathur *et al.*[186], who considered that this immunoglobulin was produced locally. Antibody in the vagina is not thought to be produced locally, according to Milne *et al.*[187], who believe its presence in vaginal secretions is derived from serum.

Serum from most individuals causes a non-immunologically mediated clumping of *C. albicans*[188]. Clumping did not occur in the serum of three patients with chronic mucocutaneous candidiasis, and these sera inhibited clumping in normal sera. The clumping inhibitor was identified as specific IgG antibody directed against *C. albicans*. The clumping factor was characterized by Smith and Louria[189] as a macroeuglobulin with a fast β-mobility. Clumping activity of rabbit sera is gradually lost during a course of immunization, antibodies presumably competing with clumping factor for binding sites on the surface of the *Candida* yeast cells.

The literature on *Candida* serology is extensive, and often contradictory. Preisler *et al.*[190] studied *Candida* agglutinating and precipitating antibodies prospectively in 154 patients with acute leukaemia. Fourteen patients developed visceral candidiasis and only seven of these showed a significant rise in agglutinin titre. Filice *et al.*[191] have claimed that no correlation exists between *Candida* antibodies and invasive candidiasis in patients with neoplastic disease. These and other reports illustrate that differences in attitude exist towards the role and value of serological testing. Apart from the differences in procedure and therefore in the results obtained, the spectrum of procedures currently available has a major omission, viz. tests for the presence of circulating antigen rather than antibody. Free antigen was first reported by Axelsen and Kirkpatrick[192] in a patient with chronic mucocutaneous candidiasis, and it was detected in the form of mannan by Weiner and Yount[193] using a patient's serum to inhibit a specific haemagglutination test. Analytical procedures of great sensitivity are now available, and an enzyme-linked immunoassay (ELISA) for detection of *Candida* mannan has been developed[20, 21]. It is anticipated that such tests will be of value in detecting the early stages of acute candidiasis. Patients with false negative serological tests may well prove to have circulating or immune-complex antigen rather than antibody.

Candida albicans is so commonly present as a commensal that sensitization is often used as a measure of the immune competence of an individual. Shannon *et al.*[195] have shown that 95% of normal subjects have positive skin tests. Alford[247] reported lymphocyte stimulation of healthy adults but reduced reactivity of lymphocytes from hospital patients without recognized immunological disorders. The lymphocyte transformation test has been proposed as an assessment *in vitro* of cell-mediated immunity[200].

(c) *Cellular hypersensitivity* – Cellular hypersensitivity to *C. albicans* increases markedly with age. Holti[194] reported that the proportion of healthy subjects with Type IV hypersensitivity cutaneous reactions rose from 14% in the 11–20 age group to 83% in subjects of 50 or older. Shannon *et al.*[195] and Hiddlestone[196] reported figures of 95%, and a skin test with *Candida* extract is frequently used as an indicator of immune responsiveness. Cellular hypersensitivity is demonstrable *in vitro*. Significant blastic response was produced to *Candida* extract in lymphocyte cultures of all 25 normal subjects tested. Of interest was the finding that 22% of hospitalized patients had reduced lymphocyte responsiveness to *Candida*, although transformation to phytohaemagglutinin was the same in both groups. The extract used for skin and studies *in vitro* is crude and the nature of the antigens eliciting the responses has received comparatively little attention. Prick tests with mannan produced a Type I response in 7.7% of controls and 45% of asthmatics studied by Faux[197]. Intracutaneous tests of hospital patients with and without precipitins produced a dual (Type I and Type III) reaction in 75% and 15% respectively. Recent studies by Gettner[198] have suggested that both physical and chemical characteristics of the antigen used for tests *in vitro* are important. Thus mannan alone seldom caused lymphocyte stimulation but commonly did so when absorbed on to latex particles. Whole cells were also found to be effective in migration inhibition[199] and they are also effective in lymphocyte transformation studies[198].

Foroozanfar[200] has defined conditions for achieving optimum transformation of lymphocytes to *Candida* immunogen. Much attention has been paid to the immune status of patients with chronic mucocutaneous candidiasis[201–207]. In this condition it is common to find defective cellular immunity expressed as a failure to respond to a *Candida* skin test. Infected patients without demonstrable Type IV cutaneous reactivity show normal lymphocyte responses to *Candida* antigen *in vitro*. Chilgren *et al.*[202] suggested that this could be explained by a failure to produce MIF, and this was later confirmed by Valdimarsson *et al.*[208]. Various patterns of immune deficiency have been recognized in such patients. Skin-test anergy may be present to *Candida* alone or to *Candida* and other reagents such as PPD and DNCB. In either case, there may be decreased or normal transformation of lymphocytes in the presence of *Candida* and other antigens together with subnormal MIF production. In some patients MIF production is normal, in which case lymphocyte transformation may or may not be reduced. In this latter category, no cellular defect is revealed by any of the tests involved. In the series of 26 patients described by Valdimarson *et al.*[206] 10 were in this category. Presumably their candidiasis was prompted by factors other than those tested. Amongst the possibilities suggested were low levels of innate immunity, deficiency of iron or vitamin A, and ineffective non-specific defence mechanisms of the skin. In some instances it has been shown that failure of lymphocytes to respond to *Candida* antigen *in vitro* is associated with a serum factor. This blocking factor[206] has a specific action and the possibility exists that it is IgG antibody. This, in turn, raises a possibility that *Candida* antibody might play a regulatory role in diminishing cellular hypersensitivity, a hypotheses which awaits definitive confirmation or rebuttal. Patients with chronic mucocutaneous candidiasis having defective MIF production have macular and scaling skin reactions, but in two patients described by Valdimarrson *et al.*[206] whose lymphocytes failed to transform, but produced MIF, the disease was characterized by granuloma formation. Patients with chronic mucocutaneous candidiasis almost always have demonstrable antibodies to *C. albicans*. Although these are not thought to be the primary protective element of the immune system, it may be that they do afford some measure of protection against dissemination. Reconstitution of the immune system has been attempted. In view of the fact that different forms of immunological defect exist in patients with this condition[209] and the possibility that deficiencies might vary both quantitatively and qualitatively with time, it is perhaps not surprising that results with immunotherapy have been erratic and usually any improvement has been short-lived. Feigin *et al.*[210] reported complete remission in a patient treated with transfer factor and amphotericin B. De Sousa *et al.*[211] administered transfer factor on three occasions and observed temporary clinical improvement after each treatment. Littman *et al.*[212] suggest that successful use of transfer factor requires prior demonstrable reactivity of the donor's lymphocytes to *Candida* antigen.

In one patient described by Buckley *et al.*[213], a girl with chronic mucocutaneous candidiasis, immunological reconstitution was attempted by allogeneic bone marrow transplant. Clinical improvement in her condition was reported 6 months after treatment. Allogeneic lymphocyte transfer in combination with transfer factor restored cell-mediated immunity in a patient with keratoconjunctivitis and superficial candidiasis[214].

Immunosuppressive therapy may interfere with lymphocyte transformation *in vitro*. Folb and Trounce[215] showed a marked reduction in 17 patients treated with high doses of predisnisone, in 21 patients receiving combined azathioprine and predisnisone, and in six patients being treated with cyclophosphamide. Apart from the patients receiving cyclophosphamide, there was no reduction in agglutinin or immunofluorescent titres to *C. albicans*. The findings are consistent with the now widely held view that impairment of cellular immunity, whether by disease or therapy, is a major causal factor in the development of candidiasis. In experiments with T-cell deficient nude mice, Cutler[34] reported that they were *more* resistant to experimental candidiasis than normal mice. It would appear that the possession by these mice of intact non-specific mechanisms of resistance such as phagocytosis and serum factors was able to compensate for the absence of T-cell associated immunity. An active role for macrophages in limiting candidiasis was suggested by Neta *et al.*[216]. Macrophages from the peritoneum of normal guinea-pigs migrated well on an agar surface and readily phagocytosed cells of *Candida*. Macrophages from animals sensitized to *C. albicans* showed a reduced migratory and phagocytic capacity. It was suggested that the initial stages of cellular immunity may be associated with a reduced activity of phagocytic macrophages, which would limit spread of the pathogen from the infected area.

2.9.8.2 *Aspergilloma*

In this condition, *Aspergillus* grows in the form of compact mycelial masses up to 5 cm in diameter, the most common cause being *A. fumigatus*. It develops in a pre-existing condition such as open healed cavities of tuberculosis, sarcoidosis, carcinoma or lung abscess. These are often sequestered and asymptomatic, only being detected on routine X-ray. In some instances, the cavity connects with the bronchi and the fungus may then be isolated from sputum. The mass of antigen, together with its chronicity, usually ensures that high levels of antibody are present. Precipitin tests are positive in over 90% of cases.

2.9.8.3 *Invasive aspergillosis*

Patients with deep-seated aspergillosis almost always have a recognizable predisposition. Meyer *et al.*[217] reviewed 93 cases seen at a cancer hospital and reported that up to 1971 41% of the patients dying with acute leukaemia had evidence of aspergillosis. Young and Bennett[218] described lack of demonstrable antibodies in 15 patients, all but one having malignant diseases, particularly acute lymphocytic or acute myelogenous leukaemia.

It is generally found, however, that antibodies are present, although seldom produced in quantity. Using a gel diffusion procedure to monitor 80 patients with acute leukaemia at 2-weekly intervals, precipitins were discovered in seven out of 10 patients who developed invasive aspergillosis. In six of these seven subjects, the antibody response was weak.

2.10 DISEASES CAUSED BY RESPIRATORY HYPERSENSITIVITY

In this category, tissue damage is brought about by hypersensitivity mechanisms. Tissue invasion is absent. As a general rule the allergens are airborne spores or mycelial fragments. When IgE antibodies are produced in an atopic subject, exposure to the allergen will elicit a Type I (immediate) hypersensitivity. Asthma is the commonest expression and many subjects with seasonal extrinsic asthma owe their condition and its provocation to clouds of airborne spores which appear in the atmosphere at different times of the year. It is noteworthy that almost all fungi known to be associated with respiratory allergy have small spores, and that the part of the respiratory system where histopathological responses are elicited is correlated with the size of the airborne particle. Common airborne spores eliciting asthma, rhinitis or conjunctivitis are from such common fungi as *Ustilago*, *Alternaria*, *Aspergillus*, *Botrytis*, *Acremonium*, *Chaetomium*, *Cladosporium*, *Sporobolomyces*, *Mucor*, *Penicillium*, *Aureobasidium*, *Fusarium*, etc. The quantities of spores produced and released by fungi can be enormous. *Aspergillus fumigatus*, for example, is common on decaying vegetation. Levels in excess of 12 million spores per m^3 have been recorded in a cowshed[219]. Austwick[220] has estimated that an active man might be expected to inhale as many as 8.4×10^7 spores during a 3-hour working session in such an environment.

2.10.1 Allergic bronchopulmonary aspergillosis

Allergic bronchopulmonary aspergillosis (ABA) is a disease of atopic subjects. Prominent clinical features include asthma which is almost always accompanied by pulmonary eosinophilia. McCarthy and Pepys[221] consider that it is responsible for more than 80% of cases seen in the United Kingdom. Other consistent findings include recurrent, transient X-ray changes and a dual skin reaction following intradermal testing with *A. fumigatus* antigen and involving both Type I and III responses. In addition *A. fumigatus* can generally be recovered from sputum and there are almost always serum precipitins to *A. fumigatus*. In practice, the presence of asthma and pulmonary eosinophilia and an immediate (Type I) response to a skin test with *A. fumigatus* is strong diagnostic evidence for ABA. Precipitins are present in 60–70% of patients, but concentration of the serum or the use of a more sensitive test for antibodies (e.g. counterimmunoelectrophoresis) shows that precipitins are almost invariably present. Plugs, consisting of compacted mycelial elements and eosinophils are formed in the proximal bronchi and are expectorated with the sputum[222]. These are present in about 75% of cases at one time or another[223], and are responsible for the transient shadowing seen in the X-rays. The histopathological response is caused by a Type III (Arthus) reaction between antigen diffusing from the mycelial elements in the plug and circulating IgG antibody.

Detection of IgG antibodies is generally achieved by precipitin tests, using culture filtrate or mycelial-extract antigens. Many different antigens are produced by *Aspergillus*, and since individual response may vary considerably, it is often helpful to use more than one isolate of *A. fumigatus* as the source of antigen. Longbottom and Pepys[224] have shown that C-substance is produced in culture media after 6–7 weeks of incubation at 37 °C, and in young mycelial extracts. Its presence can elicit false positive reactions with sera containing C-reactive protein and this must be distinguished from specific anti-*Aspergillus* antibody. In practice, antigen may be prepared in such a way as to minimize or obviate production of C-substance. It can be eliminated from gel diffusion plates by immersion in sodium citrate or phosphate solutions of high ionic strength.

Aspergillus is not a normal member of microflora of humans, and most normal sera do not contain antibodies to *A. fumigatus*. Mearns *et al.*[225] have shown that *A. fumigatus* precipitins were present in 31% of 112 patients with cystic fibrosis compared with 7% of asthmatics and 3% of patients with non-respiratory disease. In individuals without pathological lung conditions, however, antibodies to *A. fumigatus* are rare.

The contribution made by IgG antibody to pathogenesis is determined in part by the relative amounts of antigen and antibody. In moderate antigen excess, soluble immune complexes are formed. These fix and activate the C3 component of complement leading to the attraction of polymorphs and subsequent release of their lysosomal enzymes into the extracellular tissue[226]. Immunofluorescent studies show the presence of both antibody and complement. Corticosteroids minimize the effects of lysosomal enzymes and are therefore of value in the management of ABA. IgE antibody is raised in patients with ABA; in one study by Arbesman *et al.*[227] it was present in all 21 patients with ABA, but in none of 32 patients with a variety of conditions but whose sera contained *Aspergillus* precipitins. These antibodies, detected by radio-allergosorbent (RAST) tests, have some diagnostic value. Pauwels *et al.*[228] also reported elevation of total serum IgE levels in patients with ABA but these were sometimes present in other forms of aspergillosis. In contrast, specific IgE antibodies almost always correlated with ABA, and were particularly evident during acute phases of the disease. Similar findings were reported by Patterson *et al.*[229]. Using a radioimmuno-assay technique, it was shown that serum IgE was elevated in patients with ABA, but not with Bird Fancier's Disease or Farmer's Lung.

2.10.2 Farmer's lung (extrinsic allergic alveolitis)

This disease syndrome is associated with sensitization of man or animals to airborne particles and is manifested in the distal portions of the respiratory system. Several names have been proposed but the most widely used are extrinsic allergic alveolitis and hypersensitivity pneumonitis. Farmer's Lung Disease (FLD) is expressed by the development of fever, chills, dyspnoea and cough some 4–8 hours after exposure to mouldy vegetation, usually hay. Similar effects may result from the inhalation of aerosolized avian materials such as serum, feathers and faeces (Bird Fancier's Disease), vegetable dust (e.g. bagassosis), sawdust (Bark Stripper's Disease), mushroom compost (Mushroom Workers' Lung), etc. Within this group of related diseases there are clearly basic similarities in both symptoms and lung pathology, and it is likely that there is a common mechanism of pathogenesis. Similarities include interstitial and alveolar inflammation, often accompanied by non-caseating granulomas. In this section, consideration will be confined to extrinsic allergic alveolitis (EAA) caused by the inhalation of actinomycetes (FLD) or fungi (Malt Worker's Lung).

Although known since the 1930s[230], a basic understanding of the aetiology and pathogenesis of FLD was not gained until the early 1960s with publication of the studies by Pepys and his colleagues in England[231] and Kobayshi et al. in the United States[232]. Following the realization that patients with FLD usually had precipitating antibodies to mouldy hay, microbiological, clinical and pathological investigations soon provided a basic description of the disease process. Roberts and Moore[233] have recently reviewed current knowledge on the immunopathogenetic mechanisms.

Hay harvested wet is colonized sequentially by different micro-organisms, and undergoes changes in its chemical and physical nature[234]. Agricultural workers exposed to mouldy hay encounter dense aerosols of spores. The most abundant and important source of spores are those from the thermophilic actinomycetes *Micropolyspora faeni* and *Thermoactinomyces vulgaris*. These are produced in enormous numbers and being very small (about 1 μm in diameter) are liable not only to penetrate as far as the alveoli but also to be retained there. In almost all acute cases of FLD, these spores elicit precipitating antibodies, detectable by double diffusion tests. Following repeated exposure, extensive and severely debilitating pulmonary fibrosis develops and the affected subject becomes increasingly incapacitated. Once removed from the antigen source, whether by change in occupation or by inability to continue working, antibody levels decline and eventually disappear. Lung damage, however, is irreversible, except in the early stages of disease, so the decline in antibody correlates with the lack of exposure rather than clinical improvement. These antibodies are primarily IgG and may attain concentrations[235] of 300–500 μg/ml. IgM and IgA antibodies are also produced[236]. Tests routinely used to detect and in some instances quantitate antibody responses include agar gel double diffusion, counterimmunoelectrophoresis, latex agglutination, complement fixation and immunofluorescence.

Antibodies can be found in the serum of individuals exposed to dust from mouldy hay but who are without symptoms of FLD. It was originally proposed that IgG antibodies participated in the disease process by forming immune complexes with the inhaled antigens in the patient's lung[237]. Histopathological and clinical responses suggest a Type III hypersensitivity response, but it is not yet known if this operates in the absence of other pathogenic mechanisms. Skin tests have not been helpful diagnostically or in suggesting an active role for cell-mediated immunity. It has been suggested that acquired cellular responsiveness might be demonstrable *in vitro* but may be masked *in vivo* by the Type III (Arthus) reaction. Macrophage inhibition and lymphocyte transformation studies have shown unequivocal evidence of specific responsiveness to avian antigens in Bird

Fancier's Disease and correlation with symptomatic rather than asymptomatic but exposed subjects[238]. Similar attempts with peripheral lymphocytes from patients with FLD have been variable, and tests have not distinguished between affected and exposed but asymptomatic subjects[239]. It may be that better correlations would be obtained with more critically characterized antigens. Evidence for the implication of T cells is certainly suggested by the study of naturally occurring or experimentally induced allergic alveolitis in animals. Studies by Richerson[240] on guinea-pigs sensitized by different routes and with different antigens suggested that histopathological changes resembling those occurring in patients with allergic alveolitis appeared to be indicated by cellular hypersensitivity. His studies showed that when animals were treated in such a way as to favour immune-complex disease, the histopathological reaction was a haemorrhagic pneumonitis – a condition which is uncommon but which has been described for patients biopsied during acute EAA. Roska et al.[241] showed that this reaction is immunospecific and can be transferred passively with immune serum, and is suppressed by cobra venom factor, suggesting that immune complex disease occurs following inhalation of antigens. Bice et al.[242] showed that lesions produced in lungs of rabbits sensitized by intratracheal challenge with M. faeni antigen were closely associated with cellular hypersensitivity and could be transferred to normal rabbits by cells from sensitized animals.

Although the evidence for both cellular and immune-complex mediation of disease is now convincing, it is clear that other unrelated factors may contribute to the disease process. Schorlemmer et al.[8] have shown that M. faeni can activate complement by the alternative pathway and suggested that this could lead to an inflammatory reaction by a non-specific mechanism. Hollingdale[243] has reported the existence of an endotoxin-like lipopolysaccharide from M. faeni and it is possible that this might contribute to the febrile response. It may be, of course, that fever is also related to specific immunological mechanisms, and so elicited by one or more factors. Thermophilic fungi growing in the hay produce and secrete enzymes, some of which are pharmacologically active. Chymotrypsin, for example, is known to be produced by M. faeni and may itself cause an inflammatory reaction when introduced into the alveoli of non-sensitized lung tissue[244]. Individual susceptibility to airborne allergens may also be influenced by genetic and environmental factors, since only a comparatively small proportion of subjects exposed to spores of thermophili achnomycetes develop disease and an association between HLA antigens and FLD has been suggested[245]. So too has concomitant inflammation of the lung and exposure to airborne antigen, on the basis that this may promote an immune response by its adjuvant effect[233].

References

1. Hammerman, K. J. et al. (1974). The incidence of hospitalized cases of systemic mycotic infections. Sabouraudia, 12, 33

2. Baker, R. D. (1971). *Human Infections with Fungi, Actinomycetes and Algae*, p. 1 (New York: Springer-Verlag)
3. Binford, C. H. (1962). Tissue reactions elicited by fungi. In: *Fungi and Fungous Diseases* (Dalldorf, ed.), p. 220 (Springfield: Charles C. Thomas)
4. Hasenclever, H. F. and Mitchell, W. O. (1963). Acquired immunity in mice to candidiasis. *J. Bacteriol.*, **86**, 401
5. Axelsen, N. H. (1973). Quantitative immunoelectrophoretic methods as tools of polyvalent approach to standardization in the immunochemistry of *Candida albicans*. *Infect. Immun.*, **7**, 949
6. Tran van Ky, P., Vaucelle, T. and Biguet, J. (1970). Étude comparée de la structure antigénique par analyse immunoélectrophorétique et par les réactions de characterisation des activités enzymatiques des extraits antigéniques des champignons pathogenés du genre *Aspergillus (A. fumigatus, A. flavus, A. terreus*, et *A. nidulans)*. *Rev. Immunol. Thér. Antimicrob.*, **34**, 357
7. Sohnle, P. G. and Kirkpatrick, C. H. (1976). Deposition of complement in the lesions of experimental cutaneous candidiasis in guinea-pig. *J. Cutan. Pathol.*, **3**, 232
8. Schorlemmer, H. U., Edwards, J. H., Davies, P. and Allison, A. C. (1977). Macrophage responses to mouldy hay dust, *Micropolyspora faeni* and zymosan, activators of complement by the alternative pathway. *Clin. Exp. Immunol.*, **27**, 198
9. Diamond, R. D. (1974). Antibody-dependent killing of *Cryptococcus neoformans* by human peripheral blood mononuclear cells. *Nature (Lond.)*, **247**, 148
10. Yamamura, M. and Valdimarsson, H. (1978). Participation of C-3 in intracellular killing of *Candida albicans*. *Scand. J. Immunol.*, **6**, 591
11. Huppert, M., Sun, S. H. and Vukovich, K. R. (1973). Standardization of mycological reagents. In: *Proc. Int. Conf. Stand. Diagn. Mat.*, US Dpt. Hlth. Educ. Welf., p. 187
12. Goodman, N. L., Larsh, H. W. and Palmer, C. E. (1971). Cross-reactivity in skin testing with histoplasmin. *Am. Rev. Resp. Dis.*, **104**, 258
13. Hanifin, J. M., Ray, L. F. and Lobitz, W. C. Jr. (1974). Immunological reactivity in dermatophytosis. *Br. J. Dermatol.*, **90**, 1
14. Jones, H. E., Reinhardt, J. H. and Rinaldi, M. G. (1974). Model dermatophytosis in naturally infected subjects. *Arch. Dermatol.*, **110**, 369
15. Abraham, S., Pandhi, R. K., Kumar, R., Mohapatra, L. N. and Bhutani, L. K. (1975). A study of the immunological status of patients with dermatophytoses. *Dermatologica*, **151**, 281
16. Walters, B. A. J., Beardmore, G. L. and Halliday, W. J. (1976). Specific cell-mediated immunity in the laboratory diagnosis of dermatophytic infections. *Br. J. Dermatol.*, **94**, 55
17. Neill, J. M., Sugg, J. Y. and McCauley, D. W. (1951). Serologically reactive material in spinal fluid, blood and urine from a human case of cryptococcosis (torulosis). *Proc. Soc. Exp. Biol. Med.*, **77**, 775
18. Miller, G. G., Witwer, M. W., Braude, A. I. and Davis, C. E. (1974). Rapid identification of *Candida albicans* septicaemia in man by gas–liquid chromatography. *J. Clin. Invest.*, **54**, 1235
19. Weiner, M. H. and Yount, W. J. (1976). Mannan antigenaemia in the diagnosis of invasive *Candida* infections. *J. Clin. Invest.*, **58**, 1045
20. Warren, R. C. *et al.* (1977). Diagnosis of invasive candidosis by enzyme immunoassay of serum antigen. *Br. Med. J.*, 1183
21. Mackenzie, D. W. R. and Georgakopoulos, E. (1979). Use of an ELISA procedure to detect mannan antigenaemia in patients with deep-seated candidiasis. (In preparation)
22. Axelsen, N. H. and Kirkpatrick, C. H. (1973). Simultaneous characterization of free *Candida* antigens and precipitins in a patient's serum by means of crossed immunoelectrophoresis with intermediate gel. *J. Immunol. Methods*, **2**, 245

23. Young, R. C. and Bennett, J. E. (1971). Invasive aspergillosis. Absence of detectable antibody response. *Am. Rev. Resp. Dis.*, **104**, 710

24. Hiatt, J. S. Jr. and Martin, D. S. (1946). Recovery from pulmonary moniliasis following serum therapy. *J. Am. Med. Assoc.*, **130**, 205

25. Alekhin, R. M. (1974). O vnedrenii preparata TF-130. *Veterinariya (Moscow)*, **3**, 52

26. Rukhlyada, V. V., Nikolaev, S. M. and Shutyuk, V. K. (1973). Effektivnost spetsificheskoi profilaktiki trikhofitii. *Veterinariya (Moscow)*, **6**, 54

27. Kielstein, P. (1968). Immunologische Untersuchungen während der spontanen und experimentallen Rindertrichophytie. *Wiss. Z. Karl. Marx Univ.*, **17**, 177

28. Grappel, S. F., Blank, F. and Bishop, C. T. (1972). Circulating antibodies in dermatophytosis. *Dermatologica*, **144**, 1

29. Levine, H. B. and Kong, Y.-C. M. (1967). Immunologic impairment in mice treated intravenously with killed *Coccidioides immitis* spherules: suppressed response to intramuscular doses. *J. Immunol.*, **97**, 297

30. Kong, Y.-C. M. and Levine, H. B. (1967). Experimentally induced immunity in the mycoses. *Bacteriol. Rev.*, **31**, 35

31. Pappagianis, D. and Levine, H. B. (1975). The present status of vaccination against coccidioidomycosis in man. *Am. J. Epidemiol.*, **102**, 30

32. Graybill, J. R., Silva, J. Jr., Alford, R. H. and Thor. D. E. (1973). Immunological and clinical improvement of progressive coccidioidomycosis following administration of transfer factor. *Cell. Immunol.*, **8**, 120

33. Mukherji, A. K. and Mallick, K. C. B. (1972). Disseminated candidosis in cyclophosphamide-induced leucopenic state: an experimental study. *Ind. J. Med. Res.*, **60**, 1584

34. Cutler, J. E. (1976). Acute systemic candidiasis in normal and congenitally thymic-deficient (nude) mice. *J. Reticuloendotheliol. Soc.*, **19**, 121

35. Domer, J. *et al.* (1974). Pathologic and immune responses in normal and thymectomized mice to first and second infections with *Candida albicans*. *Abstr. Ann. Mtg. Am. Soc. Microbiol.*, MM4

36. Mahgoub, E. S. *et al.* (1974). Immunological status of mycetoma patients. *Bull. Soc. Pathol. Exot.*, **70**, 48

37. Bloch, B. (1908). Zur Lehre von den Dermatomykosen. *Arch. Dermatol. Syphilol.*, **93**, 157

38. Barker, S. A., Cruickshank, C. N. D., Morris, J. H. and Wood, S. R. (1962). The isolation of trichophytin glycopeptide and its structure in relation to the immediate and delayed reactions. *Immunology*, **5**, 627

39. Grappel, S. F. *et al.* (1968). Immunological studies on dermatophytes. II. Serological reactivities of mannans prepared from Galactomannans I and II of *Microsporum quinckeanum*, *Trichophyton granulosum*, *Trichophyton interdigitale*, *Trichophyton rubrum* and *Trichophyton schoenleinii*. *J. Bacteriol.*, **95**, 1238

40. Yu, R. J. *et al.* (1971). Two cell-bound keratinases of Trichophyton mentagrophytes. *J. Invest. Dermatol.*, **56**, 27

41. Basarab, O., How, M. J. and Cruickshank, C. N. D. (1968). Immunological relationships between glycopeptides of *Microsporum canis*, *Trichophyton rubrum*, *Trichophyton mentagrophytes* and other fungi. *Sabouraudia*, **6**, 119

42. Nozawa, Y. *et al.* (1971). Immunochemical studies on *Trichophyton mentagrophytes*. *Sabouraudia*, **9**, 129

43. Noguchi, T., Hattori, T., Shimonaka, H. and Ito, Y. (1971). Immunochemical studies of *Trichophyton mentagrophytes*: isolation of immunoglobulins and their immune responses. *Jap. J. Exp. Med.*, **41**, 401

44. Grappel, S. F. *et al.* (1971). Effect of antibodies on growth and structure of *Trichophyton mentagrophytes*. *Sabouraudia*, **9**, 50

45. Grappel, S. F. (1974). Immunology of dermatophytes and dermatophytosis. *Bact. Rev.*, **38**, 222

46. Eleuterio, M. K. *et al.* (1973). Role of keratinases in dermatophytosis. III. Demonstration of delayed type hypersensitivity to keratinases by the capillary tube migration test. *Dermatoligica*, **147**, 255

47. Grappel, S. F. and Blank, F. (1972). Role of keratinases in dermatophytes. I. Immune responses of guinea-pigs infected with *Trichophyton mentagrophytes* and guinea-pigs immunized with keratinases. *Dermatologica*, **145**, 245

48. Longhin, S. and Olaru, V. (1970). The value of immunotherapy in dermatophytoses. In: *Proc. 2nd Int. Symp. Med. Mycol.* (W. Sowinski, ed.), 1967, p. 181 (Poland: Poznan)

49. Huppert, M. and Keeney, E. L. (1959). Immunization against superficial fungous infection. *J. Invest. Dermatol.*, **32**, 15

50. Jones, H. E. *et al.* (1973). A clinical, mycological and immunological survey for dermatophytosis. *Arch. Dermatol.*, **108**, 61

51. Buckley, H. R. and Murray, I. G. (1966). Precipitating antibodies in chromomycosis. *Sabouraudia*, **5**, 78

52. Balina, P., Bosq, P., Negroni, P. and Quiroga, M. (1932). Un caso de Chromoblastomicosis, autoctono de Argentina. *Reb. Argent. Dermatosif*, **16**, 369

53. Martin, D. S., Baker, R. D. and Conant, N. F. (1936). A case of verrucous dermatitis caused by *Hormodendrum pedrosoi* (Chromoblastomycosis) in North Carolina. *Am. J. Trop. Med.*, **16**, 593

54. Mahgoub, E. S. (1975). Serological diagnosis of mycetoma. In: *Mycoses Proc. 3rd Int. Conf. Mycoses*, Sao Paulo, Brazil, 27–29 August, 1974, p. 154, Pan Am. Hlth. Organ., Wash. D.C.

55. Welsh, R. D. and Dolan, C. T. (1973). *Sporothrix* whole yeast agglutination test: low-titre reactions of sera of subjects not known to have sporotrichosis. *Am. J. Clin. Pathol.*, **59**, 82

56. Karlin, J. V. and Nielsen, H. S. (1970). Serologic aspects of sporotrichosis. *J. Infect. Dis.*, **121**, 316

57. Blumer, S. O., Kaufman, L., Kaplan, W., McLaughlin, D. W. and Kraft, D. E. (1973). Comparative evaluation of five serological methods for the diagnosis of sporotrichosis. *Appl. Microbiol.*, **26**, 4

58. Kaufman, L. (1976). Serodiagnosis of fungal diseases. In: *Manual of Clinical Immunology* (N. R. Rose and H. Friedman, eds.), p. 376 (Washington, D.C.: American Society of Microbiology)

59. Martins de Castro, R. (1960). Prova da esporotriquina. Contribuição para o sen estudo. *Rev. Inst. A. Lutz. (S. Paulo)*, **20**, 5

60. Gonzalez Ochoa, A. (1965). Contribuciones recientes al conocimiento de la esporotrichosis. *Gac. Méd. Méx.*, **95**, 463

61. Magalhães Pereira, A. *et al.* (1964). Estudos sôbre a immunopatologia de esporotricose. *An. Bras. Dermatol. Sif.*, **39**, 34

62. Lurie, H. (1971). Sporotrichosis. In: *Human Infections with Fungi, Actinomycetes and Algae* (R. D. Baker, ed.), p. 654 (New York: Springer-Verlag)

63. Padilha Gonçalves, A. (1962). Tratamento da esporotricose. *Brasil Med.*, **76**, 144

64. Wilson, D. E. *et al.* (1967). Clinical features of extracutaneous sporotrichosis. *Medicine (Baltimore)*, **46**, 265

65. Lynch, P. J. *et al.* (1970). Systemic sporotrichosis. *Ann. Intern. Med.*, **73**, 23

66. Mariat, F. (1968). The epidemiology of the mycosis: some comments in relation to a particular case of sporotrichosis. In: *Systemic Mycoses* (G. E. W. Wolstenholme and R. Porter, eds.), p. 144 (London: J. and A. Churchill)

67. Ingrish, F. M. and Schneidau, J. D. (1967). Cutaneous hypersensitivity to sporotrichin in Maricopa County, Arizona. *J. Invest. Dermatol.*, **49**, 146

68. Steele, R. W. *et al.* (1976). Skin test and blastogenic responses to *Sporotrichum schenckii*. *J. Clin. Invest.*, **57**, 156

69. Lloyd, K. and Travassos, L. R. (1975). Immunochemical studies on L. rhamno-D. mannans of *Sporothrix schenckii* and related fungi by use of rabbit and human antisera. *Carbohydr. Res.*, **40**, 89

70. Palmer, C. E. (1945). Geographic differences in sensitivity to histoplasmin among student nurses. *Publ. Hlth. Rep. Wash.*, **61**, 475

71. Edwards, P. Q. (1971). Histoplasmin sensitivity patterns around the world. In: *Histoplasmosis. Proc. 2nd Nat. Conf.* (L. Ajello *et al.*, eds.), p. 97 (Springfield: Charles C. Thomas)

72. Shaw, L. W. *et al.* (1950). Biological assay of lots of histoplasmin and the selection of a new working lot. *Publ. Hlth. Rep. Wash.*, **65**, 583

73. Goodman, N. L. *et al.* (1968). Histoplasmin potency as affected by culture age. *Sabouraudia*, **6**, 273

74. Sprouse, R. F. *et al.* (1969). Fractionation, isolation and chemical characterization of skin-test active components of histoplasmin. *Sabouraudia*, **7**, 1

75. Sprouse, R. F. *et al.* (1969). Purification of histoplasmin purified derivative. *Am. Rev. Resp. Dis.*, **99**, 685

76. O'Connell, E. J. *et al.* (1967). Skin-reactive antigen of *Histoplasma capsulatum*. *Proc. Soc. Exp. Biol. Med.*, **124**, 1015

77. Chick, E. W. *et al.* (1973). The use of skin tests and serological tests in histoplasmosis, coccidioidomycosis and blastomycosis. *Am. Rev. Resp. Dis.*, **108**, 156

78. United States Public Health Service (1965). Standardized diagnostic complement fixation method and adaptation to micro test. *USPHS, Monograph* No. 74

79. Heiner, D. C. (1958). Diagnosis of histoplasmosis using precipitin reactions in agar gel. *Pediatrics*, **22**, 616

80. Gordon, M. A. (1970). Practical serology of the systemic mycoses. *Int. J. Dermatol.*, **9**, 209

81. Kaufman, L. (1976). Serodiagnosis of fungal diseases. *Manual of Clinical Immunology*, p. 375 (Washington, D.C.: American Society of Microbiology)

82. Kaufman, L. *et al.* (1969). Immunological studies with an M-deficient histoplasmin skin-test antigen. *Appl. Microbiol.*, **18**, 307

83. Green, J. H. *et al.* (1976). H and M antigens of *Histoplasma capsulatum*. Preparation of antisera and location of these antigens in yeast-phase cells. *Infect. Immun.*, **14**, 826

84. Dyson, J. E. and Evans, E. E. (1955). Delayed hypersensitivity in experimental fungus infections. The skin reactivity of antigens from the yeast-phase of *Histoplasma capsulatum*. *J. Lab. Clin. Med.*, **45**, 449

85. Sorensen, L. J. and Evans, E. E. (1954). Antigenic fractions specific for *Histoplasma capsulatum* in the complement fixation reactions. *Proc. Soc. Exp. Biol. Med.*, **87**, 339

86. Kobayashi, G. (1971). Isolation and characterization of polysaccharide from *Histoplasma capsulatum*. In: *Histoplasmosis. Proc. 2nd Nat. Conf.* (L. Ajello, *et al.*, eds.), p. 38 (Springfield: Charles C. Thomas)

87. Bennett, D. E. (1966). The histoplasmin latex agglutination test: clinical evaluations and a review of the literature. *Am. J. Med. Sci.*, **251**, 85

88. Kirkpatrick, C. A. *et al.* (1971). Cellular immunologic studies in histoplasmosis. In: *Histoplasmosis, Proc. 2nd Nat. Conf.* (L. Ajello *et al.*, eds.), p. 371 (Springfield: Charles C. Thomas)

89. Garcia, J. P. and Howard, D. H. (1971). Characterization of antigens from the yeast phase of *Histoplasma capsulatum*. *Infect. Immun.*, **4**, 116

90. Howard, D. H. *et al.* (1971). Lymphocyte-mediated cellular immunity in *Histoplasmosis*. *Infect. Immun.*, **4**, 605

91. Domer, J. (1977). Comparison of cellular immune responses in guinea-pigs when immunized with cell walls of *Histoplasma capsulatum* treated by several different procedures. In: *Recent Advances in Medical Veterinary Mycology* (K. Iwata, ed.), p. 75 (Univ. Tokyo Press)

92. Alford, R. H. and Goodwin, R. A. (1973). Variation in lymphocyte reactivity to histo-

plasmin during the course of chronic pulmonary histoplasmosis. *Am. Rev. Resp. Dis.*, **108**, 85

93. Feit, C. and Tewari, R. P. (1974). Immunogenicity of ribosomal preparations from yeast cells of *Histoplasma capsulatum*. *Infect. Immun.*, **10**, 109

94. Tewari, R. *et al.* (1977). Adoptive transfer of immunity from mice immunized with ribosomes or live yeast cells of *Histoplasma capsulatum*. *Infect. Immun.*, **15**, 789

95. Smith, C. R. *et al.* (1976). Chronic pulmonary histoplasmosis; improved lymphocyte response with transfer factor. *Ann. Intern. Med.*, **84**, 708

96. Procknow, J. J. (1971). Reinfection histoplasmosis. In: *Histoplasmosis. Proc. 2nd Nat. Conf.* (L. Ajello *et al.*, eds.), p. 252 (Springfield: Charles C. Thomas)

97. Tosh, F. E. (1971). Reinfective histoplasmosis. In: *Histoplasmosis. Proc. 2nd Nat. Conf.* (L. Ajello *et al.*, eds.), p. 260 (Springfield: Charles C. Thomas)

98. Smith, C. E. (1955). Coccidioidomycosis. *Ped. Clin. N. Am.*, **2**, 109

99. Winn, W. A. (1968). A long-term study of 300 patients with cavitary-abscess lesions of the lung of coccidioidal origin. An analytical study with special reference to treatment. *Dis. Chest*, **54** (Suppl. 1), 268

100. Smith, C. E. *et al.* (1948). Histoplasmin sensitivity and coccidioidal infection. I. Occurrence of cross-reactions. *Am. J. Publ. Hlth.*, **39**, 722

101. Zweiman, B. *et al.* (1969). Coccidioidin delayed hypersensitivity: skin test and *in vitro* lymphocyte reactivities. *J. Immunol.*, **102**, 1284

102. Sinski, J. T. *et al.* (1973). Macrophage migration techniques using coccidioidin. *Infect. Immun.*, 7, 226

103. Opelz, G. and Scheer, M. I. (1975). Cutaneous sensitivity and *in vitro* responsiveness of lymphocyte in patients with disseminated coccidioidomycosis. *J. Infect. Dis.*, **132**, 250

104. Cox, R. A. *et al.* (1977). *In vitro* lymphocyte responses to coccidioidin skin test-positive and -negative persons to coccidioidin, spherulin and a Coccidioides cell wall antigen. *Infect. Immun.*, **15**, 751

105. Ibrahim, A. B. and Pappagianis, D. (1973). Experimental induction of energy to coccidioidin by antigens of *Coccidioides immitis*. *Infect. Immun.*, 7, 786

106. Pappagianis, D. *et al.* (1961). Polysaccharide of *Coccidioides immitis*. *J. Bacteriol.*, **82**, 714

107. Anderson, K. *et al.* (1971). Fractionation and composition studies of skin-test active components of sensitins from *Coccidioides immitis*. *Appl. Microbiol.*, **22**, 294

108. Huppert, M. *et al.* (1978). Antigenic analysis of coccidioidin and spherulin determined by two-dimensional immunoelectrophoresis. *Infect. Immun.*, **20**, 541

109. Levine, H. B. *et al.* (1969). Spherule coccidioidin in delayed dermal sensitivity reactions of experimental animals. *Sabouraudia*, **7**, 20

110. Scalarone, G. M. *et al.* (1973). Properties and assay of spherulins from *Coccidioides immitis* in delayed sensitivity responses of animals. *Sabouraudia*, **11**, 222

111. Levine, H. B. *et al.* (1973). Sensibilidad cutanea al *C. immitis*. Comparación entre la reacción a la esferulina y a la coccidioidina en el hombre. *Bol. Of. Sanit. Panam.*, **74**, 199

112. Stevens, D. A. *et al.* (1975). Spherulin in clinical coccidioidomycosis. Comparison with coccidioidin. *Chest*, **68**, 697

113. Smith, C. E. *et al.* (1956). Pattern of 39 500 serologic tests in coccidioidomycosis. *J. Am. Med. Assoc.*, **160**, 546

114. Smith, C. E. *et al.* (1950). Serological tests in the diagnosis and prognosis of coccidioidomycosis. *Am. J. Hyg.*, **52**, 1

115. Aguilar-Torres, F. G. *et al.* (1976). Counterimmunoelectrophoresis in the detection of antibodies against *Coccidioides immitis*. *Ann. Intern. Med.*, **85**, 740

116. Pappagianis, D. *et al.* (1972). Antibody in cerebrospinal fluid in non-meningitic coccidioidomycosis. *Sabouraudia*, **10**, 173

117. Winn, W. A. (1967). Coccidioidal meningitis: a follow-up report. In: *Coccidioidomycosis, Proc. 2nd Symposium* (L. Ajello, ed.), p. 55 (University Arizona Press)

118. Velasco Castrejon, O. *et al.* (1974). El factor de transferencia como unico recurso terapeutico, en un caso de coccidioidomicosis crónica anergica. *Rev. Latinoamer. Microbiol.*, **16**, 137
119. Cloninger, P. *et al.* (1974). Immunotherapy with transfer factor in disseminated coccidioidal osteomylitis and arthritis. *West J. Med.*, **120**, 322
120. Gerber, J. D. and Jones, R. D. (1973). Immunologic significance of aspergillin antigens of six species of *Aspergillus* in the serodiagnosis of aspergillosis. *Am. Rev. Resp. Dis.*, **108**, 1124
121. Sudman, M. S. and Kaplan, W. (1974). Antigenic relationship between American and African isolates of *Blastomyces dermatitidis* as determined by immunofluorescence. *Appl. Microbiol.*, **27**, 496
122. Azuma, I. *et al.* (1974). Chemical and immunological properties of galactomannans obtained from *Histoplasma duboisii*, *Histoplasma capsulatum*, *Paracoccidioides brasiliensis* and *Blastomyces dermatitidis*. *Mycopathol. Mycol. Appl.*, **54**, 111
123. Kaufman, L. (1975). Current status of immunology for diagnosis and prognostic evaluation of Blastomycosis, Coccidioidomycosis, and Paracoccidioidomycosis. In: *Mycoses, Proc. 3rd Int. Conf. on Mycoses*, p. 137 (Washington, D.C.: Pan. Am. Hlth. Organ.)
124. Kaufman, L. (1976). Serodiagnosis of fungal diseases. In: *Manual of Clinical Immunology*, p. 366 (Washington, D.C.: Am. Soc. Microbiol)
125. Scillian, J. J. *et al.* (1974). Passive transfer of delayed hypersensitivity to *Blastomyces dermatitidis* between mice. *Infect. Immun.*, **10**, 705
126. Spencer, H. D. and Cozad, G. C. (1973). Role of delayed hypersensitivity in blastomycosis of mice. *Infect. Immun.*, **7**, 329
127. Furcolow, M. L. and Smith, C. D. (1973). A new hypothesis on the epidemiology of blastomycosis and the ecology of *Blastomyces dermatitidis*. *Trans. N.Y. Acad. Sci.*, **35**, 421
128. Sarosi, G. A. and King, R. A. (1977). Apparent diminution of the blastomycin skin test: follow-up of an epidemic of blastomycosis. *Am. Rev. Resp. Dis.*, **116**, No. 4, p. 785
129. Lancaster, M. V. and Sprouse, R. F. (1976). Role of delayed hypersensitivities in blastomycosis of mice. *Infect. Immun.*, **14**, 623
130. Lancaster, M. V. and Sprouse, R. F. (1976). Preparative isotachophoretic separation of skin-test antigen from blastomycin purified derivative. *Infect. Immun.*, **13**, 758
131. Deighton, F. *et al.* (1977). *In vivo* and *in vitro* cell-mediated immune responses to a cell-wall antigen of *Blastomyces dermatitidis*
132. Landay, M. E. *et al.* (1972). Effect of prior vaccination on experimental blastomycosis. *Mycopathol. Mycol. Appl.*, **46**, 61
133. Purtilo, D. T. (1975). Opportunistic mycotic infections in pregnant women. *Am. J. Obstet. Gynecol.*, **122**, 607
134. Parker, J. C. Jr. *et al.* (1976). Candidosis: the most common post-mortem cerebral mycosis in an endemic fungal area. *Surg. Neurol.*, **6**, 123
135. Angulo, O. and Pollack, L. (1971). Paracoccidioidomycosis. In: *Human Infection with Fungi, Actinomycetes and Algae* (R. D. Baker, ed.), p. 507 (New York: Springer-Verlag)
136. Castro, R. M. and Negro, G. del. (1976). Particularidades clínicas da paracoccidioidomicose na criança. *Rev. Hosp. Clin.*, **31**, 194
137. Londero, A. T. (1972). The lung in paracoccidioidomycosis. In: *Paracoccidioidomycosis, Proc. 1st Pan Am. Symp. Medellin*, p. 109 (Washington, D.C.: Pan Am. Hlth. Organ.)
138. Yarzabal, L. A. (1972). Pathogenesis of paracoccidioidomycosis in man. In: *Paracoccidioidomycosis, Proc. 1st Pan Am. Symp. Medellin*, p. 261 (Washington, D.C.: Pan Am. Hlth. Organ.)
139. Borelli, D. (1972). Some ecological aspects of paracoccidioidomycosis. In: *Paracoccidioidomycosis, Proc. 1st Pan Am. Symp. Medellin*, p. 59 (Washington, D.C.: Pan Am. Hlth. Organ.)

140. Correa, A. L. and Giraldo, R. M. (1972). Study of immune mechanisms in paracoccidioidomycosis. I. Changes in immunoglobulins (IgG, IgM and IgA)

141. Fonseca, F. O. and Area Leao, A. E. (1927). Réaction cutanée specifique avec le filtrat de culture de *Coccidioides immitis*. *C. R. Soc. Biol. (Paris)*, **97**, 1796

142. Favo Netto, C. *et al.* (1976). Contribuçião ao estudo imunológico da paracoccidioidomicose. Reacões intradérmicas en pacientes com dois antígenos homologos e dois heterólogos. *Rev. Inst. Med. Trop. Sao Paulo*, **18**, 186

143. Musatti, C. C. *et al.* (1976). *In vivo* and *in vitro* evaluation of cell-mediated immunity in patients with Paracoccidioidomycosis. *Cell. Immunol.*, **24**, 365

144. Negroni, R. *et al.* (1976). Preparacion y estudio de un antigeno celular de *Paracoccidioides brasiliensis*, util para pruebas cutaneas. *Sabouraudia*, **14**, 265

145. Schneidau, J. D. (1972). A co-operative study of cross-reactivity among fungal skin-test antigens in tropical Latin America. In: *Paracoccidioidomycosis. Proc. 1st Pan Am. Symp. Medellin*, p. 233 (Washington, D.C.: Pan Am. Hlth. Organ.)

146. Greer, D. L. *et al.* (1974). Dermal sensitivity to paracoccidioidin and histoplasmin in family members of patients with paracoccidioidomycosis. *Am. J. Trop. Med. Hyg.*, **23**, 87

147. Mendes, N. F. (1975). Lymphocytes and lymph nodes in patients with paracoccidioidomycosis. In: *Mycoses, Proc. 3rd Int. Conf. Mycoses*, p. 30 (Washington, D.C.: Pan Am. Hlth. Organ.)

148. Mendes, E. (1975). Delayed hypersensitivity reaction in patients with paracoccidioidomycosis. In: *Mycoses, Proc. 3rd Int. Conf. on Mycoses*, p. 17 (Washington, D.C.: Pan Am. Hlth. Organ.)

149. Negroni, R. (1972). Serologic reactions in paracoccidioidomycosis. In: *Paracoccidioidomycosis, Proc. 1st Pan Am. Symp. Medellin*, p. 203 (Washington, D.C.: Pan Am. Hlth. Organ.)

150. Favo Netto, C. (1955). Estudos quantitativos sôbre a fixacão de complemento na blastomicose sul-americana, com antigeno polissacarido. *Arg. Cir. Clin. Exp.*, **18**, 197

151. Favo Netto, C. (1965). The immunology of South American blastomycosis. *Mycopathol. Mycol. Appl.*, **26**, 349

152. Restrepo, A. and Moncada, L. H. (1970). Serologic procedures in the diagnosis of paracoccidioidomycosis. In: *Proc. Int. Symp., Mycoses*, p. 101 (Washington, D.C.: Pan Am. Hlth. Organ.)

153. Restrepo, A. and Drouhet, E. (1970). Étude des anticorps precipitants dans la blastomycose sud-américaine par l'analyse immunoelectrophorétique des antigènes de *Paracoccidioides brasiliensis*. *Ann. Inst. Pasteur (Paris)*, **119**, 338

154. Yarzabal, L. A. (1971). Anticuerpos precipitantes especificos de la blastomicosis sudamericana, revelados por immunoelectroforesis. *Rev. Inst. Med. Trop. Sao Paulo*, **13**, 320

155. Torres, J. M. *et al.* (1974). Evaluación du un antigeno metabólico purificado de *Paracoccidioides brasiliensis*. *Rev. Asoc. Argent. Microbiol.*, **6**, 39

156. Nieto, A. *et al.* (1974). Aislamento de antigenos cationicos de *Paracoccidioides brasiliensis* mediante intercambio ionico. *Mycopathol. Mycol. Appl.*, **54**, 435

157. Yarazabal, L. A. *et al.* (1976). Isolation of a specific antigen with alkaline phosphatase activity from soluble extracts of *Paracoccidioides brasiliensis*. *Sabouraudia*, **14**, 275

158. Yarzabal, L. A. *et al.* (1977). Identification and purification of the specific antigen of *Paracoccidioides brasiliensis* responsible for immunoelectrophoretic band E. *Sabouraudia*, **15**, 79

159. Gosseye-Lissoir, F. *et al.* (1975). Cryptococcose cerebromeningée: role favorisant de la therapeutique immunosuppressive chez les transplantes renaux. *Pathol. Biol.*, **23**, 211

160. Hermans, A. P. E. (1975). Functions and malfunction of the immune system in relation to infection. In: *Mycoses, Proc. 3rd Int. Symp. Mycoses*, p. 6 (Washington, D.C.: Pan Am. Hlth. Organ.)

161. Starzl, T. E. (1976). Cryptococcosis after renal transplantation: report of 10 cases. *Surgery*, **79**, 268

162. Diamond, R. D. and Bennett, J. E. (1974). Prognostic factors in cryptococcal meningitis. A study of 111 cases. *Ann. Intern. Med.*, **80**, 176

163. Gordon, M. A. and Lapa, E. W. (1974). Elimination of rheumatoid factor in the latex test for cryptococcosis. *Am. J. Clin. Pathol.*, **61**, 488

164. Kaufman, L. (1976). Serodiagnosis of fungal diseases. In: *Manual of Clinical Immunology* (N. R. Rose and H. Friedman, eds.), p. 371 (Washington, D.C.: Am. Soc. Microbiol.)

165. Blumer, S. O. and Kaufman, L. (1972). Characterization of immunoglobulin classes of human antibodies to *Cryptococcus neoformans*. *Mycopathol. Mycol. Appl.*, **61**, 55

166. Diamond, R. D. and Bennett, J. E. (1974). Antibody-dependent killing of *Cryptococcus neoformans* by human peripheral blood mononuclear cells. *Nature (Lond.)*, **247**, 148

167. Diamond, R. D. *et al.* (1972). Factors influencing killing of *Cryptococcus neoformans* by human leukocyte *in vitro*. *J. Infect. Dis.*, **125**, 367

168. Kozel, T. R. and Mastoianni, R. P. (1976). Inhibition of phagocytosis by cryptococcal polysaccharide: dissociation of the attachment and ingestion phases of phagocytosis. *Infect. Immun.*, **14**, 62

169. Diamond, R. D. *et al.* (1973). The role of late components and the alternate complement pathway in experimental cryptococcosis. *Proc. Soc. Exp. Biol. Med.*, **144**, 312

170. Diamond, R. D. and Bennett, J. E. (1973). Disseminated cryptococcosis in man: decreased lymphocyte transformation in response to *Cryptococcus neoformans*. *J. Infect. Dis.*, **127**, 694

171. Diamond, R. D. *et al.* (1974). The role of the classical and alternative pathways in host defenses against *Cryptococcus neoformans* infection. *J. Immunol.*, **122**, 2260

172. Diamond, R. D. (1977). Effects of stimulation and suppression of cell-mediated immunity on experimental cryptococcosis. *Infect. Immun.*, **17**, 187

173. Diamond, R. D. and Bennett, J. E. (1974). Disseminated cryptococcosis in man: decreased lymphocyte transformation in response to *Cryptococcus neoformans*. *J. Infect. Dis.*, **127**, 694

174. Graybill, J. R. and Alford, R. H. (1974). Cell-mediated immunity in cryptococcosis. *Cell. Immunol.*, **14**, 14

175. Muchmore, H. G. *et al.* (1968). Delayed hypersensitivity to cryptococcin in man. *Sabouraudia*, **6**, 285

176. Atkinson, A. J. and Bennett, J. E. (1968). Experience with a new skin-test antigen prepared from *Cryptococcus neoformans*. *Am. Rev. Resp. Dis.*, **97**, 637

177. Axelsen, N. H. (1973). Quantitative immunoelectrophoretic methods as tools for a polyvalent approach to standardization in the immunochemistry of *Candida albicans*. *Infect. Immun.*, **7**, 949

178. Bacon, P. A. *et al.* (1974). Antibodies to *Candida* and autoantibodies in sub-acute bacterial endocarditis. *Q. J. Med.*, **43**, 537

179. Murray, I. G. *et al.* (1969). Serological evidence of *Candida* infection after open-heart surgery. *J. Med. Microbiol.*, **2**, 463

180. Taschdjian, C. L. *et al.* (1967). Serodiagnosis of systemic candidiasis. *J. Infect. Dis.*, **117**, 180

181. Lehner, T. (1970). Serum fluorescent antibody and immunoglobulin estimations in Candidosis. *J. Med. Microbiol.*, **3**, 475

182. Lehner, T. *et al.* (1972). The relationship between fluorescent, agglutinating, and precipitiating antibodies to *Candida albicans* and their immunoglobulin classes. *J. Clin. Pathol.*, **25**, 344

183. Müller, H. L. (1974). IgM- and IgG-antibodies against *Candida* polysaccharides in the serodiagnosis of candidiasis. *Bull. Soc. Franç. Mycol. Méd.*, **1**, 51

184. Blaker, F. *et al.* (1973). Bedentung humoraler Antikörper gegen *Candida albicans* fur den

Nachweis von Candida-Infektionen. *Dtsch. Med. Wosenschr.*, **98**, 194

185. Waldman, R. H. *et al.* (1972). Intravaginal immunization of humans with *Candida albicans. J. Immunol.*, **109**, 662

186. Mathur, S. *et al.* (1977). Humoral immunity in vaginal candidiasis. *Infect. Immun.*, **15**, 287

187. Milne, J. D. *et al.* (1977). Antibodies to *Candida albicans* in human cervicovaginal secretions. *Br. J. Vener. Dis.*, **53**, 375

188. Chilgren, R. A. *et al.* (1968). Human serum interactions with *Candida albicans. J. Immunol.*, **101**, 128

189. Smith, J. K. and Louria, D. B. (1972). Anti-*Candida* factors in serum and their inhibitors. II. Identification of a *Candida* clumping factor and the influence of the immune response on the morphology of *Candida* and anti-*Candida* activity of serum in rabbits. *J. Infect. Dis.*, **124**, 115

190. Preisler, H. D. *et al.* (1971). Anti-Candida antibodies in patients with acute leukemia. A prospective study. *Am. J. Med.*, **51**, 352

191. Filice, G. *et al.* (1977). Immunodiffusion and agglutination tests for *Candida* in patients with neoplastic disease: inconsistent correlation of results with invasive infections. *J. Infect. Dis.*, **135**, 349

192. Axelsen, N. H. and Kirkpatrick, C. H. (1973). Simultaneous characterization of free *Candida* antigens and *Candida* precipitins in a patient's serum by means of crossed immunoelectrophoresis with intermediate gel. *J. Immunol. Methods*, **2**, 245

193. Weiner, M. H. and Yount, W. J. (1976). Mannan antigenaemia in the diagnosis of invasive *Candida* infections. *J. Clin. Invest.*, **58**, 1045

194. Holti, G. (1966). Candida allergy. In: *Symposium on* Candida *Infections* (H. Winner and R. Hurley, eds.), p. 73 (Edinburgh: E. and S. Livingstone)

195. Shannon, D. C. *et al.* (1966). Cellular reactivity to *Candida albicans* antigen. *N. Engl. J. Med.*, **275**, 690

196. Hiddlestone, H. J. H. (1966). Sensitivity to *Candida albicans* antigen. *N. Z. Med. J.*, **65**, 464

197. Faux, J. (1968). Immunological studies of the antigens of *Candida albicans* in man. Ph.D. thesis, Univ. London

198. Gettner, S. (1979). Studies on the immune response to antigens of *Candida albicans*. Ph.D. thesis, Univ. London. (In preparation)

199. Budtz-Jorgensen, E. (1972). Delayed hypersensitivity to *Candida albicans* in man demonstrated *in vitro*: the capillary tube migration test. *Acta Allergologica*, **27**, 41

200. Foroozanfar, N. *et al.* (1974). Standardization of lymphocyte transformation to *Candida* immunogen. *Clin. Exp. Immunol.*, **16**, 301

201. Chilgren, R. A. *et al.* (1967). Chronic mucocutaneous candidiasis, deficiency of delayed hypersensitivity and selective local antibody defect. *Lancet, i*, 688

202. Chilgren, R. A. *et al.* (1969). The cellular immune defect in chronic mucocutaneous candidiasis. *Lancet, i*, 1286

203. Landau, J. W. (1968). Chronic mucocutaneous candidiasis-associated immunologic abnormalities. *Pediatrics*, **42**, 227

204. Kirkpatrick, C. H. *et al.* (1971). Chronic mucocutaneous candidiasis: model-building in cellular immunity. *Ann. Intern. Med.*, **74**, 955

205. Holt, P. J. L. *et al.* (1972). Chronic mucocutaneous candidiasis: a model for the investigation of cell-mediated immunity. *Br. J. Clin. Pract.*, **26**, 331

206. Valdimarsson, H. *et al.* (1973). Immune abnormalities associated with chronic mucocutaneous candidiasis. *Cell. Immunol.*, **6**, 348

207. Kirkpatrick, C. H. and Smith, T. K. (1974). Chronic mucocutaneous candidiasis: immunologic and antibiotic therapy. *Ann. Intern. Med.*, **80**, 310

208. Valdimarsson, H. (1970). Lymphocyte abnormality in chronic mucocutaneous candidiasis. *Lancet, i*, 1259

209. Hermans, P. E. (1975). Function and malfunction of the immune system in relation to infection. In: *Mycoses, Proc. 3rd Int. Conf. on Mycoses*, p. 6 (Washington, D.C.: Pan Am. Hlth. Organ.)

210. Feigin, R. D. *et al.* (1974). Treatment of mucocutaneous candidiasis with transfer factor. *Pediatrics*, **53**, 63

211. De Sousa, M. *et al.* (1976). Chronic mucocutaneous candidiasis treated with transfer factor. *Br. J. Dermatol.*, **94**, 79

212. Littman, B. H. *et al.* (1972). Transfer factor treatment of chronic mucocutaneous candidiasis: requirement for donor reactivity to *Candida* antigen. *Clin. Immunol. Immunother.*, **9**, 97

213. Buckley, R. H. *et al.* (1968). Defective cellular immunity associated with chronic mucocutaneous moniliasis and recurrent staphylococcal botryomycosis: immunological reconstitution by allogeneic bone marrow. *Clin. Exp. Immunol.*, **3**, 153

214. Wong, V. G. and Kirkpatrick, C. H. (1974). Immune reconstitution in keratoconjunctivitis and superficial candidiasis. *Arch. Ophthalmol.*, **92**, 335

215. Folb, P. I. and Trounce, J. R. (1970). Immunological aspects of Candida infection complicating steroid and immunosuppressive drug therapy. *Lancet*, **ii**, 1112

216. Neta, R. *et al.* (1971). Cellular immunity *in vitro*; migration inhibition and phagocytosis. *Infect. Immun.*, **4**, 697

217. Meyer, R. D. *et al.* (1973). Aspergillosis complicating neoplastic disease. *Am. J. Med.*, **54**, 6

218. Young, R. C. and Bennett, J. E. (1971). Invasive aspergillosis. Absence of detectable antibody response. *Am. Rev. Resp. Dis.*, **104**, 710

219. Barvah, H. K. (1961). The air spora of a cowshed. *J. Gen. Microbiol.*, **25**, 483

220. Austwick, P. K. C. (1963). Ecology of *Aspergillus fumigatus* and the pathogenic phycomycetes. *Rec. Progr. Microbiol.*, **8**, 644

221. McCarthy, D. S. and Pepys, J. (1971). Allergic broncho-pulmonary aspergillosis. Clinical immunology: (i) clinical features. *Clin. Allergy*, **1**, 261

222. Hinson, K. F. W. *et al.* (1952). Broncho-pulmonary aspergillosis. *Thorax*, **7**, 317

223. Safirstein, B. H. *et al.* (1973). Five-year follow-up of allergic bronchopulmonary aspergillosis. *Am. Rev. Resp. Dis.*, **108**, 450

224. Longbottom, J. L. and Pepys, J. (1964). Pulmonary aspergillosis: diagnostic and immunological significance of antigens and C-substance in *Aspergillus fumigatus*. *J. Pathol. Bacteriol.*, **88**, 141

225. Mearns, M. *et al.* (1967). Precipitating antibodies to *Aspergillus fumigatus* in cystic fibrosis. *Lancet*, **i**, 538

226. Pepys, J. (1973). Types of allergic reaction. In: *Clinical Immunology—Allergy—in Paediatric Medicine* (J. Brostoff, ed.), p. 1 (Oxford: Blackwell Scientific Publications)

227. Arbesman, C. E. *et al.* (1974). IgE antibodies in sera of patients with allergic broncho-pulmonary aspergillosis. *Clin. Allergy*, **4**, 349

228. Pauwels, R. *et al.* (1976). IgE antibodies in brochopulmonary aspergillosis. *Ann. Allergy*, **37**, 195

229. Patterson, R. *et al.* (1973). Serum immunoglobulin levels in pulmonary allergic aspergillosis and certain other lung diseases, with special reference to immunoglobulin E. *Am. J. Med.*, **54**, 16

230. Campbell, J. M. (1932). Acute symptoms following work with hay. *Br. Med. J.*, **2**, 1143

231. Pepys, J. and Jenkins, P. A. (1963). Farmer's lung thermophilic actinomycetes as a source of 'Farmer's Lung Hay' antigen. *Lancet*, **ii**, 607

232. Kobayashi, M. *et al.* (1963). Antigens in mouldy hay as the cause of Farmer's Lung. *Proc. Soc. Exp. Biol. Med.*, **113**, 472

233. Roberts, R. C. and Moore, V. L. (1977). Immunopathogenesis of hypersensitivity pneumonitis. *Am. Rev. Resp. Dis.*, **116**, 1075

234. Gregory, P. H. *et al.* (1963). Microbial and biochemical changes during the moulding of hay. *J. Gen. Microbiol.*, **33**, 147

235. Neilsen, K. H. *et al.* (1973). Quantitation of antibody to particulate antigens using a radio-labeled anti-immunoglobulin reagent: application to estimation of antibody in Farmer's Lung syndrome. *J. Immunol. Methods*, **3**, 301

236. Patterson, R. *et al.* (1976). Antibodies of different immunoglobulin classes against antigens causing Farmer's Lung. *Am. Rev. Resp. Dis.*, **114**, 315

237. Pepys, J. (1969). Hypersensitivity disease of the lungs due to fungi and organic dusts. *Monographs in Allergy, Vol. 4*, pp. 20–46, 59–67 (New York: S. Karger)

238. Hansen, P. J. and Penny, R. (1974). Pigeon breeders' disease. Study of the cell-mediated immune response to pigeon antigen by the lymphocyte culture technique. *Int. Arch. Allergy Appl. Immunol.*, **47**, 498

239. Marx, J. J. Jr. *et al.* (1973). Migration inhibition factor and Farmer's Lung antigen (abstract). *Clin. Res.*, **21**, 852

240. Richerson, H. B. (1972). Acute experimental hypersensitivity pneumonitis in the guinea-pig. *J. Lab. Clin. Med.*, **79**, 745

241. Roska, A. K. *et al.* (1977). Immune-complex disease in guinea-pigs. I. Elicitation by aerosol challenge, suppression with cobra venom factor, and passive transfer with serum. *Clin. Immunol. Immunopathol.*, **8**, 213

242. Bice, D. E. *et al.* (1976). Passive transfer of experimental hypersensitivity pneumonitis with lymphoid cells in the rabbit. *J. Allergy Clin. Immunol.*, **58**, 250

243. Hollingdale, M. (1975). Isolation of lipopolysaccharide from the walls of *Micropolyspora faeni*; chemical composition and serological reactivity. *J. Gen. Microbiol.*, **86**, 250

244. Nicolet, J. *et al.* (1977). Farmer's Lung: immunological response to a group of extracellular enzymes of *Micropolyspora faeni*. *Clin. Exp. Immunol.*, **27**, 401

245. Flaherty, D. K. *et al.* (1975). HL-A8 in Farmer's Lung. *Lancet*, **ii**, 507

246. Maghoub, E. S. (1976). Medical management of mycetoma. *Bull. WHO*, **54**, 303

247. Alford, R. H. (1973). Transformation of lymphocytes of normal and hospitalized adults by *Candida albicans* extract. *Proc. Soc. Exp. Biol. Med.*, **144**, 826

3
Normal Immune Responses to Protozoal Infections

J. P. ACKERS

3.1 INTRODUCTION   78

3.2 BLOOD PARASITES   78
    3.2.1 *Immune responses*   79
        3.2.1.1 *African trypanosomes*   79
        3.2.1.2 Plasmodium   81
        3.2.1.3 Trypanosoma cruzi   82
        3.2.1.4 *Non-specific defence mechanisms*   83
    3.2.2 *Conclusions*   84

3.3 INTRACELLULAR PARASITES   84
    3.3.1 Leishmania   85
        3.3.1.1 Leishmania tropica   85
        3.3.1.2 Leishmania donovani   88
        3.3.1.3 *New-World leishmaniasis*   89
    3.3.2 Toxoplasma *and other coccidia*   89
        3.3.2.1 Toxoplasma   90
        3.3.2.2 Sarcocystis   93
    3.3.3 *Conclusions*   94

3.4 PARASITES OF MUCOUS SURFACES   94
    3.4.1 Entamoeba histolytica   95
    3.4.2 Giardia intestinalis   97
    3.4.3 Trichomonas vaginalis   99
    3.4.4 *Conclusions*   101

3.5   MISCELLANEOUS EFFECTS   101

3.6   GENERAL CONCLUSIONS   103

      ACKNOWLEDGEMENTS   104

3.1   INTRODUCTION

The science of immunology was born of attempts to understand and, more importantly, cure the infectious diseases which in the past had taken so many lives. Together with public health measures and antibiotics, practical immunology, particularly in the form of vaccination, has succeeded to the point where infectious diseases have become relatively trivial as causes of death in economically advanced nations. It was natural, therefore, that immunologists should try to repeat their success when faced with the parasitic diseases which cause so much illness and death in the underdeveloped world. It is fair to say that, on balance, this aim has proved much harder to realize than was expected, and the feeling has grown that there is something special (and probably malign) about the immune response to protozoa. Although the subject has produced many fascinating surprises (such as antigenic variation) it seems wrong to base a general review on what may be special cases. It seems safer to consider briefly what is known of the immune responses to the major human protozoal parasites and then see if any general conclusions emerge. The order in which the organisms are discussed has been chosen to bring together those which occupy the same sort of habitats and which elicit the same sort of host response: thus, in this context, *Trypanosoma cruzi* is more like *Leishmania tropica* than the African trypanosomes.

3.2   BLOOD PARASITES

The parasites to be considered here fall into three groups. The first consists of the salivarian trypanosomes *Trypanosoma brucei rhodesiense* and *T. b. gambiense*, the cause, respectively, of acute and chronic African sleeping sickness in man; the related animal parasites, *T. b. brucei*, *T. congolense* and *T. vivax*, all of which infect (and cause enormous economic losses in) cattle and other domestic animals; and two parasites of laboratory rodents, *T. musculi* (mice) and *T. lewisi* (rats), which have been very largely used in experimental investigations.

The second group consists of members of the genus *Plasmodium*, the cause of malaria in man and numerous other animals and birds. Four species infect man: *P. falciparum* (the most dangerous), *P. vivax*, *P. malariae* and (rarely) *P. ovale*. Too many other species of *Plasmodium* have been used experimentally to list them all here. In addition, work with *Babesia* species has also been important. *Babesia* is closely related to *Plasmodium*; man is only rarely infected, but the genus causes economically very important diseases of cattle. Despite inclusion in this section, *Plasmodium* spp. spend most of their time multiplying within host cells, either liver cells or erythrocytes. Nevertheless, since the merozoites are exposed to the host's immune system while passing from cell to cell, and for the practical reason that very little is known of the antigenic nature of the intracellular stages in the life-cycle, they will be included here.

The third group consists of only one organism, *Trypanosoma (Schizotrypanum) cruzi*, the cause of South American trypanosomiasis (Chagas' disease). Chagas' disease clinically consists of two phases: an early acute illness during which the parasite is multiplying within tissue cells and passing into the blood-stream in easily detectable numbers, and a much longer chronic phase in which parasites are frequently undetectable in either blood or tissue.

3.2.1 Immune responses

3.2.1.1 *African trypanosomes*

The immune response to the African trypanosomes is dominated by humoral antibodies and the phenomenon of antigenic variation. This phenomenon is believed to occur in all hosts, but is perhaps most clearly seen in experimental infections of domestic animals or rodents with *T. b. brucei*. After an initial lag, parasitaemias rise rapidly, only to fall abruptly after a period of 1 or 2 weeks. Within a day or so, however, parasite numbers begin to rise again, and the process is repeated 10–20 times until (usually) the host dies. Immediately after clearing of the blood has occurred the serum can be shown to contain high titres of antibodies (agglutinins and complement-dependent lysins), but these react only with the variant which has just disappeared and have no effect on the newly appearing organisms. It thus seems clear that the trypanosome is able to persist in the blood because as one variant is eliminated a new one appears against which the host has to mount a fresh immune response.

An enormous amount of work, far more than can be summarized here, has led to the following conclusions about antigenic variation in trypanosomes. The variant antigen appears to be (as would be expected) present on the surface of the organism and to be identical with the electron-dense surface coat[1-3]. There is evidence that this coat may at times be shed in the form of filaments[4, 5], but whether this happens *in vivo* or is merely an artefact is not clear. Chemically these variant antigens are glycoproteins with a molecular weight of about 65 000; although it is easy to see that to serve their present function they must not induce cross-reacting antigens, it is nevertheless surprising to find how extensive are the differences in the amino acid sequences of the variant antigen produced successively by an infection initiated with cloned organisms[6]. It has long been known that there is a strong probability that different infections initiated by the same clone of *T. b. brucei* will lead to the formation of many of the same variants (although not always in the same order) and that transfer to the fly vector frequently leads to reversion to a 'basic antigenic type'[7]; these facts, together with the large difference in amino acid sequence between successive variant-specific antigens, make it highly unlikely that antigenic variation is brought about by random mutation[8]. It seems most probable that the trypanosome genome contains genes coding for at least 22 variant-specific antigens[9]; the nature of the switch which controls the sequential expression of these genes is not known, although induction by antibody is the obvious candidate. It should not be forgotten, however, that antigenic variants can differ ·in other properties as well as, for example, growth rate, and it is probably not true to say that antigenic variation never occurs in the absence of immunological pressure. Nevertheless, it is clear that, in evolving antigenic variation, the African trypanosomes have acquired a highly successful method of avoiding immune destruction and of enabling the infection to persist long enough for fresh vectors to be infected. Ultimately, however, for reasons which are not really understood, the host fails to respond adequately to the newly appearing variants, and complex pathological processes ensue which are ultimately fatal[10-12].

As well as the variant-specific antibodies, the host produces antibodies against many other, non-variable components of the organism, and it is these antibodies which are of most value in serodiagnosis[13,14], although there is no evidence that they play any part in protection.

Another different, and fascinating, humoral response is seen in the infection of rodents by their natural parasites, *T. lewisi* and *T. musculi*[15]. In these cases a rising parasitaemia is first controlled and then completely eliminated by two successive types of antibody: the second is trypanocidal, while the first-formed, which has been named ablastin, though not capable of killing the trypanosomes greatly slows down their multiplication. The mode of action of ablastin is not known, nor is it clear if ablastin-like activity is important in other trypanosomiases, or indeed in other protozoal infections, but the concept of a specific, division-inhibiting antibody is certainly a fascinating one; the subject has recently been the basis of a specialized workshop[16].

In contrast to the clear importance of humoral responses in African trypanosomiasis, there is at present no good evidence for the participation of cell-mediated effects in the host defences[17] although, of course, there is much evidence that T-cell participation is involved in the response[15]. Trypanosome infections also have a profound effect both on general immunoglobulin synthesis and on the response to unrelated antigens, but these will be considered below.

3.2.1.2 Plasmodium

In malaria, as in African trypanosomiasis, antibody seems to be the main effector of acquired resistance. Infection in man leads to the production of specific anti-plasmodial antibody; this antibody is present in IgM, IgG and IgA fractions[18]. However, as in trypanosomiasis, considerable amounts of non-specific immunoglobulin synthesis takes place (see below), and of the specific antibody produced probably only a small part is protective. Antibodies may be detected by agglutination of infected red cells, radio-immunoassay, indirect haemagglutination, the ELISA technique and others, and these methods form the basis of the currently used serodiagnostic procedures[14,19,20]. The effectiveness of antibody *in vivo* has been demonstrated by the passive transfer of immune IgG from adults to children with severe *P. falciparum* infection: a striking reduction in parasitaemia was produced[21]. Experimental work in both rodents[22] and rhesus monkeys infected with *P. knowlesi*[23,24] has demonstrated that one protective mechanism involves anti-merozoite antibody: this apparently agglutinates the merozoites and, more importantly, prevents their penetration into erythrocytes. A second protective mechanism, also in the rhesus monkey, has been suggested by Brown and Hills[25]: they have produced evidence for opsonic-like activity which enhances the removal of infected erythrocytes by the spleen.

Infections with *Plasmodium* persist for varying lengths of time depending on the species involved, and in particular cases of *P. malariae* can show periodic recrudescences for many years. There is, in fact, no good evidence for the commonly suggested repeated cycles of exoerythrocytic multiplication[26], and we must suppose that prolonged survival occurs in the bloodstream. To explain this survival in the face of the host's immune response, K. N. Brown has suggested that antigenic variation, similar in principle to that shown by *T. brucei*, takes place. The most direct evidence for antigenic variation comes from experiments involving *P. knowlesi*[27], but it also seems to occur in murine and avian malarias and possibly also in *P. falciparum* infections in man; the whole subject has been well reviewed recently[28]. However, the importance of antigenic variation in host resistance in human malarias is not yet clear. It is feasible to explain the occasional persistence of *P. malariae* infections for up to 30 years on this basis, even though this involves the existence of up to $2-3 \times 10^3$ distinct variants[28]; however, it is difficult to see how such an investment in structural genes could be evolutionarily advantageous. Such exceptionally prolonged infections can hardly be part of the normal transmission process, and, if not, the majority of antigen genes would not contribute to the survival of the parasite species.

Other humoral responses may well play a part in controlling the balance between host and parasite. Serum or immunoglobulin from adult donors living in areas where malaria is endemic appears to exert an inhibitory effect on the *in vitro* multiplication of *P. falciparum*[29,30].

Experiments with murine malarias have indicated that immunity could be transferred to unexposed animals far more efficiently by cells than by serum; a need for T cells has been specifically indicated[27,31-33]; on the other hand, no convincing evidence for cell-mediated cytotoxicity has yet been presented[23,26]. Some tests involving *in vitro* indicators of cell-mediated immunity have, however, given positive results (lymphocyte transformation in human *P. falciparum* malaria[34] and lymphocyte transformation and macrophage inhibition in *P. berghei*-infected rodents[35]) but their significance in the overall host response is not known. Brown has interpreted the T-cell dependence of protective immunity in terms of a 'hapten-carrier' model, in which variant-specific antigens act as haptens and a second determinant (strain-specific but common to all variants of that strain) acts as the carrier; this interesting theory is discussed by Brown[28] and Targett[26].

One of the most characteristic features of malaria is the way its incidence and severity vary with the age of the patient. Very young babies are apparently protected by maternal antibody, but between 6 months and 5 years of age the highest incidence and mortality appear. Developing immunity is manifested, firstly by a lessening of the severity of the illness, despite high parasitaemias (ascribed, without any real evidence, to immunity against toxic metabolic products of the parasite), followed later by genuine antiparasitic immunity which effectively suppresses the infection. It is also clear that this state of high immunity is only maintained by continuous challenge, and outbreaks of malaria in areas which have been free of the parasite cause epidemics affecting all ages. By contrast, there is evidence that older rats are inherently more resistant to *P. berghei* than young animals: the latter infection causes involution of the thymus, high parasitaemias and ultimately death[36].

The only antibodies mentioned so far have been directed against the merozoite or other components involved in the erythrocytic stage of development. It is generally stated that antibodies are not normally formed against other stages in the life-cycle, but this may not necessarily be true in persons exposed to repeated infections. Certainly both anti-sporozoite and anti-gamete antibody can be elicited experimentally and might have a part to play in vaccination programmes.

The immunodepressive effects of malarial infections together with the non-specific synthesis of immunoglobulin will be considered below, since these effects are common to several infection.

3.2.1.3 Trypanosoma cruzi

The natural history of infection with *T. cruzi* (an early acute phase followed by the disappearance of parasites from the blood and the onset of chronic infection) certainly suggests the operation of immune mechanisms; but in practice it has not proved easy to sort out the effector mechanisms involved.

It is also true, of course, that this immunity, if it occurs, is not completely effective and that ultimately the patient usually dies.

Specific serum antibody is formed during the acute phase of the infection and may be detected by standard methods (indirect immunofluorescence, indirect haemagglutination, etc.). Radioimmunoassay and the ELISA technique appear to be particularly sensitive; cross-reaction with sera from patients suffering from African trypanosomiasis occurs but results are lower[20]. In experimental rodent infection passive transfer of (maternal) antibody has been shown to protect against infection[37]; *in vitro* the infectivity of one of two strains tested was reduced by incubation with homologous or heterologous serum[38]. On the other hand, the value of therapeutic or prophylactic administration of immune serum is far from proved[39], and it is clear that high parasitaemias can persist in the face of equally high levels of serum antibody.

Much evidence suggests that a cell-mediated response occurs in Chagas' disease, but its importance is not clear. Delayed-type hypersensitivity reactions to skin testing have been observed[40], as have the *in vitro* indicators of a CMI response (blast transformation[41] and leukocyte migration inhibition[42]). In all cases, however, not all patients gave positive results, and, although evidence exists for cell-mediated immunity in experimental infections[43,44], no actual evidence for the killing of trypomastigotes by sensitized lymphocytes has yet been found[45]. In rats some protection against death could be transferred to newly infected animals by using spleen cells from animals which had been infected for longer periods: although the life of the recipient animals was prolonged, parasitaemia was not reduced. The nature of the cells involved was not determined[46,47].

A third component of the immune system, and one which may be of considerable importance in Chagas' disease, is the macrophage. During the course of the natural infection, initial multiplication of the parasite frequently occurs within these cells and may be demonstrated *in vitro*[48]. Macrophages from immune animals, however, may either destroy the ingested parasites[49-51] or at least limit their multiplication[52].

3.2.1.4 *Non-specific defence mechanisms*

Under this heading brief mention will be made of some host-defence mechanisms which do not involve classical immune mechanisms. In each case the importance of these mechanisms is not clear at present, but it may be very great.

Perhaps the most unexpected is the apparent ability of certain hosts to kill intraerythrocytic forms of *Plasmodium* and *Babesia*. In these hosts, damaged intraerythrocytic parasites are seen ('crisis' or 'drug' forms), particularly as the host begins to control the infection. There are many similarities (and good cross-protection) between murine infections with *P. yoelii* and *Babesia microti*, and Clark and his co-workers have shown that solid immunity may be produced either by previous infection or by injection of BCG or *Corynebacterium parvum*[53,54]. In the latter case the infection was eliminated with the formation of 'crisis' forms, but in the absence of detectable specific antibody. The same authors have suggested that protection is due to the release of non-antibody soluble mediators from lymphoid cells[55]. It is interesting that administering these agents subcutaneously is ineffective while intravenous or intraperitoneal injection is successful.

It has already been mentioned that macrophages from immune hosts may inhibit the multiplication of ingested *T. cruzi*; there is some evidence that non-specific activation of macrophages by administration of BCG may also enhance the ability to kill *T. cruzi*[51,56].

Finally, and briefly, mention should be made of the fact that in some sera some protozoa appear to be lysed by a mechanism involving the activation of complement by the alternative pathway and in the absence of specific antibody[57,58]. It is too early to judge the importance of alternative pathway activation, but it could be considerable, particularly in limiting the host range of some parasites.

3.2.2   Conclusions

Although this section is headed 'blood parasites', it is only in the case of the salivarian trypanosomes that the whole life-cycle appears to occur there, and even this has been disputed. Both *Plasmodium* and *T. cruzi* multiply intra-cellularly, but parasitaemia does occur. It is probably not coincidental that it is only in the case of African trypanosomiasis that antibody appears to be the chief factor involved in host resistance, albeit the effect is only temporary. In the case of malaria, antibodies directed against erythrocytic stages of the life-cycle also appear to be important, and, while cell-mediated responses have not, as yet, been shown to have a role, the killing of the parasite within the erythrocyte by a soluble factor (not antibody but produced by the lymphoid cells) may also be very important. In Chagas' disease a further factor in addition to antibody and cell-mediated immunity appears, and that is the ability of the host macrophage to kill ingested *T. cruzi* rather than provide it with a safe home in which to multiply. The relative importance of these three factors in the natural disease is not known, but there is evidence that antibody is relatively less important; it is thus not surprising that there is at present no good evidence for antigenic variation during infections with *T. cruzi*.

3.3   INTRACELLULAR PARASITES

Following on logically from the preceeding group are those parasites which, apart from the necessary (and often little-understood) passage from cell to cell, lead an exclusively intracellular existence. These comprise the various species of *Leishmania* which infect man, and the enormous and complex group of organisms usually referred to as the *Coccidia*.

3.3.1 Leishmania

The taxonomy of the *Leishmania* spp. is confused at present. Until recently speciation has been determined chiefly by the type of human infection produced and its geographical location, an approach which can lead to up to nine species causing human disease. Since all these leishmanias are morphologically indistinguishable, and since it is now very clear that the nature of the illness produced is very much affected by the host response, the alternative view has been to recognize only one or two species. The matter is by no means settled, but recent evidence (for example, the isoenzyme work of Al-Taqi and Evans[59]) does seem to show real differences between species that are not influenced by host responses. For convenience, the classification of Lumsden[60] is adopted here. He recognizes: (a) the *L. donovani* complex, containing three subspecies: these organisms have a predilection for infecting cells of the viscera, particularly the spleen, although it seems that they can also cause cutaneous infection; (b) the Old-World *L. tropica* complex, containing two subspecies and normally confined to cutaneous lesions; (c) the *L. mexicana* and *L. brasiliensis* complexes, each containing respectively three subspecies, and the single species of *L. peruviana*: these organisms, exclusive to the New World, cause cutaneous lesions (some of which metastasize) but they do not invade the viscera. Those authors who prefer not to split the species too finely would probably refer to (a) above as *L. donovani*, to (b) as *L. tropica* and to (c) as *L. brasiliensis* or *L. tropica brasiliensis*. Lainson and Shaw[61] have recently proposed a new classification scheme which is based on the site of multiplication within the vector; their scheme corrects what they believe to be an excessive emphasis on the difference between New- and Old-World species.

3.3.1.1 Leishmania tropica

Leishmanial infection is such a good example of the influence of host immune responses on disease processes that it has become something of a classic and the subject of several recent reviews[62-64].

The phenomenon is most clearly seen in infections with *L. tropica*. Following injection by the sandfly vector, the promastigotes invade the local macrophages and then change into the amastigote form. The parasites slowly proliferate within the macrophages, which are ultimately destroyed; the liberated amastigotes are then taken up by fresh macrophages. The lesion produced is either a 'dry' (*L. t. tropica*) or 'moist' (*L. t. major*) oriental sore, but in either case it is normally self-limiting, healing after several months. Microscopically, healing is accompanied by infiltration with lymphocytes and plasma cells and by the complete elimination of the parasite[64]. Subsequent immunity is solid and apparently life-long, but species- and sub-species-specific. The mechanism by which this is brought about is not clear however. Antibody titres in cutaneous leishmaniasis are usually low to negligible[65,66], although they may become detectable if the lymphatics are involved. Evidence for a cell-mediated response is, however, available very soon after the initial infection, in the form of a delayed-hypersensitivity reaction to skin testing with leishmanin (cultured leishmania promastigotes killed with phenol)[67]. Positive results with leishmanin (the Montenegro test) correlate well with another indicator of cell-mediated immunity, lymphoblast transformation[62]; however, the important point is that the leishmanin test becomes positive long before any protective immunity is apparent and while the lesion is full of living parasites[64]. Some understanding of the mechanisms involved in healing has been gained by examination of the infection of the guinea-pig with L. enrietti, the natural course of which closely resembles L. tropica infections in man.

Since Leishmania are obligate intramacrophage parasites, it seems logical to look there for the source of host resistance, but there is no evidence that macrophages from immune guinea-pigs can inhibit intracellular growth, although they do take up more amastigotes than macrophages from control animals[62,68]. ('Immune' guinea-pigs are those recovering from infection and which are invariably resistant to rechallenge.) Furthermore, even activated guinea-pig macrophages cannot destroy L. enrietti[69]. In one report delayed hypersensitivity was detected shortly (1–2 weeks) after infection, as in man, although spontaneous healing did not occur for 8–12 weeks[70]; in another report cell-mediated immunity was not detectable for 6 weeks[71]. Indeed, when Belehu and Turk[72] succeeded in establishing a cutaneous infection with L. enrietti in the hamster they found that, although recovery occurred and solid immunity to reinfection developed, skin-test sensitivity was never found.

In contrast to the human infection, antibody is detectable by indirect immunofluorescence early in infected guinea-pigs[62], although not by indirect haemagglutination[70]. Despite the fact that this antibody can inhibit the growth of promastigotes in culture[73], antibody does not seem to be very important in eliminating the infection; in some experimental situations pre-immunization with a soluble promastigote antigen enhances the severity of the infection[62,69].

Histological evidence strongly suggests a central role for lymphocytes in eliminating these parasites in both guinea-pigs and man. Infiltration of the lesion by lymphocyte and plasma cells is the earliest sign that healing is beginning; two mechanisms have been proposed whereby they might be effective. It has been suggested that these sensitized cells kill the amastigotes as they emerge from infected macrophages[74] and/or that they have a directly cytotoxic effect on parasitized macrophages[70]. Some evidence (which has, however, been hard to confirm) has been provided to support the second suggestion, for Bryceson and his colleagues showed that lymphocytes from convalescent guinea-pigs destroyed macrophage monolayers maintained in vitro far more rapidly than cells from control animals[68, 70]. There was some evidence that parasitized macrophages were preferentially destroyed. However, lymphocytes from animals given BCG were as destructive as those from immune animals, and Mauel[75] found no difference between normal and immune lymphocytes. Nevertheless, there is no real doubt that cell-mediated responses are central to host-resistance in cutaneous leishmaniasis, although humoral antibody (possibly produced locally by the infiltrating plasma cells[76]) may also play a part[77, 78].

The importance of cell-mediated immunity in controlling infection with L. tropica is shown by the consequences of its absence, as occurs in the condition known as diffuse cutaneous leishmaniasis (DCL). The clinical features of DCL have been described by Bryceson[79]. The primary lesion usually fails to heal, and, months or years later, metastatic lesions, presumably due to blood-borne parasites, appear on the body. Parasitized macrophages are abundant, but lymphocyte infiltration does not occur. Immunologically, studies on specific antibody production in cases of DCL have been variable, but the leishmanin test is invariably negative. Prolonged chemotherapy may result in a positive leishmanin response appearing; if this change does not occur it is very difficult to cure the patient[62]. The cause of this state of anergy is not known. Patients with DCL show no evidence of diseases known to be linked to a general failure of the immune system. Intercurrent infections run a normal course and responses to lepromin and tuberculin (although possibly not to dinitrochlorbenzene) are normal[62]. Serum immunoglobulin levels are apparently normal, although one so far unexplained finding was of elevated levels of serum IgA in four patients[79]. While host unresponsiveness is clearly important, what is not clear is whether certain strains of L. tropica are particularly prone to cause DCL. Evidence in favour of this is provided by the geographical distribution of the disease; DCL is apparently absent from the Middle East and India although cutaneous infections are common. Some authorities would regard all Old-World cases of DCL as being caused by a separate species, L. ethiopica. Although there is no definite evidence either way, Zuckerman concludes that DCL may turn out to be a consequence of peculiarities of both host and parasite[64].

One mechanism whereby the anergy might be produced has been suggested by Bryceson[80] and Dumonde[76]: if the lymphatic drainage from the site of infection was damaged this might delay the onset of protective immunity to the point where, if the parasite was growing rapidly, the antigenic mass present was sufficient to induce high-zone tolerance. In support of this idea,

Kadiva and Soulsby[81] were able to produce a DCL-like condition in guinea-pigs by inoculating *L. enrietti* into skin flaps deprived of their lymphatic drainage.

In several papers summarized in Chapter 12 Turk[62, 63] and his colleagues have discussed the concept of a spectrum of immunological responses to a particular infectious agent, different parts of the spectrum being associated with different clinical conditions. Applying the concept to leishmanias, if tropical sore occupies the centre of the spectrum with DCL at one (anergic) pole then the other pole is occupied by the condition of recidiva leishmaniasis (RL).

In RL[67] the primary lesion heals but satellite foci develop, usually on the margin. Although metastasis does not occur, the lesion is constantly growing and ultimately tissue destruction may be very extensive. Unlike the lesions of DCL, lymphocytes are abundant but amastigotes very hard to find. Specific antibody does not seem to have been looked for in RL[69] but extreme hypersensitivity to very small doses of leishmanin is present[62]. The ability of the parasite to persist (although only in small numbers) in the face of this response is not understood: indeed, it appears to be necessary to suppress the hypersensitivity (for example, with steroids) before the patient can be cured[62].

3.3.1.2   Leishmania donovani

L. donovani donovani is the causative agent of kala-azar, a disease in which the visceral macrophages (predominantly in the spleen, liver and bone-marrow) are heavily involved. In the absence of chemotherapy the illness, once established, is almost always fatal. Specific antibody is present during the infection[62, 82] but delayed hypersensitivity to leishmanin is not. The reason for this lack of cell-mediated response is not known, but successful cure with chemotherapy leads to a fall in antibody titre and the appearance of delayed hypersensitivity. Subsequently patients are immune to new infection. Kala-azar possibly corresponds immunologically to DCL following infection with *L. tropica*; however, it is difficult to place a late sequel to visceral leishmanias (post-kala-azar dermal leishmanias–PKDL) on the immunological spectrum. In PDKL relapse occurs, but affecting the skin rather than the viscera. Both antibody production and leishmanin reaction are highly variable[83] and the condition is not understood[84]. Until recently it was thought that there was no infection with members of the *L. donovani* complex analogous to oriental sore; however, it is now clear that a mild dermatropic infection with *L. d. donovani* occurs in East Africa[85, 86] and a similar condition, due to *L. d. infantum*, in France[87]. The cutaneous nature of the initial lesions may allow cell-mediated immunity to develop in time to prevent spread to the viscera; the physiological state of the host may also have a profound influence on the outcome. In any case, it is now considered possible that the majority of African infections with *L. d. donovani* may be asymptomatic.

3.3.1.3 *New-World leishmaniasis*

Leishmanial infections in the New World present a complex picture, with several species complexes involved in producing a wide variety of diseases; analogues of all the Old-World conditions exist. One of the commonest is espundia or mucocutaneous leishmaniasis, due to infection with *L. b. braziliensis.* Months or years after the primary infection the naso-pharangeal mucosa becomes involved, despite the presence of both antibody and cell-mediated responses[65,88]. The condition thus resembles PDKL and immunologically is likewise not understood. Other members of the *L. braziliensis* complex, *L. b. guyanensis* and *L. b. panamensis,* cause single or multiple lesions; they may be extremely disfiguring but do not metastasise to the nasopharynx. In contrast, the lesions produced by *L. peruviana (uta)* and the *L. mexicana* complex are normally mild, cutaneous and self-healing. Exceptions are *L. m. mexicana* lesions of the ear (Chiclero's ear: non-metastasing but chronic ulcers which may persist for many years) and cases of DCL. The latter are rarely caused by *L. m. mexicana* and *L. m. amazonesis*; *L. m. pifanoi* is known only from DCL cases. Finally there is the South American form of visceral leishmaniasis, caused by *L. d. chagasi,* and resembling the Old-World disease.

3.3.2 *Toxoplasma* and other coccidia

It has gradually become apparent, over the last 10 years, that the causative organisms of toxoplasmosis and sarcocystis (whose classification was previously uncertain) are, in fact, coccidian parasites. This has naturally led to considerably taxonomic confusion, and several new classificatory schemes have been suggested. For convenience, the following names will be used:

(a) *Toxoplasma gondii*—This is the organism long known as the cause of toxoplasmosis of almost all mammals and many birds. Despite this broad range it is now known that the definitive hosts (and the only ones in which it completes its life-cycle) are the domestic cat and related felids. The oocysts produced in the cat are identical to those previously known as the 'small race' of *Isospora bigemina.* It seems certain that the name *T. gondii* will eventually be superseded, but it is too early to say which of the many suggested alternatives will be adopted; so for the present the familiar name will be retained. For recent reviews of the subject see Jacobs[89], Tadros and Laaman[90] and Levine[91].

(b) *Sarcocystis*—The situation here is more complicated. It now seems clear that not only are members of the genus *Sarcocystis* coccidian parasites but also that they have an unusual life-cycle in which asexual reproduction takes place in a 'prey' species; this is then eaten by the 'predator' species in which the sexual part of the life-cycle occurs, resulting in the shedding of sporocysts. In this context man is a 'predator': both *S. fusiformis* of cattle and *S. miescheriana* of pigs will complete their life-cycle in man, resulting in the shedding of sporocysts identical with those of the previously known *Isospora hominis*[90,92]. Very rarely asexual reproduction occurs in man resulting in the formation of muscle cysts; Jeffrey[93], reviewing the literature of the last 100 years, was only able to find 16 cases that were probably genuine sarcosporidiosis. This infection has been attributed to *Sarcocystis lindermanni*, but there is no real evidence for the existence of a specifically human parasite[94]. As with *Toxoplasma gondii*, the nomenclature of *Sarcocystis* species seems certain to be altered in the future; for the present *S. fusiformis* will be used. Since, on present evidence, *S. fusiformis* and *S. meischeriana* behave similarly in man, it may be assumed, unless otherwise stated, that what is said about the first species applies also to the second.

(c) *Other human coccidia*—At least two other coccidia are known to infect humans, although apparently not very often. The organisms are *Isospora belli* and *I. natalensis*: little is known of their life-cycle or immunology.

3.3.2.1 Toxoplasma

Human infections with *T. gondii* appear to be acquired in three ways: (1) by ingestion of oocysts present in the faeces of the final host, the cat; (2) by the ingestion of inadequately cooked tissues of infected animals which contain pseudocysts* filled with infective bradyzoites; and (3) congenitally: in man this only appears to happen when the mother is infected during the first months of pregnancy. Although *T. gondii* is extremely common in the animals around us and in the environment in which we live, and although there is serological evidence that a significant proportion of the population has been infected (4–68% in various surveys[95]), cases of acute toxoplasmosis are far less common. Following oral ingestion the oocysts break down and the liberated sporozoites penetrate the gut mucosa and are disseminated via the blood or lymph; the same route is presumably taken by ingested bradyzoites (cystozoites). In experimental animals toxoplasmosis may easily be transmitted parenterally. The parasites penetrate into almost any type of cell and begin to divide; this is the stage of acute infection during which parasitaemia occurs. In mice the parasites are easily found at this stage in the peritoneal macrophages but are also present in many other cells. Following the first stage of intracellular multiplication, tachyzoites (endozoites) leave the ruptured cells and penetrate new ones, most commonly brain and muscle. A pseudocyst (cyst) is formed around the parasite, which slowly

---

*Nomenclature used is that of Levine[91] with common alternatives in brackets.

divides to form bradyzoites; clinically this is the stage of chronic toxo-plasmosis. This point is the end of the road for *T. gondii* in all animals except the final host in which the life-cycle is completed. Congenital toxoplasmosis is the most dangerous form, frequently resulting in severe malformation and having a high mortality. In adults various clinical patterns may be seen, including an acute febrile illness and ocular and cerebro-spinal forms, but asymptomatic infections are the most common[95].

All evidence seems to show that one attack of toxoplasmosis (whether symptomatic or not) confers solid resistance to reinfection, although rare cases of a recrudescence of parasitaemia have been reported in man and other animals[89,96,97].

Exploration of the immune response to this parasite has taken two main paths. In man, interest has centred largely on developing reliable serological tests for past and present infection, while fundamental studies of host-resistance have been largely confined to rodent infections.

It has long been known that high titres of specific antibody are usually present soon after infection. Classically, they are detected by the dye-test—a test which detects the ability of specific anti-toxoplasmal antibody (in the presence of an accessory factor) to modify the cytoplasm of the living parasite so that it no longer stains with alkaline methylene blue. The dye-test is technically difficult and not a little dangerous to carry out, but, until the development of immunofluorescence assays, it retained its place as the most reliable indicator of infection. The newer immunofluorescence tests have now largely replaced the dye-test: both become positive earlier than other anti-body assays[89], and titres remain high for many years, if not for life. Anti-bodies detected by other tests (complement fixation, indirect haemag-glutination) appear later and disappear sooner[95].

The initial response is composed of IgM, and this fact is made use of in the serodiagnosis of congenital toxoplasmosis; IgM does not cross the placenta and therefore the presence of specific anti-toxoplasma IgM in a baby is evidence for actual infection.

A rise in dye-test titre usually coincides with, and may be the cause of the disappearance of parasites from the blood. Otherwise there is little evidence to suggest that human antibodies are important in host-resistance. Mice and rabbits repeatedly vaccinated with killed *T. gondii* and possessing high levels of circulating antibody are not protected against challenge by a virulent strain of the parasite[98,99], nor could much protection be transferred by convalescent serum[100,101]. The best that has been achieved with a dead vaccine is partial protection against a small challenge[102].

Moreover, disseminated toxoplasmosis is an increasingly recognized hazard of long-term immunosuppression[89], yet these patients occasionally show high titres of anti-toxoplasma antibody[101].

Nevertheless, anti-toxoplasma antibody obtained from chronically in-fected animals is capable of killing *T. gondii in vitro* in the presence of an 'accessory factor' which appears to be complement plus properdin[103]; but it still seems probable that the major host-defence mechanisms are cell mediated. Clinically, delayed hypersensitivity to skin testing appears in man 3 to 4 weeks after exposure. However, the test usually remains negative in those with the most active disease and in infected rodents[95]. Blast transformation of peripheral lymphocytes from human patients in the presence of toxoplasma antigen has also been examined[104,105]: highest activity was found in cells from people with serological evidence of past infection, but positive results were often found in sero-negative controls, while less transformation was seen in cells from patients with acute toxoplasmosis. Frenkel[101] successfully transferred immunity to *T. gondii* infection in hamsters with spleen and lymph cells from immune animals.

It is clear that contact with living *Toxoplasma* is necessary to elicit immunity; in rodents this can be brought about either by infecting them with a strain of low virulence or by using a highly virulent strain and preventing death by chemotherapy. In either case such vaccinated animals are solidly immune from further infection. Attempts to understand the cellular basis of this resistance have concentrated on the macrophage. In a non-immune host *T. gondii* is readily taken up by the macrophages; about half the ingested organisms die but the remainder multiply unchecked: in particular they seem to be able to prevent the delivery of lysosomal enzymes to the phagocytic vacuole[106]. Macrophages non-specifically activated (by BCG) were no more able than normal ones to suppress multiplication of the parasites, but at least two mechanisms are known which might confer immunity.

Macrophages from immune animals can inhibit the intracellular multiplication of *T. gondii*[99,106,107]. Inhibitory ability is enhanced by incubating the macrophages with lymphoid cells and toxoplasma antigen; these steps may be essential if the macrophages are taken from animals several months after they became immune[106]. Although the parasites do not multiply within the macrophages, the reason is not clear; in particular the delivery of lysosomal enzymes is still blocked[106]. Both Stadtsbaeder[99] and Sethi[107] and their respective co-workers were able to confer inhibitory activity on normal macrophages by incubation with immune lymphocytes and toxoplasma antigen, but Hirsch and co-workers could not show this[106].

The second major protective mechanism apparently involves antibody. Normal macrophages cannot be successfully infected by *T. gondii* which have been pre-treated with heat-inactivated serum from immune animals. It is not clear whether antibody-coating inhibits uptake of the parasite by the macrophages[99] or whether they penetrate normally and are then destroyed[103,107]. There is some evidence that antibody-coated *Toxoplasma* are unable to prevent delivery of lysosomal enzymes to a phagocytic vacuole (Roitt, quoted in reference 106).

One feature of immunity to *T. gondii* is particularly obscure. The parasite is able to penetrate and multiply within many cells others than macrophages; yet there is little or no evidence as to how infection in these sites is brought under control. The parasite appears to have the ability to compel normally non-phagocytic cells to engulf it actively[106]; it may be significant that Lycke[108] showed that immune serum could also inhibit the penetration of *Toxoplasma* into HeLa cells.

3.3.2.2   Sarcocystis

As explained above, the life-cycle (as far as is known) of *S. fusiformis* is unusual in that the sexual and asexual stages are divided between two vertebrate hosts. Man is apparently only infected by eating meat containing viable cystozoites*: unlike *T. gondii*, infection does not follow ingestion of sporocysts[92]. When infected meat is eaten the cystozoites are liberated and penetrate the intestinal wall. In the sub-epithelial tissues they develop into macro- and micro-gametocytes, apparently without any preliminary schizogony. Oocyst formation and sporulation occurs *in situ* and mature sporocysts are discharged, steadily and for a long period, in the faeces.

The amount of work published on the immunology of *Sarcocystis* infections is minute compared with that devoted to *Toxoplasma*; nevertheless, definite differences between the two infections are clear. In experimental infection of a small number of specific-pathogen-free cats (a 'predator' host like man), one animal remained sero-negative for 6 months although it had begun shedding sporocysts 7 days after ingesting infected beef. The search for an antibody response was made using an immunofluorescence assay with cystozoites from muscle cysts as antigen. Moreover, 7 months after the first infection, this cat, together with another which had been given infected meat, was again successfully infected with cystozoites in minced beef[92]. Furthermore, in Berlin, five dogs and four cats which had all previously been infected were successfully reinfected with *S. fusiformis* (Heydorn, quoted in reference 92). Thus, two characteristic features of toxoplasmosis (high serum antibody levels and solid immunity to reinfection) are absent in the case of *Sarcocystis* infection. This minimal immune response may well be a consequence of the failure of the parasite to penetrate beyond the sub-epithelium of the gut, a feature also of some infections with *Entamoeba histolytica* (see below). Experimental evidence that man may be reinfected has been provided by Aryeetey and Piekarski[109]. Antibodies against *Sarcocystis* were found in the serum of volunteers after they had become infected, but they were also found in samples taken before the experiment and in the serum of six controls. The results of serological surveys for antibodies against *Sarcocystis* are confusing and difficult to interpret. In general, low titres of antibody (1/20–1/40) were found in a high proportion

---

*Nomenclature is that of Markus *et al.*[92].

of adults and older children (including vegetarians); only young babies seem, usually, to be sero-negative[110]. Although experimentally infected humans generally show no signs of disease, it is not clear whether or not the high proportion of sero-positive subjects means that the majority of the population has been asymptomatically infected. Other possibilities, such as the ingestion of soluble antigens in cow's milk must also be considered; one suggestion, that the test results are due to cross-reaction with *Toxoplasma* antigen, does seem to have to be eliminated (e.g. reference 109).

3.3.3 Conclusions

The parasites considered in this section, *Leishmania*, *Toxoplasma* and *Sarcocystis*, not only show similarities in the immune responses they elicit but also progressive changes. *Leishmania* species are obligate intramacrophage parasites, and serum antibody, if present, is not effective. Healing does not begin until lymphocytes and plasma cells infiltrate the lesion, but whether these cells confer on the infected macrophages the ability to kill these parasites or whether the lymphocytes directly destroy the parasitized cells is not clear. In the case of *T. gondii* infection, an almost embarassing number of mechanisms have been described whereby the parasites are killed *in vitro*; interaction between macrophages and lymphocytes is again prominent, but other systems involve antibody, and some mechanisms must eliminate the parasite from cells other than macrophages. There is a definite conflict here between the effectiveness of anti-*Toxoplasma* antibody *in vitro* and its apparent unimportance *in vivo*. *Sarcocystis fusiformis* infections, by contrast, seem to run their course without eliciting much of an immune response at all, a fact presumably linked with the shallowness of their penetration into the host.

With the exception of *T. gondii,* coccidia are rare and relatively unimportant parasites of man, but the economic damage they inflict on domestic animals and birds is enormous. Much effort has been devoted, therefore, to studying the immunology of these infections. The complexity of the response has been emphasized by Rose[111], who found that at least four separate responses may be important in fowl coccidia: early production of humoral antibody; local production of specific IgA; infiltration of lymphoid cells into the gut; and classical, delayed-type hypersensitivity. Rose concludes that synergism between humoral and cell-mediated responses is probably necessary for the full expression of immunity, and this may well be true of all the parasites in this group.

3.4 PARASITES OF MUCOUS SURFACES

The organisms considered in this section are the parasites of the alimentary and urogenital tract. They either adhere to the mucous surface or live within the lumen, but normally they do not penetrate the mucosa. Invasive amoebiasis is an exception to the last statement, but there is increasing evidence that the invasive disease is an aberrant form and that non-invasive cyst-passage is the 'normal' state of affairs. In some sense, therefore, these parasites may be regarded as being 'exterior' to their hosts; the reduced, though by no means negligible role of immunological factors in host defence is a consequence of this.

Several species of intestinal amoeba appear to be purely commensal in habit and do not ever cause disease. Others (*Dientamoeba fragilis, Pentatrichomonas hominis, Trichomonas tenax, Entamoeba gingivalis*) may possibly become mildly pathogenic, but only in rare cases. *Balantidium coli*, the only ciliate parasite in man, is definitely pathogenic, but human infections are not only relatively rare but also completely uninvestigated immunologically. In this section, therefore, only three species will be considered: *Entamoeba histolytica sensu strictu, Giardia intestinalis* and *Trichomonas vaginalis*.

3.4.1 *Entamoeba histolytica*

Infection with *E. histolytica* is acquired by ingestion of cysts, there being no evidence that the trophozoites could survive passage through the stomach. Excystment is followed by a complex series of diversions leading to a trophozoite which, on reaching the large intestine, begins to feed on bacteria and food particles[112]. In the condition of non-invasive amoebiasis the trophozoites continue to multiply until, for reasons not understood, encystment occurs. The proportion of cases of amoebiasis which consist solely of symptomless passage of cysts is not known but is certainly high*. In one survey[114], 68% of an already selected population were asymptomatic; similarly, in the Gambia, although the incidence of infection may approach 100%[115], amoebic liver abscesses are almost unknown.

It is frequently stated that anti-amoebic antibodies are not formed until penetration of the mucosa has occurred; however, it is not clear that this has been rigorously proved. Certainly 80–100% of patients with amoebic liver abscesses or amoebic dystentery will show significantly raised titres of antibody detectable by a variety of tests, of which indirect haemagglutination, immunofluorescence and gel-precipitation are the most commonly employed. However, published figures show that up to 40% of asymptomatic cyst-passers are sero-positive: although they may well have minute and otherwise undetectable amoebic ulcers, there may equally well be no penetration at all. Nevertheless, it is clear that the majority of asymptomatic cyst-passers may continue in this condition for many years without the production of humoral antibody. This is somewhat surprising, since oral administration

---

* Definitions used will be those of the World Health Organization[113]; in particular 'amoebiasis' is to be understood as indicating the condition of harbouring *Entamoeba histolytica*, with or without clinical manifestations.

of, for example, bovine serum albumin, leads firstly to a local antibody response but ultimately to a humoral response identical to that following parenteral administration of that substance[116,117]. However, a particulate antigen (sheep red-blood cells) behaved differently: oral administration to germ-free mice led to an increase in plaque-forming cells in the spleen, but this was followed by a refractory period when no response occurred, and when responsiveness returned it was in the form of a new primary response[118]. Several other reports have confirmed the lack of a secondary response to oral challenge after oral priming (see Porter[119] and McNeish[120]). It is, therefore, perhaps to be expected that the continuous presence of a small mass of a particulate antigen in the gut would not give rise to circulating antibody. In part at least, this may be due to locally produced IgA, which has now been clearly shown to inhibit the uptake of antigens from the gut[121,122]; it is interesting that one report[123] has described the detection of coproantibodies in 82% of a group of patients with amoebiasis, although it is not clear whether they were asymptomatic or not. In addition, Beinenstock[124] and Clancy and Beinenstock[125] have drawn attention to the importance of the path taken by an antigen after it has been absorbed from the gut; antigens which pass through the liver are particularly likely to elicit tolerance rather than immunity[126,127].

In a small proportion of cases, and after a variable period of time, *E. histolytica* may change from a commensal to a frankly parasitic way of life. Invasion of the mucosa leads to the formation of ulcers, with the associated clinical symptoms of colitis and dysentery. Further spread may also occur, usually to the liver but in rare cases to lung, brain and other organs. Liver abscess may occur in patients who have never had any intestinal symptoms.

The factors which cause this sudden change in the behaviour of the organism are many and complex but undoubtedly involve alteration in both the host and the parasite; the subject has been frequently reviewed (Balmuth and Siddiqui[128], Neal[129], Bos[130], Ackers[131]). There seems to be no doubt that strains of *E. histolytica* of different virulence occur and that this virulence is not immutable. The differences in this respect are most clearly shown in experimental animals but are also visible in such properties as agglutinability by concanavalin-A or surface-charge where host-response factors do not apply[132,133]. On the other hand, it is also clear that factors influencing the host, such as malnutrition and damage to the caecum or liver, may also promote invasion. There is some evidence which suggests that an impairment of the host's immune capabilities may also be important: in man, exacerbation of symptoms or an increased incidence of invasive disease has been associated with the administration of corticosteroids and immunosuppressive agents or with pregnancy[134,135]. In animals, species of amoeba normally unable to invade the tissues may do so in the presence of various agents causing immunodepression ([136,137] and Wijesundera and Targett, personal communication), and a similar phenomenon may occur in man on long-term immunosuppressive therapy[221].

Most cases of invasive amoebiasis, however, are in persons with no apparent general immunodeficiency, and invasion is promptly followed by the appearance of high levels of circulating anti-amoebic antibodies. These antibodies, detectable by a wide variety of standard procedures, provide the basis for the numerous serodiagnostic tests available, but it is clear that they are quite incapable of eliminating the invaders. *In vitro*, such antibodies have been shown to have profound effects on cultured trophozoites: immobilization[138], inhibition of phagocytosis[139] and complement-dependent killing[140] have all been reported. However, the immobilization reaction is only temporary[141]. Even more importantly, when trophozoites from dystenteric faeces are incubated with immune serum, enhancement of mobility and erythrophagocytic activity were observed[142]. Not only are these antibodies non-protective, but it is also clear, both from clinical experience and from a study of age-specific incidence-rates[143], that there is essentially no protection against repeated infections.

Delayed-type hypersensitivity reactions following skin testing have been reported in patients with invasive amoebiasis, although not in all cases[144-146]. However, one of the most notable histological features of both amoebic ulcers and amoebic liver abscesses is the marked absence of cellular infiltration around the lesion[147], and recently Ortiz-Ortiz *et al.*[148] reported depression of cell-mediated responsiveness (judged by delayed hypersensitivity and MIF production) in patients with acute amoebic liver abscesses. Responsiveness had returned when the patients were re-tested 10 days after being cured. Similar results have been reported by Landa and co-workers[149] and in experimentally infected animals[222]; in contrast Bray and Harris[115] found that lymphocyte transformation in the presence of amoebic antigen disappeared after successful treatment; however, the same authors drew attention to the enhanced lymphocyte-transformation seen in cells taken from the very small number of persons who were not infected in the presence of continuous challenge. Taken together, the results presented here are consistent with the idea that, although only certain strains of *E. histolytica* possess the ability to become invasive, those that do are restricted by host defences, among which cell-mediated immunity may be the most important[115,116].

3.4.2 *Giardia intestinalis*

Giardia are unusual among protozoa in being bilaterally symmetrical and having a large concave depression (the ventral disc) on their ventral surface. The disc apparently enables the parasite to attach itself to the duodenal and jejunal mucosa and is probably essential for survival there, as *Giardia intestinalis* is the only protozoan parasite living in the lumen of the human small intestine. As is so often the case, there is no general agreement on the taxonomy of this genus and between 3 and 40 species having been described by different authors. The human parasite will be designated *G. intestinalis* (the same organism is also called *G. lamblia* and, particularly in Eastern Europe, *Lamblia intestinalis*) and the closely related mouse parasite, *G. muris*.

Infection with *G. intestinalis* is common in warm climates, where 8–10% of an unselected population may be passing cysts. In temperate climates it has been regarded as rare, but the incidence of reported cases seems to be rising, and in 1974 *G. intestinalis* was the commonest *proved* cause of water-borne disease in the United States of America.[150]. The parasite is equally common in Britain[151].

Both clinical experience and experimental infection of volunteers[152] show that a large proportion of infections with *G. intestinalis* are asymptomatic. In other cases, however, illness may be severe, but severity is not related to the number of parasites present, and host idiosyncrasies may be important. Untreated, the acute infection may persist for weeks or months, and in a chronic form for much longer, so that efficient self-cure clearly does not happen in every case. Nevertheless, there is considerable evidence for some degree of immune response to this parasite. Most, but not all published reports describing jejunal biopsies from infected patients mention focal inflammation of the epithelium of the crypts and of the underlying lamina propria. Usually the invading cells are polymorphonuclear leukocytes, but eosinophils and occasionally lymphocytes and plasma cells may be present[153–155]. However, in other cases no inflammatory reaction could be seen[156–158]. It may be significant that the first two papers also report penetration of the *Giardia* beneath the epithelium; the majority of studies, however, show the parasite either attached to the mucosal surface or lying free in the lumen of the gut[155,159,160,161].

Circulating anti-*Giardia* antibodies have recently been found in the sera of some patients[162]. The antibodies were detected by immunofluorescence, and, perhaps surprisingly, mature cysts proved the best antigen. Positive results were obtained in 32/36 cases with malabsorption, but not from controls or from two cases of giardiasis without malabsorption. It may be true (by analogy with amoebiasis) that only cases where penetration of the epithelium has occurred would show raised serum antibody; on the other hand, damage to the epithelium, by allowing entry of parasite antigens into the body, may be the determining factor.

The role, if any, of these antibodies in host protection is not known. However, there is quite definite evidence for the importance of immune responses in preventing colonization by the parasite in the very high incidence of giardiasis among patients with various immunodeficiency syndromes[163–166], principally agammaglobulinaemia. Since most of these patients had normal or near normal cell-mediated responses, a role for antibody and particularly for locally produced antibody in host defence seems quite plausible. Indeed, Zinneman and Kaplan[167] have shown that amounts of secretory IgA in jejunal aspirates from 10 patients cured of chronic giardiasis were significantly depressed although serum IgA levels were normal; it has even been suggested that the parasite is able to suppress local synthesis of IgA[168]. It is not known how many people are repeatedly infected with *G. intestinalis*, but work with *G. muris* in the mouse has shown some acquired resistance to reinfection[169,170].

Immunological mechanisms have also been invoked to explain the mucosal damage (villous atrophy and shortening of the crypts) seen in many but not all cases of giardiasis. Similar changes have been observed in patients infected with *Strongyloides stercoralis*[171], with intestinal coccidia[172–174], with bacterial overgrowth of the normally sterile small intestine[175] and with allergies to various food antigens such as gluten (coeliac disease). Ferguson[176,177] has suggested a common mechanism whereby damage to the mucosa is a side-effect of a cell-mediated response to an antigen present in the gut: immunological deficiency, particularly in the IgA response, not only makes colonization of the gut easier but also removes the barrier that is usually capable of preventing unavoidable antigen (such as food) from eliciting this damaging response.

3.4.3 *Trichomonas vaginalis*

Trichomonas vaginalis is a frequent cause of genito-urinary-tract infections in women. Most cases are believed to be sexually transmitted, but in men the infection is not only difficult to detect but almost always asymptomatic. It is clear from clinical observation that any immune response elicited by the parasite is incapable of preventing reinfection or of reliably eliminating the parasite. Although, untreated, some women show spontaneous cure, in the majority a chronic, asymptomatic infection with periodic recrudescences occurs.

In all but the rarest cases, *T. vaginalis* is confined to the urogenital tract and causes a disease which, though exceedingly unpleasant, is not dangerous. The corresponding parasite of cattle, *Tritrichomonas foetus*, is undoubtedly more pathogenic and frequently causes abortion; following self-cure, however, the cow shows a high degree of resistance to reinfection[178], and the two infections are not, perhaps, as similar as they might seem.

Several other organisms and materials share with *T. vaginalis* the property of being confined to the urogenital system, and the immunological response to such antigens is of considerable interest. The urogenital system possesses all the attributes necessary for a local immune response[179], and evidence for such a response to *Trichomonas* is available. Microscopically, signs of an inflammatory response are frequently visible, with infiltration by lymphocytes, plasma cells and neutrophils[180]. More specifically, Chipperfield and Evans[181] showed a marked rise in the number of immunoglobulin-bearing plasma-cells in cervical biopsies of women who had been exposed to, or infected by, various sexually transmitted organisms. In all cases there was, predominantly, an increase in IgA-bearing cells; in addition, in trichomoniasis a significant increase in IgM-bearing cells also occurred.

The results of this activity are, however, harder to detect. As far as serum–antibody responses are concerned, published reports are confusing; the whole subject has been extensively reviewed by Honigberg[182]. Two problems make interpretation of the results difficult: the existence of serotypes amongst the organism, and the existence of 'natural' antibodies against T. vaginalis in the serum of animals that apparently have had no contact with the organism.

The Estonian group of Teras and his colleagues have repeatedly emphasized the importance of employing several antigenic serotypes in all attempts at serodiagnosis, and this, in part, undoubtedly accounts for the success they have had with their methods[183, 184] (for an extensive discussion and translation of much of this otherwise inaccessible work, see reference 182). As far as natural antibodies are concerned, both agglutinins and (apparently complement-dependent) lysins have been reported from the sera of many animals; the fact that they are trichomonad species – or sub-species – specific has strengthened the opinion that they are genuine antibodies[185]. At least in the case of bovine antibodies against Tri. foetus, activity is absent at birth but rises soon afterwards to adult levels, even in the absence of contact with the organism[186]. At present, contact with a normal (food?) antigen which induces cross-reacting antibodies appears to be the most likely source of these natural antibodies, but the situation is far from clear. Although there seems to be no doubt that a specific serum–antibody response does follow infection with T. vaginalis, titres are seldom more than two or four times that of the natural level and many false positive and negative results occur[182, 187–189] (and Ackers, unpublished).

An organism as localized as T. vaginalis might be expected to produce an equally localized response, and indeed such responses have been reported with Campylobacter (Vibrio) foetus in cattle[190] and uncomplicated gonorrhoea in women[191]. Not unexpectedly, there was evidence of modest amounts of specific anti-trichomonal IgA in the cervicovaginal secretion of about three-quarters of a sample of infected women, although 40% of a small group of contacts were also positive[192]. No significant amounts of antibody were detectable in semen or urine samples from male contacts of infected women[193]. The protective value of this antibody is not clear: in a small number of experiments, no effect has been demonstrated of cervicovaginal secretion (already assayed and shown to contain anti-trichomonal antibody) on the motility or viability of cultured organisms (Ackers, unpublished).

Neither local nor systemic cell-mediated immunity in trichomoniasis appears to have been properly looked for. Results of skin testing in both men and women have been published[194]: it is not clear whether immediate or delayed reactions were being sought, but reasonably promising results were obtained. The possibility of local production of IgE cannot be excluded for Kerr and Robertson[186] were able to sensitize the uterus of a cow with extracts of *Tri. foetus*, but there have apparently been no attempts to find specific IgE in human trichomoniasis.

3.4.4 Conclusions

The three parasites considered in this section occupy sites where they are less exposed to the host's immune responses than the organisms considered before. By the same token they are presumably less 'visible' to the host's immune system than blood parasites, and so, as would be expected, host-responses in general are less vigorous than those elicited by parasites in more intimate contact. A general lessening of the importance of immunological effects amongst the various factors which control the host–parasite balance might therefore be expected, and this is probably the case. Nevertheless, there is evidence, although not conclusive, that a weakening of the host's cell-mediated responses might be one factor which leads to invasive amoebiasis; it is also clear that an inability to mount an effective local antibody response in the gut aids colonization by *G. intestinalis*. In the case of *Trichomonas* there is no evidence that immunological factors are as important in determining if colonization occurs as environmental factors such as pH or the presence of oestrogenized epithelium. The fact that almost all sera contain 'natural' antibodies capable of killing *T. vaginalis* may be important in confining the organism to the urogenital system; if so, these antibodies would not be unimportant, for, if injected intraperitoneally into mice (which usually have very little, if any, natural antibody), *T. vaginalis* is more destructive and rapidly fatal than *E. histolytica*.

3.5 MISCELLANEOUS EFFECTS

No review of the immunology of protozoal infection would be complete without at least a brief mention of the effects of these infections on the host's response to other antigens and other, probably related phenomena such as the synthesis of large amounts of non-parasite-specific immunoglobulin and the production of auto-antibodies. Part or all of this triad is present in the majority of parasitic infections. All three are shown clearly in African trypanosomiasis in both man and experimental animals. Reduced immune responses to sheep red-blood cells[195–197] and nematode infections[198] in mice, and to typhoid vaccine in man[199] have been demonstrated. Responses to PPD and *Candida* were diminished and secondary bacterial infection occurred. In addition, such patients have high circulating levels of immunoglobulin (principally IgM) and high heterophile and auto-antibody titres[200].

The same three features are also present in experimental and clinical *Plasmodium* infections, except that in this case levels of both IgG and IgM are elevated[199,201,202]. Infection of mice with the related parasite *Babesia microti* also leads to a fall in the plaque-forming cell-response to sheep red-blood cells, although contact sensitization by oxazolone is unimpaired[203]. Similarly, both hamsters infected with *L. donovani*[204] and mice infected with *L. tropica*[205] show a reduced response to heterologous antigens, although the failure to respond to *L. tropica* in diffuse cutaneous leishmaniasis is confined to that organism. In patients with visceral leishmaniasis very high levels of serum immunoglobulin occur: the product is chiefly IgG and is mainly non-specific; auto-antibodies also occur[64].

In other infections the picture is not so complete. For example, in cases of Chagas' disease there may be a moderate rise in the levels of serum immunoglobulin[206], and some immunodepression has been reported in experimentally infected mice[207]. Auto-antibodies directed against heart muscle have been reported[45,208] as well as cell-mediated responses[209], but these may well be specific but cross-reacting antibodies rather than by-products of uncontrolled immunoglobulin synthesis.

Depression of the immune response to heterologous antigens has also been reported in mice infected with *T. gondii*[210] and, intraperitoneally, with *T. vaginalis*[223] (and Ackers, unpublished), while anti-colon antibodies are present in some cases of invasive amoebiasis[211].

It must be emphasized that, as discussed elsewhere in this book, immuno-depression, auto-antibodies and elevated serum globulins are not confined to parasitic infections but are found in a wide variety of viral and bacterial diseases. These phenomena have excited considerable interest, and much experimental work and theoretical speculation have been devoted to the subject, particularly in the cases of malaria and African trypanosomiasis. Discussions and further references are given in most of the papers already mentioned, as well as in Ogilvie and Wilson[212]. Three main, and several other explanations have been advanced for these phenomena, it being generally assumed that they are causally related. Since experimental evidence does not clearly favour any one explanation, all three will be presented without further comment.

Poor immune responses during infections with *T. brucei* have been ascribed to disruption of the architecture of the lymphoid organs[197], possibly brought about by release of free fatty-acids from autolysing trypano-somes[213]. Somewhat similar are those theories which suggest a defect in macrophage processing of antigens; some evidence for this in malaria-infected mice has been presented[214,215].

The second group of explanations postulates a continuous stimulation of B cells, so that, on the one hand, large amounts of non-specific immuno-globulin (inevitably including anto-antibodies) are produced and, on the other, the exhaustion of B-cell clones inhibits a specific immune response. Evidence for a B-cell mitogen has been produced in infections with *T. brucei*[200,213,216,217] and with *Babesia microti*[203].

Finally, there is now considerable evidence for the formation of suppressor T cells during murine infections with *T. brucei*[217,219,220], although not in malaria[214]. Other postulated mechanisms include failure of T-cell function[33] and the immunosuppressive effect of continuous complement activation[213]. It may well be that all these mechanisms, and others play a part in bringing about the observed effects, but, however they are brought about, this triad of changes probably contributes greatly to the damage caused by parasitic infections.

3.6   GENERAL CONCLUSIONS

From what has been said it should be clear that there is nothing unique about host immune responses to protozoa. For example, there seems to be no basis for the view, held by some, that protozoa are poor antigens, for most infections elicit fairly high antibody titres at one stage or another. Similarly, most of the immunological processes described here have parallels in bacterial, viral and mycotic infections. Classification by site is perhaps helpful in bringing this out: thus there are many similarities between the immunology of trichomoniasis and gonorrhoea, leishmaniasis and leprosy, Chagas' disease and syphilis. Depression of immune response to heterologous antigens and non-specific hypergammaglobulinaemia are also found in conditions other than parasitic infections.

One feature which seems to be characteristic of protozoal diseases is that they are usually prolonged infections. Presumably an acute illness lasting a week or two would not give sufficient time for onward transmission of the parasite. Even in acute African trypanosomiasis (caused by *T. b. rhodesiense*) the untreated patient lives for many weeks; more significantly, however, in this case, man-to-man transmission may be unimportant in the parasite's life-cycle, which may well normally involve game animals. Other human protozoal infections tend to be chronic and may persist for years.

In view of these long-lasting infections, it is natural to wonder how the parasite is able to survive in the presence of the host's defence mechanisms, and this is a problem which has led to a large amount of published work. It is clear that different parasites make use of different mechanisms.

In one group are the blood-stream parasites (African trypanosomes and *Plasmodium*) in which antibody is important in host defence: in these antigenic variation seems to be the principal parasite response to ensure survival. At the other extreme are the luminal parasites (non-invasive *Amoeba*, *Giardia* and *Trichomonas*) where restricted contact between parasite-antigen and the host immune system leads to a response inadequate to eliminate the parasite; the same appears to be true of human infection with *Sarcocystis*. Immunity may not be sterilizing, but it is probably not unimportant in these cases, as the very high incidence of giardiasis in immunodeficient patients shows.

The remaining three parasites (*Trypanosoma cruzi, Leishmania* and *Toxo-plasma*) present a more complex picture. All normally elicit both humoral and cell-mediated responses, the importance of which is not known, but if there is one common factor which enables them to persist it is the ability to grow, rather than to be destroyed, within the host macrophage, although both *T. cruzi* and *T. gondii* successfully parasitize many other types of cell as well.

It has long been felt that the immunodepression which accompanies many parasitic infections might be very important in aiding parasite survival; even more interesting than generalized immunodepression is the apparent ability of some parasites (such as *L. tropica* and *E. histolytica*) specifically to suppress cell-mediated responses against themselves. This phenomenon could clearly be of widespread significance. Indeed, we are perhaps wrong to be too surprised by the long-term survival of protozoa in an immunized host for not only chronic bacterial and viral infections but also the survival of the mammalian fetus, the presence of a normal bacterial flora on many mucous surfaces and the existence of clinically well subjects with circulating auto-antibodies all demonstrate that an immune response which leads to the total elimination of an antigen may be the exception rather than the rule.

We are just beginning to realize the complexity of the immune system and the number of alternative pathways by which a given change may be effected. At the same time, it is becoming clear that the pathological side-effects of an immune response may be very grave, and the network of controls needed to regulate this vital but dangerous system are being unravelled. At some future time it may be possible to explain why a particular infection invokes the response it does, but this will surely take a considerable time. Such knowledge ought to make possible the rational design of anti-protozoal vaccines, if, indeed, such things are possible. In practice, however, the need for them is so urgent and the fundamental problem so daunting that it may be preferable to try to develop these immunoprophylactic agents by trial-and-error methods first.

ACKNOWLEDGEMENTS

Part of the work described here was supported by a Project Grant from the Medical Research Council. I am grateful to Dr G. A. T. Targett, Miss Fiona Weir and Dr Norma Powell for their assistance in preparing the manuscript.

References

1. Vickerman, K. (1971). Morphological and physiological considerations of extracellular blood protozoa. In: *Ecology and Physiology of Parasites: a Symposium* (A. M. Fallis, ed.), p. 58 (Toronto: University Press)
2. Vickerman, K. (1974). Antigenic variation in African Trypanosomes. In: *Parasites in the*

Immunized Host: mechanisms of survival (R. Porter and J. Knight, eds.), p. 53 (Amsterdam: Associated Scientific Publishers)

3. Vickerman, K. (1974). The ultrastructure of pathogenic flagellates. In: *Trypanosomiasis and Leishmaniasis with Special Reference to Chagas' Disease* (K. Elliot, M. O'Conner and G. E. W. Wolstenholme, eds.), p. 171 (Amsterdam: Associated Scientific Publishers)

4. Wright, K. A., Lumsden, W. H. R. and Hales, H. (1970). The formation of filopodium-like processes by *Trypanosoma (Trypanozoon) brucei*. *J. Cell. Sci.*, **6**, 285

5. Ellis, D. S., Ormerod, W. E. and Lumsden, W. H. R. (1976). Filaments of *Trypanosoma brucei*: some notes on differences in original structure in two strains of *Trypanosoma (Trypanozoon) brucei rhodesiense*. *Acta Trop.*, **33**, 151

6. Cross, G. A. M. (1975). Identification, purification and properties of clone-specific glycoprotein antigen constituting the surface coat of *Trypanosoma brucei*. *Parasitology*, **71**, 393

7. Gray, A. R. (1965). Antigenic variation in a strain of *Trypanosoma brucei* transmitted by *Glossina mortitans* and *G. palpalis*. *J. Gen. Microbiol.*, **41**, 195

8. Gray, A. R. and Luckins, A. G. (1976). Antigenic variation in alivarian trypanosomes. In: *Biology of the Kinetoplastida, Vol. 1* (W. H. R. Lumsden and D. A. Evans, eds.), p. 493 (London: Academic Press)

9. Ritz, H. (1916). Über Rezidive bei experimenteller Trypanosomiasis. *Arch. Schiffs Trop. Hyg.*, **20**, 397

10. Apted, F. I. C. (1970). Clinical manifestations and diagnosis of sleeping sickness. In: *The African Trypanosomiases* (H. W. Mulligan, ed.), p. 661 (London: Allen and Unwin)

11. Ormerod, W. E. (1970). Pathogenesis and pathology of trypanosomiasis in man. In: *The African Trypanosomiases* (H. W. Mulligan, ed.), p. 587 (London: Allen and Unwin)

12. Hutt, M. S. R. and Wilks, N. E. (1971). African trypanosomiasis. In: *Pathology of Protozoal and Helminthic diseases* (R. A. Marcia-Rojas, ed.), p. 57 (Baltimore: Williams and Wilkins)

13. Kagan, I. G. (1974). Advances in the immunodiagnosis of parastic infection. *Z. Parasitenkde*, **45**, 163

14. Lumsden, W. H. R. (1978). Demonstration of antibodies to Protozoa. In: *Handbook of Experimental Immunology* (D. M. Weir, ed.), third edition (Oxford: Blackwell)

15. Targett, G. A. T. and Viens, P. (1978). Immunity to *Trypanosoma (Herpetosoma)* in rodents. In: *Biology of the Kinetoplastida, Vol. II* (W. H. R. Lumsden and D. A. Evans, eds.) (London: Academic Press) (In press)

16. D'Alesando, P. A. (1975). Ablastin, the phenomenen. *Exp. Parasitol.*, **38**, 303

17. Terry, R. J. (1976). Immunity to Africa trypanosomiasis. In: *Immunology of Parasitic Infections* (S. Cohen and E. H. Sadun, eds.), p. 203 (Oxford: Blackwell)

18. Targett, G. A. T. (1970). Antibody response to *Plasmodium falciparum* malaria: comparison of antibody titres and the antigenicity of different asexual forms of the parasite. *Clin. Exp. Immunol.*, **7**, 501

19. Voller, A., Huldt, G., Thors, C. and Engvall, E. (1975). New serological test for malaria antibodies. *Br. Med. J.*, **1**, 659

20. Voller, A., Bidwell, D. E., Bartlett, A. and Edwards, R. (1977). A comparison of isotopic and enzyme-immunoassays for tropical parasitic diseases. *Trans. R. Soc. Trop. Med. Hyg.*, **71**, 431

21. Cohen, S. and McGregor, I. A. (1963). Gammaglobulin and acquired immunity to malaria. In: *Immunity to Protozoa* (P. C. C. Garnham, A. E. Pierce and I. Roitt, eds.), p. 123 (Oxford: Blackwell)

22. Diggs, G. L. and Osler, A. G. (1975). Humoral immunity in rodent malaria. III. Studies on the site of antibody action. *J. Immunol.*, **144**, 1243

23. Cohen, S. and Butcher, G. A. (1971). Serum antibody in acquired malarial immunity. *Trans. R. Soc. Trop. Med. Hyg.*, **65**, 125

24. Miller, L. H., Aikawa, M. and Dvorak, J. A. (1975). Malaria (*Plasmodium knowlesi*) merozoites: immunity and the surface coat. *J. Immunol.*, **144**, 1237

25. Brown, K. N. and Hills, L. A. (1974). Antigenic variation and immunity to *Plasmodium knowlesi*: antibodies which induce antigenic variation and antibodies which destroy parasites. *Trans. R. Soc. Trop. Med. Hyg.*, **68**, 139

26. Targett, G. A. T. (1968). Immunological aspects of malaria infection. In: *Immunology of Human Infections, Vol. II* (A. J. Nahmias and R. O'Reilly, eds.) (New York: Plenum Press) (In press)

27. Brown, K. N. (1974). Antigenic variation and immunity to malaria. In: *Parasites in the Immunized Host: mechanisms of survival* (R. Porter and J. Knight, eds.), p. 35 (Amsterdam: Associated Scientific Publishers)

28. Brown, K. N. (1976). Resistance to malaria. In: *Immunology of Parasitic Infections* (S. Cohen and E. H. Sadun, eds.), p. 268 (Oxford: Blackwell)

29. Phillips, R. S., Trigg, P. I., Scott-Finnigan, T. J. and Bartholomew, R. K. (1972). Culture of *Plasmodium falciparum in vitro*: a subculture technique used for demonstrating antiplasmodial activity in serum from some Gambians, resident in an endemic malarious area. *Parasitology*, **65**, 525

30. Mitchell, G. H., Butcher, G. A., Voller, A. and Cohen, S. (1976). The effect of human IgG on the *in vitro* development of *Plasmodium falciparum*. *Parasitology*, **72**, 149

31. Targett, G. A. T. (1973). Thymus dependency and chronic antigenic stimulation: immunity to parasitic protozoans and helminths. In: *Contemporary Topics in Immunobiology, Vol. II* (A. J. S. Davies and R. L. Carter, eds.), p. 217 (New York: Plenum Press)

32. Clark, I. A. and Allison, A. C. (1974). *Babesia microti* and *Plasmodium berghei yoelii* infections in nude mice. *Nature (Lond.)*, **252**, 328

33. Jaywardena, A. N., Targett, G. A. T., Leuchars, E., Carter, R. L., Davies, A. J. S. and Doenhoff, M. J. (1975). T-cell activation in murine malaria. *Nature (Lond.)*, **258**, 149

34. Wyler, D. J. and Oppenheim, J. J. (1974). Lymphocyte transformation in human *Plasmodium falciparum* malaria. *J. Immunol.*, **113**, 449

35. Coleman, R. M., Bruce, A. and Rencricca, N. J. (1976). Malaria: macrophage migration inhibition factor (MIF). *J. Parasitol.*, **62**, 137

36. Graveley, S. M., Hamburger, J. and Krier, J. P. (1976). T- and B-cell population changes in young and in adult rats infected with *Plasmodium berghei*. *Infect. and Immun.*, **14**, 178

37. Miles, M. A. (1972). *Trypanosoma cruzi*: milk transmission of infection and immunity from mother to young. *Parasitology*, **65**, 1

38. Krettli, A. V. and Brener, Z. (1976). Protective effects of specific antibodies in *Trypanosoma cruzi* infections. *J. Immunol.*, **116**, 755

39. World Health Organization (1974). Immunology of Chagas' disease. *Bull. W.H.O.*, **50**, 459

40. Teixera, A. R. L. and Santos Buch, C. A. (1975). The immunology of experimental Chagas' disease. II. Delayed hypersensitivity to *Trypanosoma cruzi* antigens. *Immunology*, **28**, 401

41. Tschudi, E. I., Anziano, D. F. and Dalmasso, A. P. (1972). Lymphocyte transformation in Chagas' disease. *Infect. and Immun.*, **6**, 905

42. Camus, D., Miles, M. A., Figueredo, J. F. M., Queiroz, L. F. de, Afchain, D. and Draper, C. (1975). *In vitro* delayed hypersensitivity in Chagas' disease (chronic and acute). *Trans. R. Soc. Trop. Med. Hyg.*, **69**, 169

43. Seah, S. (1970). Delayed hypersensitivity in *Trypanosoma cruzi* infection. *Nature (Lond.)*, **225**, 1256

44. Schumis, G. A., Vattuone, H., Szarfman, A. and Pesce, V. J. (1973). Cell-mediated immunity in mice inoculated with epimastigotes or trypomastigotes of *Trypanosoma cruzi*. *Z. Tropenmed. Parasitol.*, **24**, 81

45. Teixera, A. R. L. (1975). Autoimmune mechanisms in Chagas' disease. *New Approaches in American Trypanosomiasis*, p. 98 (Washington: Pan American Health Organization)

46. Roberson, E. L. and Hanson, W. L. (1974). Transfer of immunity to *T. cruzi. Trans. R. Soc. Trop. Med. Hyg.*, **68**, 388

47. Kuhn, R. and Durum, S. K. (1973). The onset of immune protection in acute experimental Chagas' disease in C3H (HE) mice. *Int. J. Parasitol.*, **5**, 241

48. Behbehani, K. (1973). Development cycles of *Trypanosoma (Schizotrypanum) cruzi* (Chagas 1909) in mouse peritoneal macrophages in experimental acute chagasic myocarditis. *J. Reticulo. Soc.*, **11**, 604

50. Hoff, R. (1975). Recent advances in cell-mediated immunity. *New Approaches in American Trypanosomiasis*, p. 162 (Washington: Pan American Health Organization)

51. Hoff, R. (1975). Killing *in vitro* of *Trypanosoma cruzi* by macrophages from mice immunized with *T. cruzi* or BCG, and absence of cross-immunity on challenge *in vivo*. *J. Exp. Med.*, **142**, 299

52. Williams, D. M. and Remington, J. S. (1977). Effect of human monocytes and macrophages on *Trypanosoma cruzi. Immunology*, **32**, 19

53. Clark, I. A., Allison, A. C. and Cox, F. E. G. (1976). Protection of mice against *Babesia* and *Plasmodium* with BCG. *Nature (Lond.)*, **259**, 309

54. Clark, I. A., Cox, F. E. G. and Allison, A. C. (1977). Protection of mice against *Babesia* spp. and *Plasmodium* spp. with killed *Corynebacterium parvum. Parasitology*, **74**, 9

55. Clark, I. A., Richmond, J. E., Wills, E. J. and Allison, A. C. (1977). Intraerythrocytic death of the parasite in mice recovering from infection with *Babesia microti. Parasitology*, **75**, 189

56. Kress, Y., Bloom, B. R., Wittner, M., Rowen, A. and Tanowitz, H. (1975). Resistance of *Trypanosoma cruzi* to killing by macrophages. *Nature (Lond.)*, **257**, 394

57. Kierszenbaum, F., Ivanyi, J. and Budzk, D. B. (1976). Mechanisms of natural resistance to trypanosomal infection: role of complement in avian resistance to *T. cruzi* infections. *Immunology*, **30**, 1

58. Kierszenbaum, F. and Wienman, D. (1977). Antibody-independent activation of the alternative complement pathway in serum by parasite cells. *Immunology*, **32**, 245

59. Al-Taqui, M. and Evans, D. A. (1978). Characterization of *Leishmania* spp. from Kuwait by isoenzyme electrophoresis. *Trans. R. Soc. Trop. Med. Hyg.*, **72**, 56

60. Lumsden, W. H. R. (1974). Leishmaniasis and trypanosomiasis: the causative organisms compared and contrasted. In: *Trypanosomiasis and Leishmaniasis with Special Reference to Chagas' Disease* (K. Elliot, M. O'Conner and G. E. W. Wolstenholme, eds.), p. 3 (Amsterdam: Associated Scientific Publishers)

61. Lainson, R. and Shaw, J. J. (1978). The role of animals in the epidemiology of South American leishmaniasis. In: *Biology of the Kinetoplastida*, Vol. II (W. H. R. Lumsden and D. A. Evans, eds.) (London: Academic Press) (In press)

62. Turk, J. L. and Bryceson, A. D. M. (1971). Immunological phenomena in leprosy and related diseases. *Adv. Immunol.*, **13**, 209

63. Turk, J. L. and Belehu, A. (1974). Immunological spectra in infectious diseases. In: *Parasites in the Immunized Host: mechanisms of survival* (R. Porter and K. Knight, eds.), p. 101 (Amsterdam: Associated Scientific Publishers)

64. Zuckerman, A. (1975). Current status of the immunology of blood and tissue protozoa. I. *Leishmania. Exp. Parasitol.*, **38**, 370

65. Bray, R. S. and Lainson, R. (1967). Studies on the immunology and serology of leishmaniasis. V. The use of particles as vehicles in passive agglutination tests. *Trans. R. Soc. Trop. Med. Hyg.*, **61**, 490

56. Manson-Bahr, P. E. C. (1971). Leishmaniasis. *Int. Rev. Trop. Med.*, **4**, 123

57. Dostrovsky, A., Sagher, F. and Zuckerman, A. (1952). Isophasic reaction following experimental superinfection of *Leishmania tropica. Arch. Dermatol. Syph.*, **66**, 665

68. Bray, R. S. and Bryceson, A. D. M. (1968). Cutaneous leishmaniasis of the guinea-pig. Action of sensitized lymphocytes on infected macrophages. *Lancet*, **ii**, 898

69. Mauel, J., Behin, R., Biroum-Noerjasin and Doyle, J. J. (1974). Survival and death of *Leishmania* in macrophages. In: *Parasites in the Immunized Host: mechanisms of survival* (R. Porter and K. Knight, eds.), p. 385 (Amsterdam: Associated Scientific Publishers)

70. Bryceson, A. D. M., Bray, R. S., Wolstencroft, R. A. and Dumonde, D. C. (1970). Immunity in cutaneous leishmaniasis in the guinea-pig. *Clin. Exp. Immunol.*, **7**, 301

71. Blewett, T. M., Kadivar, D. M. H. and Soulsby, E. J. L. (1971). Cutaneous leishmaniasis in the guinea-pig: delayed-type hypersensitivity, lymphocyte stimulation and inhibition of macrophage migration. *Am. J. Trop. Med. Hyg.*, **20**, 546

72. Belehu, A. and Turk, J. L. (1976). Establishment of cutaneous *Leishmania enriettii* infection in hamsters. *Infect. and Immun.*, **13**, 1235

73. Rezai, H. R., Gettner, S. and Behforouz, N. (1972). Anti-leishmanial activity of immune guinea-pig serum. *J. Med. Microbiol.*, **5**, 371

74. WHO/Leish/68.7. WHO inter-regional travelling seminar on leishmaniasis. WHO/Leish/68.7, p. 1

75. Mauel, J. (1973). Mechanisms of destruction of *Leishmania* in host animals. Seminar on Leishmaniasis, King's College, Cambridge. Mimeographed Report, p. 1

76. Dumonde, D. C. (1973). Significance of *in vitro* studies of immunity in leishmaniasis. Seminar on leishmaniasis, King's College, Cambridge. Mimeographed Report, p. 1

77. Farah, F. S., Samra, S. A. and Nuwayri-Salti, N. (1975). The role of the macrophage in cutaneous leishmaniasis. *Immunology*, **29**, 755

78. Preston, P. M. and Dumonde, D. C. (1976). Experimental cutaneous leishmaniasis. V. Protective immunity in subclinical and self-healing infection in the mouse. *Clin. Exp. Immunol.*, **23**, 126

79. Bryceson, A. D. M. (1969). Diffuse cutaneous leishmaniasis in Ethiopia. I. The clinical and histological features of the disease. *Trans. R. Soc. Trop. Med. Hyg.*, **63**, 708

80. Bryceson, A. D. M. (1970). Diffuse cutaneous leishmaniasis in Ethiopia. IV. Pathogenesis of DCL. *Trans. R. Soc. Med. Hyg.*, **64**, 387

81. Kadiver, D. M. H. and Soulsby, E. J. L. (1975). Model for disseminated cutaneous leishmaniasis. *Science*, **190**, 1198

82. Walton, B. C., Brooks, W. H. and Arjona, I. (1972). Serodiagnosis of American leishmaniasis by indirect fluorescent antibody test. *Am. J. Trop. Med. Hyg.*, **21**, 296

83. Majumder, T. D. (1968). Post kala-azar dermal leishmaniasis. *Dermatol. Int.*, **6**, 174

84. Bray, R. S., Ashford, R. W., Mukherjee, A. M. and Sen Gupta, P. C. (1973). Studies on the immunology and serology of leishmaniasis. IX. Serological investigations of the parasites of Indian kala-azar and Indian post-kala-azar dermal leishmaniasis. *Trans. R. Soc. Trop. Med. Hyg.*, **67**, 125

85. Hoogstraal, H. and Heyneman, D. (1969). Leishmaniasis in the Sudan Republic. III. Leishmania species in the Patoich-Matakal area. *Am. J. Trop. Med. Hyg.*, **18**, 1133

86. Hoogstraal, H. and Heyneman, D. (1969). Leishmaniasis in the Sudan Republic. V. Infections in man with Sudanese kala-azar. *Am. J. Trop. Med. Hyg.*, **18**, 1170

87. Chance, M. L. and Peters, W. (1977). The characterization and significance of DNA and enzyme variation in the genus *Leishmania*. In: *Fifth International Congress of Protozoology*, New York. Abs. 419

88. Maekelt, G. A. (1972). Cell-mediated immunity responses in parasitic infections. In: *Immunity to Animal Parasites* (E. J. L. Soulsby, ed.), p. 343 (New York: Adademic Press)

89. Jacobs, L. (1973). New knowledge of toxoplasma and toxoplasmosis. *Adv. Parasitol.*, **11**, 631

90. Tadros, W. and Laarman, J. J. (1976). *Sarcocystis* and related coccidian parasites: a brief general review, together with a discussion on some biological aspects of their life-cycles and a new proposal for their classification. *Acta Leiden.*, **44**, 1

91. Levine, N. D. (1977). Taxonomy of *Toxoplasma*. *J. Protozool.*, **24**, 36

92. Markus, M. B., Killick-Kendrick, R. and Garnham, P. C. C. (1974). The coccidial nature and life-cycle of *Sarcocystis*. *J. Trop. Med. Hyg.*, **77**, 248

93. Jeffrey, H. C. (1974). Sarcosporidiosis in man. *Trans. R. Soc. Trop. Med. Hyg.*, **68**, 17

94. Levine, N. D. (1973). *Protozoan Parasites of Domestic Animals and of Man*, p. 293 (Minneapolis: Burgess Publishing Co.)

95. Levine, N. D. (1973). *Protozoan Parasites of Domestic Animals and of Man*, p. 294 (Minneapolis: Burgess Publishing Co.)

96. Miller, M. J., Aronson, W. J. and Remington, J. S. (1968). Late parasitaemia in asymptomatic acquired toxoplasmosis. *Ann. Intern. Med.*, **71**, 139

97. Jacobs, L. (1967). *Toxoplasma* and toxoplasmosis. *Adv. Parasitol.*, **5**, 1

98. Huldt, G. (1966). Experimental toxoplasmosis. Effect of inoculation of *Toxoplasma* in sero-positive rabbits. *Acta Pathol. Microbiol. Scand.*, **68**, 592

99. Stadtsbaeder, S., Nguyen, B. T. and Calvin-Preval, M. C. (1975). Respective role of antibodies and immune macrophages during acquired immunity against toxoplasmosis in mice. *Ann. Immunol. (Inst. Pasteur)*, **126C**, 461

100. Foster, B. G. and McCullough, W. F. (1968). Studies of active and passive immunity in animals inoculated with *Toxoplasma gondii*. *Can. J. Microbiol.*, **14**, 103

101. Frenkel, J. K. (1967). Adoptive immunity to intracellular infection. *J. Immunol.*, **98**, 1309

102. Krahenbuhl, J. L., Ruskin, J. and Remington, J. S. (1972). The use of killed vaccines in immunization against an intracellular parasite: *Toxoplasma gondii*. *J. Immunol.*, **108**, 425

103. Anderson, S. E. Jr., Bautista, S. C. and Remington, J. S. (1976). Specific antibody-dependent killing of *Toxoplasma gondii* by normal macrophages. *Clin. Expt. Immunol.*, **26**, 375

104. Tremonti, L. and Walton, B. C. (1970). Blast transformation and migration inhibition in toxoplasmosis and leishmaniasis. *Am. J. Trop. Med. Hyg.*, **19**, 49

105. Krahenbuhl, J. L., Gaines, J. D. and Remington, J. S. (1972). Lymphocyte transformation in human toxoplasmosis. *J. Infect. Dis.*, **125**, 283

106. Hirsch, J. G., Jones, T. C. and Len, L. (1974). Interaction *in vitro* between *Toxoplasma gondii* and mouse cells. In: *Parasites in the Immunized Host: mechanisms of survival* (R. Porter and J. Knight, eds.), p. 205 (Amsterdam: Associated Scientific Publishers)

107. Sethi, K. K., Pelster, B., Suzuki, N., Piekarski, G. and Brandis, H. (1975). Immunity to *Toxoplasma gondii* induced *in vitro* in non-immune mouse macrophages with specifically immune lymphocytes. *J. Immunol.*, **115**, 1151

108. Lycke, E., Lund, E., Stannegard, O. and Falsen, E. (1965). The effect of immune serum and activator on the infectivity of *Toxoplasma gondii* for cell culture. *Acta Pathol. Microbiol. Scand.*, **63**, 206

109. Aryeetey, M. E. and Piekarski, G. (1976). Serologische *Sarcocystis*-Studien and Menschen und Ratten. [Serological studies on sarcocystis in man and rats.] *Z. Parasitenkde*, **50**, 109

110. Markus, M. B. (1974). Serology of human sarcosporidosis. *Trans. R. Soc. Trop. Med. Hyg.*, **68**, 415

111. Rose, M. E. (1978). Immune responses of chickens to coccidia and coccidiosis. Proceedings of a *Symposium on Avian Coccidiosis*, Loughborough, 1977 (In press)

112. Neal, R. A. (1966). Experimental studies on *Entamoeba* with reference to speciation. *Adv. Parasitol.*, **4**, 1

113. World Health Organization (1969). Amoebiasis. *Tech. Rep. Ser.* No. 421

114. Robinson, G. L. (1968). The laboratory diagnosis of human parasitic amoeba. *Trans. R. Soc. Trop. Med. Hyg.*, **62**, 285

115. Bray, R. S. and Harris, W. G. (1977). The epidemiology of infection with *Entamoeba histolytica* in the Gambia, West Africa. *Trans. R. Soc. Trop. Med. Hyg.*, **71**, 401

116. Perlman, P. and Broberger, O. (1963). *In vitro* studies of ulcerative colitis. II. Cytotoxic action of white blood cells from patients on human fetal colon cells. *J. Exp. Med.*, **117**, 717

117. Rothberg, R. M., Kraft, S. C. and Michalek, S. M. (1973). Systemic immunity after local antigenic stimulation of the lymphoid tissue of the gastro-intestinal tract. *J. Immunol.*, **111**, 1906

118. André, C., Bazin, H. and Heremans, J. F. (1973). Influence of repeated administration of antigen by oral route on specific antibody-producing cells in the mouse spleen. *Digestion*, **9**, 166

119. Porter, P., Kenworthy, R., Noakes, D. E. and Allen, W. D. (1974). Antibody secretion in the young pig in response to oral immunization with *Escherichia coli*. *Immunology*, **27**, 841

120. McNeish, A. S., Evans, N., Gaze, H. and Rogers, K. B. (1975). The agglutinating antibody response in the duodenum in infants with enteropathogenic *E. coli* gastroenteritis. *Gut*, **16**, 727

121. Stokes, C. R., Soothill, J. F. and Turner, M. W. (1975). Immune exclusion is a function of IgA. *Nature (Lond.)*, **255**, 745

122. Walker, W. A., Isselbacher, K. J. and Bloch, K. J. (1972). Intestinal uptake of macromolecules: effect of oral immunization. *Science*, **177**, 608

123. Mahajan, R. C., Agarwal, S. C., Chuttani, P. N. and Chitkata, N. L. (1972). Coproantibodies in intestinal amoebiasis. *Indian J. Med. Res.*, **60**, 547

124. Beinenstock, J. (1974). The physiology of the local immune response and the gastrointestinal tract. In: *Progress in Immunology*, Vol. II (L. Brent and J. Holborrow, eds.), p. 197 (Amsterdam: North Holland)

125. Clancy, R. L. and Beinenstock, J. (1976). Enteric infection and immunization. In: *Immunological Aspects of the Liver and Gastro-intestinal Tract* (A. Ferguson and R. N. M. MacSween, eds.), p. 121 (Lancaster: MTP Press)

126. Battisto, J. R. and Miller, J. (1962). Immunological unresponsiveness produced in adult guinea-pigs by parenteral introduction of minute quantities of hapten or protein antigen. *Proc. Soc. Exp. Biol. Med.*, **111**, 111

127. Triger, D. R., Cynamon, M. H. and Wright, R. (1973). Studies on hepatic uptake of antigens. I. Comparison of inferior vena cava and portal vein routes of immunization. *Immunology*, **25**, 941

128. Balmuth, W. and Siddiqui, B. (1970). Amoebas and other intestinal protozoa. In: *Immunity to Parasitic Animals*, Vol. II (G. J. Jackson, R. Herman and I. Singer, eds.), p. 439 (New York: Appleton-Century-Crofts)

129. Neal, R. A. (1971). Pathogenesis of amoebiasis. *Gut*, **12**, 483

130. Bos, H. J. (1973). The problem of pathogenicity in parasitic *Entamoeba: in vitro* and *in vivo* experiments with different strains of *Entamoeba histolytica* and an *Entamoeba invadens* strain. Thesis, Leiden University (Leiden, Netherlands)

131. Ackers, J. P. (1978). Amoeba, Giardia and Trichomonas. In: *Immunology of Human Infection*, Vol. II (A. J. Nahmias and R. O'Reilly, eds.) (New York: Plenum Press) (In press)

132. Martinez-Palomo, A., Gonzalez-Robles, A. and de la Torre, M. (1973). Selective agglutination of pathogenic strain of *Entamoeba histolytica* induced by ConA. *Nature, New Biol.*, **245**, 186

133. Trissl, D., Martinez-Palomo, A., Arguello, C., de la Torre, M. and de la Hoz, R. (1977). Surface properties related to concanavalin-A induced agglutination: a comparative study of several *Entamoeba* strains. *J. Exp. Med.*, **145**, 652

134. Lewis, E. A. and Anita, A. V. (1968). Amoebic colitis: review of 295 cases. *Trans. R. Soc. Trop. Med. Hyg.*, **63**, 633

135. Kanani, S. R. and Knight, R. (1969). Relapsing amoebic colitis of 12 years' standing exacerbated by corticosteroids. *Br. Med. J.*, **2**, 613

136. Al-Dabagh, M. A. (1965). The pathogenicity of the small race of *Entamoeba histolytica* to splenectomized rats. *Trans. R. Soc. Trop. Med. Hyg.*, **59**, 545

137. Tanimoto-Weki, M., Calderón, P., de la Hoz, R. and Aguirre-García, A. (1974). Inoculacíon de tropozoítos de *E. histolytica* en hamsters bajo la acción de drogas inmunosupresoras. [Inoculation of *E. histolytica* trophozoites in hamsters on immuno-suppressive therapy.] *Arch. Invest. Med.*, **5** (Suppl. 2), 441

138. Biagi, F. F. and Buentello, L. (1961). Immobilization reaction for the diagnosis of amebiasis. *Exp. Parasitol.*, **11**, 188

139. Shaffer, J. G. and Ansfeld, A. (1956). The effect of rabbit antisera on the ability of *Entamoeba histolytica* to phagocytose red blood cells. *Am. J. Trop. Med. Hyg.*, **5**, 53

140. Chevez, A., Iturve-Allesio, I., Sepulveda, B., Segura, M. and Ortiz-Ortiz, L. (1973). Respuesta morfodinámica de los tropozoítos de *E. histolytica* a la acción del suero humano immune correspondiente. [Morphodynamic response of the trophozoites of *E. histolytica* to the action of human immune serum.] *Arch. Invest. Med.*, **4** (Suppl. 1), 71

141. Biagi, F. F., Beltran, F. H. and Ortega, P. S. (1966). Remobilization of *Entamoeba histolytica* after exposure to immobilizing antibodies. *Exp. Parasitol.*, **18**, 87

142. Pittman, F. E. and Pittman, J. C. (1973). Effects of amebic antiserum and control serum on trophozoites of *E. histolytica* in dysenteric stool. *Arch. Invest. Med.*, **4** (Suppl. 1), 93

143. Knight, R. (1975). Surveys for amoebiasis: interpretation of data and their implications. *Ann. Trop. Med. Parasitol.*, **69**, 35

144. Maddison, S. E., Kagan, I. G. and Elsdon-Dew, R. (1968). Comparison of intradermal and serologic tests for the diagnosis of amebiasis. *Am. J. Trop. Med. Hyg.*, **17**, 540

145. Kretschmer, R. R., Sepúlveda, B., Almazan, A. and Gamboa, F. (1972). Intradermal reactions to an antigen (histolyticin) obtained from axenically cultivated *Entamoeba histolytica*. *Trop. Geogr. Med.*, **24**, 275

146. Kagan, I. G. (1973). The immunology of amebiasis. *Arch. Invest. Med.*, **4** (Suppl. 1), 169

147. Brandt, H. and Perez-Tamayo, R. (1970). Pathology of human amoebiasis. *Hum. Pathol.*, **1**, 351

148. Ortiz-Ortiz, L., Zamacona, G., Sepúlveda, B. and Capín, N. R. (1975). Cell-mediated immunity in patients with amebic abscesses of the liver. *Clin. Immunol. Immunopathol.*, **4**, 127

149. Landa, L., Guerrero, M. and Capin, R. (1975). Studies on cellular immunity in invasive amoebiasis. Resumenes de la *Conferencia Internacional sobre Amibiasis*, Ciudad de Mexico, p. 104

150. Horowitz, M. A., Hughes, J. M. and Craun, G. F. (1976). Outbreaks of waterborne disease in the United States in 1974. *J. Infect. Dis.*, **133**, 588

151. British Medical Journal (1977). Giardiasis. *Br. Med. J.*, **2**, 538

152. Rentdorff, R. C. (1954). The experimental transmission of human protozoan parasites. II. *Giardia lamblia* cysts given in capsules. *Am. J. Hyg.*, **59**, 209

153. Yardley, J. H., Takano, J. and Hendrix, T. R. (1964). Epithelial and other mucosal lesions of the jejunum in giardiasis: jejunal biopsy studies. *Bull. Hopkins Hosp.*, **115**, 389

154. Cain, G. D., Moore, P. and Patterson, M. (1968). Malabsorption associated with *Giardia lamblia* infection. *South. Med. J.*, **61**, 532

155. Barbieri, D., de Brito, T., Hoshino, S., Nascimento, O. B., Campos, J. V., Quartenti, G. and Marcondes, E. (1970). Giardiasis in childhood: absorption tests and biochemistry, histochemistry, light and electron microscopy of jejunal mucosa. *Arch. Dis. Child.*, **45**, 466

156. Brandborg, L. L., Tankersley, C. B., Gottleib, S., Barancik, M. and Sartor, V. E. (1967). Histological demonstration of mucosal invasion by *Giardia lamblia* in man. *Gastroenterology*, **52**, 143

157. Morecki, R. and Parker, J. G. (1967). Ultrastructural studies of the human *Giardia lamblia* and subjacent jejunal mucosa in a subject with steatorrhea. *Gastroenterology*, **52**, 151

158. Tandon, B. N., Puri, B. K., Gandhi, P. C. and Tewari, S. G. (1974). Mucosal surface injury of jejunal mucosa in patients with giardiasis: an electron microscopic study. *Indian J. Med. Res.*, **62**, 1838

159. Takano, J. and Yardley, J. H. (1965). Jejunal lesions in patients with giardiasis and malabsorption: an electron microscopic study. *Bull. Hopkins Hosp.*, **116**, 413
160. Hoskins, L. C., Winawer, S. J., Broitman, S. A., Gottlieb, L. S. and Zamcheck, N. (1967). Clinical giardiasis and intestinal malabsorption. *Gastroenterology*, **53**, 265
161. Brooks, S. E. H., Audretsch, J., Milles, C. G. and Sparke, B. (1970). Electron microscopy of *Giardia lamblia* in human jejunal biopsies. *J. Med. Microbiol.*, **3**, 196
162. Ridley, M. J. and Ridley, D. S. (1976). Serum antibodies and jejunal histology in giardiasis associated with malabsorption. *J. Clin. Pathol.*, **29**, 30
163. Heremans, P. E., Huizenga, K. A., Hoffman, H. N., Brown, A. L. and Markowitz, H. (1966). Dysgammaglobulinaemia associated with nodular lymphoid hyperplasia of the small intestine. *Am. J. Med.*, **40**, 78
164. Ament, M. E. and Rubin, C. E. (1972). Relationship of giardiasis to abnormal intestinal structure and function in gastrointestinal immunodeficiency syndromes. *Gastroenterology*, **62**, 216
165. Ajdukiewicz, A. B., Youngs, G. R. and Bouchier, I. A. D. (1972). Nodular lymphoid hyperplasia with hypogammaglobulinaemia. *Gut*, **13**, 589
166. Ochs, H. D., Ament, M. E. and Davis, S. D. (1975). Structure and function of the gastrointestinal tract in primary immunodeficiency syndromes (IDS) and in granulocyte dysfunction. *Birth Defects*, **11**, 199
167. Zinneman, H. H. and Kaplan, A. P. (1972). The association of giardiasis with reduced intestinal secretory immunoglobulins. *Am. J. Dig. Dis.*, **17**, 793
168. Popovic, O., Paljm, A., Andic, A., Andrejevic, M., Pendic, B., Lovric, L., Jelic, S. Samovic, Z., Masic, R., Trpovic, D., Milutinovic, M. and Vukcevic, V. (1975). Immunologija lamblijaze. *Med. Istraz.*, **8**, 37
169. Roberts-Thomson, I. C., Stevens, D. P., Mahmoud, A. A. F. and Warren, K. S. (1976). Giardiasis in the mouse: an animal model. *Gastroenterology*, **71**, 57
170. Roberts-Thomson, I. C., Stevens, D. P., Mahmoud, A. A. F. and Warren, K. S. (1976). Acquired resistance to infection in an animal model of giardiasis. *J. Immunol.*, **117**, 2036
171. Stemmerman, G. N. (1967). Strongyloidosis in migrants: pathological and clinical consideration. *Gastroenterology*, **53**, 59
172. Brandborg, L. L., Goldberg, S. B. and Breidenbach, W. C. (1970). Human coccidiosis: a possible cause of malabsorption. *N. Engl. J. Med.*, **283**, 1306
173. Brandborg, L. L. (1971). Structure and function of the small intestine in some parasite diseases. *Am. J. Clin. Nutr.*, **24**, 124
174. Trier, J. S., Moxey, P. C., Schimmel, E. H. and Robles, E. (1974). Chronic intestinal coccidiosis in man: intestinal morphology and response to treatment. *Gastroenterology*, **66**, 923
175. Mortimer, D. C., Reed, P. I., Vidini, M. and Finlay, J. M. (1964). The role of the upper gastrointestinal flora in the malabsorption syndrome. *Can. Med. Assoc. J.*, **90**, 559
176. Ferguson, A. (1976). Models of intestinal hypersensitivity. *Clin. in Gastroenterology*, **5**, 271
177. MacDonald, T. T. and Ferguson, A. (1976). Hypersensitivity reactions in the small intestine. II. Effects of allograft rejection on mucosal architecture and lymphoid cell infiltrate. *Gut*, **17**, 81
178. Robertson, M. (1963). Antibody response in cattle to infection with *Trichomonas foetus*. In: *Immunity to Protozoa* (P. C. C. Garnham, A. E. Pierce and I. Roitt, eds.), p. 336 (Oxford: Blackwell)
179. B. Cinidar and A. de Weck, eds. (1976). *Immunological Response of the Female Reproductive Tract*. Based on a World Health Organization Workshop. (Copenhagen: Scriptor)
180. Nielsen, M. H. and Nielsen, R. (1975). Electron microscopy of *Trichomonas vaginalis Donné*: interaction with vaginal epithelium in human trichomoniasis. *Acta Pathol. Microbiol. Scand., Sect. B*, **83**, 305

181. Chipperfield, E. J. and Evans, D. A. (1972). The influence of local infection on immunoglobulin formation in the human endocervix. *Clin. Exp. Immunol.*, **11**, 219

182. Honigberg, B. M. (1972). Trichomonads. In: *Immunity to Parasitic Animals*, Vol. II (J. G. Jackson, R. Herman and I. Singer, eds.), p. 249 (New York: Appleton-Century-Crofts)

183. Teras, J. K. (1966). Differences in the antigenic properties within strains of *Trichomonas vaginalis*. *Wiad. Parazytol.*, **12**, 357

184. Teras, J. K., Jaakmees, H., Nigesen, U., Roigas, E. and Tompel, H. (1966). The dependence of the serologic reactions on the serotypes of *Trichomonas vaginalis*. *Wiad. Parazytol.*, **12**, 364

185. Samuels, R. and Chun-Hoon, H. (1964). Serological investigations of trichomonads. I. Comparisons of 'natural' and immune antibodies. *J. Protozool.*, **11**, 36

186. Kerr, W. R. and Robertson, M. (1953). Active and passive sensitization of the uterus of cow *in vivo* against *Trichomonas foetus* antigen and the evidence for the local production of antibodies in that site. *J. Hyg. Cambridge,* **51**, 405

187. Jaakmees, H., Teras, J., Roigas, E., Nigesen, U. and Tompel, H. (1966). Complement-fixing antibodies in the blood sera of men infected with *Trichomonas vaginalis*. *Wiad. Parazytol.*, **12**, 378

188. McEntegart, M. G. (1952). The application of a haemagglutination technique to the study of *Trichomonas vaginalis* infections. *J. Clin. Pathol.*, **5**, 275

189. Lanceley, F. and McEntegart, M. G. (1953). *Trichomonas vaginalis* in the male: the experimental infection of a few volunteers. *Lancet*, **i**, 668

190. Corbeil, L. B., Schurig, G. D., Duncan, J. R., Corbeil, R. R. and Winter, A. J. (1974). Immunoglobulin classes and biological functions of *Campylobacter (Vibrio) foetus* antibodies in serum and cervicovaginal mucus. *Infect. Immunol.*, **10**, 422

191. O'Reilly, R. J., Lee, L. and Welch, B. G. (1976). Secretory IgA antibody responses to *Neisseria gonorrhoea* in the genital secretions of infected females. *J. Infect. Dis.*, **133**, 113

192. Ackers, J. P., Lumsden, W. H. R., Catterall, R. D. and Coyle, R. (1975). Antitrichomonal antibody in the vaginal secretions of women infected with *T. vaginalis*. *Br. J. Vener. Dis.*, **51**, 319

193. Ackers, J. P., Catterall, R. D., Lumsden, W. H. R. and MacMillan, A. (1978). Absence of detectable local antibody in genito-urinary tract secretions of male contacts of women infected with *Trichomonas vaginalis*. *Br. J. Vener. Dis.*, **54**, 168

194. Jaakmees, H. and Teras, J. (1966). Intradermal reaction with specific antigens in cases of genito-urinary trichomonadosis. *Wiad. Parazytol.*, **13**, 385

195. Goodwin, L. G., Green, D. G., Guy, M. W. and Voller, A. (1972). Immunosuppression during trypanosomiasis. *Br. J. Exp. Pathol.*, **53**, 40

196. Murray, P. K., Jennings, F. W., Murray, M. and Urquhart, G. M. (1974). The nature of immunosuppression in *Trypanosoma brucei* infection in mice. I. The role of the macrophage. *Immunology*, **27**, 815

197. Murray, P. K., Jennings, F. W., Murray, M. and Urquhart, G. M. (1974). The nature of immunosuppression in *Trypanosoma brucei* infection in mice. II. The role of T and B lymphocytes. *Immunology*, **27**, 825

198. Phillips, R. S., Selby, G. R. and Wakelin, D. (1974). The effect of *Plasmodium berghei* and *Trypanosoma brucei* on the immune expulsion of the nematode *Trichuris muris* from mice. *Int. J. Parasitol.*, **4**, 409

199. Greenwood, B. N. (1974). Immunosuppression in malaria and trypanosomiasis. In: *Parasites in the Immunized Host: mechanisms of survival* (R. Porter and J. Knight, eds.), p. 137 (Amsterdam: Associated Scientific Publishers)

200. Greenwood, B. N. (1974). Possible role of B-cell mitogen in hypergammaglobulinaemia in malaria and trypanosomiasis. *Lancet*, **i**, 435

201. Wedderburn, N. (1974). Immunodepression produced by malarial infection in mice. In:

Parasites in the Immunized Host: mechanisms of survival (R. Porter and J. Knight, eds.), p. 123 (Amsterdam: Associated Scientific Publishers)

202. Cohen, S. (1974). The immune response to parasites. In: *Parasites in the Immunized Host: mechanisms of survival* (R. Porter and J. Knight, eds.), p. 3 (Amsterdam: Associated Scientific Publishers)

203. Purvis, A. C. (1977). Immunodepression to *Babesia microti* infection. *Parasitology*, 75, 197

204. Clinton, B. A., Stauber, L. A. and Palczuk, N. C. (1969). *Leishmania donovani*: antibody response to chicken ovalbumin by infected golden hamsters. *Exp. Parasitol.*, 25, 171

205. Preston, P. M. (1973). Experimental cutaneous leishmaniasis: the mouse as a model host for infection with *Leishmania tropica*. Seminar on leishmaniasis, King's College, Cambridge. Mimeographed Report, p. 1

206. Targett, G. A. T. (1978). The immunology of trypanosome infections in man. In: *Immunology of Human Infections*, Vol. II (A. J. Nahmias and R. O'Reilly, eds.) (New York: Plenum Press) (In press)

207. Clinton, B. A., Ortiz-Ortiz, L., Garcia, W., Martinez, T. and Capin, R. (1975). *Trypanosoma cruzi*: early immune responses in infected mice. *Exp. Parasitol.*, 37, 417

208. Cossio, P. M., Laguens, R. P., Diez, C., Szarfman, A., Segal, A. and Arana, R. M. (1974). Chagasic cardiopathy: antibodies reacting with plasma membrane of striated muscle and endothelial cells. *Circulation*, 50, 1252

209. de la Vega, M. J., Damilano, G. and Diez, C. (1976). Leukocyte migration inhibition test with heart antigen in American trypanosomiasis. *J. Parasitol.*, 62, 129

210. Strickland, G. T., Voller, R. A., Pettit, L. E. and Fleck, D. G. (1972). Immunodepression associated with concomitant toxoplasma and malaria infections in mice. *J. Infect. Dis.*, 126, 54

211. Salem, E., Zaki, S. A., Moneim, W. A., Kadry, S., Eisa, H. and Ezz, F. A. (1973). Autoantibodies in amoebic colitis. *J. Egypt. Med. Ass.*, 56, 113

212. Ogilvie, B. M. and Wilson, R. J. M. (1976). Evasion of the immune response by parasites. *Brit. Med. Bull.*, 32, 177

213. Assoku, R. K. G., Tizard, I. R. and Nilesen, K. H. (1977). Free fatty acids, complement activation and polyclonal B-cell stimulation as factors in the immunopathogenesis of African trypanosomiasis. *Lancet*, ii, 956

214. Warren, H. S. and Wiedanz, W. P. (1976). Malarial immunodepression *in vitro*: adherent spleen cells are functionally defective as accessory cells in the response to horse erythrocutes. *Eur. J. Immunol.*, 6, 816

215. Loose, L. D. and Di Luzio, N. R. (1976). A temporal relationship between reticuloendothelial system phagocytic alterations and antibody responses in mice infected with *Plasmodium berghei* (NYU-strain). *Am. J. Trop. Med. Hyg.*, 25, 221

216. Hudson, K. M., Freeman, J. C., Byner, C. and Terry, R. J. (1975). Immunodepression in experimental African trypanosomiasis. *Trans. R. Soc. Trop. Med. Hyg.*, 69, 273

217. Corsini, A. C., Clayton, C., Askonas, B. A. and Ogilvie, B. M. (1977). Suppressor cells and loss of B-cell potential in mice infected with *Trypanosoma brucei*. *Clin. Exp. Immunol.*, 29, 122

218. Greenwood, B. M. and Vick, R. M. (1975). Evidence for a malaria mitogen in human malaria. *Nature (Lond.)*, 257, 592

219. Jayawardena, A. and Waksman, B. H. (1977). Suppressor cells in experimental trypanosomiasis. *Nature (Lond.)*, 265, 539

220. Eardley, D. D. and Jayawardena, A. N. (1977). Suppressor cells in mice infected with *Trypanosoma brucei*. *J. Immunol.*, 119, 1029

221. Dyner, E. (1974). Les immunosuppressurs et les amibes de l'eau. [Immunosuppression and free-living amoebae.] *Ann. Soc. Belge. Med. Trop.*, 54, 405

222. Ortiz-Ortiz, L. Garmilla, C., Tanimoto-Weki, M. and Zamacona-Ravelo, G. (1973). Hipersensibilidad celular en amibiasis. I. Reacciones en hamsters inoculados con

E. histolytica. [Cellular hypersensitivity in amoebiasis. I. Reactions in hamsters inoculated with *E. histolytica.*] *Arch. Invest. Med.*, **4** (Suppl. 1), 141

223. Cappuccinelli, P., Giouarelli, M., Landolfo, S., Martinotti, G. and Vario, L. (1975). Depressione della riposta immunitaria in topi infettati con *Trypanosoma congolense* e *Trichomonas vaginalis.* [Immunodepression in mice infected with *Trypanosoma congolense* and *Trichomonas vaginalis.*] *G. Mal. Infett. Parassit.*, **27**, 788

4
Defects in Host-Defence Mechanisms

J. L. MEAKINS and N. V. CHRISTOU

4.1   INTRODUCTION   118

4.2   THE DETERMINANTS OF INFECTION   120

4.3   PRIMARY IMMUNODEFICIENCIES   122
      4.3.1   *Antibody-mediated primary immunodeficiency disease*   123
              4.3.1.1   *Sex-linked infantile hypogammaglobulinaemia*   123
              4.3.1.2   *Transient hypogammaglobulinaemia of infancy*   124
              4.3.1.3   *Sex-linked immunodeficiency with hyper-IgM*   124
              4.3.1.4   *Selective IgA deficiency*   124
              4.3.1.5   *Selective IgM deficiency*   125
              4.3.1.6   *Selective deficiency of IgG subclasses*   125
      4.3.2   *Cell-mediated immunodeficiencies*   125
              4.3.2.1   *Thymic hypoplasia with hypocalcaemia*
                        (Di George syndrome)   126
              4.3.2.2   *Chronic mucocutaneous candidiasis*   126
      4.3.3   *Neutrophil chemotactic phagocytic and bactericidal*
              disorders   126
              4.3.3.1   *Chronic granulomatous disease*   127
              4.3.3.2   *Lazy leukocyte syndrome*   127
              4.3.3.3   *Tuftsin deficiency*   128
              4.3.3.4   *Chediak–Higashi syndrome*   128
              4.3.3.5   *Glucose-6-phosphate dehydrogenase deficiency*   128
              4.3.3.6   *Myeloperoxidase deficiency*   128
              4.3.3.7   *Elevated IgE, defective chemotaxis, eczema*   129

4.3.4   *Disorders of the complement system*   129
     4.3.4.1   *Familial C5 dysfunction*   129
     4.3.4.2   *C3 deficiency*   129
     4.3.4.3   *C2 deficiency*   129
     4.3.4.4   *C1q, C1r, C1s deficiencies*   130
4.3.5   *Combined cell-mediated and humoral-mediated*
    immunodeficiency diseases   130
     4.3.5.1   *Severe combined immunodeficiency disease*   130
     4.3.5.2   *Cellular immunodeficiency with abnormal*
       immunoglobulin synthesis (Nezelof syndrome) 130
     4.3.5.3   *Combined immunodeficiency disease associated*
       with enzyme deficiencies   131
     4.3.5.4   *Immunodeficiency with thrombocytopenia, eczema,*
       and recurrent infection (the Wiskott–Aldrich
       syndrome)   131
     4.3.5.5   *Immunodeficiency with ataxia-telangiectasia* 131
     4.3.5.6   *Immunodeficiency with short-limbed dwarfism* 132
     4.3.5.7   *Episodic lymphocytopenia with lymphocytotoxin* 132

4.4   ACQUIRED DEFECTS OF HOST DEFENCE   132
    4.4.1   *Identification of patient with acquired defects of host*
     defence   134
    4.4.2   *Burns*   141
    4.4.3   *Surgery and anaesthesia*   142
    4.4.4   *Trauma and shock*   143
    4.4.5   *Immunosuppressive effect of pharmocologic agents* 143
    4.4.6   *Disease states associated with immunosuppression* 144
    4.4.7   *Malnutrition and acquired immunodeficiency*   145

4.5   SUMMARY   146

4.1   INTRODUCTION

Through the ages the practice of medicine, as many other professions, has shown a susceptibility to fashion in treatments, diseases and research. Host-defence mechanisms and their importance in infectious disease have also been subject to swings in popularity. As the twentieth century dawned many of the present-day concepts had been developed or predicted. At that time there were strongly held opinions regarding the relative importance of humoral versus cellular immunity, the interrelationships between complement (Alexin), phagocytes, opsonins and the value of vaccination and serum therapy. Each system had advocates. Shaw in *The Doctor's Dilemma* placed some of this squabbling in perspective; he pointed out how theories of disease and research come in and out of fashion.

Sir Ralph Bloomfield Bonington. 'Nature and Science are at one, Sir Patrick, believe me; though you were taught differently. *Nature has provided, in the white corpuscles as you call them – in the phagocytes as we call them – a natural means of devouring and destroying all disease germs.* There is at bottom only one genuinely scientific treatment for all diseases, and that is to *stimulate the phagocytes. Stimulate the phagocytes. Drugs are a delusion.* [Our italics.] Find the germ of the disease; prepare from it a suitable antitoxin; inject it three times a day quarter of an hour before meals; and what is the result? The phagocytes are stimulated; they devour the disease; and the patient recovers – unless, of course, he's too far gone . . .'

Sir Patrick (dreamily). 'As I sit here, I seem to hear my poor old father talking again.'

> *G. B. Shaw*
> *Act I*
> *The Doctor's Dilemma (1906)*

Since then considerable research was directed towards aspects of host defences against infection; it is only in the last 25 years and particularly the past 10 that the disparate components of the systemic response to infection have been completely dissected and their relative importance defined.

The landmark event was in 1952 when the first specific definition of the importance of host defences was described by Col. Ogden Bruton who discovered agammaglobulinaemia in a young boy with recurrent serious infections[1]. In 1968, Good[2] recounted the events leading to the discovery by Holmes[3], of the startling defect in the bactericidal function of neutrophils which was the cause of chronic granulomatous disease (CGD) in childhood. This was the first example of disease as a result of abnormal neutrophil function and also the first description of a bactericidal defect of neutrophilic dysfunction. The clinical syndrome had been described in 1957 by Berendes[4], Bridges[5], and Landing and Shirkey[6], and since 1966 it has been the prototype of neutrophilic dysfunction syndromes. Other syndromes include: Job's syndrome[7], myeloperoxidase deficiency[8], Chediak–Higashi syndrome[9] and periodic neutropenia[10]. These are only two of the wide variety of the primary, usually congenital, immunodeficiencies which are classified and discussed in Section 3 of this chapter.

The enormous value of these congenital defects is that they help delineate precise mechanisms of host defence and aid in piecing together the conceptual whole required to make a cohesive and comprehensive schema of the host's ability to protect itself in the ocean of micro-organisms in which we dwell. These congenital defects have been called experiments of nature by McQuarrie and as such usually create a pure defect, clonal in nature, the result of the incomplete expression of or lack of a gene. The acquired defect is generally not, as it were, a clonal manifestation, but rather more of a systemic, metabolic, generalized membrane or nutritional problem, and as such may present with involvement of several component parts of the immune response or portions of the function of the individual cell. It is frequently difficult to specify the particular role of the various defects which may be found to the clinical picture.

The most significant clinical feature of primary immunodeficiencies is the picture of recurrent serious infections. Any child who demonstrates this pattern must be worked up for immunologic disease. The patient who develops acquired defects secondary to a disease, its treatment, trauma, surgery, drugs, etc., is slightly more difficult to define. These patients in general present a broader range of defects and not a single defect such as that seen in CGD. It is our belief that these patients present a much more significant group for identification and treatment as they are numerous and primary defects rare. The distribution of patients with acquired defects cuts across all major disciplines. The hallmark of these patient populations susceptible to secondary immunodeficiencies is recurrent infection or a significantly increased incidence of sepsis. These points will be further developed in Section 4.

4.2 THE DETERMINANTS OF INFECTION

In order to place in perspective the role of host defences in the development of an infectious process, it is useful to examine the determinants of any infectious process[11]. These determinants are the infecting organism, the local environment in which the organism produces the infection and the systemic response to the process which are the host defences to sepsis (Figure 4.1).

The infecting organism has variable properties of virulence, therefore differences in local and systemic determinants may allow *or* prevent infection by a modestly pathogenic organism. It is apparent, however, that some bacteria are highly pathogenic in their own right and the local and systemic factors are not adequate for control. Examples include, *Clostridium tetani*, *Staphylococcus aureus*, and *Streptococcus pyogenes*.

The features that characterize the local environment (Table 4.1) are biological, mechanical and chemical forms of decontamination, and the objectives of these functions are PREVENTION OF LODGEMENT of invasive bacteria. The skin presents a mechanical barrier to invasion of bacteria, a biological control by the presence of its own abundant and entrenched local flora and a chemical barrier because of the presence of fatty acids which provide both a hostile environment for and are bactericidal to non-resident flora. The burn injury most clearly presents the breakdown of local factors and together with secondary impairment of host defences clearly identifies why the burned patient is at such risk for sepsis.

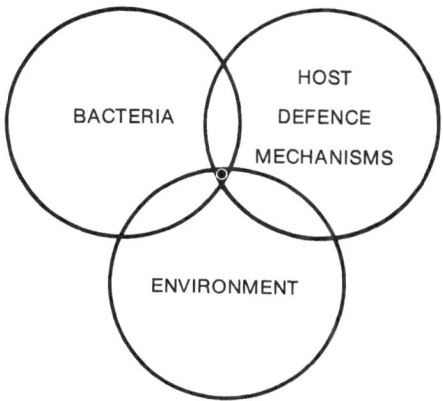

Figure 4.1 In homeostasis, the normal state, the intersection of the circles representing the relationship between the determinants of infection: bacteria, environment and host-defence mechanisms intersect at a point, indicating zero probability of sepsis

Other clear examples of the body's decontamination systems are bronchial ciliary action, tears, and the normal flora of the gastro-intestinal tract. When these basic protective measures are broken down infection usually prevails. While these features are host related they are not commonly included in discussions in host defence. We do not intend to enlarge greatly in this area but point out that, in general, these defects are acquired and often leave

Table 4.1 Environment (local factors)

Mechanical barrier	Biological decontamination
	Mechanical
	Chemical
	Microbiological
Prevention of lodgement	

uncorrectable damage. The heavy smoker who develops bronchitis virtually never has a normal tracheo-bronchial tree. Similarly the infection behind an obstruction imposed upon the biliary tree or a ureter is there until surgically corrected but is a function of an altered local environment. These features are important and can clearly be approached with preventive or therapeutic means.

The systemic response to an infecting organism or immunologic challenge is considered to be the classical host-defence mechanisms. This response is made up of a number of contributing components each of which may produce immunologic results, i.e. bacterial killing, graft rejection, etc., together with inflammation.

Host defence is made up of a humoral component, phagocytic systems, cellular immunity and complement. Each of these components has its own complexities, however, in many respects they have a final common pathway, that is, their effects are mediated by an appropriate inflammatory response. Inflammation can be thought of as a response to an irritating force, however, it is becoming clear that there are common mediators of function in these biologic responses. Thus while mechanisms of inducement are different, that is, the homograft rejection, the processes of wound healing and response to staphylococcal inoculation, in the final molecular analysis, they are similarly mediated via common mechanisms and seen as the inflammatory response. In the philosophical setting of the determinants of infections in primary immunodeficiencies, the failure of a single component as in agamma-globulinaemia or a portion of a cell function as in the final step of bacterial killing in granulomatous disease of childhood, can disrupt the response to infection. Most of these syndromes involve a single component or system and produce an altered response to infectious disease. However, it is the rare acquired or secondary immunodeficiency that produces an aberration of a single component of host defence. It is much more common for there to be a broad alteration of function in several components of host response and we would suggest that the final inflammatory response was inadequate to deal with the infectious challenge resulting in an increased incidence and/or severity of infection.

4.3 PRIMARY IMMUNODEFICIENCIES

Primary immunodeficiencies are varied and their description and classification in the literature is continuously changing. Part of the reason is that present techniques used to study the various aspects of immunity were not available to the investigators at the time that the actual cases were studied and published. Fudenberg[12] and his co-workers classified primary immunodeficiencies as those of stem cells, B cells or T cells though a cell line cannot be the end product of a defective gene. In the section that follows, primary immunodeficiency disorders are discussed under four main categories: antibody or B-cell deficiency, cellular deficiency or T-cell immunodeficiency, phagocytic dysfunction and complement deficiency. These are classified in

Table 4.2 using the terminology proposed by a Committee of the World Health Organization[12].

Table 4.2   Primary immunodeficiencies

A. *Antibody-mediated immunodeficiency disease*
  1. Sex-linked infantile hypogammaglobulinaemia
  2. Transient hypogammaglobulinaemia of infancy
  3. Sex-linked immunodeficiency with hyper-IgM
  4. Selective IgA deficiency
  5. Selective IgM deficiency
  6. Selective deficiencies of IgG subclasses

B. *Cell-mediated immunodeficiency diseases*
  1. Thymic hypoplasia with hypocalcaemia (Di George syndrome)
  2. Chronic mucocutaneous candidiasis (with or without endocrinopathy)

C. *Neutrophil chemotactic phagocytic and bactericidal dysfunction*
  1. Chronic granulomatous disease
  2. Lazy-leukocyte syndrome
  3. Tuftsin deficiency
  4. Chediak–Higashi syndrome
  5. Glucose-6-phosphate dehydrogenase deficiency
  6. Myeloperoxidase deficiency
  7. Elevated IgE, defective chemotaxis, eczema and recurrent infections

D. *Disorders of the complement system*
  1. Familial C5 dysfunction
  2. C3 deficiency (type 1, type 2)
  3. C2 deficiency
  4. C1q, C1r, C1s deficiency

E. *Combined cell-mediated and humoral-mediated immunodeficiency diseases*
  1. Severe combined immunodeficiency
  2. Cellular immunodeficiency with abnormal immunoglobulin synthesis (Nezelof syndrome)
  3. Combined immunodeficiency disease with associated enzyme deficiency
  4. Immunodeficiency with eczema and thrombocytopenia (Wiskott–Aldrich syndrome)
  5. Immunodeficiency with thymoma
  6. Immunodeficiency with ataxia telangiectasia
  7. Immunodeficiency with short-limbed dwarfism
  8. Episodic lymphocytopenia with lymphotoxin (immunological amnesia)

4.3.1   Antibody-mediated primary immunodeficiency disease

The first report in the literature of young boy with this type of deficiency was by Bruton in 1952[1]. Critlin and Janeway[13] also described a syndrome with antibody deficiency. Recognitition of such patients was at times difficult and complicated because many were of the 'mixed' variety and also had cell-mediated immunodeficiencies.

4.3.1.1   *Sex-linked infantile hypogammaglobulinaemia*[14, 15]

This is a familial disorder with an X-linked inheritance pattern affecting only males. It is estimated in the UK to have an incidence of 1/100 000 births. No estimates exist for North America. Symptoms occur at ages greater than 6 months, and consist of pyogenic infections with a predominance of Gram-positive cocci. Other associated clinical features are non-infective arthritis and intestinal malabsorption. The infections are recurrent and though there is good response to antibiotics, tissue damage such as bronchiectasis frequently develops. The IgG is less than 200 mg% with usual absence of IgA, IgM, IgE and IgD. There is absence of circulating B cells in the peripheral blood. This is felt to be secondary to complete lack of stem cells in the Bursal equivalent of man. There is failure to make antibody following antigenic stimulation. Cell-mediated immunity is intact. The mainstay of treatment is commercial γ-globulin. Patients have survived to the second and third decades of life. However, prognosis in such patients remains guarded.

4.3.1.2   Transient hypogammaglobulinaemia of infancy[13]

All infants go through a period of hypogammaglobulinaemia at approximately 5–6 months of age. The passive transfer of maternal IgG which begins at 16 weeks gestation leads to IgG levels at birth greater than that of the mother. IgG then decreases during the first 6 months of life while IgA and IgM concentrations increase. The concentration of IgG is lowest at 6 months and if the infant does not start producing its own IgG at this time, transient hypogammaglobulinaemia results. The delay may last up to 18 months and control requires γ-globulin. The cause is not known, the strongest theory being one that postulates that maternal antibodies cause suppression of endogenous immunoglobulin production in a manner similar to the suppression of normal red cell production in infants with passive transfer of antibody against Rh factors. The disorder corrects itself by 18 months.

4.3.1.3   Sex-linked immunodeficiency with hyper-IgM[16]

This is a rare disorder with X-linked inheritance in most cases. It involves a deficiency of IgG and IgA with increased levels of IgM ranging from 150–1000 mg/dl. Symptoms involve recurrent pyogenic infections with some patients showing recurrent neutropenia, haemolytic anaemia or aplastic anaemia. The cause is not known, and due to the small number of reported cases, the prognosis is not easy to determine.

4.3.1.4   Selective IgA deficiency[17]

This is the most common immunodeficiency disorder affecting 1/600 to 1/800 neonates. The most common symptom is recurrent sino-pulmonary viral and/or bacterial infections, although many patients with this disorder are entirely asymptomatic. It shows an association with reticulum cell sarcoma, squamous cell carcinoma of the oesophagus and lung, and thymoma. The incidence in atopic children is 1/200 to 1/400, and a significant number of patients have other autoimmune disorders, e.g. systemic lupus erythematosus, rheumatoid arthritis, dermatomyositis and chronic active hepatitis. There is an autosomal dominant and autosomal recessive mode of inheritance. The IgA concentration in the serum is less than 5 mg/dl and the other immunoglobulins are normal or increased. As a result of low serum IgA, levels of IgA in secretions are undetectable. The total numbers of B cells in the circulation are normal, as are IgA-bearing B cells. The disorder is probably due to decreased synthesis or release of IgA rather than absence of IgA B lymphocytes. Cell-mediated immunity including skin tests, response of peripheral blood lymphocytes to phytohaemaglutinin and allogeneic cells, and the number of circulating T lymphocytes are all normal. Treatment involves aggressive antibiotic therapy. Administration of γ-globulin is contra-indicated because it is contaminated with IgA. Since these patients can form antibodies of the other immunoglobulin classes, they are capable of forming anti IgA. IgA is recognized as foreign protein and they risk subsequent anaphylactoid transfusion reactions. Prognosis is guarded but patients can survive to the sixth or seventh decades of life with careful management.

4.3.1.5 Selective IgM deficiency[18]

This is a rare disorder characterized by the absence of IgM with normal levels of the other immunoglobulin classes and intact cell-mediated immunity. It affects both males and females and patients are susceptible to overwhelming infections with micro-organisms with polysaccharide-containing cell walls. The few cases reported do not allow generalizations about treatment and prognosis.

4.3.1.6 Selective deficiency of IgG subclasses[19]

Several patients have been described with selective defects of the serum IgG subclasses IgG_1, IgG_2, IgG_3 or IgG_4, while total serum IgG concentrations may be normal or decreased. Patients are susceptible to repeated sino-pulmonary pyogenic infections. There is good response to treatment with intramuscular γ-globulin injections.

4.3.2 Cell-mediated immunodeficiencies

Pure isolated T-cell abnormalities are rare. Usually when T-cell dysfunction occurs there are associated B-cell defects reflecting the close collaboration between T and B lymphocytes in normal immune defence mechanisms. Presently only two pure cell mediated immunodeficiencies are recognized in the literature: thymic hypoplasia with hypocalcaemia (Di George syndrome) and chronic mucocutaneous candidiasis.

4.3.2.1   *Thymic hypoplasia with hypocalcaemia (Di George syndrome)*[20]

Afflicted infants are affected immediately following birth. The syndrome involves; (a) congenital tetany secondary to hypoparathyroidism, (b) abnormal facies with 'fish-shaped' mouth, low-set ears, notched ear pinna, hypertelorism, micrognathia and antimongoloid slant of the eyes, (c) congenital heart disease, and (d) cell-mediated immunodeficiency. It affects both males and females and the mode of inheritance is not known. The thymus is absent or hypoplastic and since the parathyroids derive embryologically from the same third and fourth pharyngeal pouches, they are also involved. If the children survive the initial hypocalcaemia and heart failure, they become susceptible to recurrent infections with various viral, bacterial, fungal and protozoal infections. The diagnosis is made upon presence of all three clinical findings along with cell-mediated immune defects as measured by decreased number of the total lymphocyte count, decreased stimulation of lymphocytes by phytohaemagglutinin and allogeneic cells, and decreased number of E-rosette forming lymphocytes. It is essential to establish the diagnosis at birth because foetal thymus transplant reconstitutes CMI in 8 hours. The correction is permanent. There is no graft versus host disease which is evidence for lack of a thymic humoral factor as the cause of the cell-mediated immunodeficiency in this syndrome.

4.3.2.2   *Chronic mucocutaneous candidiasis*[21, 22]

Chronic mucocutaneous candidiasis affects both males and females and an autosomal recessive inheritance is suggested. It is characterized by persistent Candida infection of the skin, mucous membranes and nails. There is associated development of idiopathic endocrinopathy. The basic defect is unknown. There is complete anergy as measured by skin testing in the face of severe candidal infection. The response to lymphocyte transformation *in vitro* after exposure to candidal antigens is diminished. The response to PHA and allogeneic cells, however, is normal. Activation of lymphocytes and Migration Inhibiting Factor (MIF) production in response to antigens other than Candida are also normal. Autoantibodies towards the target organs may explain the cell-mediated immunodeficiency and associated endocrinopathy. Patients may survive to the second or third decade but experience extensive morbidity. Antifungal agents, transfer factor, unmatched lymphocyte transfusions and foetal thymus transplants have all been used with varying success in the treatment of this disorder.

4.3.3   Neutrophil chemotactic phagocytic and bactericidal disorders

These may be divided into extrinsic and intrinsic defects. Extrinsic deficiencies include opsonin deficiencies, suppression of total number of phagocytic cells by immunosuppressive agents, interference of phagocytic function by corticosteroids and suppression of the total number of circulating neutrophils by autoantibodies against neutrophil antigens. Intrinsic defects are related to enzyme deficiencies within the cell such as myeloperoxidase deficiency, NADH and NADPH oxidase deficiency or glucose-6-phosphate dehydrogenase deficiencies.

4.3.3.1 Chronic granulomatous disease[2-5, 23, 24]

Chronic granulomatous disease is an inherited defect of neutrophil bactericidal function. It manifests itself in the first 2 years of life with recurrent severe infections with *Staphylococcus aureus* and unusual organisms such as *S. epidermidis, Serratia marcescens,* and *Candida.* It may, however, present in the teenage years. The disorder shows sex-linked inheritance, although several females have now been described indicating an autosomal recessive form of variable penetrance may exist as well. The carrier female in the sex-linked form is asymptomatic. Studies of humoral and cell-mediated immunity show these to be intact. Phagocytosis is normal, however, bactericidal function is abnormal, with 80–90% of the bacteria remaining viable inside the neutrophils after 120 min *in vitro* as compared to 1% for normal neutrophils. The defect has been narrowed down to the cells' metabolism. There is no change in hexose monophosphate shunt activity (HMP) nor increased oxygen uptake following challenge of neutrophils with opsonized bacteria. Hydrogen peroxide production is markedly diminished. Further analysis shows affected males to lack NADP-oxidase and NADPH-oxidase whereas affected females are thought to lack glutathione peroxidase. Catalase lacking bacteria are handled normally by chronic granulomatous neutrophils since these bacteria have endogenous H_2O_2 which the neutrophil utilizes in their destruction. The quantitative nitroblue tetrazolium dye reduction test can be used in screening for this disorder. There is no dye reduction by affected cells. The diagnosis must then be proven by demonstrating a defective bactericidal curve between the patient's neutrophils and the infecting organisms or *S. aureus 502A.* Aggressive surgical management along with potent antibiotics has resulted in survivals to the second and third decades of life, however, organ dysfunction and anatomic changes secondary to recurrent chronic infection usually leads to the patients demise.

4.3.3.2 Lazy-leukocyte syndrome[25]

The lazy-leukocyte syndrome is characterized by defective chemotactic response of patient leukocytes to normal chemotactic stimuli, in association with neutropenia. Males and females are equally affected. Severe recurrent infections associated with neutropenia are observed. Rebuck window preparations show decreased polymorphonuclear leukocyte mobilization to the inflammatory focus, and there is reduced *in vitro* neutrophil chemotaxis and random migration. Stimulation of the marginal neutrophil pool by epinephrine or endotoxin is also abnormal. Cell-mediated and humoral immunity studies are normal. Treatment is with specific antibiotics. The prognosis is not known.

4.3.3.3 Tuftsin deficiency[26]

Tuftsin deficiency is characterized by a familial lack of a phagocytosis-stimulating tetrapeptide that is cleaved from a parent immunoglobulin by the spleen. Two families have been described. Tuftsin is also absent from splenectonized patients. Patients manifest both local and systemic severe bacterial infections. The diagnosis can be made by measurement of Tuftsin in special laboratories.

4.3.3.4 Chediak–Higashi syndrome[2, 23]

This syndrome is characterized by recurrent bacterial infections, partial occulocutaneous albinism, giant cytoplasmic granules, central nervous system abnormalities and a high incidence of lymphoreticular malignancy. It demonstrates a multi-system autosomal recessive inheritance. Defective neutrophil chemotaxis and intracellular killing of normally phagocytized bacteria has been described. The *rate* of bacterial killing is abnormal, for if the neutrophils are given enough time, they will kill the intracellular bacteria. Oxygen uptake, HMP activity and hydrogen peroxide production are normal. The prognosis is poor.

4.3.3.5 Glucose-6-phosphate dehydrogenase deficiency[27]

Glucose-6-phosphate (G-6-P) dehydrogenase deficiency affects both males and females of about equal frequency. The diagnosis is made by demonstrating decreased G-6-P dehydrogenase activity in peripheral blood leukocytes. Deficient cellular NADP dehydrogenase activity has also been described. As a result, the neutrophils from these patients show very little HMP activity and decreased H_2O_2 production. Consequently they cannot kill catalase-containing organisms at normal rates. The nitroblue tetrazolium reduction test is normal in these patients (mostly all have NADP/NADPH oxidase) but the killing rate is abnormal. This distinguishes G-6-P dehydrogenase deficiency from chronic granulomatous disease. Treatment and prognosis are very similar in these two immunodeficiencies.

4.3.3.6 Myeloperoxidase deficiency[28]

Several patients have been described with complete deficiency of leukocyte myeloperoxidase. Oxygen consumption, HMP activity and H_2O_2 production are normal. There is delayed intracellular killing of bacteria which becomes normal if incubation times are increased. Such patients are susceptible to recurrent infections with candidal and staphylococcal infections. The diagnosis is established by a peroxidase stain on peripheral blood, leukocytes. Antibiotics are the mainstay treatment management.

4.3.3.7 Elevated IgE, defective chemotaxis, eczema[29]

This disorder has been described in male and female patients who show an early onset of eczema, bacterial abscesses and secondary infection of the eczema associated with markedly elevated serum IgE. Humoral and cell-mediated immunity are normal. Neutrophil chemotaxis is abnormal though phagocytosis is normal.

4.3.4 Disorders of the complement system

Complement factors are necessary for normal opsonization, bacterial killing, and neutrophil chemotaxis. Despite the participation of the complement components in the phagocytic process, a number of complement deficiencies are not associated with enhanced susceptibility to infection but rather increased susceptibility to autoimmune disease.

4.3.4.1 Familial C5 dysfunction[30]

Familial C5 dysfunction is a genetic defect which results in normal C5 circulating levels which, however, does not function normally as a chemotactic stimulus. Patients present with failure to thrive, diarrhoea, seborrhoeic dermatitis, and severe sepsis with staphylococcal as well as Gram-negative enteric organisms. Males are affected as frequently as females. The chemotactic defect can be corrected by the addition of normal C5 to the *in vitro* assay. There may be leukocytosis, increased γ-globulins and defective phagocytosis as measured by the Baker's yeast assay. Cell-mediated immunity is normal.

4.3.4.2 C3 deficiency[31, 32]

A rare disorder of which two forms exist, type 1 and type 2. Type 1 is characterized by a lack of C3 proactivator, whereas in type 2 there is increased catabolism of C3. Both are associated with recurrent infections.

4.3.4.3 C2 deficiency[33]

C2 deficiency has been reported in several patients with systemic lupus erythematosus-like autoimmune disorders plus increased susceptibility to infection. An autosomal recessive mode of inheritance is suggested.

4.3.4.4   *C1q, C1r, C1s deficiencies*[34, 35]

These are again inherited defects in individual complement components. Patients are susceptible to autoimmune disease and severe infections. Total haemolytic complement is usually low. Specific diagnosis involves measurement of individual components. Treatment involves management of the autoimmune disease as well as the infection, by antibiotics and other conventional means.

4.3.5   Combined cell-mediated and humoral-mediated immunodeficiency diseases

Immunodeficiencies of both T- and B-lymphocyte systems which lead to abnormalities of both the humoral component as well as the cell-mediated component of host defence are varied and demonstrate a wide range of severity. Some of the most lethal of the immunodeficiencies are in this group.

4.3.5.1   *Severe combined immunodeficiency disease*[36]

Severe combined immunodeficiency, often abbreviated SCID, lacks both humoral immunity and cell-mediated immunity. The old term was Swiss type agammaglobulinaemia or sex-linked lymphopenic agammaglobulinaemia. The disease manifests itself by 6 months of age with viral, bacterial, fungal and protozoal infections. The patient usually dies within the first year of life secondary to infection, usually with Gram-negative organisms. Administration of immunoglobulins will protect only against pneumococcus and haemophilus influenza. Chronic *Candida* infection is also seen. *Pneumocystis carinii*, a protozoan, commonly causes infection especially in the lungs. Severe combined immunodeficiency shows both a sex-linked and autosomal forms of inheritance. Laboratory evaluation demonstrates a complete lack of B-cell and T-cell immunity. Causative theories include a defective stem cell, secondary to lymphoid hypoplasia or thymic aplasia, or failure of stem cells to differentiate secondary to a defective 'bursa' in man. Treatment with bone marrow transplants have been attempted but graft versus host disease is a common and feared complication.

4.3.5.2   *Cellular immunodeficiency with abnormal immunoglobulin synthesis (Nezelof syndrome)*[37]

The Nezelof syndrome affects both males and females with no definite inheritance pattern as yet described. It involves varying types of cellular immunity defects with lymphopenia, response to skin tests, % E-rosetting, mixed lymphocyte culture and mitogen stimulation all decreased. The level of serum immunoglobulins is normal but there is a failure of *specific* antibody synthesis. Patients are susceptible to a variety of viral, bacterial, fungal and protozoal infections. The syndrome probably involves a thymus abnormality with defective T lymphocytes as a result. There is absence of T- to B-cell co-operation required to make specific antibody. Thymosin may at times reconstitute the immune defects. Aggressive treatment of infections has led to some survivors up to 18 years of age. Chronic lung disease, chronic fungal infections and later development of malignancy are long-term complications.

4.3.5.3 Combined immunodeficiency disease associated with enzyme deficiencies[38, 39]

Combined immunodeficiency with enzyme defects demonstrates autosomal recessive inheritance. It demonstrates a complete spectrum of abnormalities in T- and B-cell immunity where this may be totally lacking or have mild aberration. There is lymphopenia, decreased, normal or elevated immunoglobulin levels and variable specific antibody response. Adenosine deaminase and nucleoside phosphorylase are the deficient enzymes so far identified. Causative theories include direct suppressive effect on lymphocytes by cyclic AMP which is elevated, or interference with cell function by inosine byproducts which accumulate secondary to the enzyme defects.

4.3.5.4 Immunodeficiency with thrombocytopenia, eczema, and recurrent infection (the Wiskott–Aldrich syndrome)[40]

The Wiskott–Aldrich syndrome is characterized by thrombocytopenia, eczema, recurrent infection and inability to form specific antibody to polysaccharide antigens. The inheritance is sex-linked. The thymus gland is normal and B cells are normal. There is a failure to process polysaccharide antigens possibly due to an abnormal macrophage–lymphocyte interaction. The macrophages are thought to lack surface receptors for IgG or IgM. IgM in the serum is low whereas IgA and IgE are elevated. The thrombocytopenia, eczema and immunodeficiency have not been linked by a unifying theory. Splenectomy is contraindicated because it is associated with fulminant infection and septicaemia.

4.3.5.5 Immunodeficiency with ataxia telangiectasia[41, 42]

This is an autosomal recessive disorder manifesting by the second year of life. Immunodeficiency with ataxia telangiectasia is diagnosed where there exists recurrent sinopulmonary infection, ataxia and telangiectasia. In 60% of patients there are abnormalities in cell-mediated immunity as measured by decreased stimulation of lymphocytes with phytohaemagglutinin and allogeneic cells, a decreased number of circulating T lymphocytes and decreased delayed hypersensitivity skin testing. Antibody-mediated immunity is also abnormal and in 40% of patients selective IgA deficiency is demonstrated. In others there is IgE deficiency. An autoantibody has been described and the defect in cell-mediated immunity is thought to be immunological attrition. Initially both cell-mediated and humoral-mediated immunity may be intact but there is progressive loss of specific antigenic response and loss of some immunoglobulins. The same is observed with cell-mediated immunity. No unifying theory linking immunodeficiency with ataxia and telangiectasia has been put forth. Some patients with this disorder have reached the fifth decade of life.

4.3.5.6 *Immunodeficiency with short-limbed dwarfism*[43, 44]

Immunodeficiency with short-limbed dwarfism affects both males and females and varies from a complete absence of B- and T-cell immunity to partial defects. There is also associated skeletal defects which seem to be inherited in an independent manner. At times the skeletal defects do not have associated immunodeficiency. Three types are described. Type 1 involves defective cell-mediated immunity only. There is lymphopenia, decreased lymphocyte stimulation *in vitro* and normal humoral immunity. Despite this, such patients fare well against viral infections, but are uniquely susceptible to varicella and smallpox. Type 2 involves defects in both humoral and cell-mediated response. Afflicted infants do not survive beyond 1 year of age. Type 3 involves defective humoral immunity. Two patients have been described who showed total hypogammaglobulinaemia. Prognosis is dependent on the type and severity of the immunodeficiency.

4.3.5.7 *Episodic lymphocytopenia with lymphocytotoxin*[45]

Twelve patients both male and female have been described with this disorder. There is lymphocytopenia associated with a lymphocytotoxin in the blood which leads to recurrent infection. There is eczema with impaired cell-mediated and humoral immunity.

4.4 ACQUIRED DEFECTS OF HOST DEFENCE

Acquired defects of host defence are by implication a result of some other influence usually secondary to a disease process, drug therapy or some other event. The list of factors which can produce these defects is an impressive and continually growing one. Characteristically they do not involve a single component but rather produce a range of abnormalities in many, if not all components of host defence. These defects tend to be variable in severity and only occasionally are they as complete as the congenital absence of a cell function. The clinical factors which may contribute to these acquired defects are common and are to be found upon all wards in any general hospital. Malnutrition, sepsis, trauma, surgery, burns, advanced age, diabetes, advanced cancer and combinations of these conditions and various clinical syndromes may all produce acquired immunodeficiency. When patients on immunosuppressive drugs and drug regimens are added to the previous group, the high incidence of nosocomial infection and deaths associated with infection is not surprising.

In those patients with acquired abnormalities, because they may not only involve the entire immune system but also because of numerous other medical and surgical problems, the role of host defences in development of sepsis may be questioned. While in a child with chronic granulomatous disease, the recurrent infections are clearly a result of abnormal neutrophil function, a burn patient who develops sepsis has an area (the burn wound) particularly suited to bacterial growth and subsequent tissue invasion, regardless of the abnormalities of host defence against infection. In a child, recurrent episodes of infection stimulates the investigation of their immune system. So too, the burn patient, because of this high incidence of sepsis has become a prototype of the patient who has major and significant acquired defects in resistance to infection. These defects will be reviewed subsequently; however at this point, it is appropriate to point out that the burn patient has been investigated immunologically because of the high and recurrent pattern of sepsis. The burn patient is easy to identify.

In the past identification of patients who appear normal physiologically but who have or may be prone to develop acquired defects of host resistance to infection has not been accomplished.

The value of identification and definition of the abnormalities of host defence becomes increasingly significant allowing not only the biological components of the immune response and their importance in development of sepsis to be identified but also at an effective clinical level the methodology for identification and description of these patients with defects of host defence mechanisms (HDM).

The subsequent discussion of acquired abnormalities of host defence has been organized on etiological grounds because most factors which disrupt host defences affect more than one component, and as a result, it becomes similarly difficult to ascribe specific infections to the patient with acquired immunodeficiencies, different from most primary immunodeficiencies. As an example, renal transplant recipients have a preponderance of viral and fungal infections in the later post-transplant period. They also have a marked increase in common bacterial pathogens throughout their course.

The control or reduction of bacterial pathogens and commensals by antibiotics also contributes to the development of bizarre infections. Patients with thermal injury, who have broad and serious alterations of host defence, only develop viral and fungal infections when the more common bacterial pathogens have been eliminated by antibiotics and topical therapy. As a final introductory note it is apparent that sepsis itself can produce alterations in host defence further confusing the situation.

4.4.1   Identification of patient with acquired defects of host defence

In practice there are a number of clinical situations where one would intuitively state that there was an increased incidence of sepsis and therefore likely to be alterations of the patient's ability to handle infection. These include advanced age, major surgery, trauma, diabetes, uraemia, severe pancreatitis, haemorrhagic shock and sepsis itself to list but a few. Not all these patients have abnormalities of host defence nor do they all develop sepsis. Identification of those likely to develop sepsis and the related mortality is therefore not only important clinically but also because it pinpoints the population who require immunological study and therefore allow description of the basic alterations in host defence. These are the first steps required before the correction and/or treatment of the abnormality can be initiated.

The patients with potential abnormalities of host defence are a large and heterogeneous group. A shot-gun approach of testing everyone has been utilized but is unrewarding and expensive. Our approach to this problem was initiated by the study of a 13-year-old boy referred to this hospital 2 months after surgery for perforated appendicitis and generalized peritonitis[46]. At that time he had high output intestinal fistulae, intra-abdominal abscesses requiring drainage, septicaemia, respiratory failure and malnutrition. Despite repeated drainage of abscesses, total parenteral nutrition at a rate of 2500–3500 cal/day, antibiotics, transfer factor and the other therapeutic efforts of modern medicine, he died 5 months after admission. The organisms grown from his blood were *S. aureus*, enterococci, *S. epidermidis* and *C. albicans*. The abscesses contained these and a variety of other Gram-negative rods. Because of his persistent inability to localize and control his various infections, aspects of his immune response were examined.

He was anergic to recall delayed hypersensitivity antigens (mumps, PPD, Varidase and Candida), accepted a skin graft without signs of rejection for 44 days, and had a serum inhibitor of the mixed lymphocyte culture (MLC) response of his own lymphocytes to allogeneic lymphocytes. Other aspects of lymphocyte and neutrophil function were normal and there were normal circulating levels of immunoglobulins. These data were pursued in a pilot study. Of 50 pre-operative and 55 seriously ill patients who were skin tested, results indicated that anergic and relatively anergic patients had a significantly increased incidence of sepsis over those whose skin tests were normal[46]. These data suggested that there was a measure of immune competence which was abnormal and related to sepsis and clinical outcome.

Utilizing the recall antigens PPD, mumps, Trichophyton, Varidase and Candida and defining the skin-test results as in Table 4.3, a prospective study of 520 patients was then carried out. Neutrophil and lymphocyte function and the effect of anergic serum on cell function was evaluated in many anergic patients and normal controls[47, 48], in whom sepsis was defined as a positive bloood culture or an abscess identified at surgery or autopsy.

Table 4.3 Responses to recall antigens

Antigens:	Candida	Trichophyton
	Mumps	
	PPD	Varidase

Normal response: 5 mm or more of induration
  at 24 or 48 hours
Anergy (A): No response (0/5)
Relative anergy (RA): Single response (1/5)
Normal (N): Two or more responses $(2^+/5)$

The patients were divided into three groups: those studied pre-operatively, those studied post-operatively or post trauma and those who did not require surgery. These data are summarized in Table 4.4. In the 322 patients studied pre-operatively those 42 patients with altered responses (either anergic or relatively anergic) had a 21.4% incidence of sepsis and a third died (Table 4.4). The surgical procedures were on the stomach, pancreas, liver, large and small intestine or major biliary tract operations. These data show that skin testing identifies a group of patients at increased risk of sepsis and mortality following surgery.

Table 4.4 Sepsis and mortality following initial skin test

Response	Number	Sepsis	Death
(a) *Pre-operative: 322 patients*			
Anergy	21	19%	33.3%
Relative anergy	21	23.8%	33.3%
Normal	280	4.6%	4.3%
(b) *Post-operative/post-trauma: 115 patients*			
Anergy	71	62%	33.8%
Relative anergy	25	60%	24·0%
Normal	19	26.3%	5.3%
(c) *Non-operative: 83 patients*			
Anergy	23	21.7%	47.8%
Relative anergy	4	25%	25%
Normal	56	0%	1.8%

The 115 patients studied in the intensive care unit (Table 4.4b) were all tested following emergency surgery, trauma (with or without operation) or the development of post-operative complications. These patients were very ill accounting for the high incidence of altered responses (83.5%) and remarkable 61.5% incidence of sepsis in patients with altered responses and 26.3% in those with normal cutaneous reactions. These are real as well as statistically significant differing rates of sepsis. The other significant difference is in the mortality rate, 5.3% for normal responders compared to 31.3% for those with altered responses.

In those 83 patients who were not operated upon, 27 had altered skin tests with a 22% sepsis rate and 44% mortality compared to no sepsis and one death in normally responsive patients. These patients were admitted with upper and lower gastro-intestinal haemorrhage, bowel obstruction not requiring surgery, pancreatitis, inflammatory bowel disease and cancer. Cancer probably contributed to mortality rate.

Table 4.5   Sequential testing in 247 patients

Skin tests	Number	Sepsis (%)	Death (%)
Anergy—anergy	41	23 (56.1)	30 (73.2)
Anergy—relative anergy	11	4 (36.4)	3 (27.3)
Anergy—normal	50	21 (42.0)	2 (4.0)
Relative anergy—anergy	7	4 (57.1)	7 (100.0)
Relative anergy—Relative anergy	6	2 (33.3)	4 (66.7)
Relative anergy—normal	44	15 (34.1)	2 (4.5)
Normal—anergy	5	5 (100.1)	5 (100.0)
Normal—relative anergy	0	0 (0.0)	0 (0.0)
Normal—normal	83	9 (10.8)	1 (1.2)

Sequential skin testing was performed two or more times in 247 patients. Based on the initial skin test, Table 4.5 shows how patient outcome seems related to the evolution of skin-test responses. It is clear that patients with abnormal or normal responses, whose skin tests become or remain normal, have a substantially better prognosis than those whose responses remain or become abnormal.

Table 4.6   Organisms in blood cultures of 91 patients

Organisms	Normal	Relative anergy	Anergy
Gram-negative rods	17	19	58
Gram-positive cocci	34	18	57
Gram-positive rods	0	0	5
Fungi	9	0	5
	51	37	125

It therefore appears that skin-test responses, a classical reflection of cell-mediated immunity (CMI) has predictive value in terms of patient sepsis and mortality and identifies a patient population unusually sensitive to major infection, i.e. septicaemia. It is of interest that the organisms which caused sepsis were common Gram-negative and Gram-positive bacteria in all patients (Table 4.6). A single patient had five positive blood cultures of Candida. These infectious problems are not usually thought to be related to CMI.

In conjunction with skin testing, numerous other aspects of host defence were assessed. Delayed hypersensitivity responses are considered a reflection of CMI, and therefore lymphocyte function was examined exhaustively. Mixed lymphocyte culture, lymphocyte response to PHA and pokeweed mitogen, cell-mediated lympholysis and lymphocyte generation of blastogenic factor were all of the same order as those of normal patients and controls. In four anergic patients there was serum inhibitor of their MLC. The only abnormal lymphocyte test was a reduction in the number of rosetting T lymphocytes as well as in the total lymphocyte count.

Table 4.7 Neutrophil chemotaxis in anergic and relatively anergic patients

Skin-test response	Stimulated migration
Anergy (40)	81.7 ± 2.3
Relative anergy (15)	$97.2 \pm 3.8*$
Normal control (19)	$117.5 \pm 1.6*$

*$P < 0.001$

Neutrophil chemotaxis has been evaluated using the leading front technique of Zigmond and Hirsch[49] which gives a distance in microns (with narrow standard errors) as the measure of chemotaxis. Table 4.7 records the chemotactic results in the 55 anergic (A) and relatively anergic (RA) patients studied. Chemotaxis is clearly reduced in patients with altered responses and

Table 4.8 Evolution of chemotaxis following restoration of normal skin-test responses

Skin-test responses	Stimulated migration
Anergic patients (14)	$78.2 \pm 5.4*$
Following restoration of cutaneous responses (14)	107.2 ± 4.0
Normal controls	117.5 ± 1.6

*$P < 0.01$

returns toward normal with recovery of normal responses (Table 4.8). This evolution of chemotaxis to normal is more clearly seen in the trauma group subsequently discussed. The influence of anergic and normal serum upon anergic and normal neutrophils shows that anergic serum inhibits chemotaxis of normal and possibly anergic neutrophils (Table 4.9). Anergic serum has been found to consistently inhibit chemotaxis of normal cells. We are in the process of characterizing the inhibitors. In a series of 12 patients, a weak but statistically significant correlation between neutrophil chemotaxis and neutrophil phagocytosis and bactericidal killing has been established.

Table 4.9   Influence of serum on neutrophil chemotaxis

	Stimulated migration
Anergic cells: normal serum	93.0 ± 3.7*
Anergic cells: anergic serum	86.2 ± 3.5*
Normal cells: normal serum	121.2 ± 1.6†
Normal cells: anergic serum	103.6 ± 2.6†

* $P < 0.01$
† $P < 0.001$

The presence of abnormal skin tests not only indicates who appears susceptible to sepsis but also those patients with abnormalities of some components of host defence which when found in patients with primary defects are related to recurrent infection. We have concluded that in the setting of these numerous but often complicated tests in patients, the failure of delayed hypersensitivity is a non-specific indicator of altered antibacterial host defences and is not related to CMI.

The pre-operative group of patients support clearly the suggestion that anergy present at time zero is associated with the subsequent development of sepsis. In other patients it becomes difficult to say that sepsis is a result of, rather than a cause of abnormal host defences. The aetiological factors listed in Table 4.10 indicate that sepsis is indeed a major aetiological factor in the

Table 4.10   Clinical association in 165 anergic patients

Sepsis	67	41%
Multiple factors	51	31%
Trauma	22	13%
Shock	14	8.5
Malnutrition	6	3.6
Unknown	5	3.0

evolution of abnormal skin tests and associated defects in host defence. Malnutrition is a much more significant factor than it appears to be, as it contributed in most of the patients with multifactorial problems and many of those with sepsis.

In an attempt to resolve which comes first, anergy and altered HDM or sepsis, a series of 53 patients with multiple injuries from blunt trauma was studied[50]. The severity of injury was assessed by assigning one point to long-bone fractures, pelvic fracture abdominal injury, chest injury and head injury (to a maximum of five). Skin tests and neutrophil chemotaxis evaluations were done as soon as possible after the accident, in some instances within hours. The development of anergy or relative anergy following injury were found to be a function of the age of the patient and the severity of injury (Figure 4.2). Patients who became A or RA did so promptly and had a significantly higher incidence of sepsis than normal responders. Mortality rate was also higher but the numbers are small.

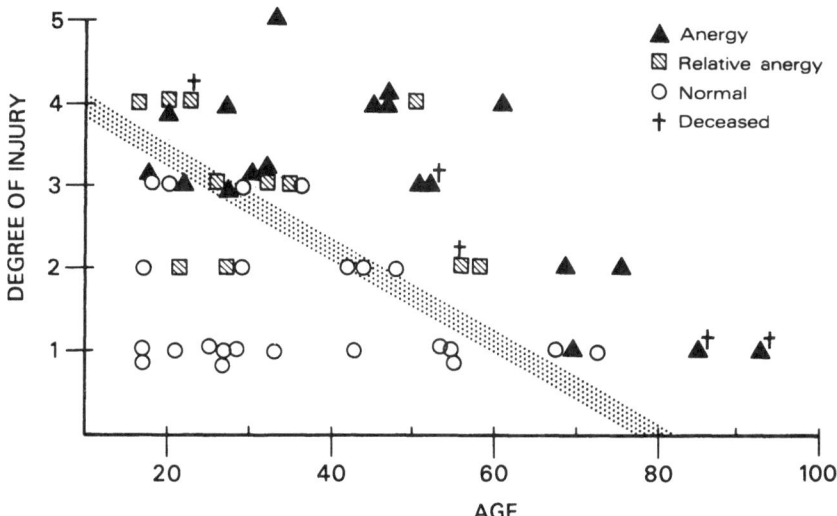

Figure 4.2 Graphic representation of relationship between patient's age, degree of injury and skin-test response. The shaded area is a hypothetical line between advancing age, degree of injury and development of anergy. Patients who died are indicated. (Reproduced by permission of authors and publishers, *J. Trauma*, 1978, **18**, 240)

Neutrophil chemotaxis was studied in 32 patients and was found reduced in both A and RA patients. Patients with minimal trauma and normal skin tests have normal chemotaxis, however, normal skin tests in presence of multiple injury, averaging 2.5 systems produces a transient abnormality of neutrophil chemotaxis. These data together with evolution and improvement of abnormal chemotaxis in all A and RA patients are seen in Figure 4.3. The evolution of chemotaxis in four patients of about the same age but differing degrees of trauma is seen in Figure 4.4. Abnormal chemotaxis was found to be a more accurate predictor of the development of sepsis than skin testing. In all anergic patients examined there is a serum inhibitor of chemotaxis of normal neutrophils.

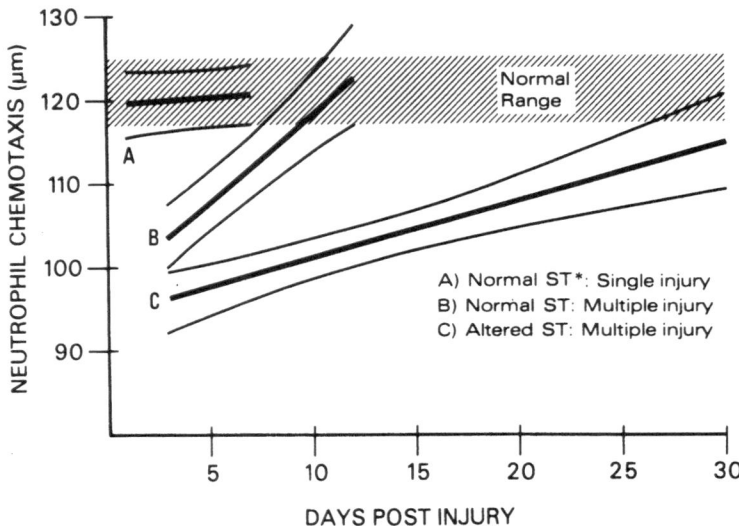

Figure 4.3   Regression of the two groups of normals and all patients with altered cutaneous responses on days post injury. (Reproduced by permission of authors and publishers, *J. Trauma,* 1978, **18**, 240) (*ST = Skin test)

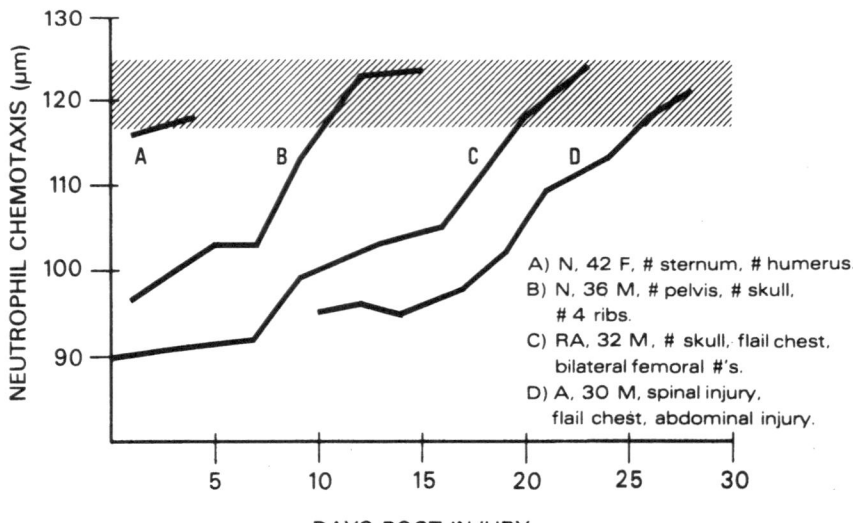

Figure 4.4   Four patients of similar age, different injury and skin-test responses showing patterns of abnormality and recovery to normal of neutrophil chemotaxis. (Reproduced by permission of authors and publishers, *J. Trauma,* 1978, **18**, 240)

In this reasonably homogeneous patient group it is clear that the injury and not sepsis are responsible for development of anergy and abnormal neutrophil function. It is therefore likely that these acquired abnormalities are also responsible at least in part for the high incidence of sepsis in the anergic patient.

4.4.2 Burns

Thermal injury is the most severe form of trauma which we manage and the survival of each patient presents a constant challenge. All components of the immune response are affected following thermal injury. This injury is the prototype of acquired derangement of host defences, all of which return to normal following resolution and healing of the burn wound.

Immunoglobulins of all classes have been found to be reduced following thermal injury in both adults and children[52,53]. The early reductions are likely to be secondary to loss as a result of generalized catabolism, leakage into burn wound and interstitial spaces and to some dilutional effect following the enormous volumes of fluids required for resuscitation. Alexander and Moncrief[53] have clearly shown that the primary humoral response to an antigen was reduced but present although the anamnestic response to tetanus was earlier and larger than in normals. The importance of these alterations might be minimal until examined in the context of all of the other abnormalities of host defence which are present in the burn injury. Complement levels are slightly reduced following thermal injury but become increasingly so, in the presence of sepsis where Alexander[54] has coined the concept and provided data for a consumptive opsonopathy.

Macrophage and reticuloendothelial system (RES) function is difficult to study in humans, and animal studies yield most data, some of which is conflicting. It does, however, appear that RES function is somewhat depressed and that there is a reduced ability to deliver monocytes to an inflammatory focus.

Cell-mediated immunity is markedly altered following thermal injury. Both man and the experimental animal suffering from thermal injuries can accept allografts from unrelated donors and occasionally multiple donors with the grafts lasting as long as 8 months[55]. Xenografts, pigskin, have been noted to survive for prolonged periods in patients with burn injury of greater than 30% of body surface[56]. We have noted, as have others, that burned patients are anergic to recall antigens. Recovery of these responses follow coverage of the burn wound.

Neutrophil function in many of its aspects is altered following a major burn injury. Bactericidal function is markedly abnormal following thermal injury and appears to be directly related to the development of septic episodes[57]. It is of interest that once the burn wound is covered bactericidal function returns to normal (Figure 4.5). Neutrophil chemotaxis was also shown to be markedly defective. These defects are usually related to the size of the burn and are important in the development of septic processes. It is of interest that improvement in neutrophil bactericidal function through nutritional support has reduced the number of septicaemias seen in one burn centre[58].

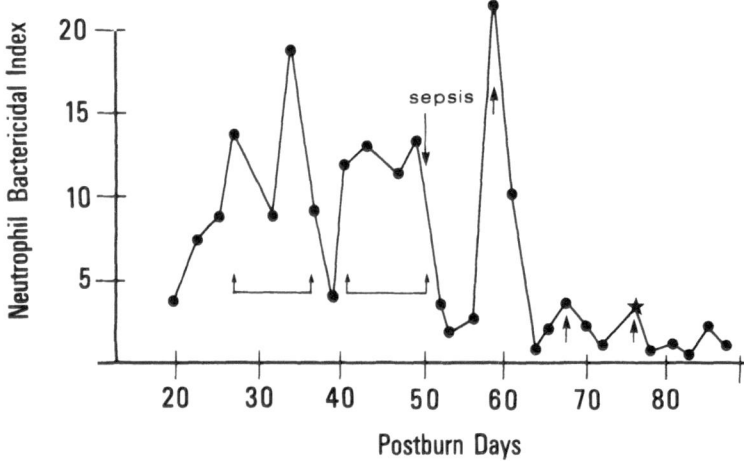

Figure 4.5   Neutrophil bactericidal index (NBI) of a 4-year-old boy with a 61% burn from 20th to 88th post-burn day. The star indicates full coverage of the burn followed by normal NBI. Abnormal NBI is 4 or greater: periodicity is shown by arrows and episodes of *Pseudomonas* sepsis followed by a period of marked abnormal NBI.

In summary, it is clear that major burn injuries (30% of body surface or greater), produce diffuse alteration in most components of host defence. The burn wound itself presents an inviting area for infection, however, the immunosuppressive effect of the thermal injury is responsible in major part for the high incidence of and mortality from sepsis.

4.4.3   Surgery and anaesthesia

It becomes very difficult to separate the effects of surgery and anaesthesia on the immune response as they are in most instances inextricably intertwined. In rats, there was a reduction in leukocyte counts and in post-operative antibody production which returned to normal by 72 hours. Phagocytosis and allergic responses may be depressed. Neutrophil chemotaxis is not affected by anaesthetics or superficial surgery but is markedly reduced by abdominal or cardiac surgery[59]. Phagocytosis is probably not affected. Slade[60] has examined many aspects of CMI and found that B and T cells are reduced and that PHA responses and MLC reactivity are reduced and do not return to normal for some time. There are many reports supporting abnormalities of CMI post-operatively. At present, these cannot be related to the development of infection although they may be important in the spread of tumour cells. Anaesthetic gases do appear to affect immune cell function, B and T cells and phagocytes; what this means for the patient is not clear.

4.4.4 Trauma and shock

Sepsis is the major cause of death and morbidity in trauma once the patient has survived the early phases of the injury. Neutrophil chemotaxis, phagocytosis and bactericidal function may all be altered following injury. Severity of injury and age of the patient are important in production of these abnormalities. The burn injury, the most severe form of trauma from which patients regularly survive demonstrates the importance of age and severity of injury on the immune system and survival. After the shock phase is over, sepsis is the principal cause of death in burned patients. There is a direct relationship between age, size of burn and mortality rate. The reticuloendothelial system may also be depressed following trauma; this defect is of short duration and is often followed by a rebound effect. There is no difference in the primary or anamnestic antibody response. Cell-mediated immunity does not appear affected by trauma.

In summary, in those clinical situations in which there is injury of a traumatic nature there are a variety of alterations in host defence. If the injury can be quantified, the acquired defects are a function of the severity of the injury and the age of the patient.

4.4.5 Immunosuppressive effect of pharmocologic agents

The immunosuppressive effect of drugs is a double-edged sword. It is clear that the development of transplantation would not have been possible and treatment of many different immunologic diseases troublesome without many of these agents but in particular 'steroids'.

The *adrenocortical steroids* have been the cornerstone of immunosuppressive therapy since their development in the 1950s. Their effects include: reduced lymphoid proliferation, lympholysis of B and T cells in high concentrations, reduction in antibody formation, inhibition of neutrophil and monocyte chemotaxis, suppression of inflammation, prolongation of tissue allografts with concomitant effects upon afferent and efferent arcs of cell-mediated immunity. Clearly one of the side effects of steroid usage is the development of infectious complications.

The purine antagonists, azothiaprine and 6-mercaptopurine, have significant immunosuppressive properties and have been, together with the corticosteroids, the agents that have allowed clinical transplantation to become a reality. Timing and dosage is important but when administered just before the antigen, delayed hypersensitivity and inflammation is reduced, primary antibody and anamnestic response abolished, and allograft survival promoted. The development of viral infection is common in these patients. If dosage is not carefully controlled, bone marrow suppression and neutropenia frequently leads to bacterial or fungal infection.

There are two classes of drugs which are extensively utilized in cancer chemotherapy, the folic acid antagonists and alkylating agents, which are effective in treating neoplastic disease and have a profound effect upon the immune system. In general, their effect is directed against actively dividing cells, therefore they may inhibit antibody response and most other lymphocyte-mediated immune reactions. Methotrexate can prolong homograft survival as well as facilitate induction of tolerance and treat graft versus host reactions. The infectious complications of these drugs are largely related to bone marrow suppression. Neutrophil function does not otherwise seem grossly affected.

Antibiotics may have immunosuppressive properties and may theoretically be working at odds with therapy. The high incidence of superinfection in patients on antibiotic therapy particularly the development of Candida infections has been ascribed in part to antibiotic-mediated immuno-suppression. The major practical difficulty relates to bone marrow sup-pression which results occasionally from many antibiotics. The tragic non-reversible idiosyncratic bone marrow aplasia from chloramphenicol is the best known of these effects.

There are other classes of drugs which may have some immunosuppressive activity of which the salicylates are the best known and most important.

4.4.6   Disease states associated with immunosuppression

Diabetic patients are well known for their increased susceptibility to infection. This predilection is a multifactorial problem which can be aggravated by infection itself. Arterial insufficiency, as seen in the extremities and in the kidneys, is more responsible for the high incidence of infections in these areas than the slightly decreased neutrophil function and otherwise slightly altered immune response. The vascular injury is such that the somewhat altered defences cannot be delivered adequately and there is a compound additive abnormality. The development of keto-acidosis compounds the problem by worsening perfusion and decreasing neutrophil function. The combination of decreased delivery of host defences together with altered local defences and slightly altered function becomes important.

Neoplastic disease may amongst its many effects alter the immune system. Hodgkin's disease has for many years been known to be associated with anergy to recall antigens and in patients with that disease the absence of delayed hypersensitivity, initially demonstrated against tuberculosis, is generally present. Abnormalities of other CMI mechanisms, particularly in the late stages, which may occur in neoplastic disease may account for the higher than expected incidence of viral infections in cancer patients. Humoral immunity is somewhat decreased in some such individuals; however, an anamnestic response to an antigen may be present while delayed hypersensitivity responses are absent.

Lymphomata other than those of Hodgkin's disease have not been as well studied, but abnormalities have also been shown to occur, particularly depressed PHA responses, prolonged homograft survival and absent delayed hypersensitivity responses. Furthermore primary and secondary humoral immune responses are abnormally low.

Chronic lymphocytic leukaemia is associated with altered B and T lymphocyte responses to specific and non-specific mitogens, abnormal delayed hypersensitivity responses, increasingly severe hypogammaglobulinaemia and altered phagocytic and bactericidal function of neutrophils. The increase in infections seen in acute leukaemia is a reflection of the marked reduction in normal circulating neutrophils and monocytes. The circulating phagocytes have altered levels of myeloperoxidase and lysozyme and in addition, carbohydrate metabolism may be altered. These defects together with immune alterations and production of neutropenia caused by chemotherapeutic induction of remission now make sepsis the major cause of death from leukaemia.

Solid tumours may be associated with a broad range of immunologic abnormalities. As with the haemotological malignancies, the stage, nature and extent of the tumour bear upon the immunological abnormalities which develop in association with cancer. All aspects of CMI are altered, the most obvious abnormality being cutaneous anergy. Delayed hypersensitivity in neoplastic disease has been shown to be related to duration of survival; those with anergy have a markedly reduced survival and decreased responsiveness to chemotherapy.

It must be pointed out that advanced cancer and chemotherapy present an increased risk to the patient with immunodeficiencies. Severe infectious problems are seen more frequently in the treatment of haematological neoplasia but are common whenever vigorous chemotherapy is utilized particularly with advanced malignancy.

Apart from the immune abnormalities which are naturally secondary to neoplastic disease, as the cancer advances there are anatomical and nutritional alterations which are associated with the development of sepsis.

4.4.7 Malnutrition and acquired immunodeficiency

The relationship between malnutrition and infection has been observed for a long time and is discussed in detail in chapter 6. A broad range of immunodeficiencies involving most components of the immune response have been described in malnutrition. Their relationship to infection seems intuitively clear but has been difficult to prove. The question has been raised as to whether malnutrition decreases the immune response or infection precipitates malnutrition. Both of these statements are probably correct and the interaction of infection, malnutrition, and immunodeficiency is probably a vicious circle each making the next stage worse.

The abnormalities of host-defence mechanisms in malnutrition include somewhat decreased phagocytic and bactericidal function, decreased lymphocyte response to mitogens, reduced or absent delayed hypersensitivity responses, generally reduced complement levels and reduced antibody responses. It is interesting that many children with protein calorie malnutrition have increased levels of immunoglobulins, a phenomenon probably related to continuous exposure to bacterial and parasitic infections. Primary antibody responses are impaired to a greater degree than secondary responses.

The incidence of malnutrition on a world-wide basis is great and has been estimated to be as high as three-quarters of the world population. In developed countries it has been found that the nutritional levels of hospital patients is decreased, particularly in cancer patients and upon surgical wards. The use of total parenteral nutrition[61,62,63] and oral hyperalimentation[58] has been shown not only to restore host defences to normal but also to reduce the associated rates of sepsis. The malnourished patients are usually anergic and restoration of body cell mass restores cutaneous responses to normal in about a third[64].

4.5 SUMMARY

The primary immunodeficiencies have led the way to definition and characterization of the importance and role of the various components of host defence in development of recurrent infections. It has become clear that the incidence of acquired defects in host resistance are a common problem in modern clinical practice and that they have major implications for the patient most particularly in the high incidence of associated infections. The aetiological factors producing these abnormalities cover a broad range of medical and surgical illnesses. The development of methods of immunomodulation is the next step in the management of these common abnormalities and will hopefully lead to reduced rates of sepsis, reduced morbidity and mortality and a longer and better quality of life for our patients.

References

1. Bruton, O. C. (1952). Agammaglobulinaemia. *Pediatrics*, **9**, 72
2. Good, R. A. (1968). Fatal (chronic) granulomatous disease of childhood: A hereditary defect of leukocyte function. *Semin. Hematol.*, **5**, 215

3. Holmes, B., Quie, P. G., Windhorst, D. B. and Good, R. A. (1966). Fatal granulomatous disease of childhood. An inborn abnormality of phagocytic function. *Lancet*, i, 1225

4. Berendes, H., Bridges, R. A. and Good, R. A. (1957). A fatal granulomatosis of childhood. *Min. Med.*, **40**, 309

5. Bridges, R. A., Berendes, H. and Good, R. A. (1957). A fatal granulomatous disease of childhood. *Am. J. Dis. Child.*, **97**, 387

6. Landing, B. H. and Shirkey, H. S. (1957). A syndrome of recurrent infection and infiltration of viscera by pigmented lipid histiocytes. *Pediatrics*, **20**, 431

7. Davis, S. D., Schaller, J. and Wedgewood, R. J. (1966). *Job's syndrome*: Recurrent 'Cold', staphylococcal abscesses. *Lancet*, i, 1013

8. Lehrer, R. I., Harifin, J. and Cline, M. J. (1969). Defective bactericidal activity in myeloperoxidase deficient human neutrophils. *Nature (Lond.)*, **223**, 78

9. Wolff, S. M., Dale, D. C., Clark, R. A., Root, R. K. and Kimball, H. R. (1972). The Chediak–Higashi syndrome: Studies on host defence. *Ann. Intern. Med.*, **76**, 293

10. Morley, A. and Stohlman, F. (1970). Cyclophosphamide-induced cyclical neutropenia: An animal model of human periodic disease. *N. Engl. J. Med.*, **282**, 642

11. Meakins, J. L. (1975). Host-defence mechanisms: Evaluation, acquired defects and immunotherapy. *Can. J. Surg.*, **18**, 259

12. Fudenberg, H. H., Good, R. A., Goodman, H. C., Hitzig, W., Kunken, H. G., Roitt, I. M., Rosen, F. S., Rowe, D. S., Seligmann, M. and Soothill, J. R. (1971). Primary immuno-deficiencies: Report of a World Health Organization Committee. *Pediatrics*, **47**, 927

13. Critlin, D. and Janeway, C. A. (1956). Agammaglobulinaemia, congenital, acquired and transient forms. *Prog. Hematol.*, I, 318

14. Good, R. A. and Zak, S. J. (1956). Disturbance in gammaglobulin/synthesis as 'Experiments of Nature'. *Pediatrics*, **18**, 109

15. Rosen, F. S. and Janeway, C. A. (1966). The gammaglobulins III. The antibody deficiency syndromes. *N. Engl. J. Med.*, **275**, 709

16. Stiehm, E. R. and Fudenberg, H. H. (1966). Clinical and immunologic features of dysgammaglobulinaemia type 1. *Am. J. Med.*, **40**, 805

17. Amman, A. J. and Hong, R. (1971). Selective IgA deficiency. Presentation of 30 cases and a review of the literature. *Medicine*, **50**, 223

18. Hobbs, J. R., Milner, R. D. G. and Watt, P. J. (1967). Gamma-M-deficiency predisposing to meningococcal septicaemia. *Br. Med. J.*, **2**, 583

19. Schur, P. H., Borel, H., Gelfand, E. W., Alper, C. A. and Rosen, F. S. (1970). Selective gamma-G-globulin deficiencies in patients with recurrent pyogenic infections. *N. Engl. J. Med.*, **283**, 631

20. Di George, A. M. (1968). Congenital absence of the thymus and its immunologic consequences. Concurrence with congenital hypoparathyroidism. In: *Immunologic Deficiency Diseases in Man* (D. Bergman and F. A. McKusick, eds.) (Baltimore: Williams and Williams)

21. Kilpatrick, C. H., Rich, R. R. and Bennet, J. E. (1971). Chronic mucocutaneous candidiasis. Model building in cellular immunity. *Ann. Intern. Med.*, **75**, 955

22. Lehner, T. (1969). Chronic candidiasis. *Trans. St John's Hosp. Dermatol. Soc.*, **50**, 8

23. Stoessel, T. P., Root, R. K. and Vaughan, M. (1972). Phagocytosis in chronic granulomatous disease and the Chediak–Higashi syndrome. *N. Engl. J. Med.*, **286**, 120

24. Johnston, R. B. and Boehner, R. L. (1971). Chronic granulomatous disease: Correlation between pathogenesis and clinical findings. *Pediatrics*, **48**, 730

25. Miller, M. E., Oski, F. A. and Harris, M. B. (1971). Lazy-leukocyte syndrome. A new disorder of neutrophil function. *Lancet*, i, 665

25. Constantopoulos, A., Najjar, V. A. and Smith, J. W. (1972). Tuftsin deficiency. A new syndrome with defective phagocytosis. *J. Pediatr.*, **80**, 564

27. Cooper, M. D., DeChatelet, L. R., McCall, C. E., La Via, M. F., Spurr, C. L. and

Baehner, R. L. (1972). Complete deficiency of leukocyte glucose-6-phosphate dehydrogenase with defective bactericidal activity. *J. Clin. Invest.*, **51**, 769

28. Lehner, R. I. and Cline, M. J. (1969). Leukocyte myeloperoxidase deficiency and disseminated candidiasis. The role of myeloperoxidase in resistance to candida infection. *J. Clin. Invest.*, **48**, 1478

29. Hill, H. R. and Quie, P. G. (1974). Raised IgE levels and defective neutrophil chemotaxis in three children with eczema, and recurrent bacterial infections. *Lancet*, **i**, 183

30. Miller, M. E. and Nilsson, N. R. (1970). A familial deficiency of the phagocytosis enhancing activity of serum related to a dysfunction of the fifth component of complement. *N. Engl. J. Med.*, **282**, 354

31. Alper, C. A., Abramson, N., Johnston, R. B., Jandl, J. H., Watson, L. and Rosen, F. S. (1970). Studies *in vitro* and *in vivo* of an abnormality in the metabolism of C3 in a patient with increased susceptibility to infection. *J. Clin. Invest.*, **49**, 1975

32. Alper, C. A., Black, K. J. and Rosen, F. S. (1973). Increased susceptibility to infection in a patient with type II essential hypercatabolism of C3. *N. Engl. J. Med.*, **288**, 601

33. Day, N. K., McLean, G. R., Michael, A. and Good, R. A. (1973). C2 deficiency. Development of lupus erythematosous. *J. Clin. Invest.*, **52**, 1601

34. Day, N. K., Stoud, G. R., DeBracio, M., Mancando, B., Windhorst, D. and Good, R. A. (1972). C1R deficiency. An unknown error associated with cutaneous and renal disease. *J. Clin. Invest.*, **51**, 1102

35. Warra, D. W., Reiter, E. O., Doyele, N. E., Gewurz, H. and Ammann, A. J. (1975). Persistent C1Q deficiency in a patient with a systemic lupus-like syndrome. *J. Pediatr.*, **86**, 743

36. Hitzig, W. H. (1973). Congenital thymus and lymphocytic deficiency disorders. In: *Immunologic Disorders in Infants and Children* (E. R. Stiehm and V. Fulgitini, eds.) (Philadelphia: W. B. Saunders)

37. Lawlar, G. J., Ammann, A. J., Wright, W. C., La Fanchi, S. H., Bilstrom, D. and Stiehm, R. E. (1974). The syndrome of cellular immunodeficiency with abnormal immunoglobulin synthesis. *J. Pediatr.*, **84**, 183

38. Giblett, E. R., Ammann, A. J., Sandman, R., Wara, D. W. and Diamond, L. K. (1975). Nucleoside phosphasylase deficiency in a child with severely defective T-cell immunity and normal B-cell immunity. *Lancet*, **i**, 1010

39. Neuwissen, H. J., Pollava, B. and Pickering, R. J. (1975). Combined immunodeficiency disease associated with adenosine deaminase deficiency. *J. Pediatr.*, **86**, 169

40. Blaese, R. M., Strober, W., Brown, R. S. and Waldman, T. A. (1968). The Wiskott–Aldrich syndrome. A disorder with a possible defect in antigen processing or recognition. *Lancet*, **i**, 1056

41. Boder, E. and Sedwick, R. P. (1975). Ataxia telangiectasia. A familial syndrome of progressive cerebellar ataxia, occulocutaneous telangiectasia and frequent pulmonary infection. *Univ. S. Calif. Med. Bull.*, **9**, 15

42. Peterson, R. D. A., Cooper, M. D. and Good, R. A. (1966). Lymphoid tissue abnormalities associated with ataxia telangiectasia. *Am. J. Med.*, **41**, 342

43. Ammann, A. J., Sutcliff, W. and Millichick, E. (1974). Antibody-mediated immunodeficiency in short-limbed dwarfism. *J. Pediatr.*, **84**, 200

44. Lux, S. E. (1970). Chronic neutropenia and abnormal cellular immunity in cartilage hair hypoplasia. *N. Engl. J. Med.*, **282**, 234

45. Kretschmer, R., August, C. S., Rosen, F. S. and Janeway, C. A. (1969). Recurrent infections episodic lymphopenia and impaired cellular immunity. *N. Engl. J. Med.*, **281**, 285

46. MacLean, L. D., Meakins, J. L., Taguchi, K., Duignan, J. P., Dhillan, K. and Gordon, J. (1975). Host resistance in sepsis and trauma. *Ann. Surg.*, **182**, 207

47. Pietsch, J. B., Meakins, J. L. and MacLean, L. D. (1977). The delayed hypersensitivity response. Application in clinical surgery. *Surgery*, **82**, 349

48. Meakins, J. L., Pietsch, J. B., Bubenik, O., Kelly, R., Rode, H., Gordon, J. and MacLean, L. D. (1977). Delayed hypersensitivity. Indicator of acquired failure of host defences in sepsis and trauma. *Ann. Surg.*, **186**, 241

49. Zigmond, S. H. and Hirsch, J. G. (1973). Leukocyte locomotion and chemotaxis. *J. Exp. Med.*, **137**, 387

50. Meakins, J. L., McLean, A. P. H., Kelly, R., Pietsch, J. B. and Bubenik, O. (1978). Delayed hypersensitivity response and neutrophil chemotaxis. Effect of trauma. *J. Trauma*, **18**, 240

51. Arteison, G., Högman, C. F., Johnson, S. G. O. and Killander, J. (1969). Changes in immunoglobulin levels in severely burned patients. *Lancet*, **i**, 546

52. Ritzmann, S. E., McLung, C. and Falls, D. (1969). Immunoglobulin levels in burned patients. *Lancet*, **i**, 1152

53. Alexander, J. W. and Moncrief, J. A. (1966). Alterations of the immune response following severe thermal injury. *Arch. Surg.*, **93**, 75

54. Alexander, J. W., McClelland, M. A., Ogle, C. K. and Ogle, J. D. (1976). Consumptive opsonopathy. Possible pathogenesis in lethal and opportunistic infections. *Ann. Surg.*, **184**, 672

55. Kay, G. D. (1957). Prolonged survival of a skin homograft in a patient with very extensive burns. *Ann. N.Y. Acad. Sci.*, **64**, 64

56. Polk, H. C. (1968). Prolongation of xenograft survival in patients with pseudomonas sepsis; a clarification. *Surg. Forum*, **19**, 514

57. Alexander, J. W. and Meakins, J. L. (1972). A physiologic basis for opportunistic infection. *Ann. Surg.*, **176**, 273

58. Alexander, J. W. (1974). Emerging concepts in control of clinical infection. *Surgery*, **75**, 934

59. Bubenik, O. and Meakins, J. L. (1976). Neutrophil chemotaxis in surgical patients. Effect of cardiopulmonary bypass. *Surg. Forum*, **27**, 267

60. Slade, M. S., Simmons, R. L., Yunis, E. J. and Greenberg, L. J. (1975). Immunodepression after major surgery in normal patients. *Surgery*, **78**, 363

61. Dionigi, R., Zonta, A., Dominioni, L., Gnes, F. and Ballabio, A. (1977). The effects of total parenteral nutrition on immunodepression due to malnutrition. *Ann. Surg.*, **185**, 467

62. Law, D. K., Dudrick, S. J. and Abdou, N. I. (1973). Immunocompetence of patients with protein–calorie malnutrition. The effects of nutritional repletion. *Ann. Intern. Med.*, **79**, 545

63. Law, D. K., Dudrich, S. J. and Abdou, N. I. (1974). The effects of dietary protein depletion on immunocompetence. The importance of nutritional repletion prior to immunologic induction. *Ann. Surg.*, **179**, 168

64. Spanier, A. H., Pietsch, J. B., Meakins, J. L., MacLean, L. D. and Shizgal, H. M. (1976). The relationship between immune competence and nutrition. *Surg. Forum*, **27**, 332

5
Immunodeficiency

A. R. HAYWARD

5.1   INTRODUCTION   153
    5.1.1   *The interdependence of immunity mechanisms*   154
    5.1.2   *The cellular basis of antibody responses*   155
    5.1.3   *Classification of immunodeficiency*   157
    5.1.4   *The cellular basis of antibody deficiency*   157

5.2   ANTIBODY DEFICIENCY   158
    5.2.1   *Introduction*   158
    5.2.2   *Classification*   159
    5.2.3   *Congenital X-linked panhypogammaglobulinaemia*   160
    5.2.4   *Congenital hypogammaglobulinaemia in girls*   161
    5.2.5   *Hypogammaglobulinaemia with IgM*   161
    5.2.6   *Transient hypogammaglobulinaemia*   162
    5.2.7   *Transcobalamin II deficiency*   162
    5.2.8   *IgA deficiency*   163
        5.2.8.1   *Clinical features*   164
        5.2.8.2   *Allergy and IgA deficiency*   164
        5.2.8.3   *Autoimmunity and IgA deficiency*   165
    5.2.9   *Primary isolated IgM deficiency*   165
    5.2.10 *Varied immunodeficiency: predominantly antibody deficiency*   165
        5.2.10.1 *IgG subclass abnormalities*   167
        5.2.10.2 *Light-chain deficiencies*   167
    5.2.11 *Treatment of antibody deficiency*   167
        5.2.11.1 *IgG replacement*   167
        5.2.11.2 *Plasma infusions*   169
        5.2.11.3 *Antibiotics*   169

5.3 SELECTIVE DEFECTS OF CELL-MEDIATED
     IMMUNITY   169
     5.3.1 *Purine nucleoside phosphorylase (PNP) deficiency*   170
     5.3.2 *Thymic hypoplasia (Di George's syndrome)*   171
     5.3.3 *Cartilage hair hypoplasia*   172
     5.3.4 *Variable immunodeficiency affecting predominantly cell-
            mediated immunity*   172
     5.3.5 *Treatment of T-cell defects*   173
            5.3.5.1 *Fetal thymus grafts*   173
            5.3.5.2 *Thymus extracts (thymosin, thymopoietin)*   173
            5.3.5.3 *Transfer factor*   173

5.4 COMBINED IMMUNODEFICIENCY   174
     5.4.1 *Severe combined immunodeficiency (SCID)*   174
     5.4.2 *SCID associated with adenosine deaminase deficiency* 175
     5.4.3 *SCID with immunoglobulins*   176
     5.4.4 *SCID with leukopenia (reticular dysgenesis)*   177
     5.4.5 *Treatment of SCID*   177
            5.4.5.1 *Marrow grafting: problems of graft versus host
                     disease*   178
            5.4.5.2 *Donor selection*   178
            5.4.5.3 *Grafts of fetal tissue or thymic epithelial cells* 179
            5.4.5.4 *Treatment of ADA deficiency by red-cell
                     transfusion*   180

5.5 MISCELLANEOUS SYNDROMES ASSOCIATED WITH
     DEFECTS OF SPECIFIC IMMUNITY   180
     5.5.1 *Ataxia telangiectasia*   180
     5.5.2 *Wiskott–Aldrich syndrome*   181
     5.5.3 *Chronic mucocutaneous candidiasis*   181
     5.5.4 *Thymoma*   182
     5.5.5 *Lymphopenia with lymphocytotoxins*   182

5.6 PRIMARY DEFECTS OF NON-SPECIFIC IMMUNITY   183
     5.6.1 *Neutropenia*   183
     5.6.2 *Qualitative defects*   184
            5.6.2.1 *Leukocyte mobility defects*   184
            5.6.2.2 *Primary cellular defects*   184
            5.6.2.3 *Defects of phagocytosis*   185
            5.6.2.4 *Bacterial killing defects*   185
     5.6.3 *Complement defects*   187
            5.6.3.1 *Defects of inactivators of activated complement
                     components*   188
     5.6.4 *Opsonizing defects*   189

5.7   SECONDARY IMMUNODEFICIENCY   189
      5.7.1   Loss of immunoglobulin   190
      5.7.2   Loss of immunoglobulin and leukocytes 190
      5.7.3   Malnutrition   190
      5.7.4   Infections   191
      5.7.5   Splenectomy   191

5.8   DIAGNOSIS   191
      5.8.1   History   191
      5.8.2   Organisms   192
      5.8.3   Investigations   192

5.9   SPECIAL HAZARDS   195
      5.9.1   Immunization   195
      5.9.2   Blood transfusion   195

5.1   INTRODUCTION

Some people experience more infections than others. While environmental factors undoubtedly contribute to this difference, direct experiments in laboratory animals indicate that resistance to infection depends on immunity and that some animals make better immune responses than others. It seems likely that normal immunity varies as much as height or longevity. Many mechanisms, some of which operate independently, contribute to the avoidance of or recovery from infections so the consequences of a partial defect in a single one may not be clinically apparent. At present most of the immunodeficiencies we can identify are severe, with either a single gene inheritance or some other characteristic phenotypic manifestation, and without treatment they are commonly fatal. Such conditions are described in the greatest detail in this chapter, because they are best characterized. Lesser degrees of immunodeficiency are certainly commoner and family studies suggest that they contribute to other immunopathological events such as allergy and auto immunity. The diversity of symptoms in patients with different types of immunodeficiency makes classifications based on clinical features less useful for understanding aetiology or giving a prognosis than those based on laboratory results and inheritance. However, since patients present with symptoms, the clinical basis on which investigations are planned is discussed in a later section of the chapter. Specific and non-specific immunity mechanisms and their interdependence are briefly reviewed next in the context of the classification of immunodeficiency, and this is followed by discussion of the cellular basis of some forms of primary defects of specific immunity.

5.1.1 The interdependence of immunity mechanisms

The avoidance of infection depends on preventing the entry of potential pathogens into the body and on disposing of those that do succeed in bypassing mechanical barriers. Purely mechanical factors as a cause of recurrent infections at the affected site are easily overlooked but their importance is exemplified by children who develop recurrent meningitis with unusual bacteria because of an occipital dermoid sinus. More common but less amenable to cure are the recurrent respiratory tract infections of patients with cystic fibrosis, where mechanical factors are again responsible. Intact immune responses are insufficient in themselves if mechanical barriers are breached, or if, as in Kartagener's syndrome, their decontamination mechanisms are interfered with[1].

Specific immune responses are characterized by an adaptive change as a result of the first experience of an antigen. That part of the response which is mediated directly by T lymphocytes (and indirectly by mononuclear phagocytes through non-antigen-specific recruitment) is called cell-mediated immunity. Antibody responses (humoral immunity) depend on the triggering of appropriate populations of B lymphocytes to differentiate into plasma cells but, for the elimination of antigen, they require complement, for opsonization, and phagocytes. Thus the effector limbs of the two main components of the specific immune response both require non-antigen-specific factors to be fully effective. This interdependence accounts in part for the similarities between the types of infection experienced by patients with defects of either antibody, complement or phagocytes. The requirement for T lymphocytes to cooperate with B lymphocytes in the course of an antibody response is also clinically important, since patients with severely impaired cell-mediated immunity commonly make poor antibody responses.

T lymphocytes are also important for the control of antibody responses. They permit the rise in affinity (a term describing the quality of fit between antigen and antibody) and the switch in isotype (or immunoglobulin heavy-chain class) from IgM to IgG or IgA.

Animals challenged with antigen to which they have been previously exposed respond more rapidly and with greater magnitude than they did on first exposure. Such differences, which distinguish secondary from primary responses, imply the existence of an immunological memory. The cellular basis of this memory is probably an expanded clone of specific antigen-responsive T and B lymphocytes which did not undergo terminal differentiation during the primary response.

Defects of specific immunity encompass antibody deficiency and impaired cell-mediated immunity in either primary or secondary responses.

Non-specific immunity differs from specific immunity in that the few adaptive changes which occur, such as elevation of polymorph count or acute phase serum reactants, are transitory. There is no memory, since this is by definition specific. Both the mechanical factors mentioned above and a range of humoral and cellular factors are involved. Examples of non-specific humoral factors are transferrin, lysozyme, interferon and complement. Transferrin acts by binding iron and so reducing the amounts of this essential element which are available to bacteria. Although there is no specific pattern of infection associated with low transferrin levels it is likely that low levels of this protein contribute to the vulnerability to infection of severely protein-deprived children. Lysozyme, which acts only on the N-acetyl glucosamine of bacterial cell walls, and the interferons, which are exclusively anti-viral, are effective in laboratory systems but it is less easy to assess their importance *in vivo*. The importance of phagocytes (polymorphs and mononuclear) and the complement system, both of which are non-specific effectors of the specific immune response, is more obvious since defects at this level result in severe infections. If elimination of antigen is interfered with, the specific component of the immune response may not be able to mature or may even be rendered ineffective, providing a further example of the interdependence of immunity mechanisms.

5.1.2   The cellular basis of antibody responses

Immunoglobulins are made by plasma cells and the precursors of plasma cells are B lymphocytes. The small amounts of immunoglobulin which the latter make are not secreted but instead are incorporated into the cell surface membrane. This cell surface immunoglobulin has the same antigen-binding specificity as the immunoglobulin made by the plasma cell descendants of the B lymphocyte. The antigen-binding specificity is determined by the amino acid sequence in the variable region of the immunoglobulin molecule and this sequence, which is also detectable as idiotype, is conserved during differentiation of the cell. The constant region sequences, which determine the immunoglobulin heavy-chain class (or isotype), are not necessarily conserved; an example of a change is the maturation of a B lymphocyte with surface IgM and IgD to a plasma cell secreting IgG. In contrast, B lymphocytes with surface IgG or IgA mature into plasma cells making these isotypes, but not IgM.

The wide range of antigens which can be distinguished by the immune system arises from an equal diversity of B lymphocyte precursors, each with a restricted specificity. The cellular basis of the specific immune response rests on the triggering of the right lymphocyte. There are two requirements for B-cell triggering for most antibody responses: one is contact with antigen and the other is contact with a soluble helper factor derived from a T lymphocyte. The requirement for antigen at a B-cell level, and usually for the T cell too, ensures specificity. When the B cell is triggered it divides, giving rise to plasma cells and also to an expanded clone of B lymphocytes which remain available for triggering by more antigen. The T lymphocyte contribution to this process is called 'help' or 'cooperation' when the outcome is antibody production, or 'suppression' when the antibody response is prevented or halted. The B cell receives the T-cell signal through a surface receptor which is separate from the antigen receptor. Experimentally the receptor for help can be artificially stimulated by antibodies raised to it and this substitutes for T-cell help.

B lymphocytes bind antigen through their surface immunoglobulin receptors. Multivalent binding is required to trigger the cell and the threshold imposed by the quality of fit between antigen and cell surface receptor is the basis of specificity. Some large molecules, such as polysaccharides, with repeating subunits can trigger B cells independently of T-cell help. Many of these 'T-independent' antigens are also non-specific stimulants to B-cell proliferation, and when they induce antibody responses these are of IgM class. It seems likely that only a restricted subpopulation of B cells can respond directly to antigen in this way, and that most are dependent on T cells for help. Under normal circumstances T-independent B-cell responses are probably largely suppressed by T cells.

About 70% of human blood lymphocytes are thymus-dependent as judged by their rosetting with sheep erythrocytes or by immunofluorescent staining with specific antisera. Proliferative responses which characterize T lymphocytes include those evoked by foreign histocompatibility antigens (in mixed lymphocyte culture, MLC) and the plant mitogens phytohaemagglutinin (PHA) and Concanavalin A (Con A). Although T cells do not have readily detectable surface immunoglobulin like that on B cells, they nevertheless probably use the variable region of the heavy chain as their antigen receptors. About 60% of human T lymphocytes have receptors for the Fc region of IgM, and up to 10% can bind IgG; few if any cells bind both. Mouse T lymphocytes express an IgG receptor following activation but the functional significance of this is obscure. IgM-binding T cells can provide both help and suppression in a number of laboratory systems.

Macrophages are essential for antibody responses *in vitro* when purified populations of T and B lymphocytes are cultured with antigen. Experimentally, mononuclear phagocytes take up antigens in a non-specific way, and, while most of the ingested material is metabolized, a small proportion is returned to the cell surface where it is accessible to lymphocytes. Macrophages act as intermediaries in the transmission of both helper and suppressor factors from T lymphocytes to B cells, and they are also important mediators of both specific and non-specific immune responses.

It is difficult to study antigen-specific responses *in vitro* because of the small clone size of the reactive lymphocytes. An alternative is to trigger most B cells to divide by using a non-specific mitogen such as pokeweed mitogen (PWM). The B-lymphocyte response to this mitogen is, like specific antigen responses, dependent on T-cell help and subject to T-cell control. Thus B lymphocytes alone do not differentiate into plasma cells following PWM stimulation unless T lymphocytes are present to provide essential helper factors. The PMW response of separated B and T lymphocytes from immunodeficient patients, healthy controls and various mixtures of these cells have been studied extensively and the results are reviewed later.

5.1.3 Classification of immunodeficiency

Defects may be primary, and congenital or acquired, or secondary, and they may affect predominantly specific or non-specific immunity mechanisms. The ever-increasing complexity which this approach invites can be self-defeating so although fuller listings are possible[2] the material in this chapter is presented in the following sequence:

(a) Defects in specific immunity affecting predominantly (i) antibody, (ii) cell-mediated immunity, and (iii) antibody and cell mediated immunity.

(b) Defects in non-specific immunity affecting (i) phagocytes, and (ii) complement.

5.1.4 The cellular basis of antibody deficiency

Boys with congenital X-linked panhypogammaglobulinaemia lack B lymphocytes in their blood, whereas they have normal numbers of T cells[3]. In general these T cells are able to help normal B cells differentiate so the lack of plasma cells in this disorder is secondary to the lack of B lymphocytes. Interestingly, affected children have B-lymphocyte precursors (pre-B cells, which have trace amounts of IgM in their cytoplasm but lack surface immunoglobulin) in their marrow[4]. Why these cells fail to develop into B lymphocytes is at present unknown, and attempts to induce their differentiation *in vitro*, using agents such as cyclic AMP and GMP, have been unsuccessful.

In contrast to the relatively rare boys mentioned above, most patients with hypogammaglobulinaemia do have B lymphocytes[5]. In some cases these cells differentiate into plasma cells when stimulated by PWM in the presence of T lymphocytes. Immunoglobulin in plasma cells is glycosylated before it is secreted. In a few patients a failure of the glycosylation appears to be associated with hypogammaglobulinaemia[6]. Recently interest has centred on patients whose B lymphocytes will differentiate when cultured with normal T cells, but not with their own T cells. Waldmann *et al.*[7] were the first to show that the T cells in some of these patients could suppress differentiation in cultures of normal blood lymphocytes, thus providing experimental support for the hypothesis that the primary defect involves too much suppression. Further studies indicate that patients with hypogammaglobulinaemia with B lymphocytes can be divided according to whether (a) PWM stimulated cultures of their blood lymphocytes generate plasma cells, (b) their isolated B cells can respond only when cultured with normal T cells, or (c) their B cells do not differentiate even in the presence of normal T cells. Family studies will be required to assess the aetiological significance of such distinctions and until they become available it would be prudent to continue to classify these patients together. Occasionally boys with X-linked congenital panhypogammaglobulinaemia have been found to have increased T-cell suppressor activity so this effect can presumably be secondary, perhaps resulting from excessive antigen stimulus without the humoral feedback by antibody. Another difficulty in interpreting the results of mixtures of patient and control lymphocytes in PWM-stimulated cultures is that different effects may be observed with different controls[8].

The importance of T cells in most antibody responses has been emphasized above, and it is not surprising that experimental animals lacking T lymphocytes (such as the nude mouse) are bad at making antibodies, especially of IgG and IgA classes. The apparently normal immunoglobulin concentrations and antibody titres of infants with De George's syndrome (congenital thymic hypoplasia) is puzzling in this respect and is discussed later.

In severe combined immunodeficiency there is congenital deficiency of both antibody- and cell-mediated immunity. These patients have very variable blood lymphocyte populations (presumably reflecting the heterogeneity of the disorder), but some have normal or high proportions of B cells. In at least one case these B lymphocytes have been found to differentiate normally into plasma cells in the presence of T lymphocytes from a healthy donor. In several other cases a fatal graft versus host disease has been accompanied by a transient rise in immunoglobulins, under circumstances where the immunoglobulin-producing cells were probably of host origin. Both observations would suggest that a lack of T cells can be a primary aetiological factor in some forms of severe combined immunodeficiency.

5.2 ANTIBODY DEFICIENCY

5.2.1 Introduction

Antibody deficiency is usually associated with low serum levels of immunoglobulins and in such cases the term 'hypogammaglobulinaemia' is appropriate. However, complete absence of all immunoglobulin from the serum, even using such relatively insensitive methods as radial immunodiffusion, is unusual and most patients have at least some IgM or IgG. A patient's ability to make antibody is a much better guide to his susceptibility to infection than the serum immunoglobulin concentration. This point is illustrated by the strong association between meningitis and isohaemagglutinin deficiency in the MRC series on hypogammaglobulinaemia[9]. Some of the patients who developed meningitis had normal or high serum IgM concentration which presumably lacked any appropriate antibody specificity.

A very few individuals have been described who failed to make antibody responses following immunization but who had completely normal serum immunoglobulin concentrations; they experienced recurrent infections typical of hypogammaglobulinaemia. Since susceptibility to infection correlates more closely with the antibody response than with the serum immunoglobulin concentrations the designation 'antibody deficiency' is clinically more useful than 'hypogammaglobulinaemia'.

5.2.2 Classification

There is no completely satisfactory basis for classifying antibody deficiency syndromes. Even the most obvious possible division, into those with or without immunoglobulin, is complicated by the presence of trace amounts of IgG in some boys with congenital X-linked panhypogammaglobulinaemia who lack B lymphocytes and plasma cells. Indeed, from the cellular considerations described earlier, the only patients one might expect to lack all immunoglobulins are those without pre-B cells, namely a few cases of severe combined immunodeficiency and some patients with thymomas[4].

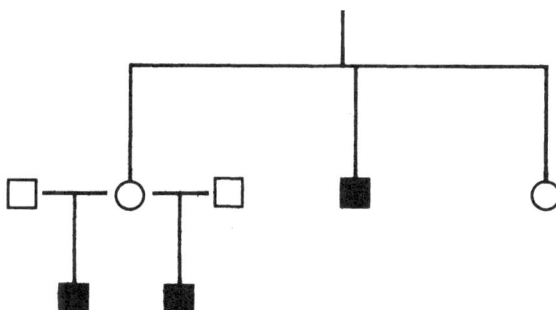

Figure 5.1 Boys with congenital X-linked hypogammaglobulinaemia (■); a family with clear evidence for X linkage

Family trees like the one in Figure 5.1 give good evidence of X-linked transmission and make it possible to recognize at least some hypogammaglobulinaemia phenotypes. Small family size limits the value of this approach for the diagnosis of individual patients. Genetic studies in particular show up the deficiencies of classifications based on serum concentrations of individual immunoglobulin isotypes because of the phenotypic variation which occurs between relatives, even in a condition as apparently well-defined as congenital X-linked panhypogammaglobulinaemia. In practice a combination of genetic, laboratory and clinical features are used to define a few antibody deficiency syndromes (Table 5.1), but most patients still have to be included under the heading 'variable immunodeficiency'. The clinical features are similar in many forms of severe antibody deficiency so, to avoid repetition, they are only described in detail for the congenital X-linked form of the disease.

Table 5.1   Primary antibody deficiency syndromes

	Inheritance
Congenital panhypogammaglobulinaemia	{ X-linked { AR
Hypogammaglobulinaemia with IgM	{ X-linked { Unknown
Transient hypogammaglobulinaemia	Unknown
Transcobalamin II deficiency	AR
Selective IgA deficiency	Unknown
Selective IgM deficiency	Unknown
Unclassified types: (1) with normal cell-mediated immunity (2) with defective cell-mediated immunity	

5.2.3   Congenital X-linked panhypogammaglobulinaemia

The transplacental passage of immunoglobulin usually provides affected infants with enough antibodies to avoid infections for the first few months of life. Subsequently, the failure of antibody synthesis generally results in recurrent bacterial infections, particularly of the respiratory tract and skin. The organisms responsible are usually streptococci, staphylococci or Gram-negative bacilli and there is a tendency for infection to spread, resulting in septicaemias and meningitis. Neither the sites of infection nor the organisms involved are unique to this form of hypogammaglobulinaemia. There is a remarkable variation in the frequency and severity of infections between patients, which presumably reflects differences in their exposure to pathogens or possibly differences in the efficiency with which non-specific immune mechanisms can compensate for the failure of antibody production.

The diagnosis rests primarily on the laboratory finding of very low levels of all classes of serum immunoglobulins together with a history of affected maternal male relatives. At present this often takes the form of maternal uncles having died in infancy of pneumonia or unexplained causes. The reduction in family size in contemporary society makes it more difficult to recognize a genetic pattern and although an affected male sibling is compatible with the diagnosis it is not diagnostic of an X-linked transmission.

Physical findings are not generally helpful in diagnosis though a relative hypoplasia of lymphoid tissue, and very small tonsils and adenoids, are typical. Other findings, such as bronchiectasis or hearing loss, are useful guides to the severity of past infections.

Investigations serve mainly to define the extent of structural damage to vulnerable sites such as the respiratory tract, and to identify any continuing infections. Haemolytic complement titres and the blood polymorph count should be normal, as should the lymphocyte count. Affected boys lack B lymphocytes in their blood, so the percentage of T lymphocytes (by the E-rosette test) is generally high. There may be an increased number of 'null' cells with IgG (Fc) and C3 receptors but without stable surface immuno-globulin or 1a antigens. Many null cells in the patients have monocyte characteristics such as positive staining with specific anti-monocyte antisera or peroxidase activity. The extent to which the absence of B lymphocytes in blood can be regarded as a diagnostic criterion for congenital X-linked pan-hypogammaglobulinaemia is uncertain. The absence is not exclusive to affected boys since it develops in some patients with thymomas and also in a few with variable hypogammaglobulinaemia. The patients possess pre-B cells in their bone marrow so their immunodeficiency is not due simply to aplasia of the entire B-lymphocyte series. Factors which normally control pre-B cell maturation are unknown and it is not impossible that some cells might follow independent pathways which bypass the block.

5.2.4   Congenital hypogammaglobulinaemia in girls

Congenital hypogammaglobulinaemia is rare in girls and when it does occur it is usually as a part of a severe combined immunodeficiency syndrome. A few girls with congenital panhypogammaglobulinaemia have resembled boys with the same condition in that they lacked B lymphocytes, but one patient we studied in London lacked pre-B cells in her marrow, suggesting a different cellular basis for her defect. Inheritance in these cases is presumably autosomal recessive (AR). On the other hand it is presumably only a matter of time until an affected boy grows up to marry a female carrier of the X-linked disease and to produce affected girl infants.

Genetically determined 'acquired' antibody deficiency is much commoner in women than the congenital form. It is discussed with other unclassified types below.

5.2.5   Hypogammaglobulinaemia with IgM

Most children with very low levels of IgG and IgA but normal or high levels of IgM are boys and, since many of them have similarly affected male relatives, at least one form of this syndrome has an X-linked recessive inheritance[10]. Little is known of the pathogenesis; as expected, the patients have B lymphocytes with surface IgM and they usually have a few with surface IgA or IgG also. The defect is of the maturation of antigen-respon-sive B lymphocytes, so the cells responsible may be T or B lymphocytes or macrophages. The IgM that the patients make gives them little protection against infection, again suggesting that the B-cell response to antigen is qualitatively as well as quantitatively defective. The serum isohaemag-glutinin titre is, as would be expected, a better correlate of susceptibility to infection than the serum IgM concentration. The very high serum IgM levels which are sometimes found at the time of diagnosis have been observed to fall following the regular administration of IgG. This suggests that 'hyper IgM' is not an intrinsic part of the syndrome, but is more likely to result from the failure of negative feedback to the immune response by IgG antibodies.

The clinical course of hypogammaglobulinaemia with IgM patients tends to be stormier than that of patients with hypogammaglobulinaemia alone. The difference is partly due to the frequent occurrence of neutropenia, or at least to a poor polymorph response to infection, in those with IgM. The prognosis in this group is poor since many develop fatal septicaemias. Thrombocytopenia also occurs, either by itself, in which case it is not usually severe, or in combination with neutropenia.

Infections with *Pneumocystis pneumoniae* or *Candida* can be a problem, and their occurrence suggests that some degree of cell-mediated immunodeficiency accompanies the antibody deficiency. Whether this is primary or secondary is not known.

5.2.6 Transient hypogammaglobulinaemia

Serum IgG concentrations are normally at their lowest 4–7 months after birth as by this time most of the maternal IgG has been catabolized or diluted and its replacement by the infant's own IgG is incomplete. The trough in IgG levels is more marked where the amount acquired from the mother was reduced, as occurs in premature or dysmature babies. The infants with the lowest IgG levels are probably the ones who are most likely to develop infections and, as a result, to have their serum immunoglobulins measured. Most of them respond to their infections with the production of increased amounts of antibody and their hypogammaglobulinaemia is appropriately called 'transient' if the immunoglobulin levels become normal within the next 3 months of life. As well as this group of patients, who probably only represent the lower end of a normal distribution curve, there are others whose low immunoglobulin concentrations at 4–7 months are likely to result from true delay in synthesis. This conclusion is based on the observations of transient hypogammaglobulinaemia in the siblings of infants with severe combined immunodeficiency, who were presumably heterozygous for the condition.

5.2.7 Transcobalamin II deficiency

A single patient described by Hitzig and Kenny[11] had transcobalamin II deficiency associated with panhypogammaglobulinaemia. The interest in this case derives more from the light it throws on the metabolic requirements for lymphocyte responses than from its uniqueness. The infant was delivered by Caesarean section and maintained in a sterile environment because two previous sons had died with neutropenia. The hypogammaglobulinaemia was recognized at 3 months and it was followed by malnutrition due to intestinal atrophy and later by pancytopenia. Treatment with vitamin B_{12} reversed all three abnormalities and subsequent challenge with previously administered antigens elicited secondary antibody responses. Subsequently the patient's neutrophils became defective in killing bacteria; this deficiency was corrected by increased B_{12} replacement together with plasma infusions.

The only established metabolic role of vitamin B_{12} in mammals is as a cofactor for methylmalonyl CoA mutase, though in bacteria it is a cofactor for transmethylation also. Since methylation is required for nucleic acid synthesis it is not surprising that methenyl folate, and so perhaps B_{12} deficiency should have adverse effects on rapidly dividing cells including those of the developing immune system. It is remarkable that the infant was able to mount delayed hypersensitivity skin responses during his period of antibody deficiency. In this respect the consequences of functional B_{12} deficiency differ from those of malnutrition, ADA deficiency and nucleoside phosphorylase deficiency, in which cell-mediated immunity is more severely impaired than antibody responses.

5.2.8 IgA deficiency

Selective lack of IgA from both serum and secretions with normal serum concentrations of other immunoglobulins occurs in about one in 700 white Caucasians, so it is the commonest primary defect of a specific immunity mechanism[12]. In most cases there is no obvious inheritance of the deficiency; in the rarer cases where the lack of IgA has been familial an autosomal recessive transmission is commoner than a dominant one. IgA deficiency is occasionally, though inconsistently, associated with abnormalities (such as deletions or ring forms) of chromosome 18. Male siblings of patients with the phenotype of X-linked panhypogammaglobulinaemia have been reported to have selective deficiency of IgA, and secondary deficiency as a result of phenytoin treatment also occurs. These observations indicate that selective IgA deficiency can have a range of causes; whether they share a common pathogenic mechanism is uncertain.

Almost all IgA deficient patients have blood lymphocytes with surface IgA and in some cases these cells have responded to pokeweed mitogen stimulation by synthesizing IgA, detectable within the cell by immunofluorescence[13]. A primary defect in the secretion of IgA by IgA-containing plasma cells has been proposed but if this were the only abnormality one might expect to find large numbers of IgA-containing plasmablasts in the lamina propria of affected patients. This does appear to be true of the majority. Another possibility is that the T cells of such patients fail to help IgA-bearing B lymphocytes respond to antigen. This hypothesis is consistent with the range of T-cell defects which have been reported in IgA deficiency, although the defects themselves have tended to be both variable and subtle. They may be secondary rather than primary.

5.2.8.1 Clinical features

These depend primarily on the method of case finding. IgA deficient individuals identified by screening blood donors are usually healthy. Those found in allergy or rheumatology clinics (these specific associations are described below) differ little from other patients with the same primary disorders but with normal IgA levels. When recurrent infections do occur they usually involve principally the respiratory tract, giving otitis, sinusitis and bronchitis. In general, upper respiratory tract symptoms predominate and there is no increased frequency of pneumonia or septicaemia. Some patients do, however, develop bronchiectasis, perhaps as a complication of upper respiratory tract infections.

The commonest gut symptom is recurrent diarrhoea, sometimes severe enough to cause malabsorbtion. It is tempting to assume that this results from small intestinal bacterial overgrowth secondary to failure of production of the main gastrointestinal antibody. However, since some boys with panhypogammaglobulinaemia are free of gut symptoms while receiving only IgG replacement, other factors must also be important.

The ability of some IgA deficient individuals to remain perfectly healthy is probably largely due to substitution of other isotypes at mucosal surfaces. In one study, IgA-deficient subjects responded to intranasal virus immunization with IgG and IgM antibodies in their nasal secretions[14]. IgM, though not IgG, can bind secretory piece and so may effectively protect both the respiratory tract and the intestine. Perhaps the morbidity of IgA-deficient patients is more closely linked to the severity of the underlying defect, such as a possible T-cell abnormality, than to the inability to produce IgA. Two associations of IgA deficiency, discussed below, indicate that the disorder has wider immunopathological features than a simple failure to make IgA.

5.2.8.2 Allergy and IgA deficiency

Both high and low levels of serum IgA are commoner in atopic patients than in controls[15]. A more specific link between a relative paucity of IgA and atopy is suggested by the observations that skin-test positive asthmatic patients have more IgE and less IgA antibody to *Dermatophagoides* antigens than a control population. In another study a relative delay in IgA production was found at 6 months of age in the atopic infants of atopic parents when compared with controls. By 1 year the difference had disappeared (see review[16]). These various observations do not necessarily imply a cause and effect relationship; it is equally possible that the T-cell mechanisms normally responsible for limiting IgE antibody production are important for helping IgA production. IgA in mucosal secretions is clearly effective in limiting the uptake of antigen and when this mechanism fails it is possible that more antigen is available to stimulate the precursors of IgE plasma cells.

Apart from hypersensitivity to environmental allergens, IgA-deficient individuals sometimes make antibodies to IgA and have adverse reactions to blood transfusions. Previous transfusion or injection with IgA-containing immunoglobulin preparations does not appear to be a prerequisite for the production of the anti-IgA antibodies which are responsible for these reactions, since they have occurred in patients who have never received either.

5.2.8.3 Autoimmunity and IgA deficiency

Rheumatoid arthritis is the commonest condition associated with auto-antibody formation to complicate IgA deficiency in Hong's series[12]. It was followed by systemic lupus erythematosus, thyroiditis, pernicious anaemia, chronic active hepatitis, pulmonary haemosiderosis and dermatomyositis[17]. In childhood the commonest association is with the polyarticular form of juvenile chronic arthritis; about 3% of these patients have low serum IgA levels. There is an impression that these patients have a somewhat milder course than those with normal IgA levels.

The aetiological basis of these relationships is obscure. Defective antigen clearance seems unlikely in patients whose IgG antibody production is normal and there is little to support the hypothesis that suppressor T cells are defective.

5.2.9 Primary isolated IgM deficiency

Primary IgM deficiency with normal concentrations of other immuno-globulins is rare. This is not surprising considering the central position of IgM-bearing B lymphocytes in the development of B cells with other immunoglobulin isotypes. The pathogenesis of selective IgM deficiency is likely to involve a failure of maturation of IgM B cells or, possibly, an excessive switch to other isotypes.

In 10 families reviewed by Hobbs[18] there were four times as many males affected as females. The IgM concentrations were mostly below 0.2 g/l but in only four of 55 individuals did they fall below 0.01 g/l. The principal symptom was infection and in 36% of cases this involved a septicaemia; 21% developed meningitis. Other conditions which occurred in the IgM-deficient patients included atopy, splenomegaly, lymphomas, Whipple's disease and Crohn's disease. 19% were asymptomatic. Because of the high frequency of septicaemia and the finding that most of the deaths were due to infection, Hobbs recommends the immediate institution of antibacterial therapy in any possible infection.

5.2.10   Varied immunodeficiency: predominantly antibody deficiency

Patients with defective antibody responses but normal cell-mediated immunity who do not fit into any of the categories described earlier are included under this provisional heading, to await further classification[2]. A number of phenotypic patterns are discernable but there is insufficient information to justify their separate classification. There is a slight excess of affected males and the onset of the condition can be at any stage. Some patients, including those in whom the onset was in adult life, have affected relatives, so there is likely to be a genetic factor in the aetiology. Autoantibody-associated diseases such as pernicious anaemia, haemolytic anaemia and rheumatoid arthritis are all more common in the patients and their relatives[19] which suggests that the hypogammaglobulinaemia may be one of several possible manifestations of a common immunopathological mechanism.

The clinical features depend more on the severity of the antibody deficiency than the actual immunoglobulin levels. The most severely affected experience the same range of infections as occurs in boys with X-linked hypogammaglobulinaemia, namely pneumonia, sinusitis, otitis and skin infections. Where pathogens are identified they are generally pyogenic bacteria. Malabsorption with diarrhoea is quite common and is very difficult to treat. Hyperplasia of the gut-associated lymphoid tissue takes place in some patients, producing the radiological appearance of nodular lymphoid hyperplasia. This complication appears to occur only in patients who have B lymphocytes; perhaps the B cells proliferate as a result of antigen stimulation but, because they do not differentiate, they do not generate any negative feedback. The predominant localization of the lymphoid hyperplasia in the gut would be consistent with the large amounts of antigen which are present there. The jejunal mucosa appears to be a site where a few lymphocytes are able to differentiate into plasma cells.

Lymphoid tissue hyperplasia can occur at other sites too and it may be mistaken for lymphoma. Since the hyperplasia can diminish following institution of immunoglobulin replacement treatment it is obviously im-

Table 5.2   Properties and activities of IgG subclasses*

	IgG_1	IgG_2	IgG_3	IgG_4
Relative proportions of adult adult serum IgG	66	23	7	4
C1q binding	+ + + +	+	+ + + +	0
Placental transport	+ + +	+ + +	+ + +	+ + +
Monocyte binding	+ + +	+	+ + + +	+ +
Antibody activity:				
Dip/tet toxoids	+ + + +	+ + +	+	±
Factor VIII	0	0	+	+ + +
Dextram and Levan	±	+ + + +	0	0

* See reference 21

portant to consider the diagnosis of immunodeficiency in patients with atypical lymphomas.

Other complications which may have an infective aetiology include dermatomyositis and a variety of neurological syndromes. Most of these have involved an encephalitis and have been slowly or rapidly progressive[20]. In several cases an ECHO virus has been isolated from the CSF or from a brain biopsy. This unusual result of ECHO virus infection, and perhaps also an increased susceptibility to vaccine strain induced poliomyelitis, are some of the few examples of impaired handling of virus infections by hypogamma-globulinaemia patients.

In some patients with variable hypogammaglobulinaemia the abnormality is more qualitative than quantitative; some examples which form recogniz-able patterns are described next.

5.2.10.1 IgG subclass abnormalities

The properties of the four subclasses of IgG are summarized in Table 5.2. IgA has two subclasses, and IgM probably has two also. The subclasses of IgG are the best characterized so discussion of subclass deficiencies is restricted to these alone. There is no reason to believe that comparable abnormalities of M or A subclasses could not exist. IgG subclass deficiencies are most often found in patients with variable hypogammaglobulinaemia, some of whom have in addition had defects of cell-mediated immunity. In the patients reviewed by Yount[21] the commonest abnormality was a relative increase in IgG_3 and in most there were also low levels of IgA or IgM. No patients had a selective absence of a single subclass, such as might be expected to result from a structural gene abnormality. The inheritance of an IgG_1 subclass deficiency in one family was compatible with inherited regulatory gene abnormality but, in most patients, defects of other control mechanisms seem more likely.

5.2.10.2 Light-chain deficiencies

The ratio of immunoglobulin molecules with κ light chains to those with λ light chains is about 2:1 in man. Other species have different ratios but there is little variation between individual members of a species. The control of light-chain synthesis is genetically determined through regulatory genes and individual B cells select one or other class at an early stage in their development. Disturbances of $\kappa : \lambda$ ratios in man are common in variable hypogammaglobulinaemia syndromes and are inevitable when there is a monoclonal immunoglobulin excess. Complete lack of κ^{22} or λ^{23} light chains is very rare and family studies in the former were more suggestive of a regulatory gene rather than a structural gene defect.

5.2.11   Treatment of antibody deficiency

5.2.11.1   *IgG replacement*

The IgG which is available for intramuscular injection is prepared from out-dated blood bank plasma by salt fractionation. It includes the antibody specificities of the donor pool and does not transmit hepatitis; it is highly effective in protecting boys with congenital hypogammaglobulinaemia from infections. The dose has to be adjusted to suit the patient. A Medical Research Council study[24] compared the frequency of infection in patients receiving 25 or 50 mg per kg body weight per week and concluded that the smaller dose was adequate for most but that some patients fared better on the larger dose. Neither dose raised the serum IgG levels of the recipients by more than about 15% and the serum levels were not very helpful in guiding treatment. IgG preparations in general contain small amounts of IgA but no IgM. There is no reason to believe that this IgA is therapeutically useful and it does not appear in secretions of the recipients. The successful management of some panhypogammaglobulinaemic patients with IgG replacement alone does not suggest that either IgA or IgM is uniquely essential. It is possible, though difficult, to prepare IgA or IgM concentrates but the short half-lives of these classes effectively precludes their use for replacement.

The main requirements of IgG replacement treatment are to give enough to prevent infections and, rarely, to deal with complications. At the lower dose level a 62 kg patient will require 10 ml i.m. weekly. Spacing the injections at 2-week intervals requires that twice the amount be given and this may be unacceptably painful. Patients in the USA are often started on injections at 3-week intervals but the amount given usually has to be reduced. More widely spaced injections would be expected to be less efficient because the catabolic rate for IgG is proportional to its serum concentration. An important aspect of management is to identify the patients who are not adequately protected by the immunoglobulin injections. A productive cough or the appearance of conjunctivitis in the days before the next injection is due should prompt a reduction in the interval between injections or an increase in the dose or the addition of antibiotics.

Reactions[25] generally occur within minutes of the injection and the symptoms include aches in the limbs or back, breathlessness and anxiety. In severe reactions there may be fever, tachycardia, hypotension and some-times death. Their treatment requires general measures for shock and adrenaline is commonly given. The reactions are almost certainly caused by kinin mediators released as a result of complement activation by IgG aggregates in the injection. Most commonly available IgG concentrates contain aggregates and the rarity of reactions following their intramuscular injection probably results from delay in their absorption and their elimin-ation by phagocytosis. Reactions are particularly rare in hypogamma-globulinaemic boys who have affected male relatives: they are almost inevitable if aggregate-containing material is given rapidly intravenously. It is possible to remove aggregates from immunoglobulin by ultracentrifugation but it is difficult to apply this on a commercial scale. The development of aggregate-free immunoglobulin is desirable because it could be given intravenously, so avoiding the need for large and painful intramuscular injections. The complement binding site on IgG is removable by enzyme treatment and the resulting $F(ab)_2$ fragments have been used to treat some patients. This material does not activate complement and can be given intravenously. It has the serious practical disadvantage of a very short half-life and the theoretical disadvantage that opsonizing activity would be expected to be abolished. Aggregate-free intact IgG preparations for intravenous use are being evaluated as they become commercially available; initial results with 100 mg per kg at 3-week intervals are very encouraging.

5.2.11.2 Plasma infusions

Infusions of 15 ml of plasma per kg body weight at 3-week intervals[26] provides about the same amount of IgG as 50 mg per kg injections at the same interval. The advantages of the large amount that can be given, and the relatively painless intravenous route, must be set against the difficulty of finding a suitable donor. Blood bank plasma is not ideal because of the risk of transmitting hepatitis, even though the donors may have been screened for HB_S antigen. If the patient is a child it may be possible to use the parents as donors and to prepare several packs of plasma for infusion at a single session of plasmaphoresis. Plasma infusions have been recommended for patients with hypogammaglobulinaemia with malabsorption since the additional protein may be beneficial: unfortunately improvement does not always follow.

5.2.11.3 Antibiotics

Every effort should be made to identify the causative organisms of infections in immunodeficient patients. When appropriate specimens have been obtained for culture it is prudent to start antibiotic treatment immediately. The choice of drug depends on the circumstances but it would include trimethoprim for a suspected upper respiratory tract infection or intravenous gentamycin, cephaloridine and metronidazole for a possible septicaemia due to enteric organisms. Antibody-deficient patients respond as promptly as other patients to appropriate antibiotics but because the antibody response is lacking it is desirable to continue effective treatment for longer.

Chronic antibiotic treatment is usually required in addition to postural drainage for patients with bronchiectasis. Rotation of ampicillin, erythromycin and cephalothin or continuous trimethoprim appear equally effective.

5.3 SELECTIVE DEFECTS OF CELL-MEDIATED IMMUNITY

Because T lymphocytes are required for most antibody responses it seems unlikely that a complete absence of T-cell function could be associated with normal antibody immunity. In 1968, when Di George first described thymic hypoplasia[27], the role of T cells in lymphocyte cooperation was not widely appreciated so a selective defect of cell-mediated immunity appeared to be a logical counterpart to hypogammaglobulinaemia. In the past decade the extreme rarity of complete thymic hypoplasia has become apparent together with the recognition of 'partial' cases in whom cell-mediated immunity was only mildly impaired. A satisfactory classification of defects of cell-mediated immunity has yet to be evolved, largely because the appropriate biochemical or cellular criteria are lacking. Nucleoside phosphorylase deficiency is described first in the following sections since, despite its rarity, it is probably the most securely established defect affecting predominantly T cells.

5.3.1 Purine nucleoside phosphorylase (PNP) deficiency

Only about ten patients have been identified; their age of presentation ranges between 3 months and 7 years. The first was a 5-year-old girl with recurrent viral infections, otitis media and diarrhoea, anaemia and lymphopenia[28]. Skin tests for delayed hypersensitivity were negative and the T-lymphocyte count in her blood was low. Her blood lymphocytes did not respond to mitogens or to histocompatibility stimuli. Antibody responses to antigens were normal, as were her serum immunoglobulin concentrations. Subsequent cases have had severe infections with Pox or Herpes viruses (one died with progressive vaccinia) but have recovered normally from RNA virus infections. Six patients became anaemic and in one the marrow was megaloblastic. In four patients the anaemia was haemolytic with a positive Coombs test. Some of the patients have developed mild spasticity; this is probably due to functional hypoxanthine–guanine phosphoribosyl transferase deficiency leading to a Lesch–Nyhan-like syndrome.

The autoimmune haemolytic anaemias and occasional presence of monoclonal IgG peaks or positive antinuclear factor tests point to poorly regulated antibody production. In most cases the immunodeficiency results from a structural gene defect for PNP (coded for on chromosome 14) but in one family a functionally defective enzyme was present. PNP converts inosine, cytosine and other nucleotides to hypoxanthine, cytidine and corresponding purines. In PNP deficiency de-oxy GTP accumulates and inhibits ribonucleotide reductase, so effectively blocking DNA synthesis[39]. T cells are affected more than B cells because they have more specific nucleoside kinase activity and, possibly, because they lack 5[1] nucleotidase. Antibody production in PNP deficient patients probably persists because helper T cells do not need to divide to function. Suppressor T cells do, however, need to divide; their failure to do so may leave the patients vulnerable to auto-antibody production.

Transfusion of red cells was thought to improve two patients, in one case de-oxycytidine (50 mg/kg) by mouth was given in addition to circumvent the ribonucleotide reductase block. If whole blood is given it should probably be irradiated (3000 rads) first since one child developed a graft-versus-host disease.

Very low levels of plasma and urine uric acid is the simplest laboratory clue to diagnosis; urinary purine excretion is a better screening test. The definitive test is PNP assay on red-cell lysates or cultured fibroblasts. Lymphocyte function tests are less likely to be useful for early diagnosis because affected infants are initially normal.

5.3.2 Thymic hypoplasia (Di George's syndrome)

The thymus originates as an epithelial outgrowth of the third and fourth pharyngeal pouches. Other structures derived from the same regions are the parathyroid glands and parts of the primitive vascular arches which subsequently contribute to the aortic arch. Di George's syndrome is characterized by abnormalities of the aortic arch with, in its most complete form, thymic and parathyroid hypoplasia[29]. The pathogenesis of the developmental failure is unknown; an intrauterine infection or drug-induced defect might be responsible but none has been incriminated. Environmental causes seem more probable than genetic ones in most cases, since there is only one report of a familial case[30]. The damage is likely to occur around the 8th week of gestation because this is the time at which the abnormal structures, which may include the philtrum and the ears, are developing. The sexes are equally affected.

Clinical presentation generally results from the cardiac abnormalities and from hypocalcaemic tetany or convulsions. It is important to distinguish between thymic hypoplasia and the much more common combination of cardiac defects and hypocalcaemia due to infection. The extent of the immunodeficiency in thymic hypoplasia is very variable; where infections have arisen they have included candidiasis, interstitial pneumonia and diarrhoea. In our experience at The Hospital for Sick Children in London the diagnosis has seemed likely in only a few patients who were found to lack a thymus during open heart surgery for truncus arteriosus or anomalous pulmonary venous drainage. These children had hypocalcaemia, though not convulsions, and infections were not a problem. Those who died did so from their cardiac abnormalities. It is unlikely that our patients had severely impaired cell-mediated immunity since graft versus host disease did not arise despite the large amount of donor blood given during bypass surgery. In other reports, infants have been investigated prior to surgery and found to have few T lymphocytes in blood with elevated B-cell numbers, giving a normal blood lymphocyte count. T-lymphocyte function as measured by skin tests for delayed hypersensitivity, or by lymphocyte responses *in vitro* to mitogens or histocompatibility antigens, has been decreased or absent. In the earlier cases described the serum immunoglobulins and antibody responses were found to be normal. Impaired antibody responses have been reported more recently.

T-cell responses have spontaneously improved in a few cases who were not specifically treated. In other patients who have been grafted with human fetal thymus the lymphocyte responses to mitogens have improved within hours or days. The striking speed of effect, and the observation in one case of laboratory improvement when the thymus graft was enclosed in a millipore diffusion chamber[30], suggest that humoral mechanisms are involved.

5.3.3   Cartilage hair hypoplasia

This rare, probably autosomal recessive, disorder was first described in Amish kindred. It is characterized by fine sparse hair, short-limbed dwarfism and hyperextensible joints[31]. A few cases have had very severe or fatal varicella infections and two developed progressive vaccinia following small-pox vaccination. Evidence for defective T-cell function includes negative delayed hypersensitivity skin tests and lymphopenia. T-lymphocyte counts in blood were low and mitogen and antigen responses *in vitro* were negative. Normal serum immunoglobulins and normal antibody responses have been reported. The immunodeficiency of cartilage hair hypoplasia has been treated with fetal thymus grafts with possible temporary benefit, and in one case with a bone marrow graft with dramatic clinical improvement claimed.

5.3.4   Variable immunodeficiency affecting predominantly cell-mediated immunity

The relative rarity of patients who might be included under this heading contrasts with the larger number who have unclassified forms of antibody deficiency. This difference probably reflects the relative insensitivity of screening tests for impaired cell-mediated immunity in comparison with tests for antibody deficiency. It is equally possible that, through faulty T–B cooperation, subtle defects of T-cell function are commonly manifested as variable forms of antibody deficiency. If patients with abnormal antibody responses (such as the cellular immunodeficiency with immunoglobulins syndrome, page 176) are excluded, then the main clinical features of patients in this group are infections with *Candida*, herpes or pox viruses or diarrhoea. Evidence for defective T-cell function has been similar to that in the previously described selective T-cell defects and in some cases has been supported by therapeutic benefit from thymus grafting or injections of thymus extract. It is now appreciated that some infants with ADA deficiency present with selective T-cell defects.

5.3.5 Treatment of T-cell defects

5.3.5.1 Fetal thymus grafts

From 10 weeks of gestational age onwards the fetal thymus contains epithelial cells, which are thought to induce the maturation of T lymphocytes by humoral factors, and mature immunocompetent T lymphocytes. The effectiveness of grafts of fetal thymus in the treatment of thymic hypoplasia is described above; therapeutic benefit has also been claimed in patients with combined immunodeficiency, ataxia telangiectasia and chronic muco-cutaneous candidiasis. Successes in treatment of thymic hypoplasia were not accompanied by engraftment with donor lymphocytes[32] so the mechanism probably depends on humoral factors released by the thymic epithelial cells. On the other hand the lymphocytes in the thymus can be dangerous through the induction of graft versus host disease. This complication is common in patients with combined immunodeficiency so, if they are to be given thymus grafts, it would seem logical to employ predominantly epithelial grafts (page 171).

5.3.5.2 Thymus extracts (thymosin, thymopoietin)

The experimental observation that incubation of immature cells with thymus extracts can induce the appearance of certain T-lymphocyte cell surface antigens has stimulated their widespread clinical use in immuno-deficient patients (see reference 33). The various techniques for thymosin preparation and the possibility that material from different sources may have different properties makes comparison of reported effects difficult. In a recent report[34] an active substance was found to be a nonapeptide with a molecular weight of about 900. In general it has been easier to obtain increased numbers of E-rosetting cells in the laboratory than to confer significant benefit on the patient. This is not entirely surprising considering that the cells of experimental animals which are 'induced' *in vitro* still tend to behave like immature cells rather than mature T cells. Perhaps a major advantage of thymus extract treatment is that it is unlikely to do harm, though a girl with nucleoside phosphorylase deficiency who was treated with it did develop asthma following the injections.

5.3.5.3 Transfer factor

Transfer factor (TF) is a dialysable extract of blood lymphocytes which confers specific immunological reactivity on an immunologically competent but previously unsensitized individual. This phenomenon is extensively reviewed elsewhere[35]. Benefit from TF treatment has been recorded in about 50% of cases of chronic mucocutaneous candidiasis or Wiskott–Aldrich syndrome[36] and, in conjunction with fetal thymus grafts, in a few cases of combined immunodeficiency. It is unclear whether improvement, in those cases where it has occurred, is due to an antigen-specific or a non-specific effect of TF. Possible adverse effects including monoclonal gammopathy and lymphoma have occurred in some patients with Wiskott–Aldrich syndrome following TF treatment.

5.4 COMBINED IMMUNODEFICIENCY

Combined immunodeficiency was originally recognized as a different condition from hypogammaglobulinaemia because affected infants had a rapidly downhill course and generally died before the age of one. As methods for testing cell-mediated immunity were developed it became apparent that the patients had severely impaired lymphocyte responses in addition to antibody deficiency – hence the term 'combined'.

Different patterns of inheritance and phenotypic variations indicate that the combined immunodeficiency syndrome is heterogeneous and in only one form has a primary enzyme defect been identified. The most severe forms of combined immunodeficiency are readily diagnosed but the more subtle forms of the syndrome merge with severe forms of variable immunodeficiency. The four main forms of the condition which are discussed here are listed in Table 5.3.

Table 5.3 Four main forms of combined immunodeficiency syndrome

Condition	Inheritance	Synonym
Severe combined immuno- deficiency (SCID)	{ AR { X-linked	Swiss type agamma- globulinaemia
SCID with ADA deficiency	AR	
SCID with immunoglobulins	{ AR { X-linked	Nezelof syndrome
SCID with leukopenia	AR	Reticular dysgenesis

5.4.1 Severe combined immunodificiency (SCID)

The clinical presentation depends mainly on environmental factors. In the UK the commonest early symptoms are diarrhoea and failure to thrive, with an onset at 2–6 months of age. The diarrhoea improves when the infant is given only clear fluids and it is not uncommon for the diagnosis to be suspected only after several bouts of 'gastroenteritis'. Candidiasis affecting the mouth or napkin area occurs in almost all infants with severe defects of cell-mediated immunity. In cases where infants are routinely immunized with BCG, cases can be expected to develop disseminated BCG infections[37];

dissemination also follows vaccination. Pneumonia is a less common presenting complaint and when it does occur opportunists such as *Pneumocystis carinii* or *Candida* are often responsible. Perhaps the relative rarity of bacterial pneumonia results from protection for the first few months of life by maternal antibody, acting with the infant's own complement and phagocytes. The effectiveness of antibiotics given after the diagnosis is made probably also contributes.

Diagnostically useful physical findings, such as a lack of palpable lymph nodes, are few. Many cases develop skin rashes, which are often transient and of unknown aetiology. Radiological abnormalities of the pelvis and long bones are present in adenosine deaminase deficiency (see below) and it would be unusual to see a thymic shadow in the chest X-ray.

The blood count is commonly normal though the finding of a persistent severe lymphopenia would strongly favour the diagnosis. Some cases develop an eosinophilia, and this is usually present in patients who have graft versus host disease following blood transfusion or marrow grafting. The immunological abnormalities on which the diagnosis is made are (1) hypogammaglobulinaemia, which ultimately affects all immunoglobulin classes, though maternal IgG will be present in infants, and (2) defective cell-mediated immunity resulting in a negative response to PHA and failure of DNCB or KLH skin sensitization.

There is little difference between the clinical features of patients from families where the inheritance is X-linked recessive compared with autosomal recessive, though survival has been described as longer in untreated affected boys. The early diagnosis of pneumocystis pneumonia, either by lung tap or open lung biopsy, and its treatment, with co-trimoxazole alone or in combination with pentamidine, appears to prolong survival considerably. Antibiotics including metronidazole have little influence on the gastrointestinal symptoms and the patients become increasingly cathectic. Death often results from septicaemia with antibiotic-resistant organisms.

5.4.2 SCID associated with adenosine deaminase deficiency

Adenosine deaminase (ADA) converts adenosine and deoxyadenosine to inosine and deoxyinosine. ADA is coded for a chromosome 20; this is the only structural locus with two allelic forms, each having a molecular weight of about 33 000. The range of isoenzyme types normally found in different tissues result from the binding of a tissue conversion factor which is a high molecular weight glycoprotein. ADA-deficient homozygotes have two null genes for ADA so transmission is autosomal recessive. The carrier state and the complete deficiency can be identified by assaying the enzyme in red-cell lysates[38]. The most toxic substrate to accumulate when ADA is absent is deoxyadenosine triphosphate. This binds to and inhibits ribonucleotide reductase[39], so blocking DNA synthesis, as does dGTP in purine nucleoside phosphorylase (PNP) deficiency. The reason why B cell responses are impaired in ADA deficiency (which is not the case in PNP deficiency) is uncertain but probably results from the relatively greater toxicity of dATP compared with dGTP. Other metabolic pathways may also be affected by ADA deficiency because S-adenosylhomocysteine also accumulates and could interfere with methylation reactions.

There is considerable phenotypic variation in ADA deficiency. Some infants are born immunologically normal (because *in utero* the mother acts as a deoxyadenosine sink) and their immunoglobulins may develop normally for a year or two. In such cases the urinary excretion of deoxyadenosine[40] is a better diagnostic clue than lymphocyte function tests. Subsequent deterioration in both clinical status and laboratory tests has been called 'immunologic attrition'. Severely affected infants die within a year unless appropriately treated. Both the rapidly and slowly progressive forms of the disease occur with complete lack of erythrocyte ADA and they contrast with the ADA deficiency without immunological abnormality which occurs in the !Kung tribe. The latter is due to a gene which is carried by over 70% of the tribe and which is associated with low levels of ADA in most tissues except red cells, in which it is almost entirely absent.

Transient hypogammaglobulinaemia has occasionally occurred in the siblings of SCID patients. This is possibly a manifestation of the heterozygous form of the condition though insufficient families have been studied to be sure of this.

Non-immunological manifestations of ADA deficiency include defective bone ossification resulting in cupping and flaring at the costochondral junctions. The bony pelvis of affected patients has been short in the vertical axis with small sacroiliac notches and broad ischia.

ADA-deficient SCID patients have been successfully reconstituted with grafts of tissue-matched sibling marrow and a small number have also improved following repeated transfusions of red cells from a healthy donor. This is more fully described in the treatment section.

5.4.3 SCID with immunoglobulins

It is the lack of normal antibody responses (rather than a lack of immunoglobulins) which justifies the inclusion of these patients under the heading of combined immunodeficiency. They are clearly a heterogeneous collection[41] and many ADA-deficient patients with immunoglobulins have probably been included in this category in the past. More recently those with low ADA levels have been excluded. The commonest isotype found is IgM but other selective deficiencies occur.

The tendency of related cases in single families to resemble each other both in their immunological findings and clinical courses strongly suggests that some cases are due to single gene defects. An X-linked form of the condition, which is possibly the only X-linked form of SCID, typically has high numbers of B cells in blood though the serum immunoglobulins are low. The B cells of one such case differentiated normally into plasma cells when cultured with normal T lymphocytes (from a healthy donor) and pokeweed mitogen[42], so the patient's defective T cells were probably responsible for the antibody deficiency.

Several infants with scaly erythroderma, eosinophilia, alopecia and reticulum cell hyperplasia have had impaired cell-mediated immunity and antibody deficiency. The clinical features superficially resemble histiocytosis X[43,44] and there are morphological similarities too since erythrophago-cytosis occurs in both. Most cases of histiocytosis X have normal immunity responses, at least in the early stages of the disease, so there is no obvious immunodeficiency basis for this group of disorders. The histiocytosis-like features of some SCID patients have been attributed to chronic graft versus host disease caused by maternal lymphocytes but direct confirmation by maternal karyotype is lacking.

5.4.4 SCID with leukopenia (reticular dysgenesis)

Affected infants have severe functional deficiencies of both lymphocytes and polymorphs and the monozygotic twins who were described in the original report died within a few days of birth. Of the few cases which have been described that of the male siblings reported by Ownby et al.[45] is the most informative. The neutrophil count of the first boy was normal at 8 days of age but fell to very low levels at 40 days. The infant died with a pseudomonas septicaemia at 52 days of age and necropsy revealed that there was a general-ized lack of granulocytes and their precursors in the marrow, the thymus was largely epithelial and there were few lymphocytes in the spleen or else-where. In the second child granulocytes were absent but the blood lympho-cyte count and the percentage of E rosettes were normal. There was no significant lymphocyte response to mitogen stimulation and IgM and IgA were not detected in cord serum. The infant died after 3 days with a cytomegalovirus pneumonia.

The pathogenesis of reticular dysgenesis is obscure. No single failure of cell development could account for the range of defects reported so it is likely that either the neutropenia or the lymphopenia is a secondary event. Neutropenia sometimes complicates hypogammaglobulinaemia but so far as is known there is no increase in frequency of unclassified immunodeficiency in the relatives of reticular dysgenesis patients.

5.4.5 Treatment of SCID

The only treatment which has resulted in permanent restoration of immune responses is grafting with bone marrow from a tissue-type matched donor[46].

The requirements for histocompatibility are stringent so they are usually only met by closely related donors – generally siblings. Tissue type is inherited as one haplotype from each parent so the chances that two siblings will have identical pairs of haplotypes are only one in four. The trend towards smaller families limits the number of cases for whom there is a suitable related donor. Of the patients who have no possible donors, those with ADA deficiency can be helped by red cell transfusions, as described below, but for the remainder there is no treatment of established value.

5.4.5.1 *Marrow grafting: problems of graft versus host disease*

Marrow grafting was introduced on the grounds that SCID patients lacked a lymphoid stem cell of a type which is normally found in the marrow. In practice, a successful response does not necessarily mean that the patient lacked a stem cell; in many cases it is more likely that the defect was of the cellular environment. Patients with severe defects of cell-mediated immunity are unable to reject foreign grafts and, as a result, are unable to protect themselves against attack by incompatible lymphocytes. The consequences of such an attack are called graft versus host disease and they feature skin rashes, diarrhoea, aplastic or haemolytic anaemia, hepatitis, pulmonary infiltrates and sometimes nephritis[47]. Mild degrees of graft versus host reactions are very common, even following grafts between siblings, and they resolve spontaneously. Chronic graft versus host disease persists most often as a scaly erythroderma and it can be incapacitating. Both transient and chronic graft versus host disease sometimes follow marrow grafts obtained from donors matched at HLA A, B, C and D loci. In such cases the antigenic stimulus is presumably due to other, as yet unrecognized, histocompatibility determinants. Since the reaction can be transient, the grafted cells must be able to acquire tolerance. Severe graft versus host disease generally develops 7 to 14 days after grafts of mismatched marrow or blood transfusion and is usually fatal. It responds little if at all to immunosuppressive drugs. The graft versus host reaction is initiated by specifically responsive T lymphocytes, and marrow preparations depleted of T lymphocytes may cause less acute forms of graft versus host disease, though this approach does not permit the use of incompatible grafts.

When blood transfusion is required the blood should first be irradiated to 3000 rad. An alternative, which is adequate for the treatment of anaemia, is to use deep-frozen, thawed and washed erythrocytes. These precautions are necessary because blood lymphocytes can cause graft versus host disease.

5.4.5.2 *Donor selection*

Donors need to be large enough to provide the 10^7–10^8 nucleated marrow cells which are commonly used; two years of age is probably the youngest used to date. The legal position in the UK concerning a non-therapeutic procedure on a minor requiring a general anaesthetic is unclear. Apart from these considerations and the exclusion of unhealthy individuals, the requirement for compatibility between donor and recipient is of paramount importance. The 6-month survival of patients given HLA A, B, C and MLC* (D locus) matched marrow is over 60%, while lesser degrees of certainty about the A and B loci matching give only a 38% survival, even when the MLC is negative[48]. In practice, the simplest approach is to tissue type any siblings and, if an identical one is found, to check that his lymphocytes are not stimulated in MLC by the cells of the patient. If there are no siblings then limited experience would suggest that uncles and aunts should be tested and any who share B locus antigens with the patient should also be tested in MLC. This preliminary selection on the basis of B antigens is justified by their closer linkage to the D locus antigens than to the A locus.

It is uncertain at present whether patients who lack suitable related donors should be offered grafts of fetal tissues or whether efforts should be made to find an unrelated donor. Access to panels of tissue-typed donors is usually based on the A and B locus antigens and compatible individuals are then tested in MLC. The number of major D locus antigens appears relatively small, and many are in linkage disequilibrium with a B locus antigen so the chance of MLC compatibility between A and B loci–identical individuals may be as high as one in 10. Despite this, only a very small number of such unrelated-donor grafts have been performed and in the single most successful case five grafts from the same donor have been required.

5.4.5.3 *Grafts of fetal tissue or thymic epithelial cells*

The hopes that fetal lymphocytes would become tolerant to the HLA antigens of an immunodeficient recipient have not materialized in that both fetal thymus and fetal liver cells have caused fatal graft versus host disease. However, some patients do appear to have been dramatically improved by fetal grafts[49]. They form two main groups: (1) those with SCID who benefited from fetal liver cells and (2) Di George's syndrome patients (described previously) who benefited from fetal thymus grafts.

The main difficulty with fetal liver grafts is to obtain a 'take'; this may result in part from the need to keep the recipient alive for 6–16 weeks until PHA-responsive cells of donor origin appear. In several patients engraftment has only been temporary and in the few where donor cells have persisted the immunological reconstitution has been predominantly of T-cell functions.

Hong *et al.*[50] have reported the successful treatment of SCID by intraperitoneal injection of fragments of thymus (from a donor undergoing

---

*Mixed lymphocyte culture (MLC).

cardiac surgery) which had been cultured *in vitro* for 18 days to reduce the number of donor lymphocytes. Several other patients have been similarly treated with encouraging results.

5.4.5.4 *Treatment of ADA deficiency by red-cell transfusion*

Erythrocytes contain ADA and consequently can be used as adenosine traps in patients with ADA deficiency. The main limitation of this approach is the need to repeat the treatment at approximately monthly intervals; in addition it is probably important to avoid giving mature responsive lymphocytes. Published reports describe the use of frozen and irradiated cells[51]. Of ten patients treated by transfusions, the five who have done best were the most immunocompetent at diagnosis. Haemolytic anaemia has developed and so accurate cross-matching is essential.

5.5 MISCELLANEOUS SYNDROMES ASSOCIATED WITH DEFECTS OF SPECIFIC IMMUNITY

5.5.1 Ataxia telangiectasia

This disorder is characterized by a predominantly cerebellar ataxia, oculo-cutaneous telangiectasia and recurrent infections[52]. The aetiology is unknown. It has an autosomal recessive transmission and the earliest symptom, which rarely appears before the age of 4, is usually unsteadiness of gait or clumsiness in picking up objects. The neurological disorder progresses over a period of years and ultimately causes pyramidal tract signs and intellectual deterioration. The characteristic telangiectasia which permit differentiation from other forms of inherited ataxia often appear 1–5 years after the onset of neurological defects. They are most prominent on the bulbar conjunctivae but also occur on the nose, ears and over the shoulders. The commonest immunological abnormality is IgE deficiency, followed by IgA deficiency[53], and these ultimately develop in about three-quarters of the patients. Many also develop defects of cell-mediated immunity, detectable as negative delayed hypersensitivity skin tests, abnormal T-lymphocyte subpopulations in the blood[54] and impaired responses to mitogens. Small morphologically immature thymuses have been found at necropsy. Infections are predominantly of the respiratory tract and it is arguable whether immunoglobulin deficiency or muscular weakness (with aspiration of saliva or impaired coughing) is more important in their causation.

Other abnormalities in ataxia telangiectasia include raised α-fetoprotein levels, skin depigmentation, impaired glucose tolerance and gonadal dysgenesis. Chromosomal abnormalities are common also and their increased frequency in PHA-stimulated lymphocyte cultures which have been exposed to low doses of irradiation is intriguing in view of the increased incidence of both epithelial and lymphoid malignancies in these patients.

No treatment which will halt the progression of the neurological disease has been established, and until this has been achieved it is doubtful whether attempts to modify the immunodeficiency are justified. The course of the disease does not appear to be influenced by the presence or absence of laboratory evidence of immunodeficiency.

5.5.2 Wiskott–Aldrich syndrome

This rare disorder is characterized by eczema, thrombocytopenia and recurrent infections. The inheritance is X-linked and recessive[55]. The eczema resembles atopic eczema in onset and distribution; since Wiskott–Aldrich syndrome (WAS) patients have high IgE levels it may well have an allergic aetiology. The platelets are small and their low number results in bleeding, which is often the most serious clinical feature. It can take the form of bloody diarrhoea or intracerebral bleeds, causing strokes. Infections often involve the skin, perhaps because it is already damaged by the eczema, or the upper respiratory tract, causing sinusitis or otitis. Survival beyond adolescence is rare in patients with the complete form of the disease. So-called incomplete forms in which the thrombocytopenia or eczema is lacking may exist but it would be difficult to distinguish such patients from those with variable immunodeficiency associated with allergy or haematological abnormalities.

The precise nature of the immunity defect in WAS is obscure. Low levels of IgM are due mainly to hypercatabolism; IgG and IgA levels are generally normal despite catabolic rates of 3 to 5 times normal respectively[56]. The blood lymphocyte count, and responses *in vitro* to mitogens and antigens, are generally normal initially but they may decline with time. Antibody responses to carbohydrate antigens are particularly poor and a lack of isohaemagglutinins may be an example of this. Impaired antigen processing seems probable but tests of macrophage function have been normal[57]. Monoclonal gammopathy and malignant lymphomas are common in WAS, perhaps as a result of the immunodeficiency.

Reduction in the frequency of infections and on occasion an increase in platelet count has been reported following transfer factor treatment[58]. The effectiveness of therapy has been associated with increases in the number of T lymphocytes in the blood. Perhaps only half of WAS patients benefit from transfer factor and response is best in patients whose monocytes lack IgG (Fc) receptors.

5.5.3 Chronic mucocutaneous candidiasis

This uncommon sporadic disorder is characterized by indolent and frequently disfiguring superficial infection with *Candida albicans*. The nails are typically dystrophic, the mouth is usually affected and the eyelid margins are thickened by blepharitis. There is great variation in the severity of lesions; some patients develop granulomas on the face and scalp while others have frequent staphylococcal abscesses in addition to the candidiasis. Associated endocrine abnormalities, including pituitary, parathyroid and adrenocortical hypofunction, are common and the presence or absence of such complications has been used for classification[59].

Immunological abnormalities have also been variable. Most patients make good antibody responses to *Candida* antigens but may lack delayed hypersensitivity to *Candida* or other antigens[60]. The lack of any consistent abnormality *in vitro* makes it difficult to formulate a unifying hypothesis to account for the disease.

Treatment with intravenous amphoteracin B or with miconazole will usually eradicate the candidiasis temporarily but relapse follows its cessation. The toxicity of most antifungal drugs prevents their long-term use. Perhaps as many as 50% of patients improve with regular injections of transfer factor[36]. In some cases the effect has been greatest when transfer factor was given immediately after a course of antifungal chemotherapy.

5.5.4   Thymoma

Disorders which may have an immunopathological basis and which are associated with thymic epithelial cell tumours include myasthenia gravis, aplastic anaemia and immunodeficiency[61]. The latter arises in 10% of cases and usually involves both humoral and cell-mediated immunity. The infections which result are mostly of the respiratory tract; some 20% of patients with thymoma have diarrhoea.

The onset of the immunodeficiency has no constant temporal relationship to the appearance of the thymoma, nor has the disorder improved following thymomectomy. The persistence of the hypogammaglobulinaemia probably results from the disappearance of pre-B cells from the patients' marrows. Since the aplastic anaemia commonly does remit following removal of the tumour it seems likely that the level of stem-cell inhibition is different in the lymphoid and erythroid series.

5.5.5   Lymphopenia with lymphocytotoxins

Antilymphocyte antibodies are potent immunosuppressive agents in experimental animals and man so it is perhaps surprising that complement-fixing lymphocytotoxins should sometimes be transiently detectable in patients recovering from virus infections, without any obvious adverse effect. Lymphocytotoxins were found in a series of immunodeficient children reported by Kretschmer *et al.*[62]. In most cases they were lymphopenic, with impaired humoral and cell-mediated immunity. Their symptoms included eczema, recurrent pneumonia and bronchiectasis. Predominant antibody deficiency was present in a 30-year-old woman who had an IgM antibody which bound to a non-immunoglobulin determinant on her own B lymphocytes and those of others[63]. The possible pathogenicity of this antibody was suggested by the increase in the blood B-lymphocyte count of the patient following its removal by plasmaphoresis.

5.6 PRIMARY DEFECTS OF NON-SPECIFIC IMMUNITY

The importance of phagocytes and complement for effective antibody-dependent immunity was emphasized earlier (page 154). Some phagocyte defects affect both polymorphs and monocytes (e.g. chronic granulomatous disease) while the actin binding deficiency appears to affect only polymorphs. Defects of phagocytes may be quantitative or qualitative and in either case may effect polymorphonuclear leukocytes alone or cells of the mononuclear phagocyte system also. Quantitative defects are described first because they are commonest; detailed information is available in standard works on haematology.

5.6.1 Neutropenia

Secondary causes of neutropenia are commoner than primary ones and those following chemotherapy for malignant disease are sufficiently familiar to provide a reference point with which the symptomatology of other neutrophil abnormalities can be compared. Increased vulnerability to infection appears when the neutrophil count falls below about $500/mm^3$, and the pathogens involved are usually bacterial, occasionally fungal. *Staphylococci, E. coli* and *Pseudomonas* spp. are particularly troublesome and the affected site is usually mucosal (especially the mouth or anus), the skin or the lung. The infections are usually at least partially localized and if dissemination occurs it results most often in metastatic foci rather than septicaemia. When the cause of neutropenia is reversible, a rise in polymorph count is accompanied by clinical improvement; the same effect follows granulocyte transfusions though the benefit is only temporary.

Primary neutropenia is rare; the congenital forms range in severity from the rapidly fatal severe ones to the much milder 'chronic benign neutropenia'. The differential diagnosis is based on the family history and the blood polymorph count. Cyclical neutropenia can be difficult to recognize but it is probably worth making every effort to diagnose such patients because it may be possible to give them antibiotic cover during their brief period of vulnerability. Experiments in collie dogs, one strain of which has a cyclical neutropenia, suggest that the underlying defect in this disease is at the marrow stem-cell level and that the increased amounts of granulopoietic colony stimulating factor which are produced during and after the neutropenic phase are an appropriate physiological response[64].

5.6.2 Qualitative defects

The principal defective mechanisms of phagocytes are:

(1) Mobility (cellular defect), e.g. actin binding deficiency;

(2) Phagocytosis, e.g. secondary defects due to steroid therapy;

(3) Bacterial killing, e.g. chronic granulomatous disease.

5.6.2.1 Leukocyte mobility defects

Mobility describes movement in any direction while chemotaxis describes a tropic response to a chemical signal, usually in the form of a complement product. Chemotactic defects are not always associated with poor mobility. The existence of primary defects in neutrophil chemotaxis was suspected originally because some patients with recurrent bacterial infections had no laboratory abnormalities other than of chemotaxis. In addition, their rate of polymorph accumulation at Rebuck skin windows was low, indicating that the abnormality was present *in vivo*. This rather slender evidence was greatly strengthened by the recognition of familial cases and, recently, by the detection of reduced chemotactic responses by neutrophils from the asymptomatic, obligate heterozygote, parents of Shwachman's disease patients[65]. The majority of patients with defects of mobility have neither affected relatives nor Shwachman's disease, so it is difficult to establish whether the abnormality is primary or secondary. The presence or absence of either raised serum IgE levels or some other metabolic disorder known to impair leukocyte mobility serves to separate out the three main groups of patients listed below.

5.6.2.2 Primary cellular defects

The patients which Miller *et al.*[66] originally described as having 'lazy leukocyte syndrome' had recurrent low-grade fevers with gingivitis, stomatitis and a neutropenia which was uninfluenced by ephedrine or endotoxin. The tendency towards low neutrophil counts is seen also in patients with Shwachman's syndrome and it may be another manifestation of the inability of neutrophils to migrate in response to stimuli. Patients with the Chediak–Higashi syndrome have poor neutrophil mobility[67], although the abnormally large lysosomal inclusions which characterize the cells may contribute to this through purely mechanical factors. The improved response following incubation of the cells with ascrobic acid suggest that there may also be a metabolic component. Patients with Chediak–Higashi syndrome have recurrent severe pyogenic infections but this may not be entirely due to defective mobility since their polymorphs are also poor at bacterial killing.

(a) *Defective chemotaxis with raised serum IgE levels* – The variable inheritance and phenotypic features[68] of these patients suggest that some of the defects are secondary. In some children, for example, severe abscesses and suppurative lymphadenopathy are associated with eczema as well as the raised IgE, and in others there is also defective cell-mediated immunity. Patients with Job's syndrome have normal cell-mediated immunity but they are distinguishable by their red hair, hyperextensible joints and the absence of the typical signs of inflammation around abscesses[69].

(b) *Defective chemotaxis associated with other metabolic abnormalities* – Some juvenile onset diabetics and their first-degree relatives have impaired chemotaxis, as have patients with mannosidosis, hypophosphataemia and severe protein calorie malnutrition[70]. It seems likely that in these conditions the polymorph disturbance is due to the underlying metabolic defect.

5.6.2.3 Defects of phagocytosis

Phagocytosis is difficult to measure so relatively little is known about its defects. The actin binding deficiency[71], which also impairs chemotaxis, is probably the best example of a primary phagocytic defect, but it is uncertain which defect is more important in the pathogenesis of the infections. The polymorphs of patients with chronic granulocytic leukaemia are relatively poor at phagocytosis but their number must compensate for this.

5.6.2.4 Bacterial killing defects

The killing of phagocytosed bacteria involves many metabolic pathways including the hexose shunt, NADPH oxidase, myeloperoxidase and the halogenation of the bacterial cell wall (see review[72]). When any one of these pathways fails, the ingested bacteria may be able to survive and proliferate in an intracellular environment free of antibodies and antibiotics. The clinical features depend more on the severity of the bactericidal defect than the biochemical abnormality, but on the basis of family studies and laboratory tests it is possible to distinguish the defects listed in Table 5.4.

Table 5.4 **Primary bactericidal defects**

Disorder	Inheritance
Chronic granulomatous disease	X-linked or autosomal recessive
Glucose-6-phosphate dehydrogenase deficiency	X-linked recessive
Myeloperoxidase deficiency	Autosomal recessive
Pyruvate kinase deficiency	?
Glutathione reductase deficiency	
Chediak–Higashi syndrome	Autosomal recessive

(a) *Chronic granulomatous disease* – This term is perhaps most appropriately reserved for the X-linked recessive form of the disease associated with a failure of peroxide or superoxide production, and which is probably due to abnormality of a newly described cytochrome[73]. The patients' cells fail to reduce the dye nitroblue tetrazolium (NBT) even following stimulation with endotoxin. The defective polymorphs are produced by the marrow in normal numbers and episodes of infection evoke a leukocytosis. The polymorphs both migrate and phagocytose bacteria normally. The commonest infecting organism is *Staphylococcus aureus* followed by a range of Gram-negative bacilli, *Serratia marcescens* and various fungi. Susceptibility to streptococcal infections is not increased, perhaps because these bacteria are catalase-negative so they are unable to destroy the small amounts of peroxide they normally produce. As a result the peroxide is available to replace that which the cell fails to make.

Chronic granulomatous disease (CGD) usually presents in the first few weeks of life with superficial skin sepsis, which may initially amount to no more than a few tiny pustules. Subsequently, groups of lymph nodes, particularly in the groin, enlarge and may suppurate. Incision usually reveals copious pus from which *Staph. aureus* is grown and it is followed by slow healing by fibrosis. The histology of the lesion commonly reveals non-caseating granulomata with giant cells and in retrospect many of these children are probably unnecessarily given anti-tuberculosis treatment. Unilateral involvement of inguinal nodes may be mistaken for a retracted testis and, on the right side, an appendix abscess may be simulated. Episodes of infection result in fever and leukocytosis and when mesenteric lymph nodes are involved they cause abdominal pain in addition. The diagnosis may be obvious from the history, especially when several sites such as the groin, axilla and neck have required incision. It is confirmed by the NBT test: for screening, the slide modification with endotoxin stimulation is adequate[74]. The more quantitative bacterial killing test or the quantitative NBT test are both suitable for identifying carriers. Interestingly, the mothers of these patients have an increased incidence of systemic lupus-like disorders.

There is no specific treatment beyond appropriate antibiotics for infections. Since antibiotics (with the exception of rifampicin) do not effectively penetrate cells it is important to continue treatment for 2–3 times as long as would be given for a comparable infection in an otherwise normal child. When abscesses form they need to be drained, following general surgical principles.

Liver abscesses, osteomyelitis and fungal infections are the most serious complications. The first two are usually caused by *Staph. aureus* and they are best treated with antibiotics and drainage. There is a strong impression that patients given continuous cloxacillin or co-trimoxazole have fewer liver abscesses. With effective anti-staphylococcal treatment, affected boys are surviving longer and some appear to resist infections better after puberty. Fungal infections are becoming more important and the limited range and effectiveness of antifungal drugs makes them difficult to treat. They generally affect the lungs and *Aspergillus* species are commonest. Annual chest X-ray and perhaps testing the serum for precipitating antibodies may permit an early diagnosis of *Aspergillus* infection, without requiring lung biopsy, and at a stage which is easier to treat.

(b) *Other bacterial killing defects* (see review[75]) – These can broadly be divided into the abnormalities of the hexose shunt (e.g. G6PD deficiency) and glutathione reductase deficiency in which the NBT test is abnormal, and the pyruvate kinase (an Embden Mayerhof pathway enzyme), myeloperoxidase or unidentified enzyme abnormalities in which the NBT test is normal. In general both types of patient are less severely affected than the boys with CGD but there is considerable variation; some of those with myeloperoxidase deficiency have been troubled only by candidiasis. The diagnosis in these patients depends on the bacterial killing test rather than the NBT test; neutrophil mobility and complement defects need to be excluded. Treatment is along the lines suggested for CGD.

5.6.3 Complement defects

Inherited complement component deficiencies result either from a failure or abnormality of synthesis or from excessive consumption. Selective deficiencies of most complement components have been identified and the patients have tended to have one of the three main groups of symptoms indicated in Table 5.5. (See review[76].)

Table 5.5 Selective complement component deficiencies

Component	Symptom
C1r C4 C2	SLE-like syndromes
C3	Recurrent bacterial infection
C5 C6 C7 C8 C9	SLE-like syndrome or gonococcal or meningococcal disease

Symptoms arise in patients homozygous for the deficiency so transmission is autosomal recessive. The heterozygous state is usually readily detectable by the low levels of the affected component. C1r and C4 deficiency are both extremely rare whereas an estimated 1% of the population in the UK and in Boston is heterozygous for C2 deficiency. Genes controlling C2 are linked with certain HLA types and C2 deficiency is associated with HLA A10, B18 and LD7a. The few C1r and C4 deficient individuals described had a systemic lupus erythematosus (SLE)-like syndrome. C2 deficiency is much commoner and its principal disease association is also SLE. C2 deficient patients with SLE tend to have lower anti-nuclear antibody titres than SLE patients with normal C2 levels. Juvenile rheumatoid arthritis is the second commonest rheumatic disease in C2 deficient individuals[77]; other conditions which have been reported include Henhoch–Schonlein purpura and dermatomyositis. Some C2 deficient individuals are perfectly healthy. Whether the association between C2 deficiency and rheumatoid diseases is due to defective antigen clearance, impaired antibody responses or other factors is unknown but family studies suggest that environmental, as well as genetic, factors are important. Activation of complement by the alternative pathway may account for the lack of susceptibility to specific infections in patients who lack components prior to C3.

Only a few individuals homozygous for C3 deficiency have been identified. One, a teenage girl, had recurrent bacterial pneumonias as well as septicaemia, otitis media and meningitis. Her susceptibility to infection closely resembled that of antibody-deficient patients, though her antibody responses were in fact normal. The similarity emphasizes the importance of C3, with its opsonizing function, for the effector mechanisms of specific immunity.

Selective deficiency of C5 is extremely rare; in one affected kindred it was associated with an SLE-like syndrome. This is different from the functional C5 deficiency described by Miller and Nilsson[78] which now appears to be clinically very heterogeneous. It is described below with other opsonizing defects. The clinical features of defects of the later 'membrane attack' complement components are much more limited since they are most consistently associated with only a susceptibility to disseminated *Neisseria* infection. This suggests that direct bacterial lysis can be an important method of defence against *Neisseria*. There is one report of a C8 deficient patient who developed lupus, with renal involvement, but was negative for antinuclear antibodies.

5.6.3.1 *Defects of inactivators of activated complement components*

(a) *C1 esterase deficiency* – Hereditary angioneurotic oedema is caused by deficiency of the serum protein which normally inactivates C1; the result is uncontrolled activation of C4 and some increase in C2 consumption. The symptoms themselves are probably due to a vasoactive peptide which is cleaved off C2 by plasmin. The disorder is symptomatic in the heterozygous state and affected individuals generally have C1 esterase levels between 5% and 30% of normal. A few patients have normal or high levels of a nonfunctional but antigenically similar protein. Although the disorder is congenital, symptoms do not generally appear until after puberty and their severity is variable. The predominant features are areas of localized swelling which are not tender and which persist for 48–72 hours. The main danger is of laryngeal airway obstruction and emergency tracheostomy can become necessary. Involvement of the jejeunum causes abdominal cramps and colonic swelling results in diarrhoea. Oral treatment with the steroid Danazol markedly reduces the frequency of attacks and is considered a therapeutic advance on tranexamic acid[79].

(b) *C3b inhibitor deficiency* – Only two families with C3b inactivator-deficient individuals have been identified. The disorder is symptomatic in the homozygous state and transmission is autosomal. Heterozygotes can be identified by low enzyme levels in their serum. The failure of C3b inactivation permits uncontrolled C3 activation and, consequently, low C3 levels in the serum. The symptoms resemble those of isolated C3 deficiency in that recurrent bacterial infections predominate. Plasma infusions temporarily increase the C3b inactivator levels but the half-life appears too short for great therapeutic benefit.

5.6.4 Opsonizing defects

Opsonization results from the binding of C3 to the surface of the particle to be phagocytosed. This may be initiated through activation of the classical pathway of complement following the binding of IgG or IgM, or, as in the case of endotoxin, through activation of the alternative pathway. Yeast particles activate the alternative pathway and it was through a failure of yeast opsonization by the serum of the patients that primary opsonizing defects were first identified[78]. Serum from as many as one in 20 of the population opsonizes poorly, whereas in children with recurrent infections but normal specific immunity the frequency is one in four[80]. Some infants with defective opsonization develop erythroderma and diarrhoea and die, while healthy adults may be unaffected by their defect. Different defective sera may opsonize normally when mixed so there are probably a number of defects identified by the test and this probably accounts, in part, for the complex genetics of transmission. The real clinical importance of opsonizing defects may lie more in their predisposition to atopy or other immunopathology[81] than to recurrent infections.

5.7 SECONDARY IMMUNODEFICIENCY

Secondary immunodeficiency is important because it is common and because it causes much avoidable morbidity. Some of the precipitating mechanisms are listed below:

(1) Loss of immunoglobulin, or of immunoglobulin and leukocytes.

(2) Malnutrition – primary, or secondary to gastrointestinal disease.

(3) Infections – primary, or in association with malnutrition.

(4) Drugs.

(5) Miscellaneous, including some malignancies, post-splenectomy syndrome, post-surgery, etc.

Examples of only a few of the above have been selected for discussion in this chapter; some other secondary immunodeficiency syndromes are described elsewhere in this volume.

5.7.1 Loss of immunoglobulin

Protein loss into the urine in the nephrotic syndrome or into the gut in protein-losing enteropathy may be sufficiently severe to cause an antibody deficiency syndrome. It is almost invariably accompanied by hypoalbuminaemia, which is diagnostically useful in distinguishing secondary from primary hypogammaglobulinaemia. In nephrotic syndrome the hypoproteinaemia may be masked by haemoconcentration, and if the proteinuria is highly selective the loss of IgG will be small compared to the loss of albumin.

It is almost impossible to achieve significant immunoglobulin replacement in the face of continued loss. Treatment therefore needs to be directed to the cause.

5.7.2 Loss of immunoglobulin and leukocytes

Although it is rare, intestinal lymphangiectasia is probably the most clear-cut example of this combination. The condition is associated with a congenital abnormality of lymphatics which renders them leaky. It may be confined to the gut or may involve an extremity also, where it causes oedema. The immunological consequences are variable in severity but they include lymphopenia, hypogammaglobulinaemia and impaired cell-mediated immunity[82]. The gut is usually too diffusely affected for resection to be useful. Loss of lymphocytes probably accompanies severe Crohn's disease but in other protein-losing enteropathies the loss is predominantly of immunoglobulin.

5.7.3 Malnutrition

This must be the commonest cause of immunodeficiency in the world. Defects of macrophage function, antibody responses and cell-mediated immunity are all found in experimental animals fed protein- or calorie-deficient diets alone or in combination (reviewed in ref. 83). Laboratory tests on malnourished humans suggest that they develop comparable defects too but the overall susceptibility to infection is influenced by additional factors such as deficiency of iron or iron-binding proteins (see Chapter 1 and ref. 84). The treatment of malnutrition is obvious but more research is needed on the extent to which infections may aggravate malnutrition and the feasibility of protecting malnourished patients by immunization. The important result of one large-scale trial of infantile BCG immunization was that the infants from the more deprived environments were less adequately protected than those from richer (and so presumably better fed) families[85]. Lesser degrees of malnutrition almost certainly cause subtle defects of specific and non-specific immune responses.

5.7.4 Infections

Von Pirquet[86] appreciated that the delayed hypersensitivity skin reaction to tuberculin became negative during the course of measles infection but reverted to positive some weeks later. Immunosuppression in this case is probably due to direct interaction between the virus and T lymphocytes, since T-lymphocyte function *in vitro* is depressed by adding measles (and some other) viruses directly to the cultures[87]. The temporary immuno-suppression is probably clinically important; von Pirquet described increased activity of pre-existing tuberculosis during measles infection and more recently the increased long-term morbidity of adenovirus pneumonia occur-ring with measles has been appreciated. An example of clinical benefit is the occasional remission of steroid-sensitive nephrotic syndrome following measles infection.

Duncan's disease[88] results from a unique susceptibility to Epstein–Barr virus (EBV). It has an X-linked recessive transmission and a range of phenotypic expressions including acquired hypogammaglobulinaemia, immunoblastic sarcoma of B cells, American Burkitt's lymphoma and an acute form which is rapidly fatal. The disease might result from a failure of T lymphocytes to eradicate B lymphocytes infected with EBV during the course of infectious mononucleosis[89].

Congenital virus infections, especially rubella, can cause hypogamma-globulinaemia as well as structural defects[90]. IgA is the commonest class to be deficient but a few infants have also been IgG deficient.

5.7.5 Splenectomy

Individuals with congenital asplenic syndromes[91] or who have been splenectomized on account of trauma or haemolytic syndromes[92] are particularly susceptible to fulminant septicaemia. Their vulnerability is such that continuous antibiotic prophylaxis has been recommended.

5.8 DIAGNOSIS

5.8.1 History

There is no clearly defined 'normal' frequency of infections so a clinical diagnosis of immunodeficiency must take into account the environment as well as the site, severity and duration of infections. Although immuno-deficient patients may be vulnerable to infection at multiple sites it is common for the respiratory tract to be most severely affected. Many primary conditions can predispose to recurrent upper or lower respiratory tract infections and some are much commoner than primary immunodeficiency. They include cystic fibrosis, aspirated foreign bodies or saliva and rarely, α_1-antitrypsin deficiency. Attention may be drawn to the respiratory tract by other disorders such as asthma and there is a strong clinical impression that all forms of atopy are associated with an increase in symptoms due to minor infections.

Other symptoms are sometimes suggestive of a particular defect: examples include the recurrent abscesses which occur with polymorph bacterial killing defects or, less commonly, with antibody deficiency. Local bacterial infections with little pus formation are found with leukocyte mobility defects. In the gut malabsorption ultimately develops in almost all infants with severe combined immunodeficiency but it is quite common in patients with defects affecting predominantly antibody or cell-mediated immunity too. Intractable diarrhoea also occurs with opsonizing defects.

Older sibling with severe congenital immunodeficiency may prompt testing of cord blood and in the case of ADA deficiency antenatal diagnosis is possible[93], though not at a stage of pregnancy suitable for termination. X-linked combined immunodeficiency may be taken as an indication for terminating a pregnancy with a male fetus; in this situation it is obviously important to discuss fully the chances of an affected infant with the parents.

In patients who present post-natally, a family history of either immuno-deficiency, allergy or auto-immune disease suggests a genetic basis for the disorder. In congenital severe immunodeficiencies affected siblings usually run similar courses unless effective treatment is possible. In the varied immunodeficiency syndromes the phenotypic expression in family members is variable.

5.8.2 Organisms

Infection by commensals or other organisms of normally low virulence such as *Mimea polymorphea* or *Serratia marcescens* gives circumstantial evidence of impaired immune responses. Sometimes recurrent infection by a restricted range of organisms gives useful clues as to the type of immunodeficiency which a patient may have. Some such associations which might alert suspicion are listed in Table 5.6.

5.8.3 Investigations

The foregoing sections may have indicated whether a defect is more likely to be in the antibody–complement–phagocyte system or in cell-mediated immunity. The efficiency of selective investigation is attractive but a lack of information often necessitates a blunderbuss approach. The investigative steps listed in Table 5.7 have been arranged on the assumption that most physicians do not have the facilities of a sophisticated immunology laboratory immediately available. Simple tests can be very informative; for example, a negative Schick test and detectable isohaemagglutinins exclude antibody deficiency and, by inference, panhypogammaglobulinaemia.

Table 5.6   Defects suggested by infecting organisms

Organism	Defective system
Bacteria	
Staph. aureus	Bacterial killing
Staphylococci and other bacteria	Antibody
	C3
	Polymorphs
Neisseria	C6–C9
Salmonellae (chronic carriage)	IgA
BCG (disseminated)	Cell-mediated immunity
Fungi	
Candida (superficial)	Cell-mediated immunity (also chronic mucocutaneous candidiasis)
Other fungi	Sometimes cell-mediated immunity
Aspergillus species	Chronic granulomatous disease
protozoa	
Pneumocystis carinii	Cell-mediated immunity
Giardia lamblia	Antibody
Viruses	
Vaccine strain poliomyelitis	Antibody
Vaccinia (disseminated)	Cell-mediated immunity (also eczema)
Varicella pneumonia	Cell-mediated immunity
Cytomegalovirus	Cell-mediated immunity

Positive delayed hypersensitivity skin tests to common antigens such as *Candida*, PPD or trichophyton virtually exclude defects of cell-mediated immunity. The rare deficiencies of single complement components can be excluded by demonstrating that fresh serum from the patient can lyse sensitized erythrocytes, and any bacteriological laboratory undertaking complement fixation tests can do this test. Unfortunately, polymorph function tests are more demanding and it is worth remembering that NBT reduction is of very limited value as a screening test since it is abnormal only in a few disorders (see page 186). Apart from the tendency of patients with neutrophil mobility defects to have lower neutrophil counts in blood, and to form less pus at sites of infection, there are no clinical clues to distinguish between bacterial killing and mobility defects. Both functions need to be tested separately.

Specialist laboratory facilities are particularly valuable in assessing possible lines of treatment in adults and establishing a primary diagnosis in

Table 5.7 A simple plan for investigating immunodeficiency*

| | Suspected defective mechanism | | | |
	Antibody	*Complement*	*Phagocyte*	*Cell-mediated immunity*
In vivo or simple laboratory test	Schick skin test Isohaemagglutinins (IgM)	—	Polymorph count and morphology Rebuck skin window†	Blood lymphocyte count Delayed hypersensitivity skin test‡
Special tests (first level)	Immunoglobulin concentrations Antibody tests *E. coli* = IgM Antistreptolysin-O = IgG	Opsonization Complement-mediated lysis C3 estimation	Bacterial killing test Leukocyte mobility test NBT test or chemo-luminescence	Lymphocyte response to mitogens
Special tests (second level)	Antibody tests: Diphtheria, tetanus, KLH, Øx174. Immunoglobulin sub-class measurement Kappa : lambda ratios Antibody heterogeneity Blood B lymphocyte count	Estimation of individual components	Leukocyte enzymes	T lymphocyte populations Functional studies: MLC and co-operation with B cells Enzyme measurement

* See reference 94 for more detailed discussion of interpretation of tests
† Interpretation may require specialist help⁹⁵
‡ Negative responses are meaningless unless prior sensitization is certain

infants. This is because tests in infants pose special problems in interpretation. Isohaemagglutinins do not normally reach adult levels until the age of 2 and response to skin tests may not appear until even later. It is obviously desirable to use the minimum quantities of blood possible, especially in infants. By using defibrinated whole blood for lymphocyte cultures and making use of the serum, lymphocyte and red cell fractions my laboratory is able to determine blood count, serum immunoglobulins, blood group and isohaemagglutinins, opsonization, C3 or haemolytic complement, PHA response and T- and B-lymphocyte populations on 3–4 ml of blood.

5.9 SPECIAL HAZARDS

5.9.1 Immunization

Infants with severe combined immunodeficiency develop progressive BCG or disseminated vaccinia following immunization with these agents. Paralysis following immunization with attenuated poliovirus is more common in antibody-deficient patients than the rest of the population[96]. These observations strongly suggest that patients with suspected or proven defects of specific immunity should not be immunized with 'live' vaccines.

A possible exception to this is the use of the bacteriophage Øx174 for antibody testing[97]; this is safe because the bacteriophage cannot infect mammalian cells. Killed bacterial antigens are generally harmless, with the exception of preparations such as TAB vaccine, which contain large amounts of endotoxin which can cause endotoxin shock in antibody-deficient patients. Healthy individuals are much less susceptible to endotoxin shock because they have cross-reactive IgM antibodies which reduce the endotoxin load.

In summary, it is prudent to advise patients with defects of specific immunity against immunization. For patients who have already started on immunoglobulin replacement injections the risk of contracting endemic exanthems appears to be very much reduced.

Patients whose immunodeficiency affects only non-specific immunity can in general be safely immunized with killed organisms or oral polio vaccine. Attenuated organisms causing local lesions such as vaccinia or BCG should be avoided in patients with polymorph defects, for fear of possible extension of the lesions.

5.9.2 Blood transfusion

Lymphocytes in banked ACD blood remain viable (as judged by responsiveness to PHA) for up to 3 weeks and so are potentially capable of causing graft versus host disease in a patient with severely impaired cell-mediated immunity. This danger can be avoided by giving the blood 3000 rad[98] or transfusing special frozen-thawed washed erythrocyte preparations. Patients with normal immunity are protected from graft versus host disease by their own lymphocytes and the cellular immune response which the transfusion evokes is manifest as an increased thymidine uptake by blood lymphocytes 4–6 days after the transfusion.

Patients with selective IgA deficiency sometimes make anti-IgA antibodies which cause mild or severe transfusion reactions[99]. This might in part be avoidable by routinely screening all IgA deficient patients for anti-IgA antibodies. Previous transfusion or injections of IgA containing immunoglobulin concentrates are not a prerequisite for anti-IgA antibody production; perhaps sensitization can take place to ruminant IgA in milk.

References

1. Afzelius, B. A. (1976). A human syndrome caused by immobile cilia. *Science*, **193**, 317
2. Cooper M. D. *et al.* (1974). Meeting report of the second international workshop on primary immunodeficiency diseases in man. *Clin. Immunol. Immunopathol.*, **2**, 416
3. Hayward, A. R. and Greaves, M. F. (1975). Central failure of B lymphocyte induction in panhypogammaglobulinaemia. *Clin. Immunol. Immunopathol.*, **3**, 461
4. Vogler, L. B. *et al.* (1976). B-lymphocyte precursors in bone marrow in immunoglobulin deficiency diseases. *Lancet*, **ii**, 376
5. Cooper, M. D. and Seligmann, M. (1976). B and T lymphocytes in immunodeficiency and lymphoproliferative diseases. In: *B and T Cells in Immune Recognition* (F. Loor and G. Rolants, eds.) (UK: Wiley and Sons)
6. Ciccimarra, F., Rosen, F. S., Schneeberger, E. and Merler, E. (1976). Failure of heavy-chain glycosylation of IgG in some patients with common variable agammaglobulinaemia. *J. Clin. Invest.*, **57**, 1386
7. Waldmann, T. A., Durm, M., Broder, S., Blackman. M., Blaese, R. M. and Strober, W. (1974). Role of suppressor T cells in pathogenesis of common variable hypogammaglobulinaemia. *Lancet*, **ii**, 609
8. Broom, B. G., de la Concha, E. G., Webster, A. D. B., Janossy, G. J. and Asherson, G. L. (1976). Intracellular immunoglobulin production *in vitro* by lymphocytes from patients with hypogammaglobulinaemia and their effect on normal lymphocytes. *Clin. Exp. Immunol.*, **23**, 73
9. M.R.C. Report (1971). Working Party on hypogammaglobulinaemia. *Special Report Series*, **310**, 55
10. Stiehm, E. R. and Fudenberg, H. H. (1966). Clinical and immunologic features of dysgammaglobulinaemia type I. *Am. J. Med.*, **40**, 805
11. Hitzig, W. H. and Kenny, A. B. (1975). The role of vitamin B12 and its transport globulins in the production of antibodies. *Clin. Exp. Immunol.*, **20**, 105
12. Buckley, R. H. (1975). Clinical and immunologic features of selective IgA deficiency. In: *Immunodeficiency in Man and Animals* (D. Bergsma *et al.*, eds.) (Sunderland: Sinauer Press)
13. Delespesse, G., Gausset, P., Cauchie, C. and Govaerts, A. (1976). Cellular aspects of selective IgA deficiency. *Clin. Exp. Immunol.*, **24**, 273
14. Ogra. P. A. *et al.* (1974). Mechanism of mucosal immunity to viral infections in A immunoglobulin deficiency syndromes. *Proc. Soc. Exp. Biol. Med.*, **145**, 811
15. Kaufman, H. S. and Hobbs, J. R. (1970). Immunoglobulin deficiencies in an atopic population. *Lancet*, **ii**, 1061
16. Soothill, J. F., Stokes, C. R., Turner, M. W., Norman, A. P. and Taylor, B. (1976). Predisposing factors and the development of reaginic allergy in infancy. *Clin. Allergy*, **6**, 305

17. Carrol, J. E., Silverman, A., Isobe, Y., Brown, W. R., Kelts, K. A. and Brooke, M. H. (1976). Inflammatory myopathy, IgA deficiency and intestinal malabsorption. *J. Pediatr.*, **89**, 216

18. Hobbs, J. R. (1975). IgM deficiency. In: *Immunodeficiency in Man and Animals* (D. Bergsma *et al.*, eds.) (Sunderland: Sinauer Press)

19. Fudenberg, H., German, J. L. and Kunkel, H. G. (1962). The occurrence of rheumatoid factor and other abnormalities in families of patients with agammaglobulinaemia. *Arthritis Rheum.*, **5**, 565

20. Webster, A. D. B. *et al.* (1978). Echovirus encephalitis and myositis in primary immuno-globulin deficiency. *Arch. Dis. Child.*, **53**, 33

21. Yount, W. J. (1975). Imbalances of IgG subclasses and gene defects in patients with primary hypogammaglobulinaemia. In: *Immunodeficiency in Man and Animals* (D. Bergsma *et al.*, eds.) (Sunderland: Sinauer Press)

22. Zegers, B. J. M., Maertsdorg, W. J., van Loghem, E., Mul, N. A. J., Stoop, J. W., van der Laag, J., Vossen, J. J. and Ballieux, R. E. (1976). Kappa chain deficiency. *N. Engl. J. Med.*, **294**, 1026

23. Barandun, S. *et al.* (1976). Deficiency of κ- or λ-type immunoglobulins. *Blood*, **47**, 79

24. MRC Report (1971). Working party on hypogammaglobulinaemia. *Special Report Series* 310

25. Soothill, J. F. (1971). Reactions to immunoglobulin. In: *Hypogammaglobulinaemia in the United Kingdom.* MRC Special Report Series 310

26. Buckley, R. H. and Durham, N. C. (1972). Plasma therapy in immunodeficiency diseases. *Am. J. Dis. Child.*, **124**, 376

27. Di George, A. M. (1968). Congenital absence of the thymus and its immunologic con-sequences. In: *Immunologic Deficiency Diseases in Man.* Birth Defects Original Article Series Vol. 4

28. Giblett, E. R., Ammann, A. J., Sandman, R., Wara, D. W. and Diamond, L. K. (1975). Nucleoside phosphorylase deficiency in a child with severely defective T-cell immunity and normal B-cell immunity. *Lancet*, **i**, 1010

29. Lischner, H. W. and Huff, D. S. (1975). T-cell deficiency in Di George syndrome. In: *Immunodeficiency in Man and Animals* (D. Bergsma *et al.*, eds.) (Sunderland: Sinauer Press)

30. Steele, R. W., Limas, C., Thurman, G. B., Schuelein, M., Bauer, H. and Bellanti, J. A. (1972). Familial thymic aplasia. (Attempted reconstruction with fetal thymus in a millipore diffusion chamber.) *N. Engl. J. Med.*, **287**, 787

31. McKusick, V. A. (1964). Metaphysical dysostosis and thin hair: a new recessively inherited syndrome? *Lancet*, **i**, 832

32. Biggar, W. D., Park, B. H., Stutman, O., Gaji-Peczalska, K. and Good, R. A. (1975). Fetal thymus transplantation: experimental and clinical observations. In: *Immunodeficiency in Man and Animals* (D. Bergsma *et al.*, eds.) (Sunderland: Sinauer Press)

33. D. W. van Bekkum (ed.) (1975). *Biological Activities of Thymic Hormones* (Rotterdam: Kooyker)

34. Bach, J.-F., Dardenne, M. and Pleau, J.-M. (1977). Biochemical characterization of a serum thymic factor. *Nature*, **266**, 55

35. Lawrence, H. S. (1969). Transfer factor. *Adv. Immunol.*, **11**, 196

36. Spitler, L. E., Levin, A. S. and Fudenberg, H. H. (1975). Transfer factor II: results of therapy. In: *Immunodeficiency in Man and Animals* (D. Bergsma *et al.*, ed.) (Sunderland: Sinauer Press)

37. Matsaniotis, N. and Economou-Mavrou, C. (1968). Fatal generalized BCG infection. In: *Immunologic Deficiency Diseases in Man* (D. Bergsma, ed.) (New York: Natl. Foundation)

38. Scott, C. R., Chen, S. H. and Giblett, E. R. (1974). Detection of the carrier state in combined immunodeficiency associated with adenosine deaminase deficiency. *J. Clin. Invest.*, **53**, 1194

39. Hirschorn, R. (1977). Defects of purine metabolism in immunodeficiency diseases. In: *Progress in Clinical Immunology* (R. Schwartz, ed.)

40. Simmonds, H. A., Panayi, G. S. and Corrigall, V. (1978). A role for purine metabolism in the immune response: adenosine deaminase activity and deoxyadenosine catabolism. *Lancet*, **i**, 60

41. Lawlor, G. J., Ammann, A. J., Wright, W. G., Lafranchi, S. H., Bilstrom, D. and Stiehm, R. (1974). The syndrome of cellular immunodeficiency with immunoglobulins. *J. Pediatr.*, **84**, 183

42. Seeger, R. C., Robins, R. A., Stevens, R. H., Klein, R. B., Waldman, D. J., Zeltzer, P. M. and Kessler, S. W. (1976). Severe combined immunodeficiency with B lymphocytes: *in vitro* correction of defective immunoglobulin production by addition of normal T lymphocytes. *Clin. Exp. Immunol.*, **26**, 1

43. Ochs, H. D., Davis, S. D., Mickelson, E., Lerner, K. G. and Wedgwood, R. J. (1974). Combined immunodeficiency and reticuloendotheliosis with eosinophilia. *J. Pediatr.*, **85**, 463

44. Cederbaum, S. D., Niwayama, G., Stiehm, E. R., Neerhout, R. C., Ammann, A. J. and Berman, W. (1974). Combined immunodeficiency presenting as the Letterer-Sieve syndrome. *J. Pediatr.*, **85**, 466

45. Ownby, D. R., Pizzo, S., Blackmon, L., Gall, S. A. and Buckley, R. H. (1976). Severe combined immunodeficiency with leukopenia (reticular dysgenesis) in siblings: immunologic and histopathologic findings. *J. Pediatr.*, **89**, 382

46. Biggar, W. D., Park, B. H. and Good, R. A. (1975). Compatible bone marrow transplantation and immunologic reconstitution of combined immunodeficiency disease. In: *Immunodeficiency in Man and Animals* (D. Bergsma *et al.*, ed.) (Sunderland: Sinauer Press)

47. Glucksberg, H. *et al.* (1974). Clinical manifestations of graft versus host disease in human recipients of marrow from HLA matched sibling donors. *Transplantation*, **18**, 295

48. Report from the ACS/NIH Bone Marrow Transplant Registry (1976)

49. Buckley, R. H. (1977). Replacement therapy in immunodeficiency. In: *Recent Advances in Clinical Immunology*, *I* (R. Thompson, ed.) (London: Churchill)

50. Hong, R., Santosham, M., Schulte-Wissermann, H., Horowitz, S., Hsu, S. H. and Winkelstein, J. A. (1976). Reconstitution of T and B lymphocyte function in severe combined immunodeficiency disease after transplantation with thymic epithelium. *Lancet*, **ii**, 1270

51. Polmar, S. H., Stern, R. C., Schwartz, A. L., Wetzler, T. M., Chase, P. A. and Hirschorn, R. (1976). Enzyme replacement therapy for adenosine deaminase deficiency and severe combined immunodeficiency. *N. Engl. J. Med.*, **295**, 1337

52. McFarlin, D. E., Strober, W. and Waldmann, T. A. (1972). Ataxia telangiectasia. *Medicine (Baltimore)*, **51**, 281

53. Polmar, S. H., Waldmann, T. A. and Terry, W. D. (1972). IgE in immunodeficiency. *Am. J. Pathol.*, **69**, 499

54. Trompeter, R. S., Layward, L. and Hayward, A. R. (1978). Primary and secondary abnormalities of T-cell subpopulations. *Clin. Exp. Immunol.*, **34**

55. Cooper, M. D., Chase, H. P., Lowman, J. T., Krivit, W. and Good, R. A. (1968). Wiskott–Aldrich syndrome: immunologic deficiency disease involving the afferent limbs of immunity. *Am. J. Med.*, **44**, 499

56. Blaese, R. M. *et al.* (1971). Hypercatabolism of IgG, IgM and albumin in the Wiskott–Aldrich syndrome. *J. Clin. Invest.*, **50**, 2331

57. Blaese, R. M., Oppenheim, J. J., Seeger, R. C. and Waldmann, T. A. (1972). Lymphocyte macrophage interaction in antigen-induced *in vitro* lymphocyte transformation in patients with the Wiskott–Aldrich syndrome and other diseases with allergy. *Cell. Immunol.*, **4**, 228

58. Spitler, L. E. *et al.* (1972). Wiskott-Aldrich syndrome: results of transfer factor therapy. *J. Clin. Invest.*, **51**, 3216

59. Wells, R. S., Higgs, J. M., MacDonald, A., Valdimarsson, H. and Holt, P. L. J. (1972). Familial chronic mucocutaneous candidiasis. *J. Med. Gen.*, **9**, 302

60. Valdimarsson, H., Higgs, J. M., Wells, R. S., Yamamura, M., Hobbs, J. R. and Holt, P. L. J. (1973). Immune abnormalities associated with chronic mucocutaneous candidiasis. *Cell. Immunol.*, **6**, 348

61. Ammann, A. J. and Hong, R. (1973). Cellular immunodeficiency disorders. In: *Immunologic Disorders in Infants and Children* (E. R. H. Stiehm and V. A. Fulginiti, eds.) (Philadelphia: Saunders)

62. Kretschmer, R., August, C. S., Rosen, F. S. and Janeway, C. A. (1969). Recurrent infections, episodic lymphopenia and impaired cellular immunity. *N. Engl. J. Med.*, **281**, 285

63. Tursz, T., Preud'homme, J.-L., La-baume, S., Matuchansky, C. and Seligmann, M. (1977). Autoantibodies to B lymphocytes in a patient with hypoimmunoglobulinaemia. *J. Clin. Invest.*, **60**, 405

64. Weiden, L., Robinett, B., Graham, T. C., Adamson, J. and Storb, R. (1974). Canine cyclic neutropenia. A stem-cell defect. *J. Clin. Invest.*, **53**, 950

65. Aggett, P. J., Harries, J. T., Harvey, B. A. M. and Soothill, J. F. (1978). An inherited defect of neutrophil mobility in Shwachman's syndrome. (Submitted)

66. Miller, M. E., Oski, F. A. and Harris, M. B. (1971). Lazy leukocyte syndrome. *Lancet*, **i**, 665

67. Boxer, L. A., Watanabe, A. M., Rister, K., Besch, H. R., Allen, J. and Baehner, R. L. (1976). Correction of leukocyte function in Chediak–Higashi syndrome by ascorbate. *N. Engl. J. Med.*, **295**, 1041

68. Hill, H. R. and Quie, P. G. (1974). Raised serum IgE levels and defective neutrophil chemotaxis in three children with eczema and recurrent bacterial infections. *Lancet*, **i**, 183

69. Davis, S. D., Schaller, J. and Wedgwood, R. J. (1966). Job's syndrome. Recurrent 'cold' staphylococcal abscesses. *Lancet*, **i**, 1013

70. Snyderman, R. and Pike, M. C. (1977). Disorders of leukocyte chemotaxis. *Pediatr. Clin. N. Am.*, **24**, 377

71. Boxer, L. A., Hedley-Whyte, E. T. and Stossel, T. (1974). Neutrophil actin dysfunction and abnormal neutrophil behaviour. *N. Engl. J. Med.*, **291**, 1093

72. Klebanoff, S. J. (1975). Antimicrobial mechanisms in neutrophilic polymorphonuclear leukocytes. *Semin. Haematol.*, **12**, 117

73. Segal, A. W., Jones, O. T. G., Webster, D. and Allison, A. C. (1978). Absence of a newly described cytochrome b from neutrophils of patients with chronic granulomatous disease. *Lancet*, **ii**, 446

74. Park, B. H., Fikrig, S. M. and Smithwick, E. M. (1968). Infection and the nitroblue tetrazolium reduction by neutrophils: a diagnostic aid. *Lancet*, **ii**, 532

75. Cline, M. J. *et al.* (1974). Granulocytes in human disease. *Ann. Intern. Med.*, **81**, 801

76. Johnston, R. B. and Stroud, R. M. (1977). Complement and host defence against infection. *J. Pediatr.*, **90**, 169

77. Glass, D., Raum, D., Gibson, D., Stillman, J. S. and Schur, P. H. (1976). Inherited deficiency of the second component of complement: rheumatic disease associations. *J. Clin. Invest.*, **58**, 853

78. Miller, M. E. and Nilsson, U. R. (1970). A familial deficiency of the phagocytosis enhancing activity of serum related to a dysfunction of the fifth component of complement (C5). *N. Engl. J. Med.*, **282**, 354

79. Gelfand, J. A., Sherins, R. J., Alling, D. W. and Frank, M. M. (1976). Treatment of hereditary angioedema with Danazol. Reversal of clinical and biochemical abnormalities. *N. Engl. J. Med.*, **295**, 1444

80. Soothill, J. F. and Harvey, B. A. M. (1976). Defective opsonization, a common immunity deficiency. *Arch. Dis. Child.*, **51**, 91

81. Soothill, J. F. (1976). Immunodeficiency and common allergic disease. In: *Proc. 12th Symposium of Advanced Medicine* (D. K. Peters, ed.) (London: Pitman Medical)

82. Strober, W. *et al.* (1967). Intestinal lymphangiectasia: a protein losing enteropathy with hypogammaglobulinaemia, lymphocytopenia and impaired homograft rejection. *J. Clin. Invest.*, **46**, 1643

83. Chandra, R. K. and Newberne, P. M. (1977). *Nutrition, Immunity and Infection* (New York and London: Plenum Press)

84. Weinberg, E. D. (1975). Iron and susceptibility to infectious disease. *Science*, **184**, 952

85. Mehta, K. P., Merchant, S. M. and Korde, U. (1976). Environmental influence on immunity due to BCG vaccination. *Indian Pediatr.*, **13**, 525

86. Von Pirquet, C. (1908). Das verhalten das kutanen tuberkulin reaktion wahrend der masern. *Dtsch. Med. Wochenschr.*, **34**, 1297

87. Wheelock, E. F., Toy, S. T. and Stjernholm, R. (1971). Interaction of viruses with human lymphocytes. In: *Progress in Immunology*

88. Purtilo, D. T. *et al.* (1975). X-linked recessive progressive combined immunodeficiency (Duncan's disease). *Lancet*, **i**, 935

89. Thorley-Lawson, D. A., Chess, L. and Strominger, J. L. (1977). Suppression of *in vitro* Epstein–Barr virus infection. *J. Exp. Med.*, **146**, 495

90. Soothill, J. F., Hayes, K. and Dudgeon, J. A. (1966). The immunoglobulins in congenital rubella. *Lancet*, **i**, 1385

91. Waldman, J. D. *et al.* (1977). Sepsis and congenital asplenia. *J. Pediatr.*, **90**, 555

92. Erickson, W. D., Burgert, E. O. and Lynn, H. B. (1968). The hazard of infection following splenectomy in children. *Am. J. Dis. Child.*, **116**, 1

93. Hirschorn, R., Beratis, N. and Rosen, F. S. (1975). Adenosine deaminase deficiency in a child diagnosed prenatally. *Lancet*, **i**, 73

94. Hayward, A. R. (1977). *Immunodeficiency.* (London: Edward Arnold)

95. Rebuck, J. W. and Crowley, J. H. (1955). A method of studying leukocytic functions *in vivo*. *Ann. N.Y. Acad. Sci.*, **59**, 757

96. Wyatt, H. V. (1973). Poliomyelitis in hypogammaglobulinaemics. *J. Infect. Dis.*, **128**, 802

97. Wedgwood, R. A., Ochs, H. D. and Davis, S. D. (1975). The recognition and classification of immunodeficiency diseases with bacteriophage Øx174. In: *Immunodeficiency in Man and Animals* (D. Bergsma *et al.*, eds.) (Sunderland: Sinauer Press)

98. Van Bekkum, D. W. (1972). Use and abuse of haemopoietic cell grafts in immune deficiency diseases. *Transplant. Rev.*, **9**, 3

99. Miller, M. V., Holland, P. V., Sugarbaker, E., Strober, W. and Waldman, T. A. (1970). Anaphylactic reactions to IgA: a difficult transfusion problem. *Am. J. Clin. Pathol.*, **54**, 618

6
Immune Status of the Malnourished Host

R. M. SUSKIND

6.1 INTRODUCTION 202

6.2 HUMORAL RESPONSE 203
   6.2.1 *Immunoglobulins and antibody response of the
       malnourished child* 203
       6.2.1.1 *B-cell enumeration* 203
       6.2.1.2 *Serum immunoglobulins* 204
       6.2.1.3 *Antibody response* 204
       6.2.1.4 *Secretory immunoglobulins (SIgA)* 204
   6.2.2 *The complement system in the malnourished child* 205
       6.2.2.1 *Complement proteins* 205
       6.2.2.2 *Haemolytic complement activity* 205

5.3 CELLULAR RESPONSE 206
   6.3.1 *The cell-mediated immune response* 206
       6.3.1.1 *Clinical and pathological changes* 206
       6.3.1.2 In vivo *skin test responsiveness* 206
       6.3.1.3 In vitro *lymphocyte function* 207
   6.3.2 *The polymorphonuclear leukocyte and macrophage in
       children with protein–calorie malnutrition* 208
       6.3.2.1 *Chemotaxis and phagocytosis* 208
       6.3.2.2 *Killing function* 208
       6.3.2.3 *Enzymatic changes* 209

6.4 CONCLUSION 210

6.1 INTRODUCTION

The severely malnourished child with marasmus or kwashiorkor has an increased morbidity and mortality secondary to his increased susceptibility to infection[1-3]. Children develop these syndromes as primary and secondary disease states. Children develop marasmus as a result of severe deprivation of both protein and calories, leading to growth retardation, weight loss, muscular atrophy and loss of subcutaneous tissue (Figure 6.1). Children develop kwashiorkor as a result of acute protein loss or deprivation. They have a clinical picture characterized by edema, skin lesions, hair changes, apathy, anorexia, an enlarged fatty liver and decreased serum total protein and albumin (Figure 6.2). These children have abundant subcutaneous fat and recover rapidly on a high-protein diet. Children with marasmus–kwashiorkor have clinical and biochemical parameters which lie somewhere between those with marasmus and those with kwashiorkor.

Children with primary and secondary protein–calorie malnutrition have nutrient deficits of protein and calories, vitamins and minerals. Their nutrient status is often confused by superimposed infection. Deficiencies of such nutrients as iron, folate, pyridoxine, vitamin A, protein and calories have been associated with alterations in the immune response. In discussing

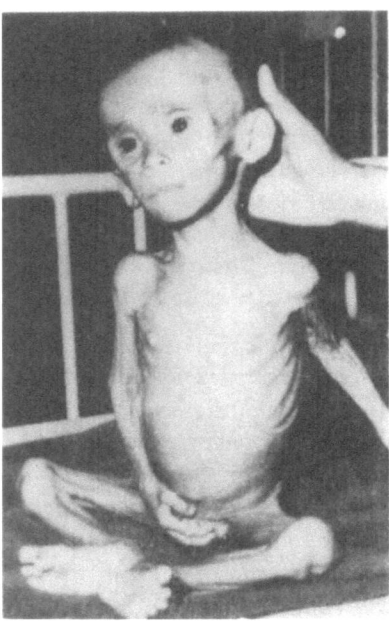

Figure 6.1   Marasmic child with evidence of growth retardation, weight loss, muscular atrophy and severe loss of subcutaneous tissue. (Courtesy of Medical Staff, Anaemia and Malnutrition Research Centre, Chiang Mai, Thailand)

the changes in the immune status of the malnourished child, one cannot readily associate these with any specific nutrient deficiency. The most one is able to do is to document the changes in the immune response and to determine whether the changes are reversible with improved nutrient intake.

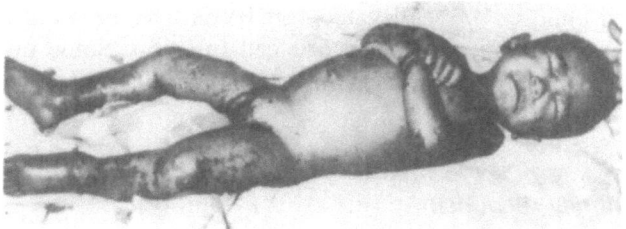

Figure 6.2   Child with kwashiorkor with evidence of oedema, skin lesions, hair changes, apathy, anorexia, an enlarged fatty liver and decreased serum total protein and albumin. (Courtesy of Medical Staff, Anaemia and Malnutrition Research Centre, Chiang Mai, Thailand)

Several host defences have been implicated as being affected in the malnourished child[4-17]. These include the humoral response (i.e. the immunoglobulin and complement systems), the cellular response (i.e. the cell-mediated immune system) and the phagocytic and killing function of leukocytes.

6.2   HUMORAL RESPONSE

6.2.1   Immunoglobulins and antibody response of the malnourished child

The bursa cell or B lymphocyte is responsible for immunoglobulin production. The competency of the B-lymphocyte system is determined by enumerating the number of B cells, by measuring circulating immunoglobulins, by measuring the antibody response to antigenic stimulation and by studying secretory immunoglobulins.

6.2.1.1   *B-cell enumeration*

While T-cell numbers are depressed in malnourished children, B-cell numbers are normal or elevated[18], accounting in part for the normal or elevated immunoglobulin titres. Several people have speculated that the elevated immunoglobulin levels of the malnourished child may be secondary to an increased exposure to various infectious agents, many of which he is not able to respond to when he becomes severely malnourished. Others have speculated that with the depressed T-cell population there may also be suppression of the T-suppressor population resulting in uncontrolled nonspecific antibody production[19].

6.2.1.2 *Serum immunoglobulins*

The majority of malnourished children have circulating IgA, IgM and IgG levels which are either normal or elevated[20-22]. Occasionally, a malnourished child without a concomitant or recent infection has decreased serum IgG, IgA and IgM[23]. Increased serum IgD and IgE have also been observed in malnourished children[24,25]. Elevated IgE levels may be secondary to an increased parasitic load or decreased T-cell function. Some investigators feel that increased IgE levels may inhibit human T-lymphocyte rosetting with sheep red cells[23].

6.2.1.3 *Antibody response*

Antibody response to antigens such as yellow fever vaccine[26], influenza vaccine[27] and typhoid vaccine[28] have been shown to be impaired in malnourished children, while antibody response to many antigens including Keyhole limpet haemocyanin, lipopolysaccharide, measles, polio virus, tetanus and diphtheria toxoid is adequate[1]. In some studies, lack of specific nutrients such as pyridoxine and pantothenic acid have been implicated in the suppression of the immune response[29,30]. In the malnourished child, it has not been determined which of the specific nutrient deficiencies is responsible for the depressed antibody response. Interpretation of the data is very difficult in most studies because of the lack of control of several critical variables such as dose of the antigen, its route of delivery, the severity of the malnutrition, the presence of infection, differences in nutritional therapy and the status of liver function[23]. The presence of associated infection may profoundly suppress antibody synthesis[27].

6.2.1.4 *Secretory immunoglobulins (SIgA)*

Recently, Chandra *et al.*[32] have demonstrated that secretory IgA antibody response to live attenuated measles and polio vaccines is reduced in malnourished children. Depressed secretory IgA has been demonstrated in the nasopharyngeal and salivary secretions of malnourished children[17,32]. Reduced mucosal immunity may permit endemic spread, thus explaining the frequent occurrence of Gram-negative septicaemia in malnutrition[23]. The increased frequency of serum antibodies to common food antigens in malnourished children may be due to defective antigen exclusion[31]. Other changes which accompany the decreased secretory immunoglobulins are an atrophied gut wall, reduced digestive enzymes and an impaired hepatic reticuloendothelial system, all of which play a role in increasing the host's susceptibility to Gram-negative organisms, especially from the gastrointestinal tract[23]. Klein *et al.*[33] have demonstrated a significantly increased prevalence of endotoxaemia in children with protein–calorie malnutrition

(PCM). This finding no doubt is related to the increased gastrointestinal tract permeability found in children with PCM.

6.2.2   The complement system in the malnourished child

6.2.2.1 *Complement proteins*

Defects in the complement system have been associated with increases in susceptibility to bacterial infection. Therefore, it is not unreasonable to expect that the complement system in the malnourished individual may be affected.

Activation of the complement system leads to production of complement fragments which are involved in host defences, including viral neutralization, chemotaxis of polymorphonuclear leukocytes, monocytes and eosinophils, opsonization of fungi, endotoxin inactivation, lysis of virus-infected cells and bacteriolysis[34]. Smythe *et al.*[4] were the first to report reduced haemolytic activity in the serum of children with protein–calorie malnutrition. In addition, many of the children they studied had C3 and C4 on the surface of their red blood cells, suggesting activation of the complement system. Other investigators who have studied the complement system in malnourished children have generally found decreased complement values when compared with well-nourished controls[24,35,36]. Munson *et al.*[37], however, failed to find any difference in the admission and discharge C3 values of malnourished Colombian patients. Sirisinha *et al.*[35] found that most of the complement components including C1q, C1s, C3, C5, C8 and C9 were significantly depressed in children with protein–calorie malnutrition. C4 was the only component which was not significantly lower than control values.

The mean complement levels in the children with kwashiorkor were lower than those with marasmus. With nutritional recovery, there was a significant increase in most of the complement components. The complement components appeared to be much more sensitive to the level of protein intake than calorie intake, with those patients receiving the higher protein intakes having a more rapid regeneration of the complement components than those having lower protein intakes[35].

6.2.2.2 *Haemolytic complement activity*

In addition to there being depression of the complement proteins, there is depression of the haemolytic complement activity in children with PCM[34]. Associated with the depression of haemolytic activity is the presence in several malnourished patients of a substance which activates serum complement (anti-complementary activity). A significant negative correlation exists between the depressed haemolytic activity and the presence of the anti-complementary activity[34]. It is well known that several substances such as insulin, polysaccharides, endotoxins and immune complexes can activate the complement system[38]. A study by Klein et al.[33] demonstrated that close to 50% of children with protein–calorie malnutrition have circulating endotoxin on admission and that, with recovery, the circulating endotoxin disappears. It appears that complement activity in malnourished children is affected not only by decreased nutrient availability, but also by an increased activation of the system.

6.3 CELLULAR RESPONSE

6.3.1 The cell-mediated immune response

6.3.1.1 Clinical and pathological changes

The cell-mediated immune response is mediated through the thymus-dependent lymphocyte (T cell) which plays a major role in host defences against most viruses, mycobacteria and fungi[39]. Malnutrition has been observed to adversely affect the host's response to tuberculosis[40]. Studies indicate that individuals given supplemental protein have a significantly lower incidence of tuberculosis than a non-supplemented, poorly nourished group of individuals[41]. In addition, individuals who are supplemented have less severe infection with tuberculosis than those who are unsupplemented. It has also been observed that the mortality rate from measles among malnourished children is four times that of well-nourished children[42]. Suskind et al.[43] observed an increased incidence of hepatitis-associated antigenaemia in children with protein–calorie malnutrition. Each of these observations would indicate that the cell-mediated immune response is compromised in the malnourished host.

Jackson first called attention to the thymic and lymphoid atrophy associated with severe protein–calorie malnutrition in 1925[44]. He noted at autopsy that children with kwashiorkor had grossly atrophied thymus glands represented by only a few strains of tissue. Microscopic examination showed that lymphoid elements and Hassel's corpuscles had been replaced by fibrous tissue[45–48]. In addition to atrophy of the thymus, peripheral lymph nodes[48], tonsils[7,49] and the spleen[4] are smaller in the malnourished children. With the lymphoid atrophy noted in malnourished children, it is not surprising that investigators have noted an increased susceptibility to those infections commonly controlled by the cell-mediated immune response[39].

6.3.1.2 In vivo skin-test responsiveness

The cell-mediated immune system is evaluated in vivo by intradermal skin testing and in vitro by enumeration of T lymphocytes and by antigen and mitogen stimulation of isolated lymphocytes. When an individual is exposed to a new antigen such as mycobacteria or BCG, his uncommitted lymphocytes become sensitized to this new antigen. Upon re-exposure to that antigen, the lymphocytes proliferate and release lymphokines, producing an inflammatory response and a positive skin test. In order to have a positive response to a skin-test antigen such as PPD or monilia, one must have lymphocytes which can be sensitized, lymphocytes which proliferate upon re-exposure to the same antigen and a normal inflammatory response[39,50].

Jayalakshmi and Gopalan[51] were the first to note that the percentage of positive tuberculin skin tests was significantly lower in children with PCM than in a control population. They were also the first to suggest that nutritional rehabilitation could lead to repair of a defective skin-test response. Other investigators have confirmed the defect in skin-test responsiveness to various antigens including monilia[52], streptococcal antigen[49], tricophyton[7], phytohaemagglutinin (PHA), mumps virus[8] and Keyhole limpet haemocyanin[49]. Most observers have noted that the degree of immunological impairment is correlated with the degree of weight loss[53]. Law et al.[8] were the first to describe a depression of delayed cutaneous hypersensitivity in malnourished adults. Following intravenous hyperalimentation of these patients, they demonstrated a significant improvement in their patients' delayed cutaneous hypersensitivity. Studies of delayed cutaneous hypersensitivity have also been done on mildly to moderately malnourished subjects. Harland et al.[54] found that the malnourished child was neither able to be sensitized when exposed to a new antigen nor able to develop a normal inflammatory response to a skin-test irritant. Both of these functions normalized with an improvement in the patient's nutritional status.

In order to confirm the in vivo demonstration of depressed cutaneous hypersensitivity, several investigators have studied the in vitro antigenic and mitogenic stimulation of isolated lymphocytes.

6.3.1.3 In vitro lymphocyte function

Peripheral blood lymphocytes from malnourished children react poorly to stimulation with such mitogens as PHA[4,49] and pokeweed[8]. Lymphocyte transformation as determined by blast cell transformation and the uptake of tritiated thymidine improves with nutritional recovery[8,50]. In addition to taking into consideration the degree and type of malnutrition, one must consider the associated infection found in malnourished children. Sellmeyer et al.[55] found that there was a fairly profound depression of lymphocyte transformation in children who had measles and gastroenteritis, but who were well nourished. One must take into consideration the possibility that there may be certain inhibitory factors in the plasma of malnourished children such as α_1 globulins[14] and C-reactive protein which are elevated in many children with protein–calorie malnutrition[4]. The malnourished child has deficiencies of protein, calories, vitamins and minerals, in addition to superimposed infection. All of these interacting factors may play roles in affecting a depression of the cell-mediated immune response. Obviously, it is impossible to determine which of these factors is responsible in the mal-nourished child. Most investigators, however, have noted recovery of the cell-mediated immune response long before complete nutritional recovery[18]. Thus the depressed skin-test reactivity in malnourished children may be explained by the depressed number and decreased responsiveness of the thymus-dependent (T) lymphocytes.

6.3.2 The polymorphonuclear leukocyte and macrophage in children with protein–calorie malnutrition

Polymorphonuclear leukocytes (PMNs) and macrophages are phagocytic cells. Phagocytic function may be divided into two major phases: (1) chemo-taxis, (2) engulfment. Post-phagocytic events include: (a) phagocytic vacuole formation and degranulation, (b) microbial killing, and (c) concomitant metabolic changes[56].

6.3.2.1 *Chemotaxis and phagocytosis*

Chemotaxis is active direct migration of polymorphonuclear leukocytes toward a chemotactic stimulus. It is a primary event early in inflammation. Using the Rebuck skin window technique, chemotactic studies have demon-strated an increased mobilization of polymorphonuclear leukocytes and a decreased migration of mononuclear cells[13,68]. The *in vitro* chemotactic response in infected and non-infected kwashiorkor children was found to be no different from that of infected or non-infected control children. However, the infected children in both groups showed a lesser response than the non-infected children[57]. Douglas *et al.*[58], using *in vitro* techniques, found an initial delay in the migratory response of cells of malnourished children. Within 3 hours, however, control values were attained.

Phagocytosis of various particles by polymorphonuclear leukocytes or monocytes from children with protein–calorie malnutrition has not been found to be adversely affected by the child's nutritional state[57,59]. In addition, the opsonic activity of plasma in malnourished children studied in India does not appear to be depressed[60]. Events which follow phagocytosis of the micro-organism include formation of a phagocytic vacuole, inclusion of phagocytic lysosomes within the phagocytic vacuole and concomitant release of the lysosomal content (degranulation)[56,61]. Electron microscopic studies of polymorphonuclear leukocytes from children with kwashiorkor using *S. aureus*, *E. coli* and *C. albicans* have demonstrated no apparent qualitative abnormality in vacuole formation or degranulation[58].

6.3.2.2 *Killing function*

Results of *in vitro* killing assays using polymorphonuclear leukocytes from malnourished children have revealed defects in the killing of *S. aureus*,

E. coli and *C. albicans*[58]. This finding has not been universal in that one report indicates defective bactericidal activity only occurred in infected children with kwashiorkor, while non-infected malnourished children had normal bactericidal activity[57]. Likewise, investigators in Thailand found that only a small percentage of malnourished children demonstrated significant defects in bactericidal killing[62].

6.3.2.3 Enzymatic changes

Activation of glycolysis and the hexomonophosphate shunt are the main metabolic events associated with particle uptake in polymorphonuclear leukocytes[58]. Lactic acid contributes to acidification of the phagosomal pH. Oxygen consumption results in the production of the superoxide radical and hydrogen peroxide. These metabolic events, as well as the release of lysosomal contents during degranulation, are of major importance in microbial killing[63].

Glycolysis is the major metabolic event providing energy for particle uptake. Particle uptake has been reported normal[57,59]. Therefore, the significance of the low lactate production and low glycolytic activity is not apparent[64]. The significance of the decreased pyruvate kinase reported by Yoshida[65] in relation to particle uptake and killing capacity of polymorphonuclear leukocytes in the malnourished children is unknown. Douglas *et al.*[58] have found normal levels of hexokinase, fructokinase, pyruvate kinase, myeloperoxidase and NADH oxidase in white cells from children with PCM. Normal levels of glucose-6-phosphate dehydrogenase and 6-phosphogluconic acid dehydrogenase have also been reported[11].

In addition to evaluating metabolites and enzyme activity in polymorphonuclear leukocytes from malnourished children, one can look at functional studies including activation of the hexomonophosphate shunt (HMS), oxygen consumption and the production of superoxide radicals and peroxides. The activity of hydrogen peroxide, myeloperoxidase and the halide-mediated killing system within the leukocyte can be assessed *in vitro* by determining the extent of incorporation of ^{131}I into trichloracetic acid (TCA) precipitable protein after phagocytosis. Decreased formation of TCA iodinated protein is associated with decreased *in vitro* microbicidal function to PMNs[66]. Degradation of thyroxine (T_4) and tri-iodothyronine (T_3) in phagocytizing polymorphonuclear leukocytes is an additional assay which can be used to assess phagocytic killing function[67]. Douglas and Schopfer[58] found high resting activity of the hexomonophosphate shunt. In addition, they found decreased iodination, low to normal T_3 and normal T_4 degradation in activated phagocytes. The majority of the investigators looking at nitro blue tetrazolium (NBT) in the phagocytes of malnourished children have noted a normal resting reduction of NBT dye[58]. The baseline levels of hexomonophosphate shunt activity and NBT scores suggest activation of the phagocytic system *in vitro*[61]. Thus, *in vitro* activation may be a consequence of the presence of infection in children with PCM and indicates relatively normal polymorphonuclear leukocyte biochemistry.

Douglas *et al.*[58], who found decreased killing function, decreased iodinization and increased basal metabolic rates in the PMNs of children with kwashiorkor, felt that, on the basis of this assessment, polymorphonuclear leukocyte function is indeed compromised in the malnourished host. However, other investigators looking at the question have found killing function abnormalities in only selected malnourished patients[62]. In their opinion, the abnormality is far from universal and one which could not be pointed to as a major factor in the malnourished child's decreased host resistance.

6.4 CONCLUSION

Children with protein–calorie malnutrition have an increased morbidity and mortality associated with infection. It has been demonstrated by several investigators that malnutrition affects several immune parameters. Several investigators have demonstrated depressed *in vivo* and *in vitro* cell-mediated immunity in the child with protein–calorie malnutrition. Although circulating immunoglobulins are elevated in PCM, the ability of the malnourished child to respond to an antigenic stimulus has been compromised in certain instances by the child's nutritional status. Secretory immunoglobulins are generally depressed in the malnourished child but recover with improved nutritional status. Individual complement proteins and haemolytic complement activity in children with protein–calorie malnutrition are significantly depressed. Investigators have also noted anti-complementary activity in the serum of the malnourished child. In contrast to the other systems, protein–calorie malnutrition does not appear to depress the chemotactic and phagocytic ability of the polymorphonuclear leukocytes. The effect of malnutrition on polymorphonuclear leukocyte killing function has been described as being depressed by some observers while others have found depressed killing function only in infected malnourished patients. Additional studies are obviously needed to clarify the effect of protein–calorie malnutrition on polymorphonuclear leukocyte activity.

ACKNOWLEDGEMENTS

I wish to thank Miss Maureen Stallings and Miss Patricia Corcoran for the editorial and typing assistance provided in the preparation of this manuscript.

References

1. Scrimshaw, N. S., Taylor, C. E. and Gordon, J. E. (1968). Interactions of nutrition and infection. W.H.O. Monograph, Series No. 57

2. Phillips, I. and Wharton, B. (1968). Acute bacterial infection in kwashiorkor and marasmus. *Br. Med. J.*, **1**, 407
3. Hutt, M. R. S. (1969). Malnutrition and infection – East African Studies. *J. Trop. Pediatr.*, **15**, 153
4. Smythe, P. M., Schonland, M., Brereton-Stiles, G. G., Coovadia, H. M., Grace, H. J., Loening, W. E. K., Mafoyane, A., Parent, M. A. and Bos, G. H. (1971). Thymolymphatic deficiency and depression. *Lancet*, **ii**, 939
5. Geefhuysen, J., Rosen, E. U., Katz, J., Ipp, T. and Metz, J. (1971). Impaired cellular immunity in kwashiorkor with improvement after therapy. *Br. Med. J.*, **4**, 527
6. Edelman, R., Suskind, R., Sirisinha, S. and Olson, R. E. (1973). Mechanisms of defective cutaneous hypersensitivity in children with protein–calorie malnutrition. *Lancet*, **ii**, 506
7. Chandra, R. K. (1972). Immunocompetence in undernutrition. *J. Pediatr.*, **81**, 1194
8. Law, D. K., Dudrick, S. J. and Abdou, N. I. (1973). Immunocompetence of patients with protein–calorie malnutrition. The effects of nutritional repletion. *Ann. Intern. Med.*, **79**, 545
9. Faulk, W. P., Samaeyer, E. M. and Davies, A. J. S. (1974). Some effects of malnutrition on the immune response in man. *Am. J. Clin. Nutr.*, **27**, 638
10. Cooper, W. C., Good, R. A. and Mariani, T. (1974). Effects of protein insufficiency on immune responsiveness. *Am. J. Clin. Nutr.*, **27**, 647
11. Selvaraj, R. J. and Bhat, K. S. (1972). Phagocytosis and leukocyte enzyme in protein–calorie malnutrition. *Biochem. J.*, **127**, 255
12. Douglas, S. D. and Schopfer, K. (1974). Phagocyte function in protein–calorie malnutrition. *Clin. Exp. Immunol.*, **17**, 121
13. Freyre, E. A., Chabes, A., Poemape, O. and Chabes, A. (1973). Abnormal rebuck skin window response in kwashiorkor. *J. Pediatr.*, **82**, 523
14. Passwell, J. H., Steward, M. W. and Soothill, J. J. (1974). The effects of protein malnutrition on macrophage function and the amount and affinity of antibody response. *Clin. Exp. Immunol.*, **17**, 491
15. Saba, T. M. and DiLuzio, N. R. (1968). Involvement of the opsonic system in starvation-induced depression of the reticuloendothelial system. *Proc. Soc. Exp. Biol. Med.*, **128**, 869
16. Tanphaichitr, P., Mekanandha, V. and Valyasevi, A. (1973). Impaired plasma opsonic activity in malnourished children. *J. Med. Assoc. Thai.*, **56**, 116
17. Sirisinha, S., Suskind, R., Edelman, R., Asvapaka, C. and Olson, R. E. (1975). Secretory and serum IgA in children with protein–calorie malnutrition. *Pediatrics*, **55**, 166
18. Kulapongs, P., Suskind, R., Vithayasai, V. and Olson, R. E. (1977). *In vitro* cell-mediated immune response in Thai children with protein–calorie malnutrition. In: *Malnutrition and the Immune Response* (R. Suskind, ed.), pp. 99–104 (New York: Raven Press)
19. Suskind, R., Sirisinha, S., Edelman, R., Vithayasai, V., Damrongsak, D., Charupatana, C. and Olson, R. E. (1977). Immunoglobulins and antibody response in Thai children with protein–calorie malnutrition. In: *Malnutrition and the Immune Response* (R. Suskind, ed.), pp. 185–90 (New York: Raven Press)
20. Aref, G. H., El-Din, K. and Hassan, A. J. (1970). Immunoglobulins in kwashiorkor. *J. Trop. Med. Hyg.*, **73**, 186
21. Keet, M. P. and Thom, H. (1969). Serum immunoglobulins in kwashiorkor. *Arch. Dis. Child.*, **44**, 600
22. Alvarado, J. and Luthringer, D. G. (1971). Serum immunoglobulins in edematous protein–calorie malnourished children. *Clin Pediatr.*, **10**, 174
23. Chandra, R. K. (1977). Immunoglobulins and antibody response in protein–calorie malnutrition. In: *Malnutrition and the Immune Response* (R. Suskind, ed.), pp. 155–68 (New York: Raven Press)
24. Neumann, C. G., Lawlor, G. J. Jr., Stiehm, E. R., Swendseid, M. E., Newton, C., Herbert, J., Ammann, A. J. and Jacob, J. (1975). Immunologic responses in malnourished children. *Am. J. Clin. Nutr.*, **89**, 104

25. Johansson, S. E. O., Mellbin, T. and Vahlquist, B. (1968). Immunoglobulin levels in Ethiopian pre-school children with special reference to high concentrations of immunoglobulin ND (gE). *Lancet*, **i**, 1118

26. Brown, R. E. and Katz, M. (1966). Failure of antibody production to yellow fever vaccine in children with kwashiorkor. *Trop. Geog. Med.*, **18**, 125

27. Jose, D. G., Welch, J. S. and Doherty, R. L. (1970). Humoral and cellular immune responses to streptococci, influenza and other antigens in Australian Aboriginal school children. *Aust. Pediatr. J.*, **6**, 192

28. Reddy, V. and Srikantia, S. G. (1964). Antibody response in kwashiorkor. *Indian J. Med. Res.*, **53**, 1154

29. Hodges, R. E., Bean, W. B., Ohlson, M. A. and Bleiler, R. E. (1962). Factors affecting human antibody response. III. Immunologic response in man deficient in pantothenic acid. *Am. J. Clin. Nutr.*, **11**, 85

30. Axelrod, A. E. (1971). Immune processes in vitamin deficiency states. *Am. J. Clin. Nutr.*, **24**, 265

31. Chandra, R. K. (1975). Food antibodies in malnutrition. *Arch. Dis. Child.*, **50**

32. Chandra, R. K. (1975). Reduced secretory antibody response to live attenuated measles and poliovirus vaccine in malnourished children. *Br. Med. J.*, **2**, 583

33. Klein, K., Suskind, R., Kulapongs, P., Mertz, G. and Olson, R. E. (1977). Endotoxemia, a possible cause of decreased complement activity in malnourished Thai children. In: *Malnutrition and the Immune Response* (R. Suskind, ed.), pp. 321–8 (New York: Raven Press)

34. Sirisinha, S., Suskind, R., Edelman, R., Kulapongs, P. and Olson, R. E. (1977). The complement system in protein–calorie malnutrition. In: *Malnutrition and the Immune Response* (R. Suskind, ed.), pp. 309–20 (New York: Raven Press)

35. Sirisinha, S., Suskind, R., Edelman, R., Charupatana, C. and Olson, R. E. (1973). Complement and C_3–proactivator levels in children with protein–calorie malnutrition and effect of dietary treatment. *Lancet*, **i**, 1016

36. Coovadia, H. M., Parent, M. A., Loening, W. E. K., Wesley, A., Burgess, B., Hallett, F., Brain, P., Grace, J., Naidoo, J., Smythe, P. M. and Vos, G. H. (1974). An evaluation of factors associated with the depression of immunity in malnutrition and in measles. *Am. J. Clin. Nutr.*, **27**, 665

37. Munson, D., Ranco, D., Arbeter, A., Velez, H. and Vitale, J. J. (1974). Serum levels of immunoglobulins, cell-mediated immunity and phagocytosis in protein–calorie malnutrition. *Am. J. Clin. Nutr.*, **27**, 625

38. Ruddy, S., Gigli, I. and Austin, R. (1972). The complement system of man. *N. Engl. J. Med.*, **287**, 489, 545, 592, 642

39. Edelman, R. (1977). Cell-mediated immune response in protein–calorie malnutrition. In: *Malnutrition of the Immune Response* (R. Suskind, ed.), pp. 47–75 (New York: Raven Press)

40. Rich, A. R. (1951). *The Pathogenesis of Tuberculosis*, second edition, pp. 374, 623 (Springfield, Ill.: Charles C. Thomas)

41. Leyton, G. B. (1946). Effects of slow starvation. *Lancet*, **ii**, 73

42. Gordon, J. E., Jansen, A. A. J. and Ascoli, W. (1965). Measles and rubella hemagglutination-inhibition antibody patterns in Mexican and Paraguayan children. *Am. J. Trop. Med. Hyg.*, **20**, 958

43. Suskind, R. M., Olson, L. C. and Olson, R. E. (1973). Malnutrition and infection with hepatitis-associated antigen. *Pediatrics*, **51**, 525

44. Jackson, C. M. (1925). *The Effects of Inanition and Malnutrition Upon Growth and Structure*, p. 285 (Philadelphia: P. Blakiston's Son and Co.)

45. Schonland, M. (1972). Depression of immunity in protein–calorie malnutrition: A post-mortem study. *J. Trop. Pediatr.*, **18**, 217

46. Vint, F. W. (1937). Post-mortem findings in natives of Kenya. *East Afr. Med. J.*, **13**, 332

47. Watts, T. (1969). Thymus weights in malnourished children. *J. Trop. Pediatr.*, **15**, 155
48. Mugerwa, J. W. (1971). The lymphoreticular system in kwashiorkor. *J. Pathol.*, **105**, 105
49. Work, T. H., Ifewunigwe, A., Jelliffe, D. B., Jelliffe, P. and Neumann, C. G. (1973). Tropical problems in nutrition. *Ann. Intern. Med.*, **79**, 701
50. Chandra, R. K. (1974). Rosette-forming T lymphocytes and cell-mediated immunity in malnutrition. *Br. Med. J.*, **3**, 608
51. Jayalakshmi, V. T. and Gopalan, C. (1958). Nutrition and tuberculosis. I. An epidemiological study. *Indian J. Med. Res.*, **46**, 87
52. Feldman, G. and Gianantonio, C. A. (1972). Aspectos immunologicos de la desnutricion en el nino. *Medicina*, **32**, 1
53. Abbassy, A. S., Badr El-Din, M. K., Hassan, A. I., Aref, G. H., Hammad, S. A., El-Araby, I. I., Badr Eli-Din, A. A., Soliman, M. H. and Hussein, M. (1974). Studies of cell-mediated immunity and allergy in protein energy malnutrition. I. Cell-mediated delayed hypersensitivity. *J. Trop. Med. Hyg.*, **77**, 13
54. Harland, P. S. E. B. (1965). Tuberculin reactions in malnourished children. *Lancet*, **ii**, 719
55. Sellmeyer, E., Bhettay, E., Truswell, A. S., Meyers, O. L. and Hansen, J. D. L. (1972). Lymphocyte transformation in malnourished children. *Arch. Dis. Child.*, **47**, 429
56. Douglas, S. D. (1970). Disorders of phagocytic function. Analytical Review. *Blood*, **35**, 851
57. Rosen, E. U., Geefhuysen, J., Anderson, R., Joffe, M. and Rabson, A. R. (1975). Leukocyte function in children with kwashiorkor. *Arch. Dis. Child.*, **50**, 220
58. Douglas, S. D. and Schopfer, K. (1977). The phagocyte in protein–calorie malnutrition. In: *Malnutrition and the Immune Response* (R. Suskind, ed.), pp. 231–43 (New York: Raven Press)
59. Tejada, C., Argueta, V., Sanchez, M. and Albertazzi, C. (1964). Phagocytic and alkaline phosphatase activity of leukocytes in kwashiorkor. *J. Pediatr.*, **64**, 753
60. Seth, V. and Chandra, R. K. (1972). Opsonic activity, phagocytosis and bactericidal capacity of polymorphs in undernutrition. *Arch. Dis. Child.*, **47**, 282
61. Douglas, S. D. and Spicer, S. S. (1971). Acid phosphatase cytochemistry of phagocytizing leukocytes from patients with chronic granulomatous disease. *Inf. Immun.*, **3**, 179
62. Leitzmann, C., Vithayasai, V., Windecker, P., Suskind, R. and Olson, R. E. (1977). Phagocytosis and killing function of polymorphonuclear leukocytes in Thai children with protein–calorie malnutrition. In: *Malnutrition and the Immune Response* (R. Suskind, ed.), pp. 253–7 (New York: Raven Press)
63. Bellanti, J. A. and Dayton, D. H., eds. (1975). *The Phagocytic Cell in Host Resistance* (New York: Raven Press)
64. Yoshida, T. and Metcoffe, J. (1967). Intermediary metabolites and adenine nucleotides in leukocytes of children with protein–calorie malnutrition. *Nature*, **214**, 525
65. Yoshida, T., Metcoffe, J. and Frenk, S. (1968). Reduced pyruvic kinase activity, altered growth patterns of ATP in leukocytes and protein–calorie malnutrition. *Am. J. Clin. Nutr.*, **21**, 162
66. Pincus, S. H. and Klebanoff, S. J. (1971). Quantitative leukocyte iodination. *N. Engl. J. Med.*, **284**, 744
67. Klebanoff, S. J. and Green, W. L. (1973). Degradation of thyroid hormones by phagocytizing human leukocytes. *J. Clin. Invest.*, **52**, 60
68. Kulapongs, P., Edelman, R., Suskind, R. M. and Olson, R. E. (1977). Defective local leukocyte mobilization in children with kwashiorkor. *Am. J. Clin. Nutr.*, **30**, 367

7
Allergy

J. PEPYS

7.1   INTRODUCTION   217

7.2   TYPES OF ALLERGIC REACTION   218
    7.2.1   *Type I – Immediate anaphylactic allergy*   218
        7.2.1.1   *Antibodies mediating Type I reactions*   219
        7.2.1.2   *Skin-test methods for Type I allergy*   220
        7.2.1.3   *Allergen-induced histamine release from*
                  circulating white cells   221
        7.2.1.4   *Radioimmunoassay for IgE antibodies*   221
        7.2.1.5   *'Elisa' test for antibodies to polysaccharide and*
                  protein allergens   221
        7.2.1.6   *Tests for IgE antibodies against whole cell-wall*
                  antigens   221
        7.2.1.7   *Passive transfer tests for IgE and STS-IgG*
                  antibody   222
    7.2.2   *Type II – Cytotoxic allergy*   222
    7.2.3   *Type III – Immune-complex complement-dependent*
              (Arthus) allergy   222
    7.2.4   *Type IV – Delayed tuberculin-type allergy*   224
        7.2.4.1   *Local persistence of the antigen at the test site*   225
        7.2.4.2   *Increased lymphatic absorption and Type IV*
                  skin-test reactions   225
        7.2.4.3   *Increased spread of the skin-test antigen*   226
        7.2.4.4   *Decreased lymphatic absorption and Type IV*
                  reactions   226
        7.2.4.5   *Effect of adrenaline-induced vasoconstriction on*
                  the epicutaneous tuberculin patch test   227

7.2.4.6   *Effect of adrenalin on the intracutaneous*
          tuberculin test   227
7.2.4.7   *Depot tuberculin tests*   227
7.2.4.8   *Effects of factors modifying the presence of*
          sensitized lymphocytes   228
7.2.4.9   *Effects of serial tests on Type IV tuberculin*
          reactions   228
7.2.4.10   *Selection of sites for repeat tests*   229
7.2.4.11   *Effects of simultaneous tests with different doses*
          on the tuberculin reaction   229
7.2.4.12   *Multiple repeat tests with increasing doses of*
          tuberculin   229
7.2.4.13   *Stability of tuberculin Type IV sensitivity*   230
7.2.4.14   *Effect of intercurrent illness on tuberculin*
          Type IV reactivity   230
7.2.5   *Association of types of allergy*   230

7.3   EXAMPLES   231
7.3.1   *Allergy and* M. tuberculosis   231
7.3.1.1   *Antigen–lymphocyte reactions*   234
7.3.1.2   *Granuloma formation, Type IV allergy*   234
7.3.1.3   *Allergy and selected infective agents*   235
7.3.1.4   *Antigenic components of* M. tuberculosis *and*
          types of allergic reaction   236
7.3.1.5   *Development of tuberculin sensitivity*   238
7.3.2   *Allergy and antigens of* M. leprae   238
7.3.3   Streptococcus pneumoniae   239
7.3.3.1   *Allergy and streptococcal antigens*   240
7.3.3.2   *Allergy skin tests with streptococcal antigens*   242
7.3.3.3   Staphylococcus aureus   242
7.3.3.4   H. influenzae   243
7.3.3.5   E. coli *allergens*   243
7.3.4   *Allergy in syphilis*   244
7.3.5   *Allergic reactions to viral allergens*   244
7.3.5.1   *Allergy and* Mycoplasma pneumoniae   246
7.3.6   *Fungal allergens*   246
7.3.6.1   *Skin tests with fungal allergens*   247
7.3.6.2   *Type I allergy to* C. albicans   248
7.3.6.3   *Specific IgE antibodies to polysaccharide*
          allergens from C. albicans *and* A. fumigatus   249
7.3.6.4   *Specific IgE antibodies to* C. albicans   249
7.3.6.5   *Allergy and* Aspergillus fumigatus   250
7.3.7   *Allergy and helminth parasitic allergens*   251
7.3.8   *Assessment of allergy to infective agents in vasculitis* 252

7.3.9   *Allergy to infective agents in eczema*   253
7.3.10   *Allergy to infective agents in local or generalized*
         erythema, papular skin reactions and the Arthus reaction   254
7.3.11   *Bacterial atopy*   255
7.3.12   *Allergic reactions to inhaled organismal particles and*
         antigens   256
         7.3.12.1 *Extrinsic allergic alveolitis*   256
         7.3.12.2 *Systemic reactions to inhaled organismal allergens*   257

7.4   GENERAL CONSIDERATIONS   258

7.1   INTRODUCTION

The term 'allergy' was introduced by von Pirquet in 1906 to describe the profound biological changes which result from adequate exposure to viable or non-viable agents so that subsequent exposure elicits an altered reaction. Used in this, its original sense, to describe the 'acquired, specific, altered capacity to react', the term 'allergy' encompasses responses, often inextricably related, ranging from no reaction at one pole to accelerated increased reactions at the other. The altered biological state, in itself, carries no implications concerning 'clinical hypersensitivity or immunity'[1]. The term 'immune' describes an end result of an infection in the course of which hypersensitivity responses which commonly persist afterwards may be evident and often are a *sine qua non* for the disease. Where hypersensitivity reactions play a part, the disease has features characteristic for the particular infecting agent and is usually named after it. The term 'allergic' is now commonly applied to hypersensitivity reactions in which the features are characteristic for the type or types of antibody involved, so that the same form of response or clinical disorder may be elicited by a wide variety of different allergens.

In this chapter examples will be given of the types of allergic reaction themselves, in relation to allergens from a number of bacteria, fungi, viruses and parasites. These reactions may be relevant, for example for diagnosis in the individual subject and prognosis in specific infections, for epidemiological and immunization studies of populations at large and also for general purposes as a means of assessing the immunological competence of the subject.

The analysis of the allergic phenomena is commonly based upon factors which are very different from those occurring in natural infection. That is, their presence is demonstrated by procedures in which components or products of the infecting agent are tested in amounts which are likely to be far in excess of those present in the body and in ways in which they are not ordinarily encountered. The reactions, however, are like those elicited by viable agents themselves when these are used for test purposes, in that they both elicit enhanced, accelerated responses.

7.2 TYPES OF ALLERGIC REACTION

There are four main types of allergic reaction[1], each with its own immunological mechanism and characteristic, well-defined features. They may be interdependent and, if sought appropriately, more than one type of allergy can often be shown to be present at the same time. The latter must be taken into account in the retrospective analysis of tissue changes in disease or elicited by deliberate tests. Tests on the skin, serum and cells provide evidence for the different types of allergy. The skin test[2], where appropriate, is the most comprehensive in this respect, throwing light not only on diagnosis and prognosis, but also on possible immunopathogenetic mechanisms for the particular disease. The principles and methods underlying skin tests are of basic importance because of their relevance to the problems of allergy and infection and they will be dealt with in some detail.

Infecting agents may be rich in potential allergens, but there are so far only a few highly purified materials available. These may not necessarily provide the same or all the information obtained with relatively crude preparations. The correlation of findings using chemically purified polysaccharide and protein materials with those obtained from the use of the infecting agents in the intact forms in which they are encountered in the body is needed, and examples of the use of bacterial and fungal cells for these purposes will be given later. It is hoped that they will give a clearer idea of what may actually be happening to the responsible agents themselves in hypersensitivity reactions in the course of infection.

7.2.1 Type I—Immediate anaphylactic allergy

The immediate skin-test reaction consists of rapidly developing urticarial-type weal and erythema, usually with itching. It starts within 60 seconds, is maximum in about 10 minutes and resolves within $1\frac{1}{2}$ to 2 hours. Such reactions are known to be mediated by two classes of antibody capable of sensitizing mast and basophil cells. Combination of the allergen with these antibodies leads to the release of potent tissue mediators, such as histamine, slow-reacting substance of anaphylaxis (SRS-A), prostaglandins and also eosinophil chemotactic reactor (ECF-A)[3]. The characteristic oedema, early neutrophil and then long-lasting eosinophil cell infiltration of the Type I skin-test weal is attributable to these mediators.

7.2.1.1 Antibodies mediating Type I reactions

The main and best-known mast cell sensitizing antibody is the immuno-globulin IgE[4]. This antibody is heat-labile, sensitizes passively for periods up to several weeks, and is termed LTS (long-term sensitizing) antibody. IgE antibody is a feature of, though not confined to, atopic subjects who produce it readily in response to the low dosage immunological challenge of ordinary environmental exposures. Highly potent allergens, such as infection with *Ascaris lumbricoides* and other parasites, induce the pro-duction of IgE antibodies in most subjects, whether atopic or not. The molecular weights of most allergens lie between 20 000 and 40 000.

There is evidence suggesting that low levels of secretory IgA may play a part in permitting allergen entry through mucosal membranes to the IgE-producing plasma cells which lie predominantly in the mucosal lymphoid tissues[5, 6, 7].

A heat-stable, short-term sensitizing (STS) antibody in the IgG, and probably IgG$_4$, subclass[8] capable of passive sensitization of mast cells for only a few hours has been described in man[9]. There is limited but growing evidence that this antibody may mediate immediate clinical reactions, e.g. to allergens from the house dust allergy mite genus *(Dermatophagoides)* in asthma[10] and to avian allergens (by passive transfer tests in man), in extrinsic allergic alveolitis in bird fanciers[11]. It has also been shown against pollen allergens[12] and against allergens from *Candida albicans*[13] and *Aspergillus fumigatus*[14]. Both IgE and STS-IgG antibodies may be present together. The reactions mediated by STS-IgG appear to be independent of comple-ment, though in a report of anaphylaxis to protamine sulphate there is suggestive evidence of a complement-dependent STS-IgG antibody re-action[15]. It is not known which IgG subclass or classes were responsible for this latter reaction.

The capacity of STS-IgG antibody to mediate release of histamine from sensitized basophils is said to be far less than that of IgE antibody[16, 17]. This would correspond with the clinical experience that in atopic subjects with IgE antibodies to avian allergens, for example, prick tests suffice to give positive reactions, whereas in individuals who are non-atopic with STS-IgG antibody intracutaneous tests with higher concentrations are usually needed[11].

Analysis of the biological activities of IgG subclass antibodies after inoculation and in disease in general[16] shows that IgG$_1$ and IgG$_3$ activate complement, IgG$_2$ is less active in this respect and IgG$_4$ does not activate it. IgG$_1$ and IgG$_3$ are cytophilic for macrophages and enhance phago-cytosis. IgG$_1$, IgG$_2$ and IgG$_4$ bind to staphylococcal protein by their FC portions. IgG$_1$, IgG$_3$ and IgG$_4$ sensitize guinea-pig skin, but their role in man in this respect has not been established and IgG$_4$ appears to be the main subclass[8, 16]. Antibodies to polysaccharide antigens such as teichoic acids from bacteria are mainly in the IgG_2 subclass and those to small molecular allergens are in the IgG_4 subclass.

7.2.1.2 Skin-test methods for Type I allergy

The skin-prick test, in which the tip of a needle (e.g. a half-inch, 26-gauge hypodermic needle) is introduced through a drop of test extract with a gentle lifting motion into the superficial layers of the epidermis, is a precise and exquisitely sensitive test. It has been calculated that it introduces a volume of 3×10^{-6} ml into the epidermis[18]. Positive immediate reactions have been elicited in tests, for example, with the chemically well-defined complex salts of platinum, by concentrations of 10^{-9} g/ml or less, that is, by an absolute skin-test dose of the order of 10^{-15} g, about 100 000 molecules[19].

The skin-prick test has a number of advantages over the intracutaneous test for eliciting Type I, IgE-mediated reactions. It is simple, safe and pain-less and readily repeatable when in doubt. No reactions at all should be elicited in control tests except in dermographic subjects. As a consequence even very small weals, 1 mm in diameter upwards with erythema, can be read as positive and it is not necessary in these tests to establish a convention whereby a reaction is regarded as positive if larger than a selected size. In a comparison of prick tests with extracts of the house dust allergy mite genus, *Dermatophagoides*, with values for specific IgE antibody in the serum, a close though not absolute correlation was found[20]. A comparison between threshold levels for reactions to tests with histamine or a histamine liberator[2], or with an irritant agent such as the enzymes of *Bacillus subtilis* used for biological detergents[21], shows that the prick test is 1000 to 10 000 times less sensitive in response to these non-specific agents than the intra-cutaneous test. Thus, while prick testing commonly employs allergen con-centrations 10 to 100 times stronger than those for intracutaneous testing, there is much leeway in the prick test for avoidance of non-specific reactions which are not uncommon in intracutaneous tests for contaminants.

The intracutaneous test for Type I allergy is made with a volume of 0.01 to 0.02 ml injected into the upper layers of the epidermis, and it requires experi-ence to inject the same volumes at each test site. Control tests often show some wealing and it is necessary to establish a convention for reading reactions, so that a positive reaction is usually taken as a weal larger than the control or more than 5 to 7 mm in diameter. This is a common source of error in the reading of borderline reactions, to which the technique also lends itself. In patients giving negative reactions to prick tests with an extract of *Dermatophagoides*, those giving reactions to intracutaneous tests with a higher concentration of extract and regarded as positive showed a poor correlation with specific IgE antibody in the serum, provocation tests and the clinical history, unlike the close correlations in the prick test positive reactors[20]. The possibility that some of these reactions to the intracutaneous tests, regarded at the time as non-specific, may have been mediated by STS-IgG must now to be considered in the light of the recent findings described above.

7.2.1.3 Allergen-induced histamine release from circulating white cells

Among other methods for demonstrating specific IgE antibodies are changes in basophil cells, and the more sensitive tests for histamine release by allergen added to whole blood, separated white blood cells or basophil cell suspensions[22]. This test correlates well with measurements of serum-specific IgE though a role for STS-IgG cannot be excluded when the tests are made on whole blood. Where washed total white cell or basophil cell suspensions are used it is likely, unless the test is made in autologous serum, that the STS-IgG antibody will have been removed, and indeed this is how this class of mast cell sensitizing antibody was first recognized in experimental animals[23].

7.2.1.4 Radioimmunoassay for IgE antibodies

The measurement of total serum IgE levels and of allergen-specific IgE by radiometric methods is a great advance[24,25]. The radioallergosorbent test (RAST) has been limited until recently to tests for specific IgE antibody to protein allergens, which are coupled to solid-phase particles or paper-discs which have been activated for this purpose by cyanogen bromide. Methods for measuring specific IgE antibody to polysaccharide allergens from *A. fumigatus* and *C. albicans* which have now been developed[26,27] should provide much impetus to the study of the allergenic properties of polysaccharide allergens from bacteria, fungi and parasites.

7.2.1.5 'Elisa' test for antibodies to polysaccharide and protein allergens

In the Elisa test the antigens, polysaccharide as well as protein, adsorb without chemical interference to polystyrene or glass surfaces, and the binding of specific antibody can be shown by the use of enzyme-linked antiserum for the particular immunoglobulin class under question. This is a highly sensitive test procedure which we have found works well for fungal polysaccharide as well as protein allergens, showing the presence of specific IgE antibody, and also of IgG and its four subclasses and IgM and IgA antibodies[28].

7.2.1.6 Tests for IgE antibodies against whole cell-wall antigens

In other tests to be discussed later, whole yeast cells of *C. albicans*[27] and bacterial bodies of *Streptococcus pneumoniae*, *Staphylococcus aureus* and

Haemophilus influenzae[29] have been used for demonstrating specific IgE antibodies to the cell-wall antigens, and, in the case of *C. albicans*, of antibody as well in IgG, its subclasses, IgM and IgA.

7.2.1.7   *Passive transfer tests for IgE and STS–IgG antibody*

Passive transfer tests in man or primates can also be used for the demonstration of specific IgE and STS-IgG antibodies, and at present this is the only method for showing specific STS-IgG antibodies[9,11]. Passive sensitization of basophil cells and of isolated tissues, skin and lung for example, can also be used for tests for specific IgE antibodies[30].

7.2.2   Type II—Cytotoxic allergy

In this form of allergy the antibodies react with antigens on the surface of cells or on non-cellular membranes or supporting tissues. The reacting antigen is either an integral component of the cell or tissue, or is an antigen that is attached to them or is formed by attachment of a hapten. Bacterial and drug products are prominent among agents capable of attachment to cells with subsequent reactions on combination with antibody. These frequently involve activation of complement with resultant cell or tissue damage. The classical example of this is nephritis in association with streptococcal infection. Furthermore, the presence in micro-organisms of antigens in common or which cross-react with cell or tissue antigens may lead to the induction of formation of antibodies capable of reacting with the cell or tissue. Bacterial polysaccharides are very relevant in this respect, the Type II allergy resulting in diseases termed auto-allergic.

7.2.3   Type III—Immune-complex complement-dependent (Arthus) allergy

The Type III skin-test reaction develops slowly after several hours, is usually maximum between 5 and 8 hours and resolves over about the next 24 hours. It is usually preceded by an introductory Type I reaction[31,32]. Reactions which are elicited after several hours, and which tend to be more indurated and lack the preceding immediate reaction, indicate that the test materials should be checked. In the author's experience such reactions are usually due to non-specific, irritant or toxic agents, so that whatever their mechanism they should not be regarded as Type III reactions. Activation of C3 component of complement by the alternative pathway may be responsible in the absence of complement-fixing antibodies.

The preceding immediate reaction plays an introductory role and illustrates the dependence of the Type III reaction on a Type I reaction. IgE antibody has been present in most patients giving the Types I and III reactions, e.g. to *A. fumigatus*[33] and to *C. albicans*[34]. In others, STS-IgG antibody mediating the Type I reaction has been found by passive transfer tests in man[11]. In yet others negative precipitin tests and the absence of precipitating antibodies in the tissue reactions have led the observers to postulate that both the Type I and Type III reactions were mediated by IgE antibody[35].

The Type III reaction, because of its slower appearance, is often referred to as 'delayed'. This is confusing because this term is commonly applied to the even more slowly developing Type IV reaction, the classical delayed allergic reaction. It is necessary therefore to avoid doubt by describing the reaction in terms of its speed of appearance and features. The reaction itself tends to be soft, often extensive, with ill-defined borders. It is itchy and accompanied by an erythematous flare. Depending upon its severity there may be a small area of central induration at which (rarely in man), some petechiae may be present. It is not uncommon with large reactions to see dependent oedema like that of Type III skin-test reactions in the guinea-pig. In experimental animals haemorrhage and necrosis are taken as criteria for the Type III (Arthus) reaction. These reactions consist of vasculitis with fibrinoid necrosis of vessel walls, platelet thrombi and perivascular infiltration with neutrophil and varying amounts of eosinophil cells, lymphoid cells, mainly mononuclear and plasma cells. The aggregates of immune-complexes formed in moderate antigen excess fix and activate complement. Clinical limitations of testing in man should preclude reactions of such severity. In the early literature on serum sickness, injections of relatively large volumes of heterologous sera were reported to cause severe reactions with necrosis, haemorrhage and extensive loss of tissue[36]. The immune-complex, complement-activated aggregates are chemotactic for neutrophil cells and are phagocytosed by them. The resultant cellular destruction leads to the liberation of tissue-damaging lysosomes. Such reactions are accompanied by release of yet another eosinophil chemotactic substance[37,38]

The amounts of allergen required to elicit a Type III reaction may be very small especially in atopic subjects giving vigorous Type I reactions to the particular allergen, e.g. to *A. fumigatus*[33]. In patients with allergic bronchopulmonary aspergillosis, all of whom give Type I reactions, about one-quarter give Type III reactions to prick tests with commercial test extracts and about one-half give reactions to protein allergens. Almost all affected subjects give Type III reactions to intracutaneous tests with commercial extracts and more vigorously to the protein materials. The clear distinction between the Type I and III components of the reaction can be seen with the prick test where the typical well-defined immediate wealing reaction resolves completely after $1\frac{1}{2}$ to 2 hours, to be followed, after a period of 1 to 2 hours of apparent normality, by the slow progressive development of the soft oedematous ill-defined Type III reaction. On rare occasions a typical Type IV reaction may make its appearance at 48 hours, long after the resolution of the

Type III reaction. It is not known whether the different sequential types of allergic reaction are mediated by the same antigenic component or by different components of the test material. In non-atopic subjects (e.g. bird fanciers with allergic alveolitis who give little or no reaction to prick tests) intracutaneous tests with larger amounts of allergen than suffice in the atopics give Type I reactions which are found to have STS-IgG antibody. This is a less potent liberator of histamine than IgE antibody[16] hence the need for the larger amounts of antigen introduced in the test.

7.2.4   Type IV—Delayed tuberculin-type allergy

This is commonly regarded as the allergy of infection and of contact dermatitis. There is, however, evidence of the participation of the other types of allergy in infection and in relation to test reactions which merit more attention than they have been given. Type IV allergy is also widely used as a criterion for cellular immune competence.

Type IV (delayed) reactions classically appear macroscopically 24 to 48 hours after the test, are maximum at 72 hours and may persist for days or weeks thereafter, often leaving areas of desquamation and pigmentation. Histological examination shows that infiltration with neutrophil and mono-nuclear cells starts within hours after the test.

The slow development of the reaction is due to the small proportion of sensitized lymphoid cells, which, in reaction with the specific antigen, liberate lymphokines which are chemotactic for and recruit other lympho-cytes, as well as other lymphokines which retard migration of cells from the test site.

The characteristic features of the histology of Type IV reactions are the epithelioid and lymphoid cell granuloma, with the lymphocytes lying in an onion-layer appearance together with plasma cells. It is common for granulomata to be regarded as synonymous with Type IV allergy. Other mechanisms for epithelioid cell granuloma formation, such as insoluble complexes which do not fix complement[39] and activation of macrophages by C3 activated by the alternative pathway[40], will be discussed in more detail under allergy to *Mycobacterium tuberculosis*.

The end picture of reactions regarded in nature as Type IV often contains evidence of Type I and III allergies. It is not difficult to show, in tests with appropriate antigens by appropriate methods, for example with *M. tuberculosis* and *C. albicans*, that Type I, III and IV allergy are present in the same subjects.

Type IV allergy may be shown by patch, prick, puncture or intra-cutaneous tests. In the case of allergy to *M. tuberculosis*, the classical model, purified protein derivative (PPD) is mainly used. Old tuberculin (OT), which contains polysaccharide as well as protein constituents, remains of interest because of its greater tendency to elicit Type I and III reactions as well. Positive reactions to intracutaneous tests are by convention, taken as areas of induration 10 mm or more in diameter. Previously 5 mm induration was regarded as positive, the present larger size being introduced for epidemiological purposes so as to make uniform reading easier. It is necessary, however, to appreciate that this convention applies to the reading of a test and not to the presence or absence of evidence of mycobacterial sensitivity. As will be shown in the discussion of allergy to *M. tuberculosis*, a single papule given to a puncture test or reactions to concentrations higher than conventional ones are regarded as evidence of so-called infra-tuberculin sensitivity and are of biological importance.

An analysis of the tuberculin skin reaction in man[2,41] shows three main factors which play predominant roles in the skin tests for Type IV allergy with this and other antigens. These are (1) the antigen must persist locally for a long enough period and in a high enough concentration, (2) the specific antibody-bearing cells must be present in the subject and available at the test site, and (3) the tissues must be capable of responding to the inflammatory stimuli[2].

There are a number of relatively simple physiological factors which exert profound effects on the persistence of antigen and availability of antibody cells. These have to be taken into account in assessing the results of tests for Type IV allergy, before bringing into consideration modification of basic mechanisms involved in cellular immune competence due to disease or immunosuppressive or stimulating agents.

7.2.4.1 Local persistence of the antigen at the test site

The local persistence of tuberculin at the test site may be decreased or increased with corresponding and very marked effects on the reaction. Lymphatic absorption of substances from normal skin is directly related to capillary blood flow. Tuberculin reactions are stronger on the upper part of the back than on the lower, owing to the upper part having a smaller capillary supply and therefore less lymphatic absorption.

7.2.4.2 Increased lymphatic absorption and Type IV skin-test reactions

Many factors strongly increase lymphatic absorption from the skin with a consequent decrease in tuberculin test reactivity[2,42,43]. Thus in erythema due to sunburn weaker reactions are obtained than on normal skin. Oedema of the skin due to local causes, including even the production of a wealing reaction by the test itself, or systemic causes such as pregnancy, malnutrition and fever, whether occurring because of disease or induced deliberately[44], all markedly increase lymphatic absorption and strongly decrease and often completely prevent tuberculin reactions.

The effects of increased lymphatic absorption can be readily observed under controlled conditions by the introduction into test sites of histamine with the production of a wealing reaction or the superinjection of saline into the test site. These procedures cause dilution, spread and enhanced absorption of the antigen. Direct visualization of the enhanced lymphatic absorption can be achieved by injection into the skin of a solution of sodium fluorescein followed by production of a weal. Its remarkably rapid disappearance within minutes may be watched under ultraviolet light through a Wood's filter. Where successive tests are modified, each at an increasing interval, by histamine or superinjected saline (it is sufficient to do this immediately after the introduction of an appropriate dose of antigen, so that a negative reaction results), it can be seen that within 10 minutes sufficient tuberculin has become 'fixed' at the site to elicit a small indurated reaction. As the interval increases between the injection of the tuberculin and the initiation of the enhanced lymphatic absorption, so the reactions elicited become larger, until no difference from the control tuberculin test is seen when the interval is $1\frac{1}{2}$ hours or longer. This shows that the 'fixation' of the reacting amount of the particular dose of tuberculin is completed within this time[43].

7.2.4.3 *Increased spread of the skin-test antigen*

Another method of assessing the effects of modifying and decreasing the local persistence of tuberculin consists of the superinjection of hyaluronidase at increasing intervals into successive sites of tuberculin injection. This serves to spread the tuberculin in the tissues so that, at the site superinjected immediately after the test, the reaction is larger than that at the control tuberculin test, but is of uniform and smaller intensity throughout and without the central induration of the control test. Thus the larger reaction is not an indication of a stronger reaction but of the spread of the antigen over a larger area, resulting in a lower but more extensively distributed concentration of tuberculin. The site superinjected after an interval of 10 minutes shows a small area of central induration, evidence of fixed tuberculin which is not capable of being spread by the hyaluronidase. When the interval between the test and the introduction of hyaluronidase is $1\frac{1}{2}$ hours or longer, the latter has no obvious effect on the reaction, which is comparable to that of the control test, showing that there has been maximum fixation of tuberculin during this time. The time intervals for commencement of and maximum fixation of the tuberculin are similar to those with the histamine superinjection[43].

7.2.4.4 *Decreased lymphatic absorption and Type IV reactions*

Agents which decrease lymphatic absorption of the antigen result in increased reactions. This may be brought about in two ways: (a) by the incorporation in the test of a vascoconstrictor such as adrenalin or (b) by incorporating the test material in a slowly absorbed vehicle.

7.2.4.5 Effect of adrenalin-induced vasoconstriction on the epicutaneous tuberculin patch test

Vasoconstriction produced by the local introduction of adrenalin has opposite effects depending upon whether it is used in epicutaneous tests, where it enhances reactions, or intracutaneous tests, where it decreases them. Von Pirquet added adrenalin to the solution of Old Tuberculin which he used for the original tuberculin scratch test and it is also added to the test material used for the multiple puncture Heaf test. The enhancing influence of vasoconstriction and decreased lymphatic absorption can be readily seen in relation to the patch test. Much more extensive and vigorous reactions are elicited on areas of skin into which adrenalin has been injected; care has to be taken to see that the injection puncture site lies well away from the patch test area since increased reactions are elicited by patch tests lying over puncture sites. The explanation for the enhanced reaction is that there is no tuberculin in the skin at the outset. The tuberculin which then penetrates into the skin has its absorption from the test site decreased because of the decreased vascular flow and lymphatic absorption resulting from the adrenalin. The vasoconstriction also decreases the availability of sensitized and other lymphocytes and of other cells at the test site. During this time the local concentration of vasoconstriction in the skin can only increase, so that higher concentrations are available for the reaction when the vasoconstriction resolves and the necessary cells become more freely available. Studies with sodium fluorescein show that its absorption from adrenalin-treated skin may take 8 or more hours in contrast to $1\frac{1}{2}$ to 2 hours from untreated skin and a matter of minutes from the weals induced by histamine.

7.2.4.6 Effect of adrenalin on the intracutaneous tuberculin test

The injection of adrenalin into intracutaneous tuberculin tests results in weaker or even completely negative reactions. Histological examination of such sites shows markedly decreased cellular infiltration from the earliest stages. In this case the vasoconstriction modifies the reaction by decreasing the availability of sensitized and other lymphocytes. During the period of vasoconstriction and in spite of the decrease in lymphatic absorption the local concentration of tuberculin can only fall since the total dose is present from the outset. As a consequence less tuberculin is likely to be available for reaction when the vasoconstriction wears off.

7.2.4.7 Depot tuberculin tests

Increased local persistence of tuberculin can also be achieved by depot materials prepared by its incorporation in an emulsion for injection or in a highly purified lanolin cream for multiple puncture tests. Both methods greatly increase the sensitivity of the test so that reactions can be elicited in subjects giving negative reactions to intracutaneous tests with the highest conventional doses of tuberculin. This demonstrates what is called 'infra-tuberculin sensitivity', and is comparable in the multiple puncture tests to tests made by the injection of BCG vaccine, the latter eliciting a greatly accelerated BCG response starting within 24 to 48 hours.

The depot preparations also persist for long periods in the skin and thus show the development at the appropriate time in previously negative reactions of mycobacterial sensitivity in response to BCG vaccination. A similar clinical phenomenon is 'revivescence' in which a previously negative tuberculin test may become positive with the subsequent development of tuberculosis[45] even some months later. The implications of the findings with depot materials will be discussed under allergy in relation to *M. tuberculosis*.

7.2.4.8   Effects of factors modifying the presence of sensitized lymphocytes

The tuberculin skin-test reaction may also be influenced by factors which modify the presence of or, as has been discussed above, the availability of sensitized lymphocytes. Certain forms of immunodeficiency affecting mainly T-lymphocyte responses are associated with decreased or absent Type IV reactions, hence the use of tests for Type IV allergy to assess cellular immune competence. The numbers of T lymphocytes can be decreased by X-ray irradiation with an inhibitory effect on the tuberculin reaction. Similarly surface active agents[46] and immunosuppressive drugs may decrease Type IV reactivity, whereas agents such as levamisole have been shown to increase it[47]. Transfer factor may also result in an increase of Type IV reactivity, presumably by restoring T-cell activity. Finally, Type IV reactivity is passively transferable by transfer factor from lymphocytes[48] and locally or systemically by sensitized lymphoid cells. Thus Type IV reactivity to tests can be modified by the availability of both antigen and antibody.

7.2.4.9   Effects of serial tests on Type IV tuberculin reactions

Serial tests in themselves may result in increased or decreased reactions. Enhanced sensitivity, for prolonged periods, to lower dosages or the production of reactions at previously negative sites may follow serial tests with increasing doses of tuberculin[49-51]. Similarly the degree of tuberculin sensitivity shows less waning in BCG vaccinated subjects in whom the tuberculin tests are repeated. The nature of the tuberculin may also play a part, because no such effect has been observed in tests with a tuberculin preparation, IP 48, which contains appreciable amounts of polysaccharide as well as protein antigens[52].

7.2.4.10 *Selection of sites for repeat tests*

The site of performance of the repeat test may have a marked effect. If the test is repeated upon a previously positive site within a few weeks, weaker or negative reactions are likely to be elicited. Such sites show greatly increased lymphatic absorption when tested by injection of sodium fluorescein and presumably the injected tuberculin is absorbed with comparable rapidity. On the other hand, repetition of tests on the same sites at longer intervals of 3 months may result in greatly accelerated, enhanced and sometimes histologically confirmed blister reactions which develop within a few hours[53]. These reactions resolve more rapidly than those on normal skin[54]. The local persistence of lymphoid cells and macrophage accumulations from the previous test is probably specifically responsible for this enhanced reactivity. It has also been reported that tuberculin reactions are enhanced at sites of non-specific inflammation[55], presumably due to the macrophage infiltration so induced[56]. These phenomena may be the basis for the Stormont test in cattle where repeated tests on the same site are used to distinguish, by virtue of increased reactions, specific mycobacterial sensitivity due to *M. johnëi* from that due to *M. tuberculosis*, which tend to cross-react.

7.2.4.11 *Effects of simultaneous tests with different doses on the tuberculin reaction*

More positive reactions were elicited in subjects tested with a single dose of 100 TU than in those tested with 10, 30 and 100 TU at the same time. However, in subjects with high degrees of sensitivity, simultaneous tests with 0.3, 1 and 3 TU give more reactions than tests with 3 TU alone. Larger reactions are also elicited by a single test with a 10 TU dose than with either 10 or 100 TU given simultaneously[57, 58].

Whatever the explanation of these differences between subjects of high and low degrees of sensitivity in response to multiple tests and the influence of the different doses on the degree of reactivity, their occurrence has to be taken into account when comparative serial studies of Type IV allergy and its implications are being made in individual subjects or groups.

7.2.4.12 *Multiple repeat tests with increasing doses of tuberculin*

Almost all infants not exposed to tuberculosis who are tested with increasing doses of PPD ranging from 0.000 001 mg (0.5 TU) up to 1.0 mg (50 000 TU) reacted to the final test[59]. The reactions elicited in those requiring high doses differed from those requiring low doses; it is possible that the repeated injections of PPD were capable of sensitization. Tuberculin is a potent anaphylactogen in its own right for guinea-pigs, a fact that has on occasion been overlooked when repeated tuberculin tests have been made in studies in experimental animals. Furthermore, precipitins to mycobacterial antigens are ubiquitous in sera from new born infants upwards[95]. The reactions elicited eventually by the high doses of tuberculin could, therefore, have been Type III and not Type IV in nature.

7.2.4.13 *Stability of tuberculin Type IV sensitivity*

Reversion to negative tests has been found over a period of 5 years in 1% of subjects who gave indurated reactions 10 mm or more in diameter to 1 TU, compared with reversion in 35% of those who gave reactions less than 10 mm in diameter or who reacted only to 100 TU[60]. Control subjects also tend to lose their sensitivity more rapidly than those in contact with tuberculous patients[45].

7.2.4.14 *Effect of intercurrent illness on tuberculin Type IV reactivity*

The degree of demonstrable tuberculin sensitivity can be markedly modified by the general effects of intercurrent diseases, in addition to their possible specific immunological effects. As described earlier, factors which increase lymphatic absorption from the test site, such as fever, oedema and irritation such as sunburn greatly decrease tuberculin reactivity. Thus tests on an oedematous limb may be negative whereas a positive and indeed very vigorous reaction might be elicited on the corresponding symmetrical non-oedematous site[42]. These factors require assessment before concluding that specific immunological mechanisms are involved or are being modified. The latter are probably involved in the depression of tuberculin sensitivity seen in tests on the fifth day after vaccination with poliomyelitis or measles vaccine and on the ninth day after yellow fever vaccination[62]. In spite of contrary claims, no depression of tuberculin reactivity has been found in response to vaccination with attenuated mumps virus[63].

The influence of the infecting dose of mycobacteria on the development of sensitivity and the relevance and clinical significance of low degrees of specific or non-specific sensitivity will be discussed further under allergy in relation to *M. tuberculosis.*

7.2.5 Association of types of allergy

The proper reading of skin tests requires observation within 15 to 20 minutes for Type I reactions, after about 5 to 8 hours for Type III reactions, at 24 to 48 hours for Type IV reactions and after some days or weeks for granulomatous reactions. Where only one or other of these responses is sought the existence of the others may be overlooked.

The coexistence of the different types of allergy and even their interdependence, for example, of Type III allergy on an introductory Type I reaction, is a challenge to their more detailed study. It is customary to regard Type IV delayed allergy as almost synonymous with allergy to infecting agents, in particular with bacterial infection.

Only limited attention has been given so far to the association of the different types of allergy to a particular infecting agent. Most has been devoted to *M. tuberculosis*, to fungi such as the dermatophytes, to *Aspergillus fumigatus* and *Candida albicans*, and with some less intensive interest to bacteria such as *Strept. pneumoniae* and *Staph. aureus* and to the various causes of parasitic disease.

The main, and indeed limited, known associations of different, chemically distinct, antigens of infecting agents in general with the demonstrable types of allergy show that polysaccharide antigens elicit Types I and III, whereas proteins are responsible mainly for Type IV allergy. Polysaccharides are on the whole ineffective for inducing allergic sensitivity, in contrast to proteins, though the former are effective in eliciting reactions in sensitized subjects. The contrasts between polysaccharide and protein allergens will be a recurring theme in the examples of the different forms of infecting agent which are discussed.

7.3 EXAMPLES

7.3.1 Allergy and *M. tuberculosis*

Prior to the introduction of effective chemotherapy for tuberculosis, the immunopathology of infection by *M. tuberculosis* was a prime object of study as it encompassed the whole field of 'allergy' in the fullest sense[61]. The description by Koch of the accelerated reaction to *M. tuberculosis* in previously infected animals, the Koch phenomenon, provided a corner-stone for the concept of allergy to infection and led von Pirquet to the introduction of the tuberculin scratch test. There are still unresolved and controversial questions concerning the relative roles and inter-relationship of hypersensitivity and immunity.

The emphasis in tuberculin sensitivity has been on delayed reactions. The failure to transfer this passively by means of serum from infected or sensitized animals led to some doubt about the allergic nature of the reaction. It is remarkable that so little attention was paid to the reports[64] of the passive transfer of sensitivity by injection into healthy recipient animals of suspensions of lymph node and splenic cells from infected animals. An effect *in vitro* of tuberculin on tissue cultures from sensitized animals was the next crucial observation[65]. This was followed much later by the discovery that delayed hypersensitivity can be passively transferred by lymphoid cells of sensitized donors[66,67], and then by the discovery that the passive transfer of delayed sensitivity by sensitized lymphocytes from subjects sensitive to tuberculin and to haemolytic streptococci could be shown to be mediated, at least in man, by soluble factors, termed transfer factor, in dialysates of leukocyte extracts[48].

Transfer factor (mol. wt. 10 000) has been found in polynucleotide-rich dialysates from human material and also in undialysable protein-rich preparations[68, 69]. It is not clear whether the action of transfer factor or factors is to sensitize unsensitized cells specifically[70, 71], to enable lymphocytes to respond, or to act as an adjuvant enhancing a previously existing level of sensitivity which was not detectable by the available tests or even perhaps in some non-specific way. Low molecular weight nucleic acids capable of transferring delayed hypersensitivity are regarded as too small to act as informational RNA[72]. It is possible that they may be highly antigenic RNA fractions[73]. Dialysable transfer factor has been used with success in patients with depressed cellular immune reactivity. It has restored the capacity to liberate migration inhibition factor[74] and has delayed skin-test reactivity and synthesis of DNA by transforming lymphocytes[75]. It has also had a beneficial therapeutic effect on chronic mucocutaneous candidiasis[75] and a refractory case of anergic mycobacterial infection[76].

A number of other potent biological properties in the expression and regulation of the responses are manifest in the lymphokines produced by sensitized lymphoid cells on challenge with specific antigen. These mediators of cellular immunity have been comprehensively reviewed[77]. They appear to be anionic glycoproteins, molecular weights 30 000 to 100 000. Their biological properties[78] include: lymphocyte mitogenic activity causing increased DNA synthesis and lymphocyte transformation; inflammatory factors responsible for delayed-type allergic reactions; cytotoxic/cytopathic factors for lymphocytes; migration inhibition factor of polymorphonuclear or macrophage cells in tissue culture; macrophage agglutination *in vitro* and *in vivo*; macrophage spreading factor; chemotactic factors for macrophages *in vivo* and *in vitro*; lymph-node activating factor evident in paracortical lymph node changes during induction of the delayed-type allergy; macrophage activating factor resulting in acquired macrophage resistance and an interferon-like factor responsible for non-specific resistance to viral infection.

The overall responses *in vivo* to the above mediators of cell-mediated allergic reactions are classified[77] into granuloma formation, allograft rejection and graft versus host reactions. They play roles as cytotoxic macrophage-activating and interferon-like products in immune surveillance (e.g. activation of macrophages and restriction of multiplication of pathogens or tumour cells) and as adjuvants by their lymph-node and macrophage activation and mitogenic effects with enhancement of antibody production, promotion of autoimmune responses and non-specific immunoglobulin synthesis. It is postulated that different subpopulations of lymphocytes may govern the generation of one or more of the mediators, with selective activation or depression, so that all the functions of lymphokines associated with delayed allergy or increased cellular resistance or both, need not necessarily be expressed together.

Certain of these biological properties could be responsible for the disappearance of macrophages from peritoneal exudates and their adherence to the peritoneum of sensitized guinea-pigs after allergic reaction to the intraperitoneal injection of antigen[79]. The full expression of Type IV allergy is the elicitation of the delayed skin-test response and this may not occur even though there is evidence of lymphocyte responses *in vitro* to the specific allergen.

A lymphokine which could be playing a part in the Type IV skin-test reaction is 'skin-reactive factor'[80]. This protein (mol. wt. 40 000) is heat stable, is generated in serum-free medium and is activated in the skin of animals depleted of C3 and of polymorphonuclear neutrophil cells, the latter being an essential component in Type III reactions. It is of lymphocytic origin as shown by the inhibition of its chemotactic effect on mononuclear cells *in vivo* by antisera to lymphocytes. Skin-reactive factors are liberated from lymphocytes by challenge with PPD as early as 7 days after immunization and increase in amount up to 4 weeks[80]. These findings correspond with the observations that accelerated skin reactions to BCG vaccine can be elicited within 3 to 4 days after oral BCG vaccine administration to infants, showing the rapid development of the allergy[81].

The skin-reactive factor elicits, in the absence of antigen, a reaction which is maximum at 3 hours and is resolving by 24 hours. It also causes a nonspecific increase in vascular permeability starting within 10 to 20 minutes, attributed to lymph node permeability factor[82]. Similar skin-reactive factors are released from non-sensitive lymphocytes by phytomitogens but not from thymus or bone-marrow lymphocytes, suggesting the possibility of a third short-lived type of lymphocyte concerned with chemical mediators for Type IV allergic reactions[80]. The reactions have features of an Arthus, Type III-like reaction and it has been suggested that there may be common lymphocyte mediators in Arthus and delayed allergic reactions particularly since immune-complexes containing IgG but not IgM antibody liberate skin-reactive factor from lymphocytes[77, 80]. These findings may be relevant to the co-existence of Type III and IV allergies in tuberculin-sensitive subjects which will be discussed later.

The evidence that the sensitized lymphocytes mediating the Type IV reactions are non-dividing[83] agrees with the fact that there is no significant lymphocyte proliferation at reaction sites. Only a minority of the donor lymphoid cells are present at sites of reaction in passive transfer tests[84] where they co-operate by virtue of their lymphokines with non-sensitive cells. An analogous situation is shown by *Listeria monocytogenes*, where the induction of cellular hypersensitivity requires cell-division, whereas when established it does not and is not affected by inhibition of mitosis.

The committed lymphocytes in cell-mediated hypersensitivity are newly formed cells with a short circulating life span. They enter readily into inflammatory reactions, such as peritoneal exudates[85] which are effective for passive transfer of Type IV allergy. Depletion of recirculating long-lived lymphocytes by thoracic duct drainage has no effect, the persisting cells effectively transferring delayed allergy. The effector cells for Type IV allergy are therefore not derived from the recirculating pool of T cells, which are responsible, however, for the induction of cell-mediated allergy[86,87].

7.3.1.1 Antigen–lymphocyte reactions

The reaction of the antigen with sensitized lymphocytes *in vitro* starts within 1 hour[88]. The synthesis and release of active products such as migration inhibition factor (MIF) occur within 6 to 7 hours[89]. MIF makes the mononuclear cells sticky and adherent so that migration is inhibited within 24 hours and the mononuclears are activated at the same time[90]. The liberation of MIF is inhibited by puromycin[91] and is thus a phenomenon associated with lymphocyte transformation. Systemic administration of tuberculin causes lymphopenia and temporary desensitization presumably either by depletion of specifically sensitized lymphoid cells or macrophage segregation or both. It is worthy of note that farmers were at one time aware of the fact that the injection of a large dose of tuberculin could make a tuberculous cow give negative tuberculin reactions for some time afterwards.

In man the injection of carefully graduated increasing doses can render highly sensitive subjects completely negative to tuberculin tests, so that reactions are not elicited by skin tests with concentrated Old Tuberculin. This procedure was based on the theory that depression of the delayed hypersensitivity, so important in the pathogenesis of tuberculosis, would improve the clinical response. This was never established and was not further tried after the introduction of effective chemotherapy. In subjects 'desensitized' in this way, relapses of diseases could be followed by severe reactions at the previous negatively reacting sites. Except for the possibilities discussed above, nothing is known of the mechanisms of this desensitization. They could, however, be of topical interest in view of the importance of delayed allergy, for example in graft rejection, and merit further study as models of allergic phenomena in their own right, irrespective of possible clinical relevance to tuberculosis.

7.3.1.2 Granuloma formation, Type IV allergy

Delayed hypersensitivity reactions induced by heat-stable components of non-viable organisms and also by infection with viable organisms result in macrophage activation and granulomatous responses which are responsible for increase in non-specific resistance and are not long-lasting in their effects. By contrast it is claimed that a labile, ribonucleic acid component of *M. tuberculosis* associated more with viable organisms is responsible for long-lasting, highly specific, lymphocyte-mediated, increased resistance without hypersensitivity[92].

The epithelioid, lymphocyte, giant cell granuloma is a characteristic feature of hypersensitivity reactions to tuberculin and of infection. The granuloma also contains immunoblasts and plasma cells together with polymorphonuclear neutrophil and eosinophil cells and fibroblasts. The factors capable of eliciting high and low turnover granulomatous responses are complex and probably associated in varying degrees[93]. The high turn-over granuloma produced by BCG, Freund's adjuvant or *B. pertussis* depends upon fresh daily supplies of bone marrow monocytes and upon mitotic division of the granuloma cells. This could be due to toxicity of the causal agents or to hypersensitivity, with the liberation of lymphokines capable of exerting these effects. Low turnover granulomata are produced by carrageenan and synthetic high molecular weight polymers and have a stable population of long-lived cells without much bone marrow monocyte recruitment or mitosis. The production of granulomata results from failure to eliminate the causal agents, which may be residues of the degraded bacteria associated with persistence of macrophages. This is supported by the finding[94] that bentonite particles coated with mycobacterial, histoplasma or schistosoma antigen elicit granulomatous reactions in specifically sensitized animals and that this reactivity is passively transferable by means of their lymphocytes but not their serum. Many non-viable and apparently inert agents can stimulate granuloma production, as well as those causing hyper-sensitivity such as beryllium and zirconium and even the tuberculin reaction itself.

Insoluble immune-complexes which do not fix complement can also induce granuloma formation[93], whereas soluble complexes of the same antigen and precipitating antibody, formed in moderate antigen excess and capable of fixing complement, mediate acute inflammatory Type III reactions. The universality of precipitins to mycobacterial antigens[95] (demonstrated by microprecipitin agar-gel tests) and the presence amongst the many antigens of *M. tuberculosis* of polysaccharides against, which high titres of precipitins may be present, shows that the production of both soluble and insoluble immune-complexes could contribute their particular immunopathogenetic effects on tissue reactions to the end picture of mycobacterial tuberculin allergy. From a review of the literature[41] there is also a suggestion requiring further study that the production of hypersensitivity granulomata may depress tuberculin reactivity.

7.3.1.3 *Allergy and selected infective agents*

Bacteria and other organisms, viruses, fungi and helminth parasites will be dealt with in terms of particular selected organisms or as part of disease processes in order to provide examples of allergy and infective agents.

7.3.1.4   *Antigenic components of* M. tuberculosis *and types of allergic reaction*

Type I, III and IV allergic reactions are present together and can be elicited in animals and man sensitized to *M. tuberculosis*[41]. Immediate, Type I and Arthus, Type III reactions are elicited mainly, though not exclusively, by polysaccharide antigens as in other bacteria, fungi and parasites[96,97]. Type I skin reactions are demonstrable in experimental animals by the immediate exudation of dye injected intravenously[41,97]. High titres of precipitating antibody are also found in animals sensitized to *M. tuberculosis* against polysaccharide antigens. These polysaccharides are capable of eliciting immediate Type I and Type III reactions. It is not known in this context whether the antibody mediating the Type I reaction is IgE or STS-IgG antibody or both. The passive transfer of Type I allergy[97] suggests that IgE antibody is present but this has yet to be demonstrated by tests *in vivo*. As will be described with polysaccharide antigens of *C. albicans* and *A. fumigatus* this should now be possible.

Tuberculo-polysaccharide[96] elicited immediate reactions in man lasting for 2 hours followed by a second reaction which appeared at 4 hours and lasted for 24 hours, at which time the reaction to tuberculoprotein was beginning to show. Arthus-like reactions developing after 2 hours and maximum between 4 and 8 hours have also been reported to fractions of *M. tuberculosis* H37Ra[97]. Similar reactions to higher doses of tuberculin, 10 to 250 TU, have been observed[98]. It is not uncommon for tests with Old Tuberculin which contains polysaccharide antigens to give Type III followed by Type IV reactions. The Type III reactions have to be sought at about 5 to 8 hours after the test and are fully resolved by 48 to 72 hours, the conventional time for reading Type IV reactions.

Four polysaccharides have been isolated[101] from *M. tuberculosis:* mannan, glucan, arabinomannan and arabinogalactan. The arabinogalactan has been identified as containing the immunoreactive sugar, which need not necessarily be the terminal sugar, responsible for high degrees of specific, immediate, anaphylactic Type I and Type III reactions. The arabinomannan was less active. Neither polysaccharide elicited Type IV reactions. In sensitized animals they elicited reactions which developed after 1 hour and were maximum at 5 hours, whereas by comparison the reaction to a tuberculin-active peptide started after 3 hours and was maximum between 24 and 48 hours. In tests in experimental animals, the potent anaphylactogenic properties of PPD have to be taken into account where animals may be retested later for Type I allergy.

The amounts of polysaccharide used for eliciting Type I and III reactions are greater than those of tuberculoprotein used for showing Type IV allergy. In man at least, the possible severity of reactions precludes the use of much larger doses of protein as they could possibly also elicit Type III reactions.

Tuberculin peptides capable of eliciting reactions in sensitized subjects and almost as potent as PPD-S have been prepared[99] and are claimed to be specific for human or bovine bacilli[100]. Unlike PPD-S they did not induce anaphylactic sensitivity in guinea-pigs. Peptides with molecular weights of 5000 to 10 000 have been prepared and 0.2 μg is equivalent to 50 TU of Old Tuberculin[101].

Other test preparations include extracts of living organisms disrupted by ultrasonic disintegration[102]. Comparison of 16 such preparations from different mycobacteria with PPD-RT23 showed no differences in positive and negative reactions read at 72 hours in residents of countries with endemic tuberculosis and leprosy. In healthy subjects, tuberculin-positive reactors also reacted to all the mycobacterial preparations except to one from an unidentified slow-growing species resembling *M. avium*. In Burma, however, sensitization was more evident to mycobacterial species, especially the slow growers other than *M. tuberculosis*. More vigorous reactions were given where the prevalence of mycobacterial species was low as in Libya. Where they are common, as in Burma where there is a high incidence of the *M. avium*-like species, the reactions were weaker to the other mycobacteria. The suggestion is made that there may be a threshold for cell-mediated immunity in relation to skin-test responses. If this is exceeded the skin test becomes negative so that there are among the non-reactors subjects who are either excessively sensitized or non-sensitized. In spite of this a greater percentage of tuberculous patients in each country reacted more vigorously to the specific preparation than the controls. In Burma, 13% were non-reactors to PPD and the other preparations suggesting an apparent anergy to all the test materials. In lepromatous leprosy, by contrast, there is anergy to the specific organism and less so to related species. In *M. ulcerans* infection anergy was found to both the specific antigen and to PPD-RT23. These findings suggest that there is a spectrum of tuberculosis, as in leprosy and *M. ulcerans* infection.

In patients given BCG vaccinations, those who become tuberculin positive react to the other preparations, but not those who remain tuberculin negative. In *M. ulcerans* infection the skin test returns to positivity following effective chemotherapy and it is during the anergic phase that there is tissue damage, suggesting that anergy may have a bad effect in tuberculosis.

The use of living or dead BCG vaccine to show 'infratuberculin' sensitivity may result in positive reactions where tuberculin-negative tests have previously been found[41, 103]. Others using parallel tests with tuberculin and BCG suggest that in subjects who are tuberculin negative and BCG positive, the hypersensitivity is directed against the mycobacterium rather than the tuberculin[104].

Low degrees of mycobacterial allergy have previously been attributed to mycobacteria other than *M. tuberculosis*[105] and comparative tests have shown specific reactions to tuberculins produced from the different mycobacteria[106,107]. Low degrees of sensitivity, the sources of which are not necessarily known, are associated with resistance to infection[108]. In view of the high incidence of infratuberculin sensitivity shown by depot tuberculins in subjects regarded as negative to conventional tuberculin test doses and therefore suitable for BCG vaccination, an appreciable number could be expected to and do give accelerated reactions to BCG vaccination[109]. Whilst it may be desirable to raise the degree of tuberculin allergy to levels measurable by conventional tests, it seems likely that the beneficial effects of BCG vaccination would be more readily shown by subjecting negative reactors to depot tuberculin tests to study of its efficacy. Multiple puncture tests with a depot tuberculin (5 mg PPD/g anhydrous wool alcohol) gave an incidence of positive reactions in 92% of non-exposed subjects who had given negative reactions to intracutaneous tests with 100 TU PPD[109]: this is comparable to the finding that positive reactions could be elicited with PPD in 77–88% of non-contact subjects tested intracutaneously with doses up to 1000 TU[57]. The depot tuberculin has the advantage over BCG in such tests in that it does not convert the subject to tuberculin positivity as does BCG vaccination, so that observation of the immunological progress of the subject is not hindered by the tests done.

7.3.1.5 *Development of tuberculin sensitivity*

The larger the infecting dose of *M. tuberculosis* the earlier is the appearance of tuberculin sensitivity, being evident in experimental animals from the fifth day[49]. In man a linear relationship between the dose of BCG and the area of induration to tuberculin tests was found[110]. In infants undergoing oral BCG vaccination accelerated reactions to a BCG skin test were present as early as the third or fourth day[81]. A similar phenomenon is seen in the allergic reactions in the skin of rats infected with *Sporotrichum* spp. before the appearance of response at the primary inoculation site[111].

7.3.2 Allergy and antigens of *M. leprae*

Skin tests for leprosy in the past have been diagnostic of the form of disease, lepromatous or tuberculoid, rather than of the disease, the lepromatous group being anergic. 'Protein' preparations (Fernandez) give reactions at 24 to 48 hours, whereas lepromin prepared from tissues rich in organisms gives a nodular (Mitsuada) reaction appearing at about 7 days and maximum at 3 to 4 weeks. Grinding of the organisms increases the proportion of reactions at 24 to 48 hours, and decreases those at 7 days.

The recent discovery of the growth of *M. leprae* in the armadillo[112] has provided a better source of organisms, which when prepared by ultrasonic disintegration give reactions at 30 days comparable to the Mitsuda antigen from human leprosy tested at the same time, the lepromatous subjects giving negative and the tuberculoid lepers giving positive reactions[113].

Tests with a depot lepromin (Mitsuada type) like those with depot tuberculin, show much enhanced potency as well as economy of test material[114]. The depot lepromin persists at the test site so that, at about 4 weeks after BCG vaccination, positive reactions appear at previously negative sites. This confirms the presence of related antigens in BCG and *M. leprae*. The demonstration of allergy to *M. leprae* by the depot lepromin test has advantages such as economy, ease of administration, lack of severity of reactions and provision of immunological information of value for clinical and epidemiological purposes. Similar procedures with more precise preparations from organisms which grow in the armadillo would be of interest.

7.3.3 *Streptococcus pneumoniae*

As with tuberculosis, interest in the immunology of pneumonia due to *Streptococcus pneumoniae* flourished until the introduction of effective chemotherapy. A role for anaphylactic sensitization as a contributory factor in the development of lobar pneumoniae in subjects sensitized to pneumococci by previous exposure was suggested[115]. This theory was supported by observations in guinea-pigs[116].

The incidence of allergy to *S. pneumoniae* antigens as shown by positive skin tests was first reported with alcohol-precipitated 'protein' fractions in some patients with pneumonia[117]. The supernatants of autolysed pneumococci were found[118] to give immediate reactions to intracutaneous tests from 1 to 21 days after the crisis, but not during the acute stage. This was confirmed[119] with polysaccharide and purified somatic protein antigens. Immediate reactions to type-specific polysaccharides were elicited only in the post-crisis and convalescent periods. A failure to react was taken as a bad prognostic sign. The type-specific polysaccharides are of capsular origin in smooth strains. There are also polysaccharide allergens in non-capsulated rough strains. The protein fractions were not type-specific and elicited Type IV reactions. The immediate reaction was passively transferable[120], and positive reactions were observed only rarely in subjects who did not have pneumonia[121]. The elicitation by type-specific polysaccharides of immediate reactions followed by extensive 'puffed-up' swellings which were resolving by 24 hours was reported[122], the swellings having features of a Type III reaction.

The skin-test reaction to pneumococcal (polysaccharide)-specific soluble substance has been used as a guide to antiserum therapy for pneumonia[119], and free capsular polysaccharide was also found in the blood stream. Repeated intracutaneous injections of the pneumococcal polysaccharide induces Type I allergy in normal subjects[123] thus illustrating the potent allergenicity of polysaccharide allergens. A similar potent enhancing effect on sensitivity is observed with fungal polysaccharides, such as the mannan of

C. albicans[34]. This is relevant to the use of repeated tests with such materials for assessment of immunological status in relation to particular sources of the polysaccharide, and also to a possible mechanism whereby growth of the agent and liberation of such polysaccharides can enhance sensitivity to the point where allergic reactions and their consequences in their own right make their appearance, such as vasculitis, urticaria and angio-oedema, or where actual infection with its allergic mechanisms appears.

There are a number of polysaccharides in *Strept. pneumoniae*, including a somatic polysaccharide pneumococcal C-substance which combines with C-reactive protein. C-substance has closely related chemical determinants to capsular material and cross-reacts with it. Polysaccharides of a similar or possibly identical nature, with the appropriate phosphatidyl choline determinant which is responsible for the reaction with C-reactive protein, are widely distributed in nature, being found in fungi such as *A. fumigatus*, the dermatophyte species, helminths of the nematode, trematode and cestode species and even in a wide range of vegetable materials, a prime example of this being the kernel of the palm-nut[124]. The polysaccharides are mainly glucogalactomannan peptides. All of these C-substance-like materials appear to have common allergenicity in that they can all give Type I skin-test reactions in patients with allergic aspergillosis. They also have common precipitinogenic sugars in that they can combine with certain of the precipitating antibodies in the sera of patients with pulmonary aspergilloma. Degradation of the sugar moiety destroys this precipitinogenic activity, which is probably dependent upon one or more immunoreactive sugars, but not the capacity to combine with C-reactive protein[125].

7.3.3.1 *Allergy and streptococcal antigens*

Skin tests with cellular and extracellular products of group A streptococci, which are far from pure[126], cause fewer reactions in the general population than in affected subjects[127]. Lymphocytic transformation by 'streptolysin S' is decreased in rheumatic fever and in systemic streptococcal infections[128] and appears to be due to a streptococcal product other than the streptolysin.

In an analysis of these problems[129] the following suggestions as to how allergic disease may be produced by streptococcal infections have been put forward:

(1) A serum-sickness-like illness in which combination of antibody and circulating antigen is a model.

(2) Reactions to streptococcal antigen fixed in the tissues, analogous to nephrotoxic serum nephritis mediated by circulating antibody, sensitized lymphocytes or both. No evidence has been found of the bacterial antigen in the heart, but more intensive search along the lines of studies in allergic vasculitis[130] may yet do so.

(3) The production of autoantibodies resulting from the toxic tissue damage. Streptolysins S and O disrupt lysosomes and local altered host antigens may induce autoantibodies. Whether these in turn cause tissue damage is not known.

(4) A possible role for lymphocyte activation by streptococcal products at the site of infection with liberation of tissue-damaging lymphokines has not been established.

(5) Allergic reactions resulting from cross-reactivity between streptococcal and tissue antigens (e.g. cardiac antigens) are possible. There is, however, an abundance of cross-reacting systems, the immunopathological relevance of which is not known.

(6) Tissue damage by streptococcal toxins has to be considered.

In this context the work of toxins and their enhancing effect on deposition of complexes, cited in the studies on vasculitis, may be important[130]. Antibodies may be produced against 'irrelevant' antigens rather than the toxins, thus enabling the toxins to prepare the way for the otherwise non-harmful antigen–antibody complexes to assume a damaging role.

Bacterial cellular substances include endotoxins and exotoxins (e.g. from streptococci, staphylococci and C. diphtheriae) which predispose vessels to penetration by complexes which might otherwise remain harmlessly in the circulation[131]. Failure to produce antibodies to an exotoxin may predispose to tissue damage by otherwise non-toxic antigens released during infection. For example, diphtheria toxin enhances penetration of the blood vessels of guinea-pigs by unrelated antigen–antibody complexes which does not occur in previously immunized animals.

The introductory role of Type I allergy in the development of the Type III, immune-complex complement dependent reaction[31] appears similar to the effects of the toxins discussed above, and it would seem that a similar 'helper' factor or mechanism may be required for bacterial complex-induced disease. For example, in rats with intraperitoneal diffusion chambers containing living cultures of either group A streptococci from a case of human glomerulonephritis or a non-nephritic strain, both induced similar levels of antibody but nephritis occurred only with the former type. Eluates from the diseased kidneys, but not the unaffected ones, contained type-specific antibodies. This raises the question of whether an agent was produced which acted on the glomerular membrane or whether an appropriate antibody or other agent capable of mediating a Type I-like reaction, or possibly both, were present and favoured deposition of the immune-complexes. It is necessary[130] to distinguish cytotoxic nephritis due to toxins in which tubules are affected soon after infection from the glomerular damage in glomerulonephritis which appears several weeks later.

In patients with acute post-streptococcal glomerulonephritis there is evidence of a relationship between tissue damage and serum antibody.

Serum complement is also decreased in acute nephritis, in contrast to rheumatic fever. Antibody and complement can be found in the glomeruli giving rise to the 'lumpy' deposits on the epithelial side of the basement membrane. The tissue damage may, however, not necessarily be complement dependent.

In studies on experimental glomerulonephritis the administration of a single dose of protein antigens results in acute disease whereas multiple small doses are associated with the development of chronic disease. With other bacterial antigens, repeated subcutaneous injection of *Proteus mirabilis* into mice causes acute or subacute glomerulonephritis[132]. High levels of agglutinin to the O and H antigens are produced but bear no relationship to the development of nephritis. Antigen of *P. mirabilis* is found on immunofluorescence examination in the affected glomeruli where it can persist for 3 weeks. The appearance of the renal lesions is associated with the appearance of antibodies. Repeated injections of formalin-killed *Escherichia coli* into rabbits induce high levels of agglutinins at 4 to 6 weeks, the appearance of a rheumatoid-like factor at 10 weeks and mild glomerulonephritis at 21 weeks[133].

7.3.3.2 Allergy skin-tests with streptococcal antigens

Preparations such as streptokinase-streptodornase are part of a battery of bacterial, fungal and viral antigens used for skin tests for Type IV allergy in the assessment of cellular immune competence because of the frequent presence of sensitization. M antigen of group A haemolytic streptococcus and other streptococcal antigens have been used for the study in man of passive transfer of delayed Type IV allergy[48].

In patients with recurrent aphthous stomatitis positive delayed skin-test reactions have been elicited with a killed vaccine of pleomorphic transitional α-form cultures of α-haemolytic streptococcus isolated from the lesions. A few of these patients also gave immediate reactions[134].

7.3.3.3 Staphylococcus aureus

The capacity of protein A of *Staph. aureus* to combine non-specifically with the Fc piece of IgG and of such combinations to elicit Type III reactions in rabbits raises problems in distinguishing this from antibody-mediated reactions[135,136]. The property of non-specific fixation is used for removal or separation of IgG from serum. Most coagulase-positive strains have two major groups of antigen, protein A and cell-wall polysaccharide-type ribitol teichoic acids[137]. Earlier workers showed the capacity of *Staph. aureus* culture filtrates to cause release of histamine from perfused lung and liver and directly from human leukocytes[138], whereas the latter did not occur with teichoic acid preparations[139]. In our own experience[140] teichoic acid preparations can, in a small proportion of subjects, elicit Type I prick-test reactions, and the presence of specific IgE antibody against the bacterial cell wall, shown by tests using whole killed, slide-fixed organisms, suggests that it may be responsible[29]. We have, furthermore, shown that 70% of sera of UK subjects have precipitins to the *Staph. aureus* teichoic acid and that this reaction can be blocked by absorption of the sera with N-acetyl-glucosamine[142]. Such teichoic acids are widely present in extracts of different vegetable dusts, e.g. coffee bean, bagasse, mouldy hay, etc., probably due to bacterial contamination by *Staph. aureus*. Whilst specific enough in their own right, these precipitin reactions are not specifically related to the source material under study.

The presence of specific IgE and precipitating antibodies provides a basis for Type I and III allergies which may have been obscured by the effects of the various toxins in this organism.

7.3.3.4 H. influenzae

Skin tests with specific H_1 and H_2 allergens (and H_3 to H_5 which are non-specific and are shared with other Gram-negative bacteria) showed that some patients gave immediate reactions to intracutaneous tests and all developed indurated reactions at 5 hours which were maximum at 24 hours, with or without a preceding immediate reaction[143]. All the preparations contained endotoxin. Typical Type III reactions are almost invariably preceded by a Type I 'introductory' reaction and this could be used as a criterion for trying to separate specific allergic reactions from the non-specific effects of endotoxin. Endotoxin preparations elicited reactions resembling Type III reactions in 90% of subjects[144]. The endotoxins activate the C3 component of complement by the alternative pathway with the production of C3a which has tissue-damaging and anaphylatoxin activity causing histamine release from mast cells[145].

7.3.3.5 E. coli *allergens*

General sensitization to *E. coli* polysaccharides is considered a possible cause of oedema and haemorrhagic gastroenteritis in young pigs, a disease in which antibodies may be acquired across the placenta or through maternal colostrum. These animals may die suddenly due to proliferation of the organism with sudden absorption of large amounts of antigen. This resembles the anaphylactic-like death in fowl typhoid due to *Salmonella gallinarum* in which there are high levels of circulating antibody and large amounts of polysaccharide antigen in the organs. Allergic reactions of Type I and III and possibly Type II by virtue of polysaccharide attachment to the red blood cells could all be present[146]. Enterotoxin formation by related serotypes is another possible factor. Mechanisms of a similar nature have been proposed in bacillary dysentery[147]. *E. coli* 013 and *Shigella flexneri* have common antigenic determinants and since most humans are normally sensitized and have antibodies to *E. coli* vigorous reactions may be elicited by *Shigella flexneri*. The fulminating disease known in Japan as Ekiri could be produced by such mechanisms or by Schwartzman reactions or both. Animals are not susceptible to this organism but become so if sensitized to the antigens of *E. coli*.

Protein preparations of *E. coli* have also been used for Type IV skin-test reactions as a measure of cellular immune competence because of its ubiquitous presence in the body.

7.3.4 Allergy in syphilis

Allergic mechanisms are postulated for the different aspects of syphilis at different stages of development. Thus the histology of the primary chancre consists of plasma cells, lymphoid cells and macrophages with appearances suggestive of an allergic granuloma. In the secondary stage the lymphadenopathy and skin eruptions are attributed to allergic reactions to disseminated treponemata, whereas in the tertiary stage with severe damage few organisms are present, resembling findings in tuberculosis. In congenital syphilis[148] it is suggested that the appearance of the lesions at the 5th to 6th month may be related to the development of immunological competence.

Treponema pallidum contains phospholipid antigenic determinants common to the cardiolipins of the inner membrane of the mitochondria of all living cells, thus providing a basis for autoantibodies induced by and cross-reacting with these haptens. Autoantibodies to brain, erythrocyte and mitochondrial cardiolipins are present[149].

Antitreponemal antibodies, distinct from those to cardiolipins, are also formed during infection[150]. These may contribute to resistance and possibly also by the formation of complexes with soluble antigen to allergic tissue-damaging reactions, such as the manifestations of secondary syphilis.

The lymphoid cells in syphilis show decreased reactivity to stimulation by phytohaemagglutinin as compared with those of healthy subjects. A factor is present in the serum which reduces the response of normal lymphocytes to this stimulus[151,152]. As in lepromatous leprosy where decreased delayed allergy is associated with extensive lesions rich in organisms, so it is thought the decreased lymphocyte responsiveness in syphilis may be related to the widespread distribution of the treponemes in primary and secondary syphilis.

7.3.5 Allergic reactions to viral allergens

All the types of allergic reaction can be elicited by viral allergens. Where allergy is minimal or absent a carrier state is likely to be present. There are a variety of sources of viral allergens and reasons for reactions. The allergens may be present in budding viruses or may be virus-determined antigens, such as enzymes; they may multiply in the vascular endothelium and may be liberated by cell destruction due to allergic reactions. Where there is failure of cell-mediated responses the virus may persist and immune-complex formation take place. Other mechanisms for prolonged viraemia include the production in terms of immunity of antibodies to irrelevant antigens such as non-structural proteins or internal ribonucleoprotein. These antigens can, however, participate in the formation of immune-complexes and cause disease. The production of low-affinity antibodies may also result in poor elimination of the virus, as may certain deficiencies in complement related to clearance of immune-complexes[153].

Examples of the influence of allergic mechanisms are provided by the virus of lymphocytic chorio-meningitis. A large proportion of mice are infected shortly after birth and many become life-long carriers. Where there are high titres of antibody in the blood, brain and tissue manifestations of disease are absent. Where there are low levels of antibody, immune-complexes are formed and glomerulonephritis results. In immunocompetent mice with Type IV allergy, encephalitis is produced, whereas non-competent mice develop the carrier state.

The production of immune-complex disease is genetically determined by factors influencing the rate of multiplication, the affinity of antigen for antibody, the response of macrophages, and the sharing of antigens between host and virus. Similar phenomena are observed with hepatitis B antigen. This may be responsible for a serum-sickness-like disease, or polyarteritis in which the antigen, IgM and C3 are present in the vessel walls, or for glomerulonephritis. Arthritis may precede the hepatitis and subside with the appearance of antibodies and the disappearance of the antigen from the circulation.

The roles of allergy in the response to hepatitis B antigen are shown by subjects infected in the handling of renal dialysis equipment[154]. In those with depressed Type IV allergy, mild hepatitis with persistent antigenaemia is found. In immunologically normal subjects acute hepatitis with rapid clearance of the antigen from the blood occurs. The antigen also persists in patients with other diseases such as lepromatous leprosy where Type IV allergy, i.e. the cell-mediated response, is depressed. These phenomena are important in pathogenesis and in terminating the production of the antigen. This determines whether the infection is self-limiting or persists and causes liver damage. Autoantibody production also correlates with the amounts of hepatitis B antigen and is used as an indicator of persistent disease or relapse.

Dengue haemorrhagic fever is an example of the role of sensitization to viruses by a primary infection so that the disease develops in a second infection. There are usually several viruses endemic and present concurrently with a rate of infection of over 5% per annum. On second infection there is a vigorous anamnestic antibody response which can result in a shock syndrome with massive activation and fall in circulating complement[155]. The viraemia is greater in the second infection associated with levels of reactive but poorly neutralizing antibody. The virus buds through the cell membrane thus making possible a Type II cytolytic allergic reaction.

Respiratory syncytial virus is a common and most important cause of acute respiratory disease in children. Infants may have high levels of passively acquired antibody and the disease is most severe in the first two months of life[156, 157]. Children given poorly immunogenic vaccine may as a consequence have more severe disease with natural infections. The bronchiolitis has been attributed to Type I allergy[158] but the presence of deposits of IgG in the same distribution of the virus and the severity of the tissue reaction is suggestive of Type III allergy and possibly Type II to the viral buds.

Measles has its allergic component in the form of the rash which is probably due to Type IV allergy. The disease follows its normal course in agammaglobulinaemia, but where there is depression of T-cell system there may be a fatal giant cell pneumonia without a rash[159]. Abnormally severe and clinically abnormal disease occurs in children who become infected after vaccination with inactivated vaccine[160].

Mumps virus gives delayed reactions which are of epidemiological rather than diagnostic value and are also used for assessment of cellular immune competence, because the majority of subjects give a positive reaction even though in 25% of them there is no history of the disease and many of these reactions are possibly attributable to a subclinical infection[161]. In infected subjects reactions can be elicited by the 4th or 5th day after infection in 50% of the subjects and at the 9th or 10th day by 80%.

7.3.5.1 *Allergy and* Mycoplasma pneumoniae

A role for allergic reactions rather than direct pathogenicity is postulated for infections by *M. pneumoniae*. Fever and pneumonitis occur only after the second exposure and the presence of erythema nodosum and the Stevens-Johnson syndrome are suggestive of allergy.

Inactivated vaccines do not induce growth-inhibiting antibody and as a consequence vaccinated subjects are more severely affected on challenge than non-vaccinated subjects[162]. Autoantibodies to antigen I of the erythrocytes are also induced and these may react not with the *Mycoplasma* itself, but with the erythrocytes and possibly also with tissue cells, thus being the probable cause of the often associated haemolytic anaemia.

7.3.6 Fungal allergens

In fungal as with bacterial allergy the polysaccharide allergens are potent allergenically in eliciting reactions in sensitized subjects and give Type I and III but not Type IV reactions, whereas protein allergens can elicit all three. It is also because of the affinity of polysaccharides for cell membranes that they may mediate Type II allergy. Fungal polysaccharides, like those from pneumococci with which they may be closely related, are type-specific while the proteins show broad species specificity. The purified poly-saccharides are haptenic and react well with antisera, but they fail to induce antibody production in experimental animals or do so only weakly[163-165]. A β-naphthol polysaccharide from *C. albicans* has been found to induce a good antibody response when injected together with Freund's adjuvant[166].

There is a great variety of polysaccharides in fungi cultured from the same slope even when grown in the same medium and under the same conditions, let alone all the possible variations in these. Most fungal polysaccharides are branched-chain molecules with usually three or more different mono-saccharides, most commonly mannose, galactose and glucose[165-172].

They often contain a small amount of bound N, not detectable by tests for protein. The polysaccharides may be fabricated into the structural framework or capsular sheath; others serve as reserve foods and yet others appear to be products of metabolism without any apparent definite function. Some of the polysaccharides have, however, other biological actions besides being potent allergens, such as the capacity to combine with C-reactive protein in the same way as pneumococcal C-substance[124]. In order to assess the differences between the polysaccharide and protein allergens, it is necessary to obtain them in as chemically pure forms as possible, as for example from *Candida albicans* and *Aspergillus fumigatus*, to be discussed later. Study of the allergenic potential of whole fungal cells, e.g. the yeast cells of *C. albicans*, provides a useful source of the whole spectrum of cell-wall allergens, protein, polysaccharides, etc., very similar to their occurrence in the body. This may clarify the relative importance and roles of the chemically separated allergens which are tested in forms and amounts often very different from those encountered *in vivo*.

7.3.6.1 *Skin tests with fungal allergens*

The importance of the different chemical components and unstandardized nature of test preparations, in relation here to fungi, can be seen from comparison of their contents of polysaccharide and protein antigens. In the case of *Candida albicans* a commercial preparation, similar to those widely used as representative of protein antigens for skin and *in vitro* tests, was found to contain mainly polysaccharide mannan antigens with a very limited amount of protein. By contrast our preparation of cytoplasmic proteins contains a large number, 40 to 50 or more, of distinct antigens[27,173]. This protein preparation has been purified by passage through a Concanavalin A column to remove the residual mannan antigens[13]. Such procedures make it possible to assess the relative roles of the polysaccharide and protein allergens and provide a basis for reproducible preparation of test materials rather than the unknown combinations available at present. The correct interpretation of skin-test reactions is complicated by the mixture of poly-saccharide and protein antigens, because both the polysaccharide mannan and protein components of *C. albicans* can elicit Type I reactions in which, as far as the polysaccharide is concerned, both IgE and STS-IgG are present. As far as is now known, at least IgE antibody is present against the protein[13,173].

Type IV reactions are elicited mainly by protein allergens, though these can also elicit Type I and III reactions. Polysaccharide allergens are not associated with Type IV reactions[174] and elicit mainly Type I and III reactions. In the *Trichophyton* spp.[175] a glucan has been found to elicit Type I reactions and a glycopeptide fraction to give stronger Type I and in addition Type IV reactions.

Examples of the main differences in terms of Type IV allergy and the nature of the fungal allergens are shown by dermatophytes, such as the *Trichophyton* genus[175] and by *Candida albicans*. Though this has been less well studied, with results on the whole of a similar nature, both immediate and delayed reactions have been elicited by extracts of other fungi, such as *Histoplasma capsulatum*, *Coccidioides immitis*, *Blastomyces dermatitidis*, *Nocardia brasiliensis*, *Actinomyces* and *Sporothrix schenckii*. There is much cross-reactivity between the preparations of the latter fungi, the homologous antigen tending to give stronger reactions[177,178]. Cross-reactivity between polysaccharides is more likely by virtue of the commonness of the sugars they contain, and preparations of proteins free of polysaccharide and of the polysaccharides themselves may help to improve the specificity of the tests.

7.3.6.2 *Type I allergy to* C. albicans

The problems associated with the different chemical components becomes even more complex with opportunist fungal pathogens which are present universally, such as *C. albicans*, when the question is to decide whether the findings are clinically relevant. The fungus, however, provides a good model for the assessment of the different types of allergic reaction to its different chemical components[13,173] and in serological tests for the appropriate antibodies to the whole yeast cells[27].

Immediate Type I reactions to prick tests with the polysaccharide can be mediated by specific STS-IgG antibody, demonstrable by PCA tests in the monkey[13], and also by specific IgE antibody to insolubilized mannan (to which reference will be made later) or possibly by both since both may be present together[27,173]. Type I reactions are also given by the protein, polysaccharide-free, allergen and specific IgE antibody is present. It is probable that STS-IgG antibody will also be found, but whatever the case there are at least three and possibly four mechanisms for Type I reactions in relation to these two chemical components. The available commercial or other preparations contain both polysaccharide and protein antigens, thus making interpretation of the reaction difficult.

7.3.6.3 Specific IgE antibodies to polysaccharide allergens from C. albicans and A. fumigatus

The demonstration of specific IgE antibodies in the serum is relevant to assessment of the main mechanism for Type I allergy. The conventional radioallergosorbent test (RAST) in which the allergen is coupled to a solid phase immunosorbent, such as cellulose or sepharose particles, or paper discs after activation by cyanogen bromide[24], is used for protein antigens which can be coupled in this way. Polysaccharides cannot be coupled in the same way and tests have been devised in which the polysaccharide preparation is polymerized[26], e.g. from *A. fumigatus* which contained about 5% protein and *C. albicans* in which no protein was detectable or insolubilized[27,173], or linked to a sepharose epoxy resin preparation, e.g. from *C. albicans*. In these first two methods the insolubilized polysaccharide acts as its own solid-phase immunosorbent. These methods are likely to prove of value for the study of IgE antibodies against polysaccharides from a wide range of infective agents.

7.3.6.4 Specific IgE antibodies to C. albicans

Comparisons have been made of measurements of specific IgE antibodies to the cytoplasmic polysaccharide-free protein, to the insolubilized mannan and whole yeast cells of *C. albicans* and to antigens of *A. fumigatus*[27,173]. The test sera were derived from patients with a soft-tissue *C. albicans* granuloma, Kimura's disease occurring in young Japanese males, and patients with asthma and allergic broncho-pulmonary aspergillosis. At least some of the sera of each group showed the presence of IgE antibodies to the whole range of antigens, with the highest incidence in Kimura's disease and allergic broncho-pulmonary aspergillosis. There were, however, differences in that most of the sera from patients with Kimura's disease had IgE to all of the allergens but little to *A. fumigatus*, and the sera of the aspergillosis patients had little IgE antibody to the mannan whilst most had IgE antibody to all of the other allergens including *A. fumigatus*. The sera from the patients with the specific *C. albicans* granuloma had more IgE antibodies to the mannan, which is a feature of yeast-cell wall, and in which form they probably encountered it. Tests with the whole yeast cells gave comparable IgE results for Kimura's disease and aspergillosis though this may have been due to different cell-membrane antigenic components. The use of the whole intact killed fungal cells for this purpose provides a model for the study of IgE antibodies against other infective agents in the forms in which they are likely to be present *in vivo*. The yeast cells also reacted well with antibodies in the different immunoglobulin classes: IgA, IgM and IgG and its subclasses[173].

The ubiquity of *C. albicans* precipitins is shown by their presence against the cell-wall mannan in almost all patients if the sera are sufficiently concentrated. When the precipitin test is made to measure about 0.2 mg antibody N/ml about 20% of control sera give positive reactions, compared with 50% of sera from asthmatics and 75% of sera from patients with allergic aspergillosis[34]. The differences here appear to be clinically relevant because skin tests with the mannan in allergic aspergillosis elicit Type I and III reactions in almost all cases. There is very little cross-reactivity between *C. albicans* and *A. fumigatus* and it is possible that *C. albicans* is participating in the allergic pulmonary reactions of this disease. The potency of the polysaccharide allergens is shown by the fact that healthy subjects giving negative skin reactions and precipitin tests at the 0.2 mg antibody N/ml level all give Type I and III reactions and positive precipitin tests on retesting 3 to 4 weeks later. A similar phenomenon has been described with repeated injections in man of pneumococcal polysaccharide[123]. In view of the presence of polysaccharides in the cell membrane of many infective agents, the possibility that they may, like *C. albicans* mannan, enhance Type I and III hypersensitivity may be brought into play when they multiply in the body, and a vicious circle could be established in which hypersensitivity and growth of the agent increase in parallel. In skin tests with *Histoplasma capsulatum* allergens, for example, it has long been known that blood should be taken before the skin test because of its enhancing effect on the serological tests.

7.3.6.5   *Allergy and* Aspergillus fumigatus

A. fumigatus is a ubiquitous fungus widely distributed in nature. It too is of some importance for the study of immunopathology in man because it provides evidence of the associated effects of Type I and III allergies to an agent capable of growing in the bronchi. It can induce Type I allergy, especially in atopic subjects, like any other of the common inhalant fungal allergens, and positive skin-test reactions are elicited with commercial extracts in about 10–15% of uncomplicated extrinsic asthmatics. It plays a different role in pulmonary eosinophilia, almost always associated with asthma which is complicated by the transitory pulmonary collapse-consolidations seen on X-ray and a higher blood eosinophilia than is usual in uncomplicated asthma. About 80% of asthmatics with pulmonary eosinophilia in the UK have evidence of allergic broncho-pulmonary aspergillosis[33,179] with Type I allergy to the fungus, and markedly raised levels of, specific IgE antibody, accompanied by positive precipitin tests in most cases capable of mediating Type I and II reactions. An essential feature of the diagnosis is the presence of Type I allergy upon which the development of the Type III allergy depends. Skin-prick tests with commercial extracts giving Type I reactions elicit Type III reactions in about 25% of the cases, whereas a protein preparation elicits them in about 50% of the cases. Intracutaneous tests elicit Type I and III reactions in almost all cases and inhalation tests also give an analogous pattern of immediate and non-immediate asthmatic reactions.

The bronchial changes associated with the pulmonary shadows are characteristic and are attributable to a Type III reaction to antigen from the fungus growing in the respiratory tract. At some time or other most patients cough up tough rubbery sputum plugs which tend to be in the proximal bronchi in relation to the sites of the lung shadows. These plugs contain growing fungal hyphae of *A. fumigatus*, the antigens of which can elicit Type I and III reactions. The characteristic proximal cylindrical or saccular bronchiectasis which will appear at these sites is attributed to the tissue-damaging effects of the Type III allergic reaction. It is possible that Type III reactions to *C. albicans* already described may produce effects of a similar nature if circumstances permit.

7.3.7   Allergy and helminth parasitic allergens

Features of Type I allergy with high serum levels of IgE and eosinophilia are common in parasitic infections. The antigens from *Echinococcus granulosus, Trichinella spiralis, Dirofilaria immitis* and *Ascaris lumbricoides* elicit more immediate than delayed reactions. This is probably attributable to the polysaccharides which can be readily extracted from the parasites. By analogy with the potent allergenic effect of the mannan polysaccharide of *C. albicans* it is probable that the parasitic polysaccharides enhance the degree of sensitivity thus giving rise to the high degree of allergy so commonly found.

Among the polysaccharides of the nematode, cestode and trematode parasites is one which reacts with C-reactive protein like pneumococcal C-substance[124]. This can also give Type I prick-test reactions in patients with allergic broncho-pulmonary aspergillosis. *A. fumigatus* has a polysaccharide – a glucogalactomannan peptide – which has similar properties. Cross-reactions are common in helminth infections[180]. These polysaccharides have not been studied in any detail for their capacity to elicit not only Type I but also Type III reactions. Precipitins against *Ascaris* for example are commonly present in association with high degrees of Type I allergy.

The granulomata of certain parasitic diseases such as schistosomiasis probably have a Type IV component. It has been shown that bentonite particles coated with schistosoma antigen elicit granulomatous reactions in sensitized animals, and that this form of reaction can be passively transferred with the lymphoid cells but not the serum[94]. Insoluble immune-complexes formed by the diffusible or shed antigens could also be playing a part in the granuloma formation[39].

In the analysis of the immunopathology of parasitic diseases, Type I, III and IV allergies, at least, have all to be considered for their contribution, as is the case with *M. tuberculosis* described earlier[43].

7.3.8   Assessment of allergy to infective agents in vasculitis

The allergic mechanisms responsible for vasculitis are relevant to allergic reactions in other diseases[181].

A role for allergy to bacteria and fungi in vasculitis has been intensively studied[182-186]. Antigens derived from streptococci, *Staph. aureus*, *M. tuberculosis* and *C. albicans* have been found in the lesions, sometimes as complexes in combination with IgG antibody. Indirect evidence of such complex formation is provided by the increased presence of rheumatoid factor, in response to the complexing of IgG molecules, and of immuno-conglutinin, in response to activated complement.

Immunofluorescence studies in 67 subjects with vasculitis showed the presence of antigen from *Streptococcus* group A in 12, *C. albicans* in eight and occasionally *Streptococcus* group D, *Staph. aureus* and *M. tuberculosis*. The soluble antigens gave a finely granular appearance in 10% of cases distinguishable from the occasional finding of larger particulate antigens, probably whole organisms. IgG, IgM and B-1-C component of complement were frequently present in the same lesions, especially in cutaneous vasculitis. In those subjects with vasculitis following on streptococcal infection, antibodies were found to both protein and polysaccharide antigens, capable of forming complement-fixing complexes *in vitro*. The sera of patients with streptococcal infection but without vasculitis were more effective in forming such complexes. The lesser activity in this context of the sera of the vasculitis patients was attributed to the removal of the relevant antibodies during the production of the lesions. It was noted that the complexes formed with some bacterial antigens penetrate more easily into the vascular endo-thelium than complexes containing the bland proteins usually used in experimental vasculitis.

The sera of normal persons and of those convalescing from streptococcal infections contain precipitins to extracellular agents, some of these being enzymes or toxins[187]. The sera of patients with post-streptococcal vasculitis tend to have less neutralizing antibodies to some of the streptococcal enzymes, e.g. proteinase, and to toxins than in the subjects without vasculitis[184].

In the assessment of the finding of antigen–antibody complexes in the vasculitis lesions it is emphasized that such complexes are common in the circulation and their presence in the lesions may be fortuitous. The uptake of intravascular complexes in skin lesions induced by adjuvants or delayed allergic reactions has been observed in guinea-pigs. Also the presence of antigen or antibody in the lesions is not necessarily evidence of complex formation.

The reasons for the persistence of 'spontaneous' vascular lesions for weeks or months are obscure. In the classical Arthus reaction the antigens are relatively rapidly degraded. These are usually protein antigens and the same fate may not necessarily be met by polysaccharide antigens. The author has observed cyclical recurrences at intervals of 2 to 3 days for 1 to 2 weeks at the sites of Type III reactions elicited with the cell-wall polysaccharide mannan of *C. albicans*. In serum sickness the breakdown of complexes and their reconstitution is regarded as the mechanism for the recurrent nature of this disorder. Similarly drug allergic disorders may persist and recur for very long periods after cessation of the drug.

The histological appearances in allergic vasculitis consist mainly of in-filtration with mononuclear cells – possibly due to a Type IV reaction. They could also be due, for example, to deposition of group A streptococcal poly-saccharide complexes with antibody which have been shown[188] to induce nodular lesions in the skin of non-sensitized animals.

7.3.9 Allergy to infective agents in eczema

The possible roles of bacterial allergens in the production and/or mainten-ance of generalized and nummular eczema has been examined in detail[189–192]. The allergens from *Staph. aureus* which were tested were polysaccharide, lipopolysaccharide, teichoic and nucleic acid preparations and a commercial particulate extract. The phenol lipopolysaccharide and the cell-wall teichoic acid preparations adsorbed readily to monolayers of skin, embryo or amnion, showing the affinity of polysaccharides for cells and their potential role in Type II allergic reactions. Specific allergic damage was produced in the presence of antibody and complement. Delayed necrosis can be elicited by teichoic acid preparations in the skin of patients with high levels of antibody, associated with the release of lysosomes from leukocytes in the presence of antibody[193].

Immediate Type I and non-immediate 4-hour (Type III or Type III-like) reactions were elicited by skin tests with the above materials in 21.8% of patients with generalized eczema, in 55.2% with nummular eczema, in 75% with other forms of skin disease and in 10% of controls. There were few isolated 4-hour or delayed Type IV allergic reactions. No correlation was found between agglutinins or titre of complement fixing antibodies in patients giving immediate and 4-hour reactions[191,192]. The duality of the combined reactions resembles that of the Type III reaction with its depen-dence upon a preceding Type I reaction[31]. Differences in appearance of the reactions from those usually elicited with fungal and other allergens may be related to the nature of the antigens or antibodies involved. No evidence of specific IgE antibody was found, though this may now be possible using whole killed fixed cells of *Staph. aureus, Strept. pneumoniae* and *H. influenzae* as the source of solid-phase immunosorbent[29].

7.3.10   Allergy to infective agents in local or generalized erythema, papular skin reactions and the Arthus reaction

A possible role for bacterial allergy in fixed reactions and generalized erythema has been sought[191]. Such reactions are regarded as being due to bacterial toxaemia. The problems here are once again those of assessing the clinical relevance of ubiquitous common commensal organisms with frequent evidence of antibodies and allergic sensitivity.

Drug allergy is the recognized mechanism for 'fixed' eruptions, the response usually being localized and its immunological basis unknown. The re-introduction of an antigen in man or guinea-pigs may elicit an erythematous reaction at the site of previous delayed skin-test reactions[130]. This appears to be an Arthus-like response to antigen combining with cell-bound antibody. Thus in guinea-pigs with contact sensitivity induced by topical application the sites of previous delayed type reactions may respond to re-exposure by another route with an erythematous reaction and there may even be generalized erythema. It is suggested that this may be a modified Arthus-like reaction because the speed of appearance of the erythema is 4 to 6 hours, though its duration is somewhat longer, about 48 hours. Slight thickening of the skin and desquamation may persist for 1 to 2 weeks and is accompanied by histological evidence of congestion, oedema and infiltration by neutrophil and a few eosinophil cells. This reaction is not like the soft oedematous, ill-defined swelling of Type III reactions elicited by fungal and other allergens. It is not materially modified by antihistamine drugs which are so effective for anaphylactic reactions in the guinea-pig, nor by the use of antilymphocytic sera which inhibit Type IV contact reactions. Decrease in the polymorphonuclear neutrophil cells inhibits the reaction as it does the Arthus reaction which is dependent upon them. The antigens are found fixed to small mononuclear and plasma cells suggestive of cell-bound antibody, and more cells fix antigen 2 hours after challenge than before, indicating fresh antibody synthesis. A possible fungal cause of this form of allergic reaction is infection with *Trichophyton mentagrophytes* without adjuvants[130] whereas these are required for *Staph. aureus*. Injection of these antigens in Freund's adjuvant induces Type IV allergy but not the flare response.

The frequent application of live cultures of *Staph. aureus* in water and oil emulsion to abraded skin or its application to a small area near a site into which Freund's adjuvant has been injected induces delayed allergy and also the capacity for the specific flare response to its lipopolysaccharide. Epidermal desquamation of remote sites persists for 10 to 14 days. A similar skin response without desquamation occurs in guinea-pigs after injection with streptococcal erythrogenic toxin but desquamation occurs at the sites of previous delayed-type skin-test reactions. This is not a specific response, occurring at sites previously tested with and reacting to chemicals, tuberculin, trichophytin and *Staph. aureus* extracts. Skin tests show delayed sensitivity only, as occurs in response to common commensal bacteria in healthy subjects, unless enough antigen is injected to induce the rash. No serum precipitins, however, are demonstrable[189].

In eczema the bacterial antigens are present on the skin surface and there is evidence of percutaneous absorption and binding to epidermal cells[189-192]. It has still to be established whether or not the various reactions associated with these antigens are relevant to allergic mechanisms in eczema, possibly mediated by the capacity of protein A from *Staph. aureus* and by similar proteins in other organisms to combine with the Fc portion of the IgG molecule, or whether the various findings are simply epiphenomena in tissues damaged by other mechanisms.

7.3.11 Bacterial atopy

The role of bacteria in respiratory tract allergy is a controversial subject requiring clarification. Bacterial antigens have been used for skin tests in asthma, namely 'protein' extracts of common respiratory tract commensal organisms, since 1916[194, 195]. Positive reactions were then elicited to *Staph. aureus* in 18% and *S. albus* in 6% with 1–2% reacting to *Strept. viridans*, *Strept. haemolyticus*, *C. diphtheriae*, *Micrococcus tetragenus* and *M. cararrhalis*, but no controls were tested. Later tests[196] with nucleoproteins from the commensals, including *H. influenzae*, were made. *Staph. aureus* gave positive reactions in 25% and a number gave an erythematous reaction at 6 hours with oedema. The same incidence of reactions was obtained in atopic and non-atopic subjects[197].

In tests with fragmented bacteria, *Staph. aureus* gave positive reactions in 31% of allergic and 8% of non-allergic subjects. Tests with 34 crude poly-saccharide and nucleoprotein fractions of *Staph. aureus* and *Staph. faecalis* gave immediate reactions to the polysaccharide and delayed reactions to the protein bacterial allergens. The latter were maximum at 20 hours and seldom occurred without a preceding immediate reaction[198]. This suggests that they may have been Type III reactions. Tests with nucleoprotein type-specific fractions from 10 strains of *Staph. aureus* cultured from nasal swabs of asthmatics gave delayed reactions with no differences between allergic subjects and controls. Purified polysaccharide fraction gave immediate reactions and no delayed reactions with 73% positive in allergics and 32% in controls[200].

A distinction was found between type-specific polysaccharides from pathogenic and non-pathogenic *Staph. aureus*[199]. Positive reactions were elicited in 12% of normal children and 65 to 70% of normal adults with the polysaccharide from the pathogenic strain but seldom with that from the non-pathogenic strain. All patients with staphylococcal infection gave immediate reactions. The higher incidence of reaction in the allergics has to be treated with caution because of the enhanced reactivity of atopic subjects to what may be non-specific wealing agents[20]. Furthermore, staphylococcal preparations may contain wealing agents. Intracutaneous tests with cell-wall teichoic acid preparations from *Staph. aureus* gave immediate reactions in normal subjects[200,201] and we have observed a small number of positive prick-test reactions with an α-teichoic acid preparation.

The complexity of polysaccharide and protein antigens in bacteria and their presence in usually unknown amounts in most test materials requires resolution of the sort discussed earlier in terms of similar chemical allergens of *C. albicans*. The identification of the different classes of antibody to the bacterial antigens is also necessary for assessment of possible allergic reactions. The demonstration of specific IgE antibody to the intact cells of common commensals[29] as with *C. albicans* yeast cells[27] may be more relevant clinically as the organisms are likely to be met *in vivo* in this form. Tests with purified fractions are necessary for basic immunological assessments but they are likely to be tested in amounts far in excess of those occurring in the body.

The use of bacterial vaccines for treatment of allergic disease has to be seen in the context of the above points requiring clarification, and it is not surprising that no evidence has yet been provided of beneficial effects from such vaccines. With improved allergens and better understanding of the possible immunological mechanisms further trials of specific treatment under properly controlled conditions would be justified.

7.3.12 Allergic reactions to inhaled organismal particles and antigens

7.3.12.1 *Extrinsic allergic alveolitis*

The inhalation of spores of commonly non-pathogenic organisms can cause extrinsic allergic alveolitis of the farmer's lung or bird fancier's lung type[202]. Amongst the causal agents are: thermophilic actinomycetes such as *Micropolyspora faeni*, *Thermoactinomyces vulgaris* and *T. sacchari*, fungi such as *Cryptostroma corticale*, *Penicillium casei* and *P. frequentans*, *Aspergillus clavatus* and *A. fumigatus*, *Aureobasidium pullulans*, *Graphium* sp. and others, and free living amoebae[203] such as *Acanthamoeba polyphaga* and *A. castellani*.

This is a disease mainly of non-atopic subjects in whom the inhalation of particles of organic materials of a size small enough to penetrate to the peripheral gas-exchanging tissues of the lungs leads to sensitization with the production of precipitins and of sensitized lymphocytes. Where the materials are appropriate for mainly intracutaneous tests, Type I and III allergic reactions are elicited. IgE antibody is usually not present and there is evidence of STS-IgG antibody which could be mediating the Type I introductory reaction for the Type III response[14].

Many of the features of this disease are compatible with a Type III immune-complex reaction to the inhaled allergens, such as Type III skin-test reactions and the development of pulmonary reactions 3 to 4 hours after deliberate exposure. The characteristic pathological changes are patchy infiltration of alveolar walls with lymphoid, plasma, histiocytic and giant cells with inclusions and in particular of epithelioid granulomata. The latter have been interpreted by some as evidence of Type IV allergy but, as has been pointed out earlier in relation to M. tuberculosis, granuloma formation may have several mechanisms, such as insoluble immune-complex formation[39], the effect of particles such as spores coated with antigen along the lines of the antigen-coated bentonite particles[94] in which sensitized lymphocytes are involved, and also the capacity of a number of the causes of this disorder to activate complement by the alternative pathway with consequent macrophage activation[40,204]. This in turn could be associated with granuloma formation. Thus more than one mechanism may be involved in the pathological changes. In practice the identification of the many organic dusts causing this disease has been made by the precipitin test. This provides evidence of exposure and sensitization though it is not necessarily diagnostic of the disease.

7.3.12.2 Systemic reactions to inhaled organismal allergens

Subjects exposed to organismal allergens or their products in microbiological laboratories or industry may give systemic allergic reactions to them. Examples of this are the induction of systemic manifestations with fever in tuberculin-sensitive subjects following inhalation of tuberculin in its preparation. Similarly workers engaged in the manufacture of biological detergents in which the enzymes of B. subtilis are used may develop allergic respiratory disease in which both IgE and IgG antibodies are demonstrable[205]. Atopic subjects are sensitized more frequently and more rapidly. In those without a clinical history which would exclude them from the particular occupational exposure, assessment of atopic status by, for example, prick tests with a small battery of extracts of common allergens or the use of the RAST on the serum can be of use for selection for employment in the particular environment.

Exposure to non-viable organisms may have similar effects. For example, in subjects who have suffered from brucellosis, it can reproduce all the manifestations of the acute disease within a few hours with fever, chills, malaise and myalgia, lasting for many hours[206]. This raises questions as to whether recurrences of this and other diseases without known re-infection or possibly even specific re-exposure may be due to exposure to other organisms containing cross-reacting antigens.

In laboratory workers handling helminths such as *Ascaris*, reactions may also be elicited by inhalation of the emanations.

7.4 GENERAL CONSIDERATIONS

The examples given here of the patterns of allergic sensitivity in their own right to infecting agents and their products shows that, for completeness, information is required on the class or classes of antibody relevant to purified chemical components and also to the intact organism, the form in which it occurs in the body. The reactions elicited have to be distinguished, for example, from the effects of toxins or of agents capable of mimicking allergic reactions by activation of complement via the alternative pathway.

Much is known about the participation of hypersensitivity to infective agents in the production of certain diseases, but this can certainly be amplified by the application of information gained concerning specific antibody classes, the responsible agents, and the corresponding tissue reactions they can elicit.

Attention has mainly been paid to the diagnostic use of antigens from infective agents prepared in a few instances by protein fractionation and consisting usually of relatively crude materials. These may contain a mixture of protein, polysaccharide, glycopeptide, lipoprotein, lipopolysaccharide, etc. The role of polysaccharide allergens has on the whole not been studied as intensively as that of proteins. Their importance cannot be underestimated as shown by their potent effects in enhancing Type I and III allergies and as they are mainly present in the cell membrane of the organisms they are likely to be even more relevant than the proteins usually studied which are usually of cytoplasmic origin. These polysaccharides may show a wide degree of cross-reactivity of immunoreactive sugars. Their capacity to fix to tissue cells makes them candidates for Type II cytotoxic allergy as well as their role in Type I and III, but not, it would seem, in Type IV allergies. Protein antigens can also elicit Type I and III allergies, and, even more pertinently perhaps, Type IV allergy.

The final assessment of the clinical value of the findings with crude materials, with chemically separated and if possible purified allergens and with intact organisms depends upon their relevance to well-defined disorders. Where the organism is pathogenic and not ubiquitously present as with the common skin, respiratory tract and gut commensals, the allergic reactivity has most interest in diagnostic terms. Where, however, the agent is a common opportunistic pathogen or even a non-pathogen the clinical relevance is more difficult to determine and would appear to be most closely related to diseases described as 'allergic'.

References

1. Gell, P. G. H., Coombs, R. R. A. and Lachmann, P. J. (1975). *Clinical Aspects of Immunology*, p. 762 (Oxford: Blackwell Scientific Publications)
2. Pepys, J. (1975). Skin tests in diagnosis. In: *Clinical Aspects of Immunology* (P. G. H. Gell, R. R. A. Coombs and P. J. Lachmann, eds.), pp. 55–80 (Oxford: Blackwell Scientific Publications)
3. Kay, A. B. and Austen, K. F. (1971). The IgE mediated release of an eosinophil chemotactic factor from human lung. *J. Immunol.*, **107**, 899
4. Ishizaka, K. and Ishizaka, T. (1971). Mechanisms of reaginic hypersensitivity: a review. *Clin. Allergy*, **1**, 9
5. Kaufman, H. S. and Hobbs, J. R. (1970). Immunologic defects in an atopic population. *Lancet*, **ii**, 1061
6. Taylor, B., Norman, A. P., Orgel, H. A., Stokes, C. R., Turner, M. W. and Soothill, J. F. (1973). Transient IgA deficiency and pathogenicity of infantile atopy. *Lancet*, **ii**, 111
7. Tada, T. and Ishizaka, K. (1970). Distribution of IgE-forming cells in lymphoid tissues of the human and monkey. *J. Immunol.*, **104**, 377
8. Stanworth, D. R. and Smith, A. K. (1973). Inhibition of reagin-mediated PCA reactions in baboons by IgG_4 subclass. *Clin Allergy*, **3**, 37
9. Parish, W. E. (1970). Short-term anaphylactic IgG antibodies in human sera. *Lancet*, **ii**, 791
10. Bryant, D. H., Burns, M. W. and Lazarus, L. (1975). Identification of IgG antibody as a carrier of reaginic activity in asthmatic subjects. *J. Allergy Clin. Immunol.*, **56**, 417
11. Warren, C. P. W., Cherniack, R. M. and Tse, K. (1977). Extrinsic allergic alveolitis from bird exposure. *Clin. Allergy*, **7**, 303
12. Berry, J. B. and Brighton, W. D. (1977). Familial human, short-term sensitizing (IgG-STS) antibody. *Clin. Allergy*, **7**, 401
13. Longbottom, J. L., Brighton, W. D., Edge, G. and Pepys, J. (1976). Antibodies mediating Type I skin-test reactions to polysaccharide and protein antigens of *Candida albicans*. *Clin. Allergy*, **6**, 41
14. Pepys, J., Parish, W. E., Stenius, B. and Wide, L. (1975). Long-term and short-term sensitizing antibodies to common allergens in extrinsic and cryptogenic asthma. *Clin. Allergy*, **5**, 237 (Abstract)
15. Lakin, J. D., Thomas, J. B., Strong, D. M. and Yocum, M. W. (1978). Anaphylaxis to protamine sulphate mediated by a complement dependent IgG antibody. *J. Allergy Clin. Immunol.*, **61**, 102
16. Parish, W. E. (1975). Some biological activities of IgG subclass antibodies after inoculation and in disease. In: *Allergy '74. Proc. 9th Eur. Congr. of Allerg. & Clin. Immunol.* (M. A. Ganderton and A. W. Frankland, eds.), p. 153 (London: Pitman Medical)
17. Grant, J. A. and Lichtenstein, L. M. (1972). Reversed *in vitro* anaphylaxis induced by anti-IgG: Specificity of the reaction and comparison with antigen-induced histamine release. *J. Immunol.*, **109**, 20
18. Squire, J. R. (1952). Tissue reactions to protein sensitization. *Br. Med. J.*, **1**, 1
19. Cleare, M. J., Hughes, E. G., Jacoby, B. and Pepys, J. (1976). Immediate (Type I) allergic responses to platinum compounds. *Clin. Allergy*, **6**, 183
20. Stenius, B., Wide, L., Seymour, W. M., Holford-Strevens, V. and Pepys, J. (1971). Clinical significance of specific IgE to common allergens. (1) Relationship of specific IgE against *Dermatophagoides* species and grass pollen to skin and nasal tests and history. *Clin. Allergy*, **1**, 37
21. Belin, L. G. and Norman, P. S. (1977). Diagnostic tests in the skin and serum of workers sensitized to *Bacillus subtilis* enzymes. *Clin. Allergy*, **7**, 55
22. Siraganian, R. P. and Brodsky, M. J. (1976). Automated histamine analysis for *in vitro*

allergy testing. I. A method utilizing allergen-induced histamine release from whole blood. *J. Allergy Clin. Immunol.*, **57**, 525

23. Prouvost-Danon, A., Peixoto, J. M. and Queiroz Javierre, M. (1967). Reagin-like antibody mediated passive anaphylactic reaction. *Life Sci.*, **6**, 1793

24. Johansson, S. G. O. (1967). Raised levels of a new immunoglobulin (IgND) in asthma. *Lancet*, **ii**, 951

25. Wide, L., Bennich, H. and Johansson, S. G. O. (1967). Diagnosis of allergy by an *in vitro* test for allergen antibodies. *Lancet*, **ii**, 1105

26. Baldo, B. A. and Pepys, J. (1976). Radioallergosorbent (RAST) studies with insolubilized polysaccharides. *Clin. Allergy*, **6**, 563

27. Edge, G. and Pepys, J. (1976). RAST tests avec des antigenes polysaccharidiques et des cellules lavees. *Rev. Franc. Allerg.*, **16**, 251

28. Sepulveda, R., Longbottom, J. L. and Pepys, J. (1978). Enzyme-linked immunosorbent assay (ELISA) for antibodies to *A. fumigatus*, an alternative for antibody detection. (In prep.)

29. Tee, R. and Pepys, J. (1977). Specific IgE antibodies to whole killed cells of *Staph. aureus, Strept. pneumoniae* and *H. influenzae*. (In prep.)

30. Augustin, R. (1973). Techniques for the study and assay of reagins in allergic subjects. In: *Handbook of Experimental Immunology*, 2nd Edition (D. M. Weir, ed.) (Oxford: Blackwell Scientific Publications)

31. Cochrane, C. G. (1971). Mechanisms involved in the deposition of immune-complexes in tissues. *J. Exp. Med.*, **134** (Suppl. 75)

32. Pepys, J. (1969). Hypersensitivity diseases of the lungs due to fungi and organic dusts. *Monogr. Allergy*, Vol. 4 (Basel: Karger)

33. McCarthy, D. S. and Pepys, J. (1971). Allergic broncho-pulmonary aspergillosis. Clinical Immunology. (1) Clinical features. (2) Skin, nasal and bronchial tests. *Clin. Allergy*, **1**, 261, 415

34. Pepys, J., Faux, J. A., Longbottom, J. L., McCarthy, D. S. and Hargreave, F. E. (1968). *Candida albicans* precipitins in respiratory disease in man. *J. Allergy*, **41**, 305

35. Dolovich, J., Hargreave, F. E., Chalmers, K., Shier, K. J., Gouldie, J. and Bienenstock, J. (1973). Late cutaneous allergic responses in isolated IgE-dependent reactors. *J. Allergy Clin. Immunol.*, **52**, 83

36. Ratner, B. (1943). *Allergy, Anaphylaxis and Immunotherapy*, p. 487 (Baltimore: Williams and Wilkins)

37. Kay, A. B. (1970). Studies on eosinophil leukocyte migration. II. Factors specifically chemotactic for eosinophils and neutrophils generated from guinea-pig serum by antigen/antibody complexes. *Clin. Exp. Immunol.*, **107**, 899

38. Kay, A. B. and Austen, E. K. (1971). The IgE mediated release of an eosinophil leukocyte chemotactic factor from human lung. *J. Immunol.*, **107**, 899

39. Spector, W. G. and Heesom, N. (1969). The production of granulomata by antigen–antibody complexes. *J. Pathol.*, **98**, 31

40. Schorlemmer, H. U., Edwards, J. H., Davies, P. and Allison, A. W. (1977). Macrophage responses to mouldy hay dust, *Micropolyspora faeni* and *Zymosan*, activators of complement by the alternative pathway. *Clin. Exp. Immunol.*, **27**, 198

41. Pepys, J. (1976). Allergic manifestations in tuberculosis. In: *Textbook of Immunopathology*, (P. A. Miescher and H. J. Muller-Eberhard, eds.), Ch. 27, p. 453 (New York: Grune and Stratton)

42. Seeberg, G. (1947). Intradermal reactions of the delayed type in relation to the absorptive behaviour of the skin. *Acta Derm. Vener.*, **27** (Suppl.), 18

43. Pepys, J. (1955). The relationship of non-specific and specific factors in the tuberculin reaction. *Am. Rev. Tuberc.*, **71**, 49

44. Gernez, Ch. and Marchandise, Ch. (1935). La specificte des reactions cutanées tuberculinques. *Rev. Immunol.*, **1**, 315

45. Daniels, M., Ridehalgh, F., Springett, V. H. and Hall, I. M. (1948). *Tuberculosis in Young Adults*. Rophit Tuberculosis Survey 1935–1944 (London: H. K. Lewis)

46. Hart, P. D'A., Long, D. A., Rees, R. J. W. (1952). Depression of tuberculin sensitivity in guinea-pigs by certain antituberculous surface-active agents. *Br. Med. J.*, i, 680

47. Faenes, R. B., Dillon, P. and Choi, Y. S. (1976). Levamisole augments the cytotoxic T-cell response depending on the dose of drugs and antigen administered. *Clin. Exp. Immunol.*, 27, 502

48. Lawrence, H. S. (1955). Transfer in humans of delayed skin-test sensitivity to streptococcal M substance and to tuberculin with disrupted leucocytes. *J. Clin. Invest.*, 34, 219

49. Canetti, G. (1946). L'allergie tuberculeuse chez l'homme. *Collection de l'Institut Pasteur* (Flammarion: Editions Medicales)

50. O'Grady, F. (1956). Mantoux reaction patterns in active and arrested tuberculosis. *Br. J. Tuberc.*, 50, 159

51. O'Grady, F. (1957). Tuberculin sensitization in man. *Br. J. Tuberc.*, 51, 74

52. Gernez-Rieuz, Ch., Tacquet, A., Gervois, M., Voisin, C. and Macquet, V. (1961). Valeur theorique et pratique des reactions cutanées tuberculiniques. *XIIIe Congres de la Tuberculose*

53. Bachi, J. (1959). Studies on tuberculin reactions repeated in the same site (Report II) Histological study in human skin. *Kakhaku*, 34, 879

54. WHO Tuberculosis Research Office (1955). Repeated tuberculin tests in the same site. *Bull. WHO*, 12, 197

55. Hill, W. C. (1969). The influence of the cellular infiltration on the evolution and intensity of delayed hypersensitivity reactions. *J. Exp. Med.*, 129, 363

56. Goldman, A. S. and Walker, B. E. (1962). The origin of cells in the infiltrates at the sites of foreign protein injection. *Lab. Invest.*, 11, 808

57. Pollock, T. M., Sutherland, I. and Hart, P. D'Arcy (1959). The specificity of the tuberculin reaction in man in Great Britain. *Tubercle (Lond.)*, 68, 678

58. Rosenthal, S. R. and Libby, J. E. P. (1960). Simultaneous multiple tuberculin testing. *Bull. WHO*, 23, 689

59. Furculow, M. I., Hewell, B., Nelson, W. E. and Palmer, C. E. (1941). Quantitative studies of the tuberculin reaction. I. Titration of tuberculin sensitivity and its relation to tuberculous infection. *Publ. Hlth. Rep. (Wash.)*, 56, 1082

60. Dahlstrom, A. W. (1940). The instability of the tuberculin reaction: observations on dispensary patients with special reference to the existence of demonstrable tuberculosis lesions and the degree of exposure to tubercle bacilli. *Am. Rev. Tuberc.*, 42, 471

61. Rich, A. R. (1951). The pathogenesis of tuberculosis. (Springfield: C. C. Thomas)

62. Brody, J. A., Overfield, T. and Hammes, L. M. (1964). Depression of the tuberculin reaction by viral vaccines. *N. Engl. J. Med.*, 271, 1294

63. Berkovich, S., Fiking, S., Brunell, P. A., Portugalaza, C. and Steiner, M. (1972). Effects of mumps vaccine on tuberculin sensitivity. *Pediatrics*, 80, 84

64. Bail, O. (1910). Uebertragung der Tuberkulnenifindlichkeit. *Z. Immunitatsforsch. Exp. Therap.*, 1, 470

65. Rich, A. R. and Lewis, M. R. (1927). Mechanisms of allergy in tuberculosis. *Proc. Soc. Exp. Biol. Med.*, 25, 596

66. Landsteiner, K. and Chase, M. W. (1942). Experiments on transfer of cutaneous sensitivity to simple compounds. *Proc. Soc. Exp. Biol. Med.*, 49, 688

67. Chase, M. W. (1945). The cellular transfer of cutaneous hypersensitivity to tuberculin. *Proc. Soc. Exp. Biol. Med.*, 59, 134

68. H. S. Lawrence and M. Landy, eds. (1969). *Mediators of Cellular Immunity* (New York: Academic Press)

69. B. R. Bloom and P. R. Glade, eds. (1971). In vitro *Methods in Cell-mediated Immunity* (New York: Academic Press)

70. Mannick, J. A. and Egdahl, R. H. (1962). Transformation of non-immune lymph node cells to state of transplantation immunity by RNA. A preliminary report. *Ann. Surg.*, **156**, 356

71. Thor, D. E. and Dray, S. (1968). The cell migration-inhibition correlate of delayed hypersensitivity. Conversion of human non-sensitive lymph node cells to sensitive cells with RNA extract. *J. Immunol.*, **101**, 469

72. Arala-Chaves, M. P., Lebacq, E. G. and Heremans, J. F. (1967). Fractionation of human leukocyte extracts transferring delayed hypersensitivity to tuberculin. *Int. Arch. Allergy*, **31**, 353

73. Fishman, M. and Adler, F. L. (1963). Antibody formation initiated *in vitro*. II. Antibody synthesis in x-irradiated recipients of diffusion chambers containing nucleic acid derived from macrophages incubated with antigen. *J. Exp. Med.*, **117**, 595

74. Rocklin, R. E., Chilgren, R. A., Hong, R. and David, J. R. (1970). Transfer of cellular hypersensitivity in chronic mucocutaneous candidiasis monitored *in vivo* and *in vitro*. *Cell. Immunol.*, **1**, 290

75. Valdimarsson, H., Wood, C. B. S., Hobbs, J. R. and Holt, P. J. L. (1972). Immunological factors in a case of chronic granulomatous candidiasis and its treatment with transfer factor. *Clin. Exp. Immunol.*, **11**, 151

76. Kind, Ch. *et al.* (1970). Transfer factor therapy in a patient with anergic pulmonary tuberculosis. *Schweiz Med. Wochenschr.*, **107**, 1742

77. Dumonde, D. C. and Maini, R. N. (1971). The clinical significance of mediators of cellular immunity. *Clin. Allergy*, **1**, 123

78. Morley, J., Wolstencroft, R. A. and Dumonde, D. C. (1973). The measurement of lymphokines. In: *Handbook of Experimental Immunology*, ch. 28 (Oxford: Blackwell Scientific Publications)

79. Nelson, D. S. and Boyden, S. V. (1963). The loss of macrophages from peritoneal exudates following the injection of antigen into guinea-pigs with delayed type hypersensitivity. *Immunology*, **6**, 264

80. Turk, J. L. (1971). Mechanisms in cell-mediated immunity. *Ann. Sclavo*, **13**, 748

81. Saye, L. (1953). Contribution a l'étude de la reaction de reinfection et de la sensibilité a la tuberculine chez les enfants vaccines avec le BCG sec par voie digestive. *Presse Med.*, **61**, 524

82. Willoughby, D. A., Boughton, B. and Schild, H. O. (1963). A factor capable of increasing vascular permeability present in lymph node cells. A possible mediator of the delayed reaction. *Immunology*, **6**, 480

83. Bloom, B. R. (1971). The number and nature of tuberculin hypersensitive lymphocytes. *Ann. Sclavo*, **13**, 758

84. Turk, J. L. (1967). Delayed hypersensitivity: specific cell-mediated immunity. *Br. Med. Bull.*, **23**, 1

85. McGregor, D. D., Kester, F. T. and Mackaness, G. B. (1971). The mediator of cellular immunity. I. The life-span and circulation dynamics of the immunologically committed lymphocyte. *J. Exp. Med.*, **133**, 389

86. Coe, J. E., Feldman, J. D. and Lee, S. (1966). Immunologic competence of thoracic duct cells. I. Delayed hypersensitivity. *J. Exp. Med.*, **123**, 267

87. Mackaness, G. B. (1971). Delayed hypersensitivity and the mechanism of cellular resistance to infection. *Progr. Immunol.*, **413**,

88. David, J. R., Lawrence, H. S. and Thomas, L. (1964). The *in vitro* desensitization of sensitive cells by trypsin. *J. Exp. Med.*, **120**, 1189

89. Bennett, B. and Bloom, B. R. (1967). Studies on the migration inhibitory factor associated with delayed-type hypersensitivity, cytodynamics and specificity. *Transplant*, **5**: *Suppl.*, 996

90. Blanden, R. V. (1968). Modification of macrophage production. *J. Reticuloendothel. Soc.*, **5**, 179

91. David, J. R. (1965). Suppression of delayed hypersensitivity *in vitro* by inhibition of protein synthesis. *J. Exp. Med.*, **122**, 1125

92. Youmans, G. P. and Youmans, A. S. (1971). 'Mycobacterium tuberculosis' immunogens. *Ann. Sclavo*, **13**, 706

93. Spector, W. G. (1971). The mechanism of granuloma formation. *Ann. Sclavo*, **13**, 788

94. Boros, D. I. and Warren, K. S. (1973). The bentonite granuloma: characterization of a model system for infection and foreign body granulomatous inflammation, using soluble mycobacterial, histoplasma and schistosoma antigens. *Immunology*, **24**, 511

95. Pepys, J. (1962). Precipitins against mycobacterial and other extracts in sarcoidosis. *Thorax*, **17**, 284 (Abstract)

96. Cournand, A. and Lester, M. S. (1939). Skin reactions due to tubercle bacillus polysaccharides. *Prod. 3rd Internat. Congr. Microbiol. N.Y.*, p. 621

97. Glenchur, H., Fossieck, B. E. C. T. and Silverman, M. (1965). An immediate skin test for the diagnosis of active pulmonary tuberculosis. *Am. Rev. Resp. Dis.*, **92**, 74

98. Duboczy, B. O. (1965). Non-specific early type of tuberculin reaction. *Am. Rev. Resp. Dis.*, **92**, 55

99. Morisawa, S. A., Tanaka, A., Shajima, K. and Yamamura, K. (1960). Studies on tuberculin-active peptide. *Biochem. Biophys. Acta*, **8**, 252

100. Yasuda, A. (1968). Specificity of skin tests with purified peptides from various strains of Mycobacterium and *Nocardia asteroides*. *Fukuoka Acta Med.*, **51**, 778

101. Yamamura, Y., Onove, K. and Azuma, I. (1968). Chemical and immunological studies in peptides and polysaccharides from tubercle bacilli. *Ann. N.Y. Acad. Sci.*, **154**, 88

102. Shield, M. J., Stanford, J. L., Paul, R. C. and Carswell, J. W. (1977). Multiple skin testing of tuberculosis patients using a wide range of new tuberculins and a comparison with leprosy and *Mycobacterium ulcerans* infection. *J. Hyg.*, **78**, 331

103. Assis, A. and Carvalho, A. de (1942). Da alergia infra-tuberculinica (alergia latente de Willis). *Hospital*, Rio de Janeiro, **22**, 173

104. Fourestier, M. and Blacque-Belair, A. (1957). *Études sur l'Allergie et l'Immunité dans l'Infection Tuberculeuse.* (Paris: Vigot Freres)

105. Edwards, L. B. and Palmer, C. E. (1958). Epidemiologic studies of tuberculin hypersensitivity. I. Preliminary results with purified protein derivatives prepared from atypical acid fast organisms. *Am. J. Hyg.*, **68**, 213

106. Edwards, P. Q. and Edwards, L. B. (1960). Story of the tuberculin test, from an epidemiologic viewpoint. *Am. Rev. Resp. Dis.*, **81**, 1

107. Keay, A. J. and Edmond, E. (1966). Differential Mantoux testing in the testing of atypical mycobacterial infection in children. *Lancet*, **ii**, 1425

108. Medical Research Council Report (1956). BCG and vole bacillus vaccines in the prevention of tuberculosis in adolescents. *Br. Med. J.*, **1**, 413

109. Pepys, J., Bruce, R. A. and James, D. G. (1958). Multiple puncture depot tuberculin (PPD) cream tests in man. *Tubercle (Lond.)*, **39**, 283

110. Bruce, R. A. (1961). Observations on the measurement of skin sensitivity to tuberculin. *Tubercle (Lond.)*, **42**, 199

111. Sulzberger, M. (1940). *Dermatologic Allergy*, p. 319 (Springfield: Charles C. Thomas)

112. Kirchheimer, W. F. and Storrs, E. E. (1971). Attempts to establish the Armadillo (*Dasyptus novemcinctus* Linn) as a model for the study of leprosy. I. Report of lepromatoid leprosy in an experimentally infected Armadillo. *Int. J. Leprosy*, **39**, 693

113. Convit, J. and Pinardi, M. E. (1974). Leprosy. Confirmation in the armadillo. *Science*, **184**, 1191

114. Kinnear-Brown, J. A. and Stone, M. M. (1961). The multipuncture depot lepromin test. *Int. J. Leprosy*, **29**, 1

115. Lauche, A. (1927). Uber die lobare Pneumonie der Neugeborenen. Ein Beitrag zum

Studium der Beziehungen zwischen Enzundungsablauf und Immunität olage. *Z. Geburtsch. Gynak.*, **91**, 627

116. Lindau, A. (1933). Studies on varying responses to pneumococcal infections especially lobar pneumonia. *Acta Path. Microbiol. Scand.*, **10**, 1

117. Clough, P. W. (1915). Some observations on hypersensitiveness to pneumococcus protein, with special reference to its relation to immunity. *Bull. Johns Hop. Hosp.*, **26**, 37

118. Weil, R. (1916). Note on a skin reaction in pneumonia. *J. Exp. Med.*, **23**, 11

119. Tillett, W. S. and Francis, T. (1929). Cutaneous reactions to the polysaccharide and proteins of pneumococcus in lobar pneumonia. *J. Exp. Med.*, **50**, 687

120. Finland, M. and Sutliff, W. D. (1931). Specific cutaneous reactions and circulating antibodies in the course of lobar pneumonia. I. Cases receiving no serum therapy. II. Cases treated with antipneumococcic sera. *J. Exp. Med.*, **54**, 637, 653

121. Sutliff, W. D. and Finland, M. (1932). Anti-pneumococcic immunity reactions in individuals of different ages. *J. Exp. Med.*, **55**, 837

122. Finland, M. and Brown, J. W. (1938). Reactions of human subjects to the injection of purified type specific pneumococcus polysaccharide. *J. Clin. Invest.*, **17**, 479

123. Finland, M. and Dawling, H. F. (1935). Cutaneous reactions and antibody response to intracutaneous injections of pneumococcus polysaccharides. *J. Immunol.*, **29**, 285

124. Pepys, J. and Longbottom, J. L. (1971). Antigenic and C-substance activities of related glycopeptides from fungal, parasitic and vegetable sources. *Int. Arch. Allergy*, **41**, 219

125. Longbottom, J. L. (1964). Immunological investigation of *Aspergillus fumigatus* in relation to disease in man. (Ph D thesis, University of London)

126. Beachy, E. G., Alberti, H. and Stollerman, G. H. (1969). Delayed hypersensitivity to purified streptococcal M protein in guinea-pigs and man. *J. Immunol.*, **102**, 42

127. Lawrence, H. S. (1954). Transfer of skin reactivity to Streptococcal Products. In: *Streptococcal Infections* (M. McCarty, ed.) (New York: Columbia University Press)

128. Hirschhorn, K., Schreibman, R. R., Verbo, S. and Gruskin, R. H. (1964). The action of streptolysin S on peripheral lymphocytes of normal subjects and patients with rheumatic fever. *Proc. Nat. Acad. Sci. (USA)*, **52**, 1151

129. Taranta, A. and Uhr, J. W. (1971). In: *Immunological Diseases* (M. Samter, D. W. Talmage, B. Rose, W. B. Sherman and J. H. Vaughan, eds.), 2nd ed. p. 607 (Boston: Little, Brown and Co.)

130. Parish, W. E. (1972). Host damage resulting from hypersensitivity to bacteria. *Symp. Soc. Gen. Microbiol.*, **22**, 157

131. Parish, W. E. (1970). Complexes of bacterial antigens with IgG and IgM antibodies in cutaneous vasculitis. *International Symposium on Immune-complex Diseases, Spoleto, Italy*, p. 98 (Milan: C. Erba)

132. Wood, C. and White, R. G. (1956). Experimental glomerulo-nephritis produced in mice by subcutaneous injections of heat-killed *Proteus mirabilis. Br. J. Exp. Pathol.*, **37**, 49

133. Howes, E. L. Jr. and Pincus, T. (1963). The development of a combined glomerulo-nephritis and amyloidosis following the injection of formalin-killed *B. coli. Fed. Proc.*, **22**, 257

134. Graykowski, E. A., Barile, M. F., Lee, W. B. and Stanley, H. R. (1966). Recurrent aphthous stomatitis. Clinical, therapeutic, histologic and hypersensitivity aspects. *J. Am. Med. Assoc.*, **196**, 637

135. Forsgren, A. and Sjoquist, J. (1966). 'Protein A' from *S. aureus*. I. Pseudo-immune reaction with human γ-globulin. *J. Immunol.*, **97**, 822

136. Sjoquist, J. and Stalenheim, G. (1969). 'Protein A' from *Staphylococcus aureus*. IV. Complement fixing activity of protein A-IgG complexes. *J. Immunol.*, **103**, 467

137. Oeding, P. (1965). Antigenic properties of staphylococci. *Ann. N.Y. Acad. Sci.*, **128**, 183

138. Feldberg, W. and Keogh, E. V. (1937). Liberation of histamine from perfused lung by staphylococcal toxin. *J. Physiol.*, **90**, 280

139. Martin, R. R. and White, A. (1969). The *in vitro* release of leukocyte histamine by staphylococcal antigens. *J. Immunol.*, **102**, 437

140. Davies, R. J. (1978). Serological and skin test responses to allergens from *Staphylococcus aureus, Streptococcus pneumoniae* and *Haemophilus influenzae* in asthma and chronic bronchitis. (MD thesis, University of Cambridge)

141. Davies, R. J., Holford-Strevens, V. C., Wells, I. D. and Pepys, J. (1976). Bacterial precipitins and their immunoglobulin class in atopic asthma, non-atopic asthma and chronic bronchitis. *Thorax*, **31**, 419

142. Faux, J. A., Holford-Strevens, V., Wells, I. D. and Pepys, J. (1970). 'False positive' precipitation reactions to extracts of organic dusts due to a teichoic acid from *S. aureus*. *Clin. Exp. Immunol.*, **7**, 897

143. Van der Zwan, J. C., Orie, N. G. M. and de Vries, K. (1975). Biphasic reaction after inhalation of *Haemophilus influenzae* in patients with chronic non-specific lung disease. *Clin. Exp. Immunol.*, **7**, 897

144. Thomas, L. (1959). Mechanisms involved in tissue damage by endotoxins of gram-negative bacteria. In: *Cellular and Humeral Aspects of the Hypersensitive States* (H. S. Lawrence, ed.) (New York: Hoeber)

145. Gewurz, H., Skin, H. S. and Mergenhagen, S. E. (1968). Interactions of the complement system with endotoxin lipopolysaccharides: consumption of each of the six terminal complement components. *J. Exp. Med.*, **128**, 1049

146. Thomlinson, J. R. and Buxton, A. (1963). Anaphylaxis in pigs and its relationship to the pathogenesis of oedema, disease and gastroenteritis associated with *Escherichia coli*. *Immunology*, **6**, 2

147. Matsumura, T. (1962). Studies on bacterial cross-allergic reaction on the basis of natural sensitization by intestinal flora. *Gunma J. Med. Sci.*, **11**, 4

148. Silverstein, A. M. (1962). Congenital syphilis and the timing of immunogenesis in the human foetus. *Nature*, **194**, 196

149. Wright, D. J. M. and Doniach, D. (1971). The significance of cardiolysin immuno-fluorescence (CLF). *Proc. R. Soc. Med.*, **64**, 419

150. Banffer, J. R. J. (1972). Demonstration of precipitins against a treponemal antigen by counter-immunoelectrophoresis. *Lancet*, i, 996

151. Levene, G. M., Turk, J. L., Wright, D. J. M. and Grimble, A. G. S. (1969). Reduced lymphocyte transformation due to a plasma factor in patients with active syphilis. *Lancet*, ii, 246

152. Levene, G. M., Wright, D. J. M. and Turk, J. L. (1971). Cell-mediated immunity and lymphocyte transformation in syphilis. *Proc. R. Soc. Med.*, **64**, 426

153. Takahashi, M., Coop, J., Ferreira, A. and Nussenzureg, H. (1976). *Transplantation Rev.*, **32**, 121

154. Dudley, F. J., Fox, R. H. and Sherlock, S. (1972). Cellular immunity and hepatitis associated Australian antigen liver disease. *Lancet*, i, 723

155. Fischer, D. B. and Halstead, S. B. (1970). Observations related to pathogenesis of dengue haemorrhagic fever. V. Examination of age specific sequential infection rates using a mathematical model. *Yale J. Biol. Med.*, **42**, 329

156. Channock, R. M., Smith, C. B., Friedewald, W. T., Parrott, R. H., Forsyth, B. R., Coats, H. V., Kapikian, A. Z. and Charpure, M. A. (1967). In: *Vaccines against Viral and Rickettsial Diseases of Man*, No. 147, p. 53 (Washington: Pan American Hlth. Org. Scientific Publ.)

157. Blandford, G. (1970). Arthus reaction and pneumonia. *Br. Med. J.*, **1**, 758

158. Gardner, P. S., McQuillin, J. and Court, D. S. M. (1970). Speculation on pathogenesis in death from respiratory syncytial virus infection. *Br. Med. J.*, **1**, 327

159. Burnett, F. M. (1968). Measles as an index of immunological functions. *Lancet*, ii, 610

160. Fulgitini, W. C., Eller, J. J., Downie, A. W. and Kempe, C. H. (1967). Altered reactivity to measles virus. Atypical measles in children previously immunised with inactivated measles virus vaccines. *J. Am. Med. Assoc.*, **202**, 1075

161. Enders, J. F., Kane, L. W., Maris, E. P. and Stokes, J. C. Jr. (1946). Immunity in mumps and correlation of the presence of dermal hypersensitivity and resistance to mumps. *J. Exp. Med.*, **84**, 341

162. Smith, C. B., Friedwald, W. T. and Chanock, R. M. (1967). Inactivated *Mycoplasma pneumoniae* vaccine. *J. Am. Med. Assoc.*, **199**, 353

163. Thijøtta, T., Rasch, S. and Urdal, K. (1951). Preparation of fungus antigens for immunization and for serological reaction. A preliminary report. *Acta Path. Microbiol. Scand.*, **28**, 132

164. Elinov, N. P. and Zaikina, N. A. (1959). The precipitin test in the serological diagnosis of moniliasis. *Zh. Mikrobiol. (Mosk)*, **30**, 42

165. Seeliger, H. P. R. (1964). Immunochemistry of fungi. *Mykosen*, **7**, 71

166. Summers, D. F., Grollman, A. P. and Hasenclever, H. F. (1964). Polysaccharide antigens of *Candida* cell-wall. *J. Immunol.*, **92**, 491

167. Whistler, R. L. (1965). *Methods in Carbohydrate Chemistry*. V. General Polysaccharides. (New York and London: Academic Press)

168. Peat, S., Whelan, W. J. and Edwards, T. E. (1961). Polysaccharides of Baker's yeast. *J. Chem. Soc.*, 29

169. Hasenclever, H. F. and Mitchell, W. O. (1964). Immunochemical studies on polysaccharides of yeasts. *J. Immunol.*, **93**, 763

170. Biguet, J., Havez, R., Tran van Ky, P. and Degaey, R. (1961). Étude electrophoretique chromatographique et immunologique des antigenes de *Candida albicans*. Characterization de deux antigenes specifiques. *Ann. Inst. Pasteur*, **100**, 13

171. Barker, S. A., Cruickshank, C. N. D. and Morris, J. H. (1963). Structure of a galacto-mannan-peptide allergen from *Trichophyton mentagrophytes*. *Biochim. Biophys. Acta*, **74**, 239

172. Bishop, C. T., Blanki, F. and Hranisavljevic-Jakovljevic, M. (1962). The water-soluble polysaccharides of dermatophytes. I. A galactomannan from *Trichophyton granulosum*. *Can. J. Chem.*, **40**, 1816

173. Edge, G. (1978). Antibodies to antigens of *Candida albicans* in allergic respiratory disease. PhD Thesis, Univ. London

174. Chaparas, S. D., Thor, D. E., Godfrey, H. P., Baer, H. and Hedrich, Sally R. (1970). Tuberculin active carbohydrate that induces inhibition of macrophage migration but not lymphocyte transformation. *Science*, **170**, 637

175. Barker, S. A., Cruickshank, C. N. D., Morris, J. H. and Wood, S. R. (1962). The isolation of trichophyton glycopeptide and its structure in relation to immediate and delayed reactions. *Immunology*, **5**, 672

176. How, M. J., Whitnall, M. T. and Somers, P. J. (1973). Allergenic glucans from dermatophytes. II. Enzymic degradation. *Carbohydrate Res.*, **26**, 21

177. Wilson, J. W. (1957). *Clinical and Immunologic Aspects of Fungous Diseases*. (Springfield: Charles C. Thomas)

178. Lewis, C. E., Hopper, M. E., Wilson, J. W. and Plunkett, O. A. (1958). *An Introduction to Mycology*, p. 229 (Chicago: The Year Book Publishers Inc.)

179. Malo, J.-L., Longbottom, J. L., Mitchell, J., Hawkins, R. and Pepys, J. (1977). Studies in chronic allergic bronchopulmonary aspergillosis. III. Immunological findings. *Thorax*, **32**, 209

180. Baer, R. L. and Yanowitz, M. (1950). Skin tests in various infectious and parasitic diseases. *Arch. Dermatol. Syph.*, **62**, 491

181. Parish, W. E. and Rhodes, E. L. (1967). Bacterial antigens and aggregated gamma-globulin in the lesions of nodular vasculitis. *Br. J. Dermatol.*, **79**, 131

182. Parish, W. E. (1972). Cutaneous vasculitis: antigen-antibody complexes and prolonged fibrinolysis. *Proc. R. Soc. Med.*, **65**, 276

183. Parish, W. E. (1971). Studies on vasculitis. II. Some properties of complexes formed of antibacterial antibodies from persons with or without cutaneous vasculitis. *Clin. Allergy*, **1**, 111

184. Parish, W. E. (1971). Studies on vasculitis. III. Decreased formation of antibody to M protein, group A polysaccharide and to some exotoxins in persons with cutaneous vasculitis after streptococcal infections. *Clin. Allergy*, **1**, 295

185. Parish, W. E. (1971). Studies on vasculitis. IV. The low incidence of antibacterial anaphylactic antibodies in the sera of persons with cutaneous vasculitis following bacterial infection. *Clin. Allergy*, **1**, 433

186. Parish, W. E. (1976). Studies on vasculitis. VI. Antiglobulins or rheumatoid-like factors in cutaneous vasculitis lesions detected by an improved immunofluorescent procedure. *Clin. Allergy*, **6**, 553

187. Halbert, S. P. (1964). Analysis of human streptococcal infections by immuno-diffusion studies of the antibody response. In: *The Streptococcus, Rheumatic Fever and Glomerulonephritis* (J. W. Uhr, ed.), p. 83 (Baltimore: Williams and Wilkins)

188. Schwab, J. A. (1964). Analysis of the experimental lesion of connective tissue produced by a complex of C-polysaccharide from group A streptococci. II. Influence of age and hypersensitivity. *J. Exp. Med.*, **119**, 401

189. Welbourn, E., Champion, R. H. and Parish, W. E. (1976). Hypersensitivity to bacteria in eczema. Bacterial culture, skin tests and immunofluorescent detections of immunoglobulins and bacterial antigens. *Br. J. Dermatol.*, **94**, 619

190. Parish, W. E., Welbourn, E. and Champion, R. H. (1976). Hypersensitivity to bacteria in eczema. II. Yitre and immunoglobulin class of antibodies to staphylococci and micrococci. *Br. J. Dermatol.*, **95**, 285

191. Welbourn, E., Champion, R. H. and Parish, W. E. (1976). Hypersensitivity to bacteria in eczema. III. Arthus-like responses to bacterial antigens without specific antibody. *Br. J. Dermatol.*, **95**, 379

192. Parish, W. E., Welbourn, E. and Champion, R. H. (1976). Hypersensitivity to bacteria in eczema. IV. Cytotoxic effect of antibacterial antibody on skin cells acquiring bacterial antigens. *Br. J. Dermatol.*, **95**, 493

193. Martin, R. R., Crowder, J. G. and White, A. (1967). Human reactions to staphylococcal antigens. A possible role of leukocyte lysosomal enzymes. *Immunology*, **99**, 269

194. Walker, I. C. (1916). Studies on the sensitization of patients with bronchial asthma to bacterial proteins as demonstrated by the skin reaction and the methods employed in the preparation of these proteins. *J. Med. Res.*, **35**, 487

195. Cooke, R. A. (1932). Infective asthma: indication of its allergic nature. *Am. J. Med. Sci.*, **183**, 309

196. Strevens, F. A. and Jordani, L. (1936). Reactions to intracutaneous injections of nucleoproteins of the upper respiratory pathogenic bacteria in asthmatic patients. *J. Allergy*, **7**, 443

197. Kraft, B., Mothersill, M. H. and Nestman, R. (1949). Immediate urticarial reactions to intradermal injections of bacterial antigens: preliminary report. *Ann. Allergy*, **7**, 162

198. Swineford, O. and Holman, J. (1949). Studies in bacterial allergy: results of 3860 cutaneous tests with 34 crude polysaccharide and nucleoprotein fractions of 14 different bacteria. *J. Allergy*, **20**, 420

199. Julianelle, L. A. and Hartmann, A. F. (1936). The immunological specificity of staphylococci. IV. Cutaneous reactions to the type specific carbohydrate. *J. Exp. Med.*, **64**, 149

200. Strominger, J. L. (1962). Biosynthesis of bacterial cell-walls. *Fed. Proc.*, **21**, 134

201. Toru, M., Jabat, E. A. and Bezer, A. E. (1964). Separation of teichoic acid of *Staphylococcus aureus* into two immunologically distinct specific polysaccharides with alpha and

beta-N acetyl glucosaminyl linkages respectively. Antigenicity of teichoic acids in man. *J. Exp. Med.*, **120**, 13

202. Pepys, J. and Turner-Warwick, M. (1975). The lung in allergic disease. In: *Clinical Aspects of Immunology*, 3rd ed. (P. G. H. Gell, R. R. A. Coombs and P. J. Lachmann, eds.), p. 1217 (Oxford: Blackwell Scientific Publications)

203. Edwards, J. H., Griffiths, A. J. and Mullins, J. (1976). Protozoa as sources of antigen in 'humidifier' fever. *Nature*, **264**, 438

204. Edwards, J. H. (1976). A quantitative study on the activation of the alternative pathway of complement by mouldy hay dust and thermophilic actinomycetes. *Clin. Allergy*, **6**, 19

205. Pepys, J., Wells, I. D., De Souza, M. F. and Greenberg, M. (1973). Clinical and immunological responses to enzymes of *B. subtilis* in factory workers and consumers. *Clin. Allergy*, **3**,143

206. Spinks, W. W. (1957). Significance of bacterial hypersensitivity in human brucellosis. *Ann. Intern. Med.*, **47**, 861

8
Mechanisms of Anergy in Infectious Diseases

W. E. BULLOCK

8.1   INTRODUCTION   270

8.2   CLINICAL CONDITIONS COMMONLY ASSOCIATED
      WITH ANERGY   271
      8.2.1   *Sarcoidosis and Hodgkin's disease*   271
      8.2.2   *Viral infections*   272
      8.2.3   *Infection by micro-organisms that induce a granulomatous
              inflammatory response*   273

8.3   MODULATORS OF THE IMMUNE RESPONSE IN
      GRANULOMATOUS INFECTION   277
      8.3.1   *Immunosuppressive serum factors*   277
      8.3.2   *Disturbances of lymphocyte traffic*   279
      8.3.3   *Suppressor cells and anergy*   283

8.4   SYNTHESIS AND SUMMARY   285

I call this clinical phenomenon of lessening of reactivity 'anergy' (lack of reactivity), in contrast to the term 'allergy'. I apply this name quite generally to the absence of clinical manifestation of reaction . . .

C. E. Von Pirquet, 1911[1]

8.1 INTRODUCTION

From the moment that Von Pirquet first defined anergy as the antipode of allergy, this 'lack of reactivity' generally has been regarded as a rather curious kind of failure of immune function that may be observed in a variety of disease states. Understandably, a clinical phenomenon defined only by the *absence* of reactivity, is not one likely to be approached with great enthusiasm by most clinical investigators. Hence, anergy remains as one of the most poorly understood aspects of clinical immunology today. Nevertheless, some of the advances in cellular immunology during the past decade have provided new insights into the possible mechanisms of anergy and have stimulated considerable interest in this topic. Most significant in this respect has been the recent conceptualization and demonstration of an immunoregulatory control system in mammals that exerts potent negative feedback or suppressor effects upon the immune response.

Given this newer knowledge of inhibitory feedback control mechanisms, it is now possible to view anergy not simply as an absence of reactivity but rather as a state resulting in some cases from stimulation of an immune response that functions actively in a suppressor mode. Indeed, this modern concept of active suppression is similar in some ways to the speculations of Jadassohn who envisaged a 'positive' form of anergy over 50 years ago[2]. Rather than accepting the lack of skin-test reactivity to tuberculin that he observed among patients with sarcoidosis as an absence of immunological reactivity, he considered anergy to be a positive clinical state in which a type of equilibrium between antigen and 'antibodies' had been reached. Thus, he held a remarkably 'modern' view that the presence or absence of a skin-test response depended upon a *dynamic* relationship between an antigen and the immune defences. There is in fact, much in the newer knowledge of cellular immunology to suggest that the clinical expression of either anergy or a 'positive' immune response does represent the algebraic sum of both helper and suppressor effector activities.

It is the purpose of this chapter to discuss anergy with specific reference to infectious diseases and to review possible mechanisms by which this state is induced and maintained. Particular attention will be directed to anergy as it applies to the clinical phenomenon of delayed type hypersensitivity (DTH) and cell-mediated immunity (CMI) respectively. The term CMI will be used in the context of infectious diseases and herewith, is defined as the acquired enhancement of resistance to infection caused by living micro-organisms of the obligate or facultative intracellular type. Throughout the chapter, DTH and CMI are viewed as being functionally interrelated. Although historically, there has been a conceptual hiatus in our under-standing of the relationship between DTH to various microbial antigens and the functions of CMI, clear evidence for an operational link between DTH and CMI has been derived from two major lines of evidence. First, a series of experiments in mice by Mackaness and co-workers[3] demonstrated that control of infection by *Listeria monocytogenes* and elimination of viable bacteria from the liver and spleen coincided chronologically with the acquisition of DTH to *Listeria* and the activation of host macrophages. This work therefore suggested a strong causal relationship between T-lymphocyte function and macrophage activation in both the DTH and the cell-mediated immune responses. The second line of evidence linking DTH to CMI derives from clinical observations, notably of the syndromes of congenital thymic deficiency in which the absence of DTH and CMI consistently is associated with high mortality rates caused by intracellular micro-organisms[4].

8.2 CLINICAL CONDITIONS COMMONLY ASSOCIATED WITH ANERGY

8.2.1 Sarcoidosis and Hodgkin's disease

Once the use of tuberculin skin testing became widespread for detection of DTH to the tubercle bacillus, disease states associated with diminished DTH to tuberculin were soon identified. As early as 1905, it was recognized that a high percentage of patients with sarcoidosis failed to react to tuberculin[5] and 19 years later, Hodgkin's disease also was reported to impose a state of anergy to tuberculin. Subsequently, it was recognized that a substantial proportion of patients with these diseases may be anergic to a variety of skin-test antigens including those prepared from *Candida albicans*, *Trichophyton gypseum*, and mumps virus[7,8]. Furthermore, there is impairment in the capacity of these patients to respond to challenge with simple chemical allergens following attempted sensitization. Although application of haptens such as 2,4–dinitrochlorobenzene (DNCB) to the skin can induce sensitization to a challenge dose in approximately 85–90% of normals, the response is poor among patients with active sarcoidosis and may be totally absent in active Hodgkin's disease[9,10]. *In vitro*, T lymphocytes from the peripheral blood of sarcoid patients may or may not respond well to mitogenic stimulation with phytohaemagglutinin (PHA) or other lectins[11,12] whereas the response is usually severely reduced in active Hodgkin's disease[13].

The more profound anergy of active Hodgkin's disease is accompanied by a deficiency of CMI which is reflected clinically by increased susceptibility to primary infections or, more commonly, to reactivation of latent infection with micro-organisms which are usually controlled by CMI. Characteristically, these infections are caused by fungi (*Candida*, *Aspergillus*, *Histoplasma* and *Cryptococcus*), *Mycobacterium tuberculosis*, protozoa (*Pneumocystis carinii* and *Toxoplasma gondii*), and the herpes viruses (varicella and cytomegalovirus). Patients with active Hodgkin's disease are more prone to these infections than patients with sarcoidosis, not only because the abnormalities of T-lymphocyte function are more severe but also because immunosuppressive therapy and cachexia further compromise host defences. Upon recovery from sarcoidosis, delayed-type reactivity to skin-test antigens and lymphocyte responses to mitogens usually improve although persistent abnormalities of these immune functions have been reported[14].

8.2.2 Viral infections

It has been known for many years that measles infection frequently abrogates the DTH response to skin testing with tuberculin and other antigens[15,16]. Depression of the response to tuberculin may be observed during the late incubation period, and for as long as 42 days after appearance of the rash. There is limited evidence that measles may compromise cell-mediated immune defence mechanisms to the extent that quiescent pulmonary tuberculosis can become active and already active cases may worsen during the period of anergy[18]. Administration of measles vaccine also suppresses the reaction to tuberculin, but less severely and for a shorter period than do natural infections[17].

The mechanism by which the measles virus interferes with host immune responses is unclear. However, it is known that the virus replicates within both B and T lymphocytes as well as within monocytes[19]. Furthermore, if live, or killed virus is added to lymphocyte cultures, the blastogenic response to antigens and PHA is abolished. Since direct cytotoxic damage to lymphoid cells by measles virus has not been established[21], some workers suggest that the inhibition of immune responses *in vitro* may be secondary to an effect of measles infection upon the accessory function of monocytes[22]. Alternatively, the extracellular interferon produced by infected lymphocytes may itself exert an immunodepressive effect[23].

Influenza is a second major viral illness that consistently induces clinical anergy. Marked reduction in, or loss of, pre-existing DTH to a variety of skin-test antigens has been observed during peak infection with a return to normal reactivity approximately 2–4 weeks later[24,25]. Likewise, the lymphocyte blastogenic response to mitogens and antigens may be depressed *in vitro*, again with return to normal during a 4-week period after infection[26]. Addition of influenza virus to cultures of normal lymphocytes suppresses the response to PHA but the mechanism by which this occurs is speculative[25]. In contradistinction to the measles virus, interaction of influenza virus with lymphocytes results in a loss of infectivity possibly because the cycle of viral replication within lymphocytes is incomplete[27]. Thus, inhibition of mitogen-induced DNA synthesis does not appear to be caused by viral replication and/or cell death[21].

Infection by other common viruses may also depress the DTH response; among these are rubella, varicella, Epstein–Barr virus, hepatitis, mumps, and the vaccine strain of type I poliovirus[28-31]. There is no good evidence that these or the influenza viruses are capable of suppressing host CMI to such a degree that superinfection or reactivation of latent infections become a problem.

8.2.3   Infection by micro-organisms that induce a granulomatous inflammatory response

A number of non-viral infections of humans and experimental animals are now known to perturb the DTH response *in vivo* as well as the *in vitro* correlates thereof. Salient features of the anergic state induced by these infections are outlined in Table 8.1. The table does not list all of the infections in which depression of the immune response has been observed, but rather it represents a selection based on the amount of clinical data available and the basic similarity of animal models to human infections associated with anergy. Not listed are two additional human infections in which the evidence for an association with anergy is still limited. The first is disseminated infection by *Histoplasma capsulatum*. Among patients with disseminated histoplasmosis, the DTH response to intradermal (i.d.) injection of histoplasmin tends to be weak or absent[53,54]. However, adequately controlled studies of these patients are needed to establish both the prevalence of anergy and the extent to which responses to specific and non-specific antigens are impaired. The second infection is trypanosomiasis. The evidence linking this infection to disturbances of the DTH response is based primarily on a single publication[55] in which significant depression of skin-test responses to purified protein derivative (PPD) of *M. tuberculosis* and *Candida* antigens were reported among patients infected with *Trypanosoma gambiense* as compared with control subjects. Likewise, the response of patients to challenge with DNCB following sensitization with this hapten (42%) was considerably lower than that of a control group (81%). Unfortunately, at the time of testing, all patients were receiving arsenical therapy that could have affected these test results considerably.

A truly remarkable example of the complex relationship between cellular immune responses of the host and facultative or obligate intracellular pathogens is found in human leprosy. For nearly 60 years it has been known that leprosy patients capable of mounting a DTH response to skin testing with antigens of *Mycobacterium leprae* are likely to restrict the growth of leprosy bacilli within their tissues[56]. Moreover, the lymphocytes of these patients with so-called 'tuberculoid' leprosy respond to *M. leprae* antigens *in vitro* by blastogenic transformation[57]. The histopathology of tuberculoid lesions is characterized by well-developed granulomatous inflammation composed predominantly of epithelioid cells, giant cells, and large numbers of lymphocytes. Acid-fast staining bacilli are seen infrequently in such lesions.

As well described by Ridley and Jopling[58] (see chapter 12), infection with *M. leprae* may result in a wide spectrum of disease, one pole of which is

Table 8.1 Non-viral infections commonly associated with anergy

Microbial agent	Clinical expression	Host	Skin-test anergy to:		Hyporesponsiveness in vitro to:			Selected references
			Specific antigens	Other antigens	Specific antigens	Other antigens	Mitogens	
Mycobacterium leprae	lepromatous leprosy	human	yes	yes	yes	yes	yes	32, 33
Mycobacterium lepraemurium	disseminated infection	rodent	yes	yes	yes	yes	yes	34, 35
Mycobacterium tuberculosis	miliary tuberculosis	human	yes	yes	yes	NE*	yes	36, 37, 38
Coccidioides immitis	disseminated coccidioidomycosis	human	yes	yes	yes	NE	NE	39, 40, 41
Paracoccidiodes brasiliensis	South American blastomycosis	human	yes	yes	yes	yes	yes	42, 43
Cryptococcus neoformans	cryptococcosis	human	NE	NE	yes	no	NE	44, 45
Treponema pallidum	secondary syphilis	human	NE	NE	yes	NE	NE	46, 47
Leishmania aethiopica	diffuse cutaneous leishmaniasis	human	yes	NE	NE	NE	NE	48
Leishmania enrietii	experimental cutaneous leishmaniasis	guinea-pig	yes	NE	yes	NE	NE	49, 50
Trypanosoma congolense	experimental trypanosomiasis	rabbit	yes	yes	NE	yes	yes	51, 52

* NE: not established

recognized clinically as tuberculoid leprosy. At the opposite pole is the form of disease commonly known as lepromatous leprosy. Patients with lepromatous leprosy with few exceptions, are anergic to antigens of *M. leprae* by skin testing. This is true whether tests are performed with integral lepromin (a heat-killed suspension of *M. leprae* plus tissue components prepared from lepromatous nodules) or with more purified bacillary antigens (Dharmendra preparation). Some individuals may regain skin-test reactivity to *M. leprae* after long-term therapy; the majority, however, remain anergic even though bacilli may no longer be identifiable in tissue biopsies. Clinical anergy is paralleled *in vitro* as shown by the fact that lymphocytes from lepromatous patients mount a poor blastogenic response to *M. leprae*[57]. In addition, lymphocytes from these donors fail to produce migratory inhibitory factor (MIF) when stimulated by *M. leprae* whereas the cells from tuberculoid patients can do so[59].

The histopathology of polar lepromatous leprosy differs strikingly from tuberculoid infection in that the inflammatory infiltrate consists largely of histiocytes or macrophages with a foamy appearance resulting from an accumulation of bacterial lipids. Not only are epithelioid and giant cells absent but lymphocytes also are scant and rather diffusely distributed. Macrophages contain aggregates (globi) of acid-fast staining organisms and up to 1×10^9 bacilli per gram of tissue may be present; in some cases the total body burden may be as high as 10^{12} lepra bacilli[60]. Pathological involvement of the dermis is widespread. It is, however, important to note that the lymphoreticular organs and nerves also are extensively invaded by poorly differentiated granulomatous inflammation[61-63].

In addition to anergy specific for *M. leprae* there is a generalized, non-specific impairment of the DTH response in many patients with lepromatous leprosy. Clinically, this deficiency is reflected by hyporeactivity to skin testing with several microbial antigens[32,64] and by impaired responses to sensitizing haptens as compared with control groups[32]. Significant prolongation of skin homograft survival has been observed as well[65]. *In vitro*, lymphocytes from lepromatous patients frequently respond poorly to PHA[33,65-67], to PPD[33], to the Bacillus Calmette-Guérin (BCG), and to antigens of *Streptococcus*[33,70], respectively. Non-specific impairment of DTH is not restricted entirely to lepromatous forms of leprosy since a similar abnormality has been described in tuberculoid leprosy (BT type) although it is of lesser degree and is detected less consistently[32,64,71].

The non-specific impairment of DTH in lepromatous patients is generally less severe than the specific anergy to *M. leprae*. Current evidence suggests that the non-specific component of anergy is of approximately the same magnitude as that observed in active sarcoidosis but weaker than that associated with Hodgkin's disease. Thus, in both sarcoidosis and leprosy, the non-specific component does not appear to block skin-test responses to PPD in patients who have, or recently have had active tuberculosis. Although a number of factors, including nutritional status[72], may modulate the intensity of non-specific anergy, the size of the 'antigen load' may be especially important as indicated by the fact that effective antimicrobial therapy over a period of several months or years can reverse the non-specific component of anergy[32,70,73,74]. In addition, preliminary evidence suggests that the non-specific component of anergy may be less severe among patients who experience erythema nodosum leprosum (ENL), an acute or chronic inflammatory response which is presumed to be an Arthus-like reaction[68,70,75].

The non-specific anergy of leprosy does not grossly predispose patients to infection by other pathogens that challenge the cell-mediated defences. Neither do the limited studies of mortality experience point to an increased frequency of malignancy[76,77]. However, it must be emphasized that carefully controlled, long-range studies have not been conducted on the frequency and severity of other infectious diseases among leprosy patients. Therefore, the very high prevalence of tuberculosis observed among these patients[61] may stem in part from non-specific impairment of CMI, notwithstanding the obvious epidemiological factors which undoubtedly contribute to the high rate of infection among institutionalized patients. The need for careful studies of susceptibility to other infections is underscored by the currently unresolved question as to whether there truly is a higher prevalence of hepatitis B surface antigenaemia among lepromatous patients than among normal individuals of similar socio-economic background[78,79]. Furthermore, clinical reports of a high prevalence of necrosis and retarded resolution at the sites of smallpox vaccination[80,81] suggest that non-specific anergy in lepromatous patients may be of clinical significance.

Studies on the nature of anergy are conducted more easily in leprosy than in many intracellular infections (Table 8.1) because of its extraordinary chronicity and wide spectrum of activity. Response to therapy in the other infections is usually more rapid, and the clinical course is often less chronic. Therefore, interpretation of immunological studies on patients with these infections is more subject to the variables of time and therapy. Nevertheless, these studies have provided far better definition of the immunopathological spectrum for a variety of infections. As a result, it is now possible to assign individual cases to a position within the spectrum of a given infection with reasonable accuracy thereby aiding the physician in prognosis and the approach to therapy. Indeed, as one scans the various spectra of these infections, a remarkably consistent phenomenon becomes apparent: as a facultative or obligate intracellular pathogen becomes more widely disseminated with involvement of the secondary lymphoid organs, there is an increasing impairment in the capacity to express specific DTH and CMI to this organism. In advanced (i.e. polar) stages of dissemination, specific anergy is virtually absolute. Moreover, immune mechanisms resulting in *non-specific* impairment of cellular immunity become increasingly active as dissemination of infection progresses. Conversely, humoral immunity tends to respond in a reciprocal fashion. Thus, if the effector mechanisms of CMI can localize the infecting agent successfully, titres of specific serum antibody are low as a rule. With dissemination however, antibody titres are usually elevated in association with polyclonal hypergammaglobulinaemia.

Our understanding of the factors governing this general behaviour of disseminated granulomatous infections is rudimentary at best. Nevertheless, the rapid advances of cellular immunology have greatly expanded our concepts of these infections and have laid to rest any notion that the immunopathology involved can be explained meaningfully by a single mechanism. The remainder of this chapter, therefore, will be directed, in so far as current information will permit, to a consideration of some elements in the mosaic of factors that may affect immunological responsiveness in these infections.

8.3 MODULATORS OF THE IMMUNE RESPONSE IN GRANULOMATOUS INFECTION

8.3.1 Immunosuppressive serum factors

The sera from a substantial proportion of patients with the infections listed in Table 9.1 contain factors that depress in vitro tests of cellular immunity. Among the infections reported to induce these serum factors are tuberculosis[82], histoplasmosis[83], leprosy[33], and secondary syphilis[84]. These inhibitors are heterogeneous in that some may depress reactivity only to antigens of the infecting agent whereas others non-specifically suppress the responses of sensitized lymphocytes to multiple antigens and to mitogens. For example, inhibition by sera from patients with tuberculosis and histoplasmosis is said to be antigen specific[82,83]. On the other hand, sera from lepromatous patients often contain a factor or factors that non-specifically depress the blast response of both autologous and normal allogeneic lymphocytes to PHA and specific antigens. In addition, sera from untreated patients may severely depress the mixed lymphocyte reaction (MLR) between normal cell populations[85]. To date, the factor(s) has been characterized only partially as being heat-stable, non-dialysable, and present at low concentrations in serum or plasma[33].

Several substances have been detected in human serum, any one of which is capable of suppressing in vitro tests of cellular immunity if added in sufficient concentration. One of these is an α-globulin rich protein extractable from normal human serum. Most of the activity of this protein appears to reside in a low-molecular weight polypeptide fraction that is capable of suppressing the proliferative response of lymphocytes to specific antigens and to mitogens[86]. If given to experimental animals, this fraction can prolong survival of skin allografts[87]. Although it is tempting to regard the α-globulin associated peptide as a product of the normal immunoregulatory mechanisms, high concentrations of the purified material are required to effect suppression in culture systems. Currently, there is little published evidence that levels of this fraction are unusually high in the infections under discussion. Even if elevated levels can be demonstrated, the proof that they are causally related to immunosuppression *in vivo* will be difficult.

Another component of normal human serum that may exert an immunoregulatory function is a sub-species of low-density lipoprotein (LDL) identified by electrophoretic mobility as a beta lipoprotein[88]. Purified LDL is a potent suppressor of the primary inductive phase of lymphocyte stimulation by lectins and antigens; given to mice, human LDL markedly suppresses T-cell dependent antibody responses to sheep red blood cells (SRBC)[89]. Significantly, the dose of LDL required to induce suppression both *in vitro* and *in vivo* is considerably less than required with other normal 'immunoregulatory' proteins such as the α-globulin associated polypeptide and α-fetoprotein[90]. The molar concentrations required for suppression are, in fact, within physiologic range. An abnormal, but closely related species of LDL, has been identified in the serum of some patients with viral hepatitis and post-viral chronic hepatocellular injury[91]. In view of these findings, it would be useful to screen sera from patients with granulomatous infections commonly inducing hepatic pathology to determine if elevated levels of LDL or the abnormal variant are present. If so, detailed studies to ascertain whether elevated levels of LDL bear a high degree of correlation with anergy would be of interest though not definitive of causality.

One of the well-characterized serum factors that may suppress the response of immunocompetent cells is C-reactive protein (CRP). It is an acute phase protein synthesized rapidly and in large quantities by the liver[92] in response to a wide range of inflammatory stimuli, including infections listed in Table 9.1[93]. CRP exists in serum as a pentamer of 23 000 molecular weight subunits and *in vitro*, is capable of suppressing several types of immune reactions. Purified human CRP binds primarily to both human and mouse T lymphocytes with resultant reduction in the response of these cells to allogeneic cells in a MLR[94]. CRP also suppresses T-cell blastogenic responses to antigens as well as antigen- and mitogen-induced MIF production[95]. The effect of elevated CRP levels on T-cell kinetics and function *in vivo* are unknown and must await further study before the relative importance of this protein as an 'immunoregulator' can be determined.

A rather different species of humoral factor may contribute to the anergy of infectious diseases by interfering with the chemotactic response of cells to inflammatory stimuli. One well-studied protein of this type, so-called 'chemotactic factor inactivator' (CFI), is present in trace amounts in normal serum. CFI has a broad spectrum of activity as indicated by its ability to inactivate the chemotactic fragments of human C3 and C5, and the bacterial chemotactic factor derived from *Escherichia coli*[96]. The serum concentration of CFI is greatly increased in patients with Hodgkin's disease and leprosy, among others[97,98]. Moreover, there is a direct correlation between increased levels of CFI activity and depressed DTH to a panel of skin-test antigens in patients with lepromatous leprosy[98]. Indeed, the elevated levels of CFI may be relevant to the observation that there is a quantitative defect in the migration of inflammatory cells to sites of experimental skin abrasion in lepromatous patients. The number of leukocytes migrating into quantitative collection chambers applied to skin abrasions during a 24-hour period is approximately one-half the number counted among normal controls and patients with tuberculoid leprosy[99]. These findings suggest that in lepromatous patients, there may be defects in the expression of inflammation which are not restricted to the reactions of CMI but are of a more general nature. If it is assumed that dermal inflammatory reactions are mediated by leukotactic factors, then the elevated levels of CFI may, in part, explain the abnormal cell migration.

The list of humoral factors discussed above is far from complete, and considerable work remains to assess the possible immunosuppressor activity of other moieties that may be present in the serum of patients with infection-induced anergy. These include α-fetoprotein[90], circulating antigen–antibody complexes[100] and antibody that may be directly cytotoxic to immunocompetent cells or capable of cell binding, thereby obscuring cell surface structures necessary for the usual stimulatory reaction[101]. The fact that there are several immunoinhibitory fractions in human serum which are quite heterogeneous as determined by commonly utilized separation methods, promises to make the task of sorting most difficult[102].

8.3.2 Disturbances of lymphocyte traffic

Granulomatous pathology of the lymph nodes and spleen is a prominent feature of many disseminated intracellular infections (Table 8.1). The nature of this pathology has been described best in the lymph nodes of patients with lepromatous leprosy. Typically, the paracortical regions of lymph nodes are infiltrated by masses of cells belonging to the histiocytic–macrophage series that contain many acid-fast bacilli. Although lymphocytes appear to be displaced from the paracortical areas, the germinal centres are normal or increased in size and number. As patients improve with antimicrobial therapy, the histiocytic infiltrates within paracortical areas begin to regress with a concomitant increase in the relative number of lymphocytes. Occasionally, however, clusters of macrophages may persist for several years[62].

Within the spleen, sinusoids of the red pulp are infiltrated by foamy macrophages containing lepra bacilli, and the white pulp (Malphigian corpuscles) is damaged by granulomata quite consistently[61]; lymphocytes normally abundant within the periarteriolar lymphocyte sheaths of the white pulp may be replaced extensively by aggregates of macrophages[103].

Very similar pathology is present within the lymph nodes and spleens of *M. lepraemurium*-infected rats and in experimental histoplasmosis of mice[104,105]. The immunopathology of lymphoid organs in patients with disseminated histoplasmosis or coccidioidomycosis has not been well described. However, it is likely that the same type and location of granulomatous pathology within the splenic white pulp and lymph node-paracortical regions will be recognized with increasing frequency[106-108].

A highly significant feature of the lymphoid pathology described centres in the fact that it encroaches directly upon the anatomical regions which are normally composed predominantly of T lymphocytes. Furthermore, these T-cell domains are precisely the areas through which a vital and extensive recirculation of lymphocytes takes place in mammals. In rats, for example, the recirculating pool of lymphocytes is estimated to contain 1.75×10^9 cells (approximately 80–85% T lymphocytes) of which 4.5×10^8 may be in the spleen and 1.2×10^9 in the lymph nodes at any moment in time[109]. Radiolabelled small lymphocytes appear to migrate through the splenic compartment with a modal transit time of 5–6 hours whereas transit time through lymph nodes is 12–18 hours[109].

Recirculation of lymphocytes through the lymph nodes is accomplished by passage of cells from blood into the paracortical areas via post-capillary venules. Complementary recognition sites on the specialized endothelium of these venules most probably attract recirculating lymphocytes which then migrate through the vessel wall[110]. T cells percolate through the paracortex and medulla to efferent lymphatics from which they are returned to blood via the thoracic duct. The route of lymphocyte recirculation within the spleen is less well defined. It is generally agreed, however, that after i.v. injection, radiolabelled T cells localize initially in the marginal zone around the splenic white pulp and then migrate into the periarteriolar lymphocyte sheath. Lymphocytes probably return to venous sinuses of the red pulp by means of bridging channels across the marginal zone between white and red pulp[111]. The rate at which lymphocytes migrate through normal lymph nodes and spleen appears to depend largely upon the intrinsic amoeboid activity of the cells themselves although other factors, not fully understood, undoubtedly play a role.

It is widely held that the extensive recirculation of small lymphocytes through lymphoid organs in normal animals serves to facilitate the interaction of these cells with antigens and other cells active in the generation of an immune response. A critical question then, is whether involvement of the pathways for lymphocyte migration in lymphoid organs by granulomatous pathology can significantly perturb the traffic of immunocompetent cells and the immune functions subserved by this traffic. Recently, this issue has been addressed using an experimental model of murine leprosy, the pathology of which consistently involves the splenic white pulp and paracortical areas of lymph nodes[104].

In paired experiments, the thoracic ducts of *M. lepraemurium*-infected rats and age-matched controls were cannulated and the recirculating lymphocytes drained for 3 days to reduce the net hourly output of cells to low levels. On the 3rd day, pooled thoracic duct (TD) lymphocytes collected from normal syngeneic donors were labelled with [³H]5-uridine and an average of 1.6×10^6 cells/g body weight given to infected and control rats. After cell infusion, TD lymph was collected at 4-hour intervals for 52 hours to quantitate the output of recirculating T cells per hour. As expected, there was no increase in the cell output from the TD during the first 4 hours since most donor lymphocytes could not have traversed the lymph nodes in so short a time. However, by the 8th hour, some of the infused lymphocytes did reach the TD effluent in normal animals. Lymphocyte output peaked between the 12th and 24th hour and declined to background levels as TD drainage continued. By contrast, there was little increase in cell output from the TDs of infected rats during the entire 52-hour post-infusion period. Comparative radio-autographic studies of cells collected from the TD lymph of normal and infected rats indicated that a large proportion of the labelled lymphocytes had failed to migrate into efferent lymph.

To investigate the possibility that a factor in the serum of infected rats could have disturbed the traffic of infused lymphocytes by altering their surface properties or other functions, reverse experiments were performed in which lymphocytes from *infected* donor rats were given to *normal* recipients which had been injected with pooled serum from infected rats. No impairment of migration by lymphocytes from *infected* donors was detected[104]. It was shown in other experiments that the impaired migration of chromium-51 labelled lymphocytes within infected animals could not be explained by failure of these cells to gain entry to lymph nodes because of extensive pathology within the paracortical areas. To the contrary, lymphocytes readily entered lymphoid organs but were then sequestered for an unknown period[112]. Splenectomy of infected animals resulted in a significant increase in the number of cells appearing in TD lymph as compared to infected animals with intact spleens. This and other experiments confirmed the presence of extensive trapping activity by the spleen, however, substantial numbers of cells also were trapped by the lymph nodes and possibly some by the liver as well[112]. Cell trapping could not be demonstrated at other sites and there was no evidence for rapid destruction of labelled cells with excretion of soluble label in the urine or stool.

Additional evidence for impaired egress of lymphocytes from the lymphoid organs has been obtained by studies of lymphocyte mobilization in *M. lepraemurium*-infected mice following injection of the synthetic polyanion polymethacrylic acid (PMAA). This substance produces an absolute lymphocytosis in normal mice 3–4 hours after i.v. injection by mobilizing lymphocytes to blood from the splenic white pulp and paracortical areas of lymph nodes; within 24–48 hours blood lymphocyte levels return to normal[113]. When 'leprous' mice are injected with PMAA, lymphocyte mobilization to peripheral blood is significantly less than in PMAA injected controls. Moreover, if radiolabelled lymph node cells from syngeneic donors are given i.v. to infected and control mice and allowed to 'home' to the lymphoid organs, the number of these cells mobilized by subsequent injection of PMAA is also reduced significantly in infected animals[114].

The mechanism by which recirculating TD lymphocytes or lymph node cells are retained within the lymphoid organs of infected animals is unclear. It is conceivable that granulomata may obstruct a sufficient number of delicate channels within the reticulin network of spleen and lymph nodes to render the migration of lymphocytes more circuitous. On the other hand, reactive swelling of endothelial cells lining the lymph channels may slow cell traffic. It seems more likely, however, that the large population of macrophages within lymphoid organs play a role in retaining lymphocytes either by direct cell to cell interaction or by local production of factors that could act upon lymphocytes to slow amoeboid activity and/or alter surface properties. Circumstantial evidence that macrophages do play a role in lymphocyte trapping has been provided by experimental studies of the adjuvant, *Corynebacterium parvum*. Thus, i.v. administration of *C. parvum* causes the number of macrophages within the spleen to increase greatly and in addition, lymphocyte trapping activity is significantly enhanced[115]. In studies on the nature of the trapping activity induced by *C. parvum*, Frost and Lance[116] found that selective depletion of B- or T-lymphocyte populations as well as indiscriminant ablation of lymphocytes by lethal, total-body radiation or corticosteroids did not reduce trapping activity. The fact that particulate or high molecular-weight substances which were non-immunogenic could also induce trapping further suggested that this activity may be a macrophage-dependent phenomenon.

The immunobiological significance of lymphocyte entrapment by infected animals remains to be determined. Certainly, it is possible that extensive, non-specific trapping of recirculating cells may reduce the number available for migration to peripheral sites in response to antigenic stimuli. Of interest in this regard is the demonstration by Schlossman et al.[117] that guinea-pigs previously sensitized to dinitrophenyl-substituted oligolysine peptides in complete Freund's adjuvant could be given a single i.v. injection of the antigen and rendered unreactive to subsequent intradermal challenge with the same antigen for a period of 3–10 days. Furthermore, the DTH response of desensitized animals to an *unrelated* antigen (PPD) was diminished slightly although this non-specific depression was short-lived and incomplete. Fairly conclusive evidence was obtained that the lack of skin reactivity to DNP–peptide resulted from entrapment of antigen-reactive lymphocytes within the lymph nodes of desensitized animals. Unfortunately, however, the mechanism of the depressed response to PPD was not explored. In any event, these findings suggest that if a single injection of one antigen can induce transient anergy in peripheral tissues, then exposure of lymphoid organs to multiple antigens during chronic infection may induce a *prolonged* state of hyporesponsiveness by similar means. Indeed, there is some indication that trapping of antigen-specific lymphocytes in lymphoid tissues may contribute to the anergic state often observed in patients with disseminated tuberculosis[118].

8.3.3 Suppressor cells and anergy

The recognition of a suppressor component within the immunoregulatory mechanism has been of great importance in understanding how responses to foreign and autoantigens are controlled. Although the suppressor functions of T lymphocytes have been studied most extensively, there is good evidence that all major cell types known to co-operate in augmenting the immune response can function as inhibitors. Thus, under appropriate conditions, B lymphocytes and macrophages may be immunosuppressive[119,120]. In normal animals living under 'average' conditions of antigenic stimulation, the immunostimulatory and suppressor activities of these cells are presumably in equilibrium. However, the balance between these immunoregulatory functions may be severely disturbed by prolonged and intense antigenic stimulation of the type encountered in certain infectious diseases.

That intense suppressor activity of a complex nature can be generated during chronic infection has been shown by recent work in which a T-cell dependent antibody response by spleen cells from *M. lepraemurium*-infected mice was measured repetitively until death at 22–25 weeks[121]. Spleen cells from infected and control mice were stimulated with SRBC in the Mishell– Dutton culture system[122] and the primary antibody response assayed by counting the number of plaque-forming cells (PFC) per culture after the method of Cunningham and Szenberg[123]. Forty-eight hours after i.v. inoculation of *M. lepraemurium*, the primary IgM response to SRBC by spleen cells from infected mice was equal to that of normal splenocytes. By the 6th week, the response had fallen to 25% of control values and from the 11th week onward, the PFC response was always less than 10% of that in spleen cell cultures from age-matched controls. These results suggested activation of suppressor cells in the spleens of infected mice. Therefore, spleen cells were collected at serial intervals throughout the course of infection and added to one of two sets of splenocyte cultures from normal litter mates; the second set of cultures served as a control.

In Figure 8.1 it can be seen that 5×10^6 infected spleen cells did not suppress the PFC response of 1×10^7 normal splenocytes during the first 4 weeks of infection; however they did so consistently thereafter. From the 5th through 10th week, the suppression was mild with reductions in PFC per culture ranging from 24% to 48%. Suppressor activity increased greatly at 10–11 weeks, and after the 14th week 'leprous' spleen cells always reduced the response of normal splenocytes by at least 90%. It is unlikely that immunodepression was caused by the presence of *M. lepraemurium* itself since addition of an equivalent number of these bacilli to normal spleen cell cultures induced only slight reduction in the PFC response. Interestingly, cells from the peripheral lymph nodes of 'leprous' mice did not suppress normal lymph node cells until the infection was terminal at which time the PFC response was reduced by only 29% (Figure 8.1). Thus, the spleen appeared to be the principal domicile of suppressor cells throughout most of the infection.

Characterization of the splenic suppressor cells during early infection (5–10 weeks) revealed a sub-population with the properties of macrophages, i.e. they were adherant to nylon-wool columns and glass, 95% phagocytized latex particles, and 91% stained positively for non-specific esterase activity. Nylon-passed splenic T lymphocytes were not suppressive during this early stage. In addition to these macrophage-like cells, a *second* sub-population of splenic suppressor cells was identified during the 10th–11th week of infection and throughout the remaining life-span[121]. These cells were T lymphocytes since they readily passed nylon–wool columns, and treatment with anti-Thy 1.2 serum plus complement abolished most of the suppressor activity, whereas sham anti-Thy 1.2 treatment did not.

It is of note that the *M. lepraemurium* infection is held in check by C3H mice until the 10th–11th week at which time the spleen begins to enlarge rapidly and organ counts of *M. lepraemurium* increase steadily. Whereas 4-week infected mice can express DTH to proteins of *M. lepraemurium* or to SRBC after immunization, they become anergic at approximately 10–11 weeks of infection (Bullock, W. E., unpublished observations). It appears,

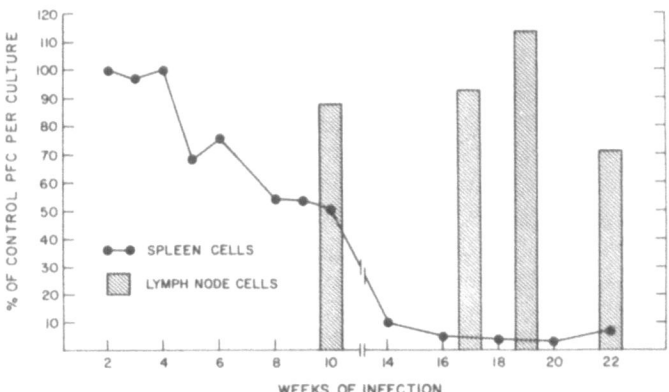

Figure 8.1   Effect of 5×10^6 spleen or lymph node cells from infected mice on the primary antibody response to SRBC *in vitro* by 10^7 lymph node or spleen cells from age-matched, normal control mice. (Reproduced by permission of Williams and Wilkins Co., Baltimore, Md.)

therefore, that the antigenic stimulation of early infection effectively activates 'helper' T lymphocytes which in turn stimulate the antimicrobial activity of macrophages. However, under the constant stimulus of proliferating helper T cells, activated macrophages may acquire suppressor properties, perhaps secondary to an increase in surface area. Thus, the macrophage may present more surface receptors capable of adsorbing putative helper factors produced by T lymphocytes. Activated macrophages might also inhibit immunocompetent cells by direct contact or by producing a soluble suppressor substance.

An important sub-population of lymphocytes with the capacity to function in a bi-directional manner is present in the spleen and thymus but not in lymph nodes[124,125]. The immunoregulatory function of these cells depends largely upon the activity of the cells being regulated. When the latter are responding at a high level, the activity of regulatory lymphocytes tends to be *suppressive*; conversely, it *enhances* when immune activity is low. As a group, the immunoregulatory lymphocytes appear to be less mature, i.e. have not achieved terminal differentiation, are thymus-dependent, and are relatively short-lived[126]. By means of alloantisera that define cell-surface differentiation components called Ly antigens, these cells have been shown to bear the phenotype Ly-1+, 2+, 3+[127,128]. Possibly, it is this regulatory sub-population that is driven to function in a suppressor rather than helper mode by the continuing immunostimulation of chronic *M. lepraemurium* infection. Thus, the appearance of suppressor T cells at 10–11 weeks, when suppressor activity begins to increase greatly in infected mice may signal a 'switch-over' by the Ly-1+, 2+, 3+ sub-population to generation of suppressor T cells as a critical level of maximal helper immune function is reached.

Although this construction of events is speculative, current advances in the characterization of T-lymphocyte sub-populations according to Ly phenotype clearly will permit the hypothesis to be tested. Indeed, there is already considerable evidence that the immune response is highly regulated by a series of interactions among distinct T lymphocyte sub-classes of different Ly phenotype[129]. The great importance of this T to T-cell interaction in normal regulation of the immune system is further underscored by the recent finding that a major disorder in NZB mice (an inbred strain which develops a lupus erythematosus-like autoimmune disorder) is the absence or malfunction of the Ly-1+, 2+, 3+ T-lymphocyte subset responsible for feedback inhibition of immune function[130].

8.4 SYNTHESIS AND SUMMARY

The granulomatous pathology in most of the disseminated infections discussed here is characterized by common elements that must be considered in seeking explanations for the associated states of anergy. Of paramount importance is the fact that the secondary lymphoid organs are likely to contain high concentrations of antigens in intimate relationship to aggregates of inflammatory cells composed predominantly of cells in the monocyte–macrophage series and lymphocytes in varying proportions. Almost certainly, it is the dynamic interplay among these elements especially within the microenvironment of the spleen, that ultimately determines the intensity and specificity of an immune response as well as its predominant mode of expression, i.e. as either helper or suppressor function.

Infection with large numbers of micro-organisms generally enhances splenic suppressor cell activity as has been demonstrated in several animal models. Among the organisms used for this purpose are *Listeria monocytogenes,*Trichinella spiralis, Plasmodium berghei yoelli, Trypansoma brucei*, killed *C. parvum* and Freund adjuvant[131–136]. Smaller inocula, on the other hand, clearly augment the immune response in some cases[131,137]. Furthermore, successful resolution of antigen-cell aggregates in self-limiting infections such as those caused by *Listeria* and *Plasmodium berghei yoelli*, is associated with reversal of suppressor activity[131,133]. Likewise, in most disseminated intracellular infections of man, resolution (i.e. healing) of these pathological aggregates with therapeutic assistance usually is associated with recovery of the capacity to express specific cellular immunity to the invading organism as well as the ability to respond to non-specific antigens. Lepromatous leprosy represents a significant exception to this generalization since full recovery of specific CMI to *M. leprae* is uncommon even after years of therapy. In this case, however, sufficient quantities of *M. leprae* antigens may well remain deposited within the secondary lymphoid tissues to chronically stimulate a suppressor arm of the immunoregulatory control mechanism.

Although the recognition of immunoregulatory suppressor functions has opened enormous new areas of research, years will be required to determine the full significance of these functions in the complex phenomenon of anergy. As a matter of fact, it still is too early to judge the relative importance of two other hypothetical mechanisms that have been invoked for many years to explain the anergy of lepromatous patients.

The first of these is tolerance induction. By tolerance is meant a state of specific immunological unresponsiveness induced through exposure to antigen such that further challenge with the tolerance-inducing antigen evokes no response. According to the clonal selection theory, tolerance should result from clonal deletion and/or abortion of antigen-specific cells[138]. Evidence for clonal deletion has been obtained in certain highly controlled experimental systems employing single, highly purified antigens[139]. In other systems, however, it has not been possible to demonstrate clonal deletion and in some, activation of suppressor cells may actually constitute the mechanism by which tolerance is induced and maintained[140]. Furthermore, in the complicated milieu of systemic infection, it has been impossible to gain control of a sufficient number of variables to support the contention that anergy to *M. leprae* in experimental animals or in man is the result of clonal deletion[69].

The second mechanism by which some have sought to explain anergy in certain infections is antigenic competition. Antigenic competition may be defined as the *non-specific* depression of the immune response to one antigen by administration of another antigen. This type of immunodepression is often observed when two antigens are given in sequence. Unfortunately, little is known concerning the mechanism of this phenomenon[141]. As is true in some models of tolerance, however, there is preliminary evidence that antigenic competition can be mediated by suppressor cell activity[142, 143]. Although antigenic competition might better explain the *non-specific* suppression of CMI that is observed frequently in disseminated infection, there is currently no solid data to support or refute this hypothesis.

Heretofore, it has been common practice to view infections associated with anergy as examples of failure or deficiency of the cell-mediated immune response. Strict adherence to this approach is no longer tenable. For as we have seen, granulomatous pathology within secondary lymphoid organs may impose a rather prolonged exposure of recirculating immunocompetent cells to an intricate microenvironment in which the outcome of exposure to antigen may be one of net suppression or augmentation as determined by highly structured interrelationships among immunoregulatory cell sub-populations. It becomes imperative, therefore, that we explore an alternate hypothesis, namely, that impairment of the host response to certain infecting agents may result at least in part from intense stimulation of immuno-suppressor regulatory mechanisms. In humans, such investigation is extra-ordinarily difficult since outbreeding is likely to remain high on nearly everyone's list of favourite sporting events. In addition, reliable markers have not been available that would permit recognition of distinct T-cell subclasses.

Recently, however, Moretta *et al.*[144] have determined that the peripheral blood T lymphocytes of man are separable into distinct sub-populations with cell surface receptors for the Fc portion of either IgG or IgM. Most circulating T lymphocytes bear receptors for IgM; these cells appear to help B lymphocytes to respond well to stimulation by pokeweed mitogen (PWM) with proliferation and differentiation into plasma cells. Conversely, up to 20% of blood T cells carry receptors for IgG and, following exposure to IgG-containing antigen–antibody complexes, they can suppress the B-cell response to PWM. In rapid succession to this discovery, imbalances between these T-cell sub-populations have been observed in immuno-deficiency syndromes[145] and in chronic fungal infection[144], one of the first non-viral infectious diseases of humans in which the presence of suppressor cell activity has been claimed[146]. This, of course, is but an exciting beginning and the future promises much by way of new markers specific for various sub-populations of human T cells[147].

The implications of current research for future approaches to the immunotherapy of 'anergic' infectious diseases may be considerable; for if in some cases, it is now regarded as desirable to augment T-cell helper activity by giving such therapeutic modalities as transfer factor, thymic hormones, etc. then in others, it may prove to be of value to abrogate certain immunoregulatory functions, particularly of suppressor cell populations. In any event, continued investigations of the interrelationships among antigens, lymphocytes and macrophages will most certainly be rewarding, and in the long run, may lead us to conclude that the concept of 'positive anergy' expressed decades ago by Jadassohn was a most remarkable vision of things to come.

ACKNOWLEDGEMENT

The author thanks Mrs Dee Steinforth for assistance in typing the manuscript. This work was supported by United States Public Health Service Grant Number AI-10094.

References

1. Von Pirquet, C. E. (1911). Allergy. *Arch. Intern. Med.*, **7**, 258
2. Jadassohn, J. (1914). Die Tuberkulide. *Arch. Dermatol. Syph.*, **119**, 10
3. Mackaness, G. B. (1962). Cellular resistance to infection. *J. Exp. Med.*, **116**, 381
4. Good, R. A., Biggars, W. D. and Park, B. H. (1971). Immunodeficiency Diseases of Man. In: *Progress in Immunology* (B. Amos, ed.), p. 669 (New York: Academic Press)
5. Boeck, C. (1905). Fortgesetzte Untersuchungen über das multiple begigne Sarkoid. *Arch. Dermatol. Syph.*, **73**, 71
6. Bastai, P. (1928). Über die klinische Bedeutung der tuberkulin Anergie bei Malignem-lymphogranulom. *Klin. Wochenschr.*, **7**, 1606
7. Friou, G. J. (1952). A study of the cutaneous reactions to oidiomycin, trichophyton, and mumps skin-test antigens in patients with sarcoidosis. *Yale J. Biol. Med.*, **24**, 533
8. Schier, W. W., Roth, A., Ostroff, G. and Schrift, M. H. (1956). Hodgkin's disease and immunity. *Am. J. Med.*, **20**, 94
9. Verrier Jones, J. (1967). Development of sensitivity to dinitrochlorobenzene in patients with sarcoidosis. *Clin. Exp. Immunol.*, **2**, 447
10. Aisenberg, A. C. (1962). Studies on delayed hypersensitivity in Hodgkin's disease. *J. Clin. Invest.*, **41**, 1964
11. Hedfors, E. (1974). Activation of peripheral T cells of sarcoidosis patients and healthy controls. *Clin. Exp. Immunol.*, **18**, 379
12. Topilsky, M., Williams, M., Siltzbach, L. E. and Glade, P. R. (1972). Lymphocyte response in sarcoidosis. *Lancet*, **i**, 117
13. Hersh, E. M. and Oppenheim, J. J. (1965). Impaired *in vitro* lymphocyte transformation in Hodgkin's disease. *N. Engl. J. Med.*, **273**, 1006
14. Israel, H. L. and Sones, M. (1965). Immunologic defect in patients recovered from sarcoidosis. *N. Engl. J. Med.*, **273**, 1003
15. Von Pirquet, C. E. (1908). Das Verhalten der kutanen Tuberkulin-reaktion während der Masern. *Dtsch. Med. Wochenschr.*, **34**, 1297

16. Starr, S. and Berkovich, S. (1964). Effects of measles, gamma-globulin-modified measles and vaccine measles on the tuberculin test. *N. Engl. J. Med.*, **270**, 386

17. Fireman, P., Friday, G. and Kumante, J. (1969). Effect of measles vaccine on immunological responsiveness. *Pediatrics*, **43**, 264

18. Kohn, J. L. and Koiransky, H. (1932). Relation of measles and tuberculosis in young child. Clinical and roentgenographic study. *Am. J. Dis. Child.*, **44**, 1187

19. Sullivan, J. L., Barry, D. W., Lucas, S. J. and Albrecht, P. (1975). Measles infection of mononuclear cells. I. Acute infection of peripheral blood lymphocytes and monocytes. *J. Exp. Med.*, **142**, 773

20. Lucas, C. J., Galama, J. M. D. and Ubels-Postma, J. (1977). Measles virus-infected suppression of lymphocyte reactivity *in vitro*. *Cell Immunol.*, **32**, 70

21. Willems, F. Th. C., Melnick, J. L. and Rawls, W. E. (1969). Viral inhibition of the phytohemagglutinin response of human lymphocytes and application to viral hepatitis. *Proc. Soc. Exp. Biol. Med.*, **130**, 652

22. Finkel, A. and Dent, P. B. (1973). Abnormalities in lymphocyte proliferation in classical and atypical measles. *Cell. Immunol.*, **6**, 41

23. Lindahl-Magnusson, P., Leary, P. and Gresser, I. (1972). Interferon inhibits DNA synthesis induced in mouse lymphocyte suspensions by phytohaemagglutinin or by allogeneic cells. *Nature (New Biol.)*, **237**, 120

24. Bloomfield, A. J. and Mateer, J. G. (1919). Changes in skin sensitivities to tuberculin during epidemic influenza. *Am. Rev. Tuber.*, **3**, 166

25. Kantzler, G. B., Lauteria, S. F., Cusumano, C. L., Lee, J. D., Ganguly, R. and Waldman, R. H. (1973). Immunosuppression during influenza virus infection. *Infect. Immun.*, **10**, 996

26. Dolin, R., Richmand, D. D., Murphay, B. R. and Fauci, A. S. (1977). Cell-mediated immune responses in humans after induced infection with influenza A virus. *J. Infect. Dis.*, **135**, 714

27. Zisman, B. and Denman, A. M. (1973). Inactivation of myxoviruses by lymphoid cells. *J. Gen. Virol.*, **20**, 1

28. Kauffman, C. A., Phair, J. P., Linnemann, C. C., Jr. and Schiff, G. M. (1974). Cell-mediated immunity in humans during viral infection. I. Effect of rubella on dermal hypersensitivity, phytohemagglutinin responses and T lymphocyte numbers. *Infect. Immun.*, **10**, 212

29. Mangi, R. J., Niederman, J. C., Kelleher, J. E. Jr., Dwyer, J. M., Evans, A. S. and Kantor, F. S. (1974). Depression of cell-mediated immunity during active infectious mononucleosis. *N. Engl. J. Med.*, **291**, 1149

30. Berkovich, S. and Starr, S. (1966). Effects of live type I poliovirus vaccine and other viruses on the tuberculin test. *N. Engl. J. Med.*, **274**, 67

31. Notkins, A. L., Mergenhagen, S. E. and Howard, R. J. (1970). Effect of virus infections on the function of the immune system. *Annu. Rev. Microbiol.*, **24**, 525

32. Bullock, W. E. (1968). Studies of immune mechanisms in leprosy. I. Depression of delayed allergic response to skin-test antigens. *N. Engl. J. Med.*, **278**, 298

33. Bullock, W. E. and Fasal, P. F. (1971). Studies of immune mechanisms in leprosy. III. The role of cellular and humoral factors in impairment of the *in vitro* immune response. *J. Immunol.*, **106**, 888

34. Ptak, W., Gaugas, J. M., Rees, R. J. W., Allison, A. C. (1970). Immune responses in mice with murine leprosy. *Clin. Exp. Immunol.*, **6**, 117

35. Bullock, W. E., Evans, P. E. and Filomeno, A. R. (1977). Impairment of cell-mediated immune responses by infection with *Mycobacterium lepraemurium*. *Infect. Immun.*, **18**, 157

36. Waxman, J. and Lockshin, M. (1973). *In vitro* and *in vivo* cellular immunity in miliary tuberculosis. *Am. Rev. Resp. Dis.*, **107**, 661

37. Zeitz, S. J., Ostrow, J. H. and Van Arsdel, P. P. (1974). Humoral and cellular immunity in the anergic tuberculosis patient: A prospective study. *J. Allergy Clin. Immunol.*, **53**, 20

38. Uberoi, S., Malaviya, A. N., Chattopadhyay, C., Kumar, R. and Shrinivas. (1975). Secondary immunodeficiency in miliary tuberculosis. *Clin. Exp. Immunol.*, **22**, 404

39. Catanzaro, A., Spitler, L. E. and Moser, K. M. (1975). Cellular immune response in coccidioidomycosis. *Cell. Immunol.*, **15**, 360

40. Opelz, G. and Scheer, M. I. (1975). Cutaneous sensitivity and *in vitro* responsiveness of lymphocytes in patients with disseminated coccidioidomycosis. *J. Infec. Dis.*, **132**, 250

41. Cox, R. A. and Vivas, J. R. (1977). Spectrum of *in vivo* and *in vitro* cell-mediated immune responses in coccidioidomycosis. *Cell. Immunol.*, **31**, 130

42. Mendes, E. and Raphael, A. (1970). Impaired delayed hypersensitivity in patients with South American blastomycosis. *J. Allergy.*, **47**, 17

43. Musatti, C. C. (1975). Cell-mediated immunity in patients with paracoccidioidomycosis. Mycoses: Proc. Third Int. Conf. on the Mycoses. *PAHO Sci. Publ.*, **304**, 23

44. Diamond, R. D. and Bennet, J. E. (1973). Disseminated cryptococcosis in man. Decreased lymphocyte transformation in response to *Cryptococcus neoformans. J. Infect. Dis.*, **127**, 694

45. Graybill, J. R. and Alford, R. H. (1974). Cell-mediated immunity in cryptococcosis. *Cell. Immunol.*, **14**, 12

46. Musher, D. M., Schell, R. F. and Knox, J. M. (1974). *In vitro* lymphocyte response to *Treponema refringens* in human syphilis. *Infect. Immun.*, **9**, 654

47. Friedman, P. S. and Turk, J. L. (1975). A spectrum of lymphocyte responsiveness in human syphilis. *Clin. Exp. Immunol.*, **21**, 59

48. Bryceson, A. D. M. (1970). Diffuse cutaneous leishmaniasis in Ethiopia. III. Immunological studies. *Trans. R. Soc. Trop. Med. Hyg.*, **64**, 380

49. Bryceson, A. P. M., Bray, R. S. and Dumonde, D. C. (1974). Experimental cutaneous leishmaniasis. IV. Selective suppression of cell-mediated immunity during the response of guinea-pigs to infection with *Leishmania enriettii. Clin. Exp. Immunol.*, **16**, 189

50. Kadivar, D. M. and Soulsby, E. J. L. (1975). Model for disseminated cutaneous leishmaniasis. *Science*, **190**, 1198

51. Mansfield, J. M. and Kreier, J. P. (1972). Tests for antibody and cell-mediated hypersensitivity to trypanosome antigens in rabbits infected with *Trypanosome congolense. Infect. Immun.*, **6**, 62

52. Mansfield, J. M. and Wallace, J. H. (1974). Suppression of cell-mediated immunity in experimental African trypanosomiasis. *Infect. Immun.*, **10**, 335

53. Reddy, P., Gorelick, D. F., Brasher, C. A. and Larsh, H. (1970). Progressive disseminated histoplasmosis as seen in adults. *Am. J. Med.*, **48**, 629

54. Smith, J. W. and Utz, J. P. (1972). Progressive disseminated histoplasmosis. A prospective study of 26 patients. *Ann. Intern. Med.*, **76**, 557

55. Greenwood, B. M., Whittle, H. C. and Molyneux, D. H. (1973). Immunosuppression in Gambian trypanosomiasis. *Trans. R. Soc. Trop. Med. Hyg.*, **67**, 846

56. Mitsuda, H. (1919). On the value of a skin reaction to a suspension of leprous nodules. *Hifuka Hinyôka Zasshi.*, **19**, 697; reprinted in English (1953). *Int. J. Leprosy*, **21**, 347

57. Myrvang, B., Godal, T., Ridley, D. S., Froland, S. S. and Song, Y. K. (1973). Immune responsiveness to *Mycobacterium leprae* and other mycobacterial antigens throughout the clinical and histopathological spectrum of leprosy. *Clin. Exp. Immunol.*, **14**, 541

58. Ridley, D. S. and Jopling, W. H. (1966). Classification of leprosy according to immunity. *Int. J. Leprosy*, **34**, 255

59. Han, S. H., Weiser, R. S., Wang, J. J., Tsai, L. C. and Lin, P. P. (1974). The behaviour of leprous lymphocytes and macrophages in the macrophage migration–inhibition test. *Int. J. Leprosy*, **42**, 186

60. Shepard, C. C. (1961). Discussion. In: *Transactions of Leonard Wood Memorial John Hopkins University Symposium on Research in Leprosy, Baltimore*, p. 230

61. Desikan, K. V. and Job, C. K. (1968). A review of post-mortem findings in 37 cases of leprosy. *Int. J. Leprosy*, **36**, 32

62. Turk, J. L. and Waters, M. F. R. (1971). Immunological significance of changes in lymph nodes across the leprosy spectrum. *Clin. Exp. Immunol.*, **8**, 363

63. Job, C. K. (1971). Pathology of peripheral nerve lesions in lepromatous leprosy – A light and electron microscopic study. *Int. J. Leprosy*, **39**, 251

64. Buck, A. A. and Hasenclever, H. F. (1963). Influence of leprosy on delayed-type skin reactions and serum agglutination titres to *Candida albicans*. *Am. J. Hyg.*, **77**, 305

65. Han, S. H., Weiser, R. S. and Kau, S. T. (1971). Prolonged survival of skin allografts in leprosy patients. *Int. J. Leprosy*, **39**, 1

66. Dierks, R. E. and Shepard, C. C. (1968). Effect of phytohemagglutinin and various mycobacterial antigens on lymphocyte cultures from leprosy patients. *Proc. Soc. Exp. Biol. Med.*, **127**, 391

67. Mehra, V. L., Talwar, G. P., Balakrishnan, K. and Bhutani, L. K. (1972). Influence of chemotherapy and serum factors on the mitogenic response of peripheral leukocytes of leprosy patients to phytohemagglutinin. *Clin. Exp. Immunol.*, **12**, 205

68. Lim, S. D., Jacobson, R. R., Park, B. H. and Good, R. A. (1975). Leprosy. XII. Quantitative analysis of thymus-derived lymphocyte response to phytohemagglutinin in leprosy. *Int. J. Leprosy*, **43**, 95

69. Godal, T., Myrvang, B., Fröland, S. S., Shao, J. and Melaku, G. (1972). Evidence that the mechanism of immunological tolerance ('central failure') is operative in the lack of host resistance in lepromatous leprosy. *Scand. J. Immunol.*, **1**, 311

70. Sheagren, J. N., Block, J. B., Trautman, J. R. and Wolff, S. M. (1969). Immunologic reactivity in patients with leprosy. *Ann. Intern. Med.*, **70**, 295

71. Guinto, R. S. and Mabalay, M. A. (1962). Note on tuberculin reaction in leprosy *Int. J. Leprosy*, **30**, 278

72. Suskind, R. M., ed. (1977). *Malnutrition and the Immune Response.* (New York: Raven Press)

73. Sher, R., Holm, G., Kok, S. H., Koornhof, H. J. and Glover, A. (1976). T and CR⁺ lymphocyte profile in leprosy and the effect of treatment. *Infect. Immun.*, **13**, 31

74. Nath, I., Curtiss, J., Sharma, A. K. and Talwar, G. P. (1977). Circulating T-cell numbers and their mitogenic potential in leprosy – correlation with mycobacterial load. *Clin. Exp. Immunol.*, **29**, 393

75. Rea, T. H., Quismorio, F. P., Harding, B., Nies, K. M., Di Saia, P. J., Levan, N. E. and Friou, G. J. (1976). Immunologic responses in patients with lepromatous leprosy. *Arch. Dermatol.*, **112**, 791

76. Oleinick, A. (1969). Altered immunity and cancer risk: a review of the problem and analysis of the cancer mortality experience of leprosy patients. *J. Nat. Cancer Inst.*, **43**, 775

77. Purtilo, D. T. and Pangi, C. (1975). Incidence of cancer in patients with leprosy. *Cancer*, **35**, 1259

78. Blumberg, B. S., Melartin, L., Lechat, M. and Guinto, R. S. (1967). Association between lepromatous leprosy and Australia antigen. *Lancet*, **ii**, 173

79. Sher, R., Mackay, M. E., Macnab, G. M., Kok, S. M. and Koornhof, H. J. (1977). Hepatitis B antigen, hepatitis B antibody, and subtypes in leprosy. *Infect. Immun.*, **17**, 1

80. Denney, O. E. (1922). Specific leprous reactions and abnormal vaccinia induced in lepers by small-pox vaccination. *Publ. Health Rep.*, **37**, 3141

81. Saha, K., Mittal, M. M. and Ray, L. S. N. (1973). Consequences of small-pox vaccination in leprosy patients. *Infect. Immun.*, **8**, 301

82. Heilman, D. H. and McFarland, W. (1966). Inhibition of tuberculin-induced mitogenesis in cultures of lymphocytes from tuberculous donors. *Int. Arch. Allergy Appl. Immunol.*, **30**, 58

83. Newberry, W. M. Jr., Chandler, J. W. Jr., Chin, T. D. Y. and Kirkpatrick, C. H. (1968). Immunology of the mycoses. I. Depressed lymphocyte transformation in chronic histoplasmosis. *J. Immunol.*, **100**, 436

84. Levene, G. M., Turk, J. L., Wright, D. J. M. and Grimble, A. G. S. (1969). Reduced lymphocyte transformation due to a plasma factor in patients with active syphilis. *Lancet*, ii, 246

85. Nelson, D. S., Penrose, J. M., Waters, M. F. R., Pearson, J. M. H. and Nelson, M. (1975). Depressive effect of serum from patients with leprosy on mixed lymphocyte reactions. *Clin. Exp. Immunol.*, 22, 388

86. Occhino, J. C., Glasgow, A. H., Cooperband, S. R., Mannick, J. A. and Schmid, K. (1973). Isolation of an immunosuppressive peptide fraction from human plasma. *J. Immunol.*, 110, 685

87. Mannick, J. A. and Schmid, K. (1967). Prolongation of allograft survival by an alpha globulin isolated from normal blood. *Transplantation*, 5, 1231

88. Curtiss, L. K. and Edgington, T. S. (1976). Regulatory serum lipoproteins. Regulation of lymphocyte stimulation by a species of low-density lipoprotein. *J. Immunol.*, 116, 1452

89. Curtiss, L. K., DeHeer, D. H. and Edgington, T. S. (1977). *In vivo* suppression of the primary immune response by a species of low-density lipoprotein. *J. Immunol.*, 118, 652

90. Yachnin, S. (1976). Demonstration of the inhibitory effect of human alpha-fetoprotein on *in vitro* transformation of human lymphocytes. *Proc. Natl. Acad. Sci.*, 73, 2857

91. Chisari, F. V. and Edgington, T. S. (1975). Lymphocyte E-rosette inhibitory factor. A regulatory serum lipoprotein. *J. Exp. Med.*, 142, 1092

92. Hurlimann, J., Thorbecke, G. J. and Hochwald, J. M. (1966). The liver as the site of C-reactive protein formation. *J. Exp. Med.*, 123, 365

93. Bush, O. B. Jr. (1958). C-reactive protein in leprosy. *Int. J. Leprosy*, 26, 123

94. Mortensen, R. F., Osmand, A. P. and Gewurz, H. (1975). Effects of C-reactive protein on the lymphoid system. I. Binding to thymus-dependent lymphocytes and alteration of their functions. *J. Exp. Med.*, 141, 821

95. Mortensen, R. F., Braun, D., Gewurz, H. (1977). Effects of C-reactive protein on lymphocyte functions. III. Inhibition of antigen-induced lymphocyte stimulation and lymphokine production. *Cell. Immunol.*, 28, 59

96. Berenberg, J. L. and Ward, P. A. (1973). Chemotactic factor inactivator in normal human serum. *J. Clin. Invest.*, 52, 1200

97. Ward, P. A. and Berenberg, J. L. (1974). Defective regulation of inflammatory mediators in Hodgkin's disease. *N. Engl. J. Med.*, 290, 76

98. Ward, P. A., Goralnick, S. J., Bullock, W. E. (1976). Defective leukotaxis in patients with lepromatous leprosy. *J. Lab. Clin. Med.*, 87, 1025

99. Bullock, W. E., Ho, M. F., Chen, M. J. (1974). Quantitative and qualitative studies of the local cellular exudative response in leprosy. *J. Reticuloendothelial Soc.*, 16, 259

100. Ryan, J. L., Arbeit, R. D., Dichler, H. B. and Henkart, P. A. (1975). Inhibition of lymphocyte mitogenesis by immobilized antigen-antibody complexes. *J. Exp. Med.*, 142, 814

101. Williams, R. C. Jr., Emmons, J. D. and Yunis, E. J. (1970). Studies of human sera with cytotoxic activity. *J. Clin. Invest.*, 50, 1514

102. Voorting-Hawking, M. and Gabriel Michael, J. (1977). Isolation and characterization of immunoregulatory factors from normal human serum. I. Preliminary biochemical and biological characterization of immunosuppressive factors. *J. Immunol.*, 118, 505

103. Bullock, W. E. (1978). Leprosy as a model of immunological perturbation. *J. Infect. Dis.*, 137, 341

104. Bullock, W. E. (1976). Perturbation of lymphocyte circulation in experimental murine leprosy. I. Description of the defect. *J. Immunol.*, 117, 1164

105. Artz, R. P. and Bullock, W. E. (1978). Immunosuppressor activity in experimental disseminated histoplasmosis. Presented at The First International Histoplasmosis Conference, April 10–12, Atlanta, Georgia

106. Parsons, R. J. and Zarafonetis, C. J. D. (1945). Histoplasmosis in man – report of 7 cases and review of 71 cases. *Arch. Int. Med.*, 75, 1

107. Salfelder, K., Brass, K., Doehnert, G., Doehnert, R. and Sauerteig, E. (1970). Fatal disseminated histoplasmosis – Anatomic study of autopsy cases. *Virch. Arch. Abt. A Path. Anat.*, **350**, 303

108. Forbus, W. D. and Bestebreurtje, A. M. (1946). Coccidioidomycosis: A study of 95 cases of the disseminated type with special reference to the pathogenesis of the disease. *Military Surgeon*, **99**, 653

109. Ford, W. L. and Gowans, J. L. (1969). The traffic of lymphocytes. *Semin. Hematol.*, **6**, 68

110. Ford, W. L. (1975). Lymphocyte migration and immune responses. *Prog. Allergy*, **19**, 1

111. Mitchell, J. (1973). Lymphocyte circulation in the spleen. Marginal zone bridging channels and their possible role in cell traffic. *Immunol., Lond.*, **24**, 93

112. Bullock, W. E. (1976). Perturbation of lymphocyte circulation in experimental murine leprosy. II. Nature of the defect. *J. Immunol.*, **117**, 1171

113. Ormai, S., Hagenbeek, A., Palkovits, M., van Bekkum, D. W. (1973). Changes of lymphocyte kinetics in the normal rat, induced by the lymphocyte mobilizing agent polymethacrylic acid. *Cell Tiss. Kinet.*, **6**, 407

114. Bullock, W. E., Vergamini, M. S. (1977). The impairment of lymphocyte mobilization from lymphoid organs by granulomatous infection. *Cell. Immunol.*, **29**, 337

115. Frost, P. and Lance, E. M. (1974). The relation of lymphocyte trapping to the mode of action of adjuvants. In: *Immunopotentiation Ciba Found. Symp. No. 18* (new series), p. 29

116. Frost, P. and Lance, E. M. (1974). The cellular origin of the lymphocyte trap. *Immunol., Lond.*, **26**, 175

117. Schlossman, S. F., Levin, H. A., Rocklin, R. E. and David, J. R. (1971). The comparmentalization of antigen-reactive lymphocytes in desensitized guinea-pigs. *J. Exp. Med.*, **134**, 741

118. Rook, G. A. W., Carswell, J. W. and Stanford, J. L. (1976). Preliminary evidence for the trapping of antigen-specific lymphocytes in the lymphoid tissue of 'anergic' tuberculosis patients. *Clin. Exp. Immunol.*, **26**, 129

119. Gershon, R. K. (1974). T-cell control of antibody production. *Contemp. Topics in Immunbiol.*, **3**, 1

120. Waldman, T. A. and Broder, S. (1977). Suppressor cells in the regulation of the immune response. *Clin. Immunol.*, **3**, 155

121. Bullock, W. E., Carlson, E. M. and Gershon, R. K. (1978). The evolution of immunosuppressive cell populations in experimental mycobacterial infection. *J. Immunol.*, **120**, 1709

122. Mishell, R. I. and Dutton, R. W. (1967). Immunization of dissociated spleen cell cultures from normal mice. *J. Exp. Med.*, **126**, 423

123. Cunningham, A. J. and Szenberg, A. (1968). Further improvements in the plaque technique for detecting single antibody-forming cells. *Immunology*, **14**, 599

124. Gershon, R. K., Lance, E. M. and Kondo, K. (1974). Immunoregulatory role of spleen localizing thymocytes. *J. Immunol.*, **112**, 546

125. Wu, C.-Y. and Lance, E. M. (1974). Immunoregulation by spleen-seeking thymocytes. II. Role in the response to sheep erythrocytes. *Cell. Immunol.*, **13**, 1

126. Gershon, R. K., Eardley, D. D., Naidorf, K. F. and Ptak, W. (1977). The Hermaphrocyte: A suppressor–helper T cell. Cold Spring Harbor Symposia on Quant. Biol. **XLI**, 85

127. Feldman, M., Beverly, P. C. L., Woody, J. D. and McKenzie, I. F. C. (1977). T–T interactions in the induction of suppressor and helper T cells: analysis of membrane phenotype of precursor and amplifier cells. *J. Exp. Med.*, **145**, 793

128. Cantor, H. and Boyse, E. A. (1977). Regulation of cellular and humoral immune response by T-cell subclasses. Cold Spring Harbor Symposia on Quant. Biol., **XLI**, 23

129. Eardley, P. D., Hugenberger, J., McVay-Boudreau, L., Shen, F. W., Gershon, R. K. and Cantor, H. (1978). Immunoregulatory circuits among T-cell sets. I. T-helper cells induce other T-cell sets to exert feedback inhibition. *J. Exp. Med.*, **147**, 1106

130. Cantor, H., McVay-Bourdreau, L., Hugenberg, J., Naidorf, K., Shen, F. W. and Gershon, R. K. (1978). Immunoregulatory circuits among T-cell sets. II. Physiologic role of feedback inhibition *in vivo*: Absence in NZB mice. *J. Exp. Med.*, **147**, 1116

131. Kongshavn, R. A. L., Hoc, A. and Sebaldt, R. J. (1977). Suppression of *in vitro* antibody responses by *Listeria* primed spleen cells. *Cell. Immunol.*, **28**, 284

132. Jones, J. F., Crandall, C. A. and Crandall, R. B. (1976). T-dependent suppression of the primary antibody response to sheep erythrocytes in mice infected with *Trinchinella spiralis*. *Cell. Immunol.*, **27**, 102

133. Weinbaum, F. I., Evans, C. B., Baker, P. J. and Tigelaar, R. E. (1976). Immunologic states of BALB/c mice during the course of a non-lethal malaria infection. *Fed. Proc.*, **35**, 416 (ABST.)

134. Jayawardena, A. N. and Waksman, B. H. (1977). Suppressor cells in experimental trypanosomiasis. *Nature*, **265**, 539

135. Scott, M. T. (1974). Depression of delayed-type hypersensitivity by *Corynebacterium parvum*: mandatory role of the spleen. *Cell. Immunol.*, **13**, 251

136. Reinisch, C. L., Gleiner, N. A. and Schlossman, S. F. (1976). Adjuvant regulation of T-cell function. *J. Immunol.*, **116**, 710

137. Wiener, E. (1975). The role of macrophages in the amplified *in vitro* response to sheep red blood cells by spleen cells from *Corynebacterium parvum* treated mice. *Cell. Immunol.*, **19**, 1

138. Burnet, F. M. (1959). *The Clonal Selection Theory of Acquired Immunity*, p. 208 (Cambridge: University Press)

139. Howard, J. G. and Mitchison, N. A. (1975). Immunological tolerance. *Prog. Allergy.*, **18**, 43

140. Stumpf, R., Heuer, J. and Kölsch, E. (1977). Suppressor T cells in low-zone tolerance. I. Mode of action of suppressor cells. *Eur. J. Immunol.*, **7**, 74

141. Pross, H. F. and Eidinger, D. (1974). Antigenic competition: A review of non-specific antigen induced suppression. *Adv. in Immunol.*, **18**, 133

142. Radovich, J. and Talmage, D. W. (1967). Antigenic competition: Cellular or humoral. *Science*, **158**, 512

143. Gershon, R. K. and Kondo, K. (1971). Antigenic competition between heterologous erythrocytes. *J. Immunol.*, **106**, 1524

144. Moretta, L., Webb, S. R., Grossi, C. E., Lydyard, P. M. and Cooper, M. D. (1977). Functional analysis of two human T-cell sub-populations: Help and suppression of B-cell responses by T cells bearing receptors of IgM or IgG. *J. Exp. Med.*, **146**, 184

145. Moretta, L. Mingari, M. C., Webb, S. R., Pearl, E. R., Lydyard, P. M., Grossi, C. E., Lawton, A. R. and Cooper, M. D. (1977). Imbalances in T cell sub-populations associated with immunodeficiency and autoimmune syndromes. *Eur. J. Immunol.*, **7**, 696

146. Stobo, J. D., Paul, S., Van Scoy, R. E. and Hermans, P. E. (1976). Suppressor thymus-derived lymphocytes in fungal infection. *J. Clin. Invest.*, **57**, 319

147. Evans, R. L., Breard, J. M., Lazarus, H., Schlossman, S. F. and Chess, L. (1977). Detection, isolation and functional characteristics of two human T-cell subclasses bearing unique differentiation antigens. *J. Exp. Med.*, **145**, 221

9
Immune Complexes and Tissue Injury

P. CASALI, L. H. PERRIN and P.-H. LAMBERT

9.1	INTRODUCTION		296
	9.1.1	*The nature of immune complexes*	297
	9.1.2	*The site of formation and the fate of immune complexes*	297
	9.1.3	*Biological activities of immune complexes*	299
		9.1.3.1 *Activation of complement*	300
		(a) *Solubilization of the antigen–antibody complexes*	300
		(b) *C3 immune adherence*	301
		(c) *Chemotaxis*	301
		(d) *Exocytosis of neutrophil granules*	301
		(e) *Anaphylatoxin activity*	301
		(f) *Lysis of cells*	301
		9.1.3.2 *Interactions with cells*	301
		(a) *Platelets*	302
		(b) *Neutrophils*	302
		(c) *Eosinophils*	302
		(d) *Basophils and mast cells*	303
		(e) *Mononuclear phagocytes*	303
		(f) *Lymphocytes*	304
	9.1.4	*Tissue injury induced by immune complexes*	306
9.2	DETECTION OF IMMUNE COMPLEXES		307
	9.2.1	*Detection of immune complexes in tissues*	308
	9.2.2	*Detection of immune complexes in biological fluids*	308
		9.2.2.1 *Antigen-specific methods*	308

9.2.2.2   *Antigen non-specific methods*   309
            (a)   *Methods based on the physical.properties*
                    of immune complexes   309
            (b)   *Methods based on the biological properties*
                    of immune complexes   314
    9.2.3   *Indirect evidence for the presence of immune complexes*   316

9.3   ROLE OF IMMUNE COMPLEXES IN INFECTIOUS
      DISEASES   317
    9.3.1   *Immune complexes associated with virus infections*   317
            9.3.1.1   *Animal models*   318
            9.3.1.2   *Virus-induced immune complexes diseases*
                        in man   319
                    (a)   *Hepatitis B infection*   319
                    (b)   *Dengue haemorrhagic fever (DHF)*   319
                    (c)   *Epstein–Barr virus infections*   320
                    (d)   *Measles virus infection*   320
    9.3.2   *Immune complexes associated with bacterial infections*   320
            9.3.2.1   *Infections with Gram-positive and Gram-*
                        negative cocci   320
            9.3.2.2   *Leprosy*   322
    9.3.3   *Immune complexes occurring during parasitic diseases*   323
            9.3.3.1   *Protozoal infections*   323
                    (a)   *Malaria*   323
                    (b)   *Trypanosomiasis*   325
                    (c)   *Leishmaniasis*   329
            9.3.3.2   *Helminthic infections*   329
                    (a)   *Schistosomiasis*   329
                    (b)   *Onchocerciasis*   330

9.4   CONCLUSIONS   330

9.1   INTRODUCTION

The development of tissue injury during infectious diseases may result from
at least two major mechanisms, which are often combined. First, infectious
agents can induce cell damage, directly or through the release of toxic
products. Secondly, the cellular and humoral immune responses directed
against antigens of the infectious agent, can also result in tissue injury.
In vivo, the formation of immune complexes represents a major pathway for
the pathological expression of such humoral immune responses. Indeed,

immune complexes are formed when antibodies are produced and react with antigen molecules which are persisting in the host or which are released from cells into extracellular fluids. In addition, some infectious agents can induce a polyclonal antibody synthesis, resulting in the production of antibodies with a broad spectrum of specificity, including auto-antibodies, and possibly leading to the formation of immune complexes involving auto-antigens[1].

9.1.1 The nature of immune complexes

The formation, the structure and the properties of immune complexes depend on the nature of the antigen, of the antibody, of their interaction and on the secondary binding of immune complex-reactive molecules. The size, the charge and the possible reactivity of the *antigen* with various biological structures influence the size and the biological activities of immune complexes. For example, antigens which display some affinity for C1q can react more efficiently with C1q when presented in an aggregated form in complexes. Polymeric antigens which carry a single determinant in repetitive representation can induce the formation of immune complexes involving antibodies with a restricted specificity. Alternatively, immune complexes involving antibodies with multiple specificities can be formed when antigens carrying several different determinants are involved. Evidently, a molecule with a single antigenic determinant can only form complexes containing a single antibody molecule. The *antibody* involved in the immune complex can be of various immunoglobulin classes and subclasses thus having different types of biological activity. The *avidity* of antibody for antigens in the complexes will also determine and critically influence the biological activity of immune complexes. The *ratio* of the antigen to the antibody molecules and their relative *concentrations* determine the size, the solubility and the reactivity of complexes. Finally, according to the nature of the complexes, different types of molecules can be secondarily bound to immune complexes: complement components, such as C1q, C1r, C1s, and C3; antibodies with anti-immunoglobulin activity, either with anti-Fc activity (7S antiglobulins or rheumatoid factor) or with anti-antibody activity; antibodies against fixed C3 and C4 (immunoconglutinins). The binding of these molecules to a small-size complex results in the formation of a larger-size complex, with new physical and biological properties.

9.1.2 The site of formation and the fate of immune complexes

In vivo the fate and the effects of immune complexes are directly dependent on the site of their formation and on the nature of the antigens and the antibodies as well as their relative concentrations. In extracellular fluids, immune complexes can be formed following the binding of an antibody with either a cell-free antigen or with an antigen present on the cell membrane.

The binding of antibody to cell-free antigen results in the formation of cell-free immune complex and is likely a major mechanism of formation of immune complexes during bacterial and parasitic infections (antigens can be constituted by materials actively released from micro-organisms or derived from micro-organisms destruction). In general, the reaction of antibody with antigens present on cell surface results in formation of cell-bound immune complexes. The cell surface-associated antigens can be either attached to the membrane (infectious agents or infectious products, such as bacterial lipopolysaccharides[2], with some cytophilic activity), or newly formed as new surface structure following the infection of the cells by micro-organisms. It has been shown in some virus infections that the formation of cell-bound immune complexes can result in a subsequent release of immune complexes. For example, antibodies can bind to new antigenic determinants expressed on the surface of cells infected by measles virus. After a polar redistribution (capping) of these determinants and of the bound antibodies, the surface-bound immune complexes are released into the extracellular cell-free medium[3] (Figure 9.1).

In vivo, extracellular immune complexes involving cell-free or cell-bound antigens can be formed in circulation or in extravascular fluids, or in both compartments (Figure 9.2). The fate of the immune complexes in circulating blood depends mainly on the size of the complexes. Large-size complexes, either complement or non-complement fixing, are almost completely cleared from circulation within a few minutes[4, 5]. The cleared complexes are actively concentrated in the liver by Kuppfer cells. Small size, and particularly non-complement fixing, immune complexes are poorly cleared from the circulation, and, in some instances, can be fixed in vessels walls or in filtering membranes such as renal glomeruli[5] or choroid plexus[6]. Immune complexes have been found in renal glomeruli following a variety of infections such as

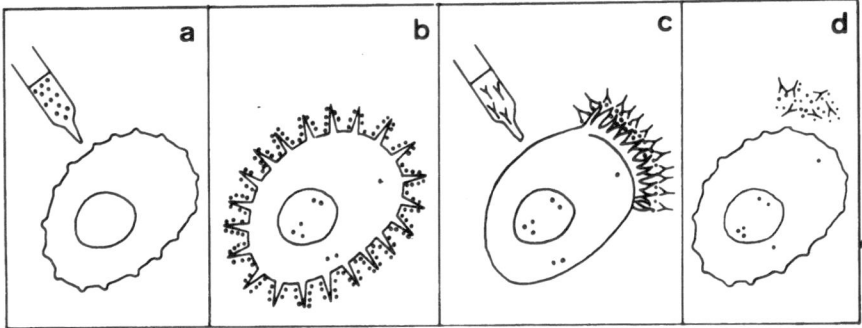

Figure 9.1 Formation and release of immune complexes at the surface of Hela cells infected with measles virus after incubation of the infected cells with human anti-measles virus antibodies. Cells were infected with measles virus (a), measles virus antigen are expressed at the surface of the infected cells 6 h after infection (b), antibodies are added in the medium and at 37 °C cap the measles virus antigen (c), immune complexes are released in the medium (d)

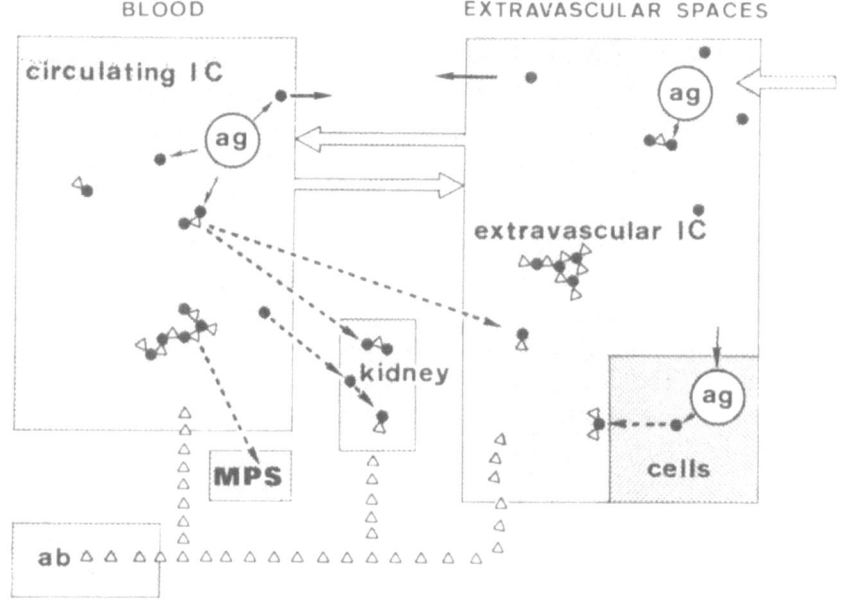

Figure 9.2 Possible sites of formation of immune complexes (IC) *in vivo*: these may be formed in blood or in extravascular spaces, according to the localization of the antigens at the time when antibodies appear (ag represents a source of antigen, e.g. a micro-organism). The fate of the complexes is dependent on the site of their formation. MPS represents the mononuclear phagocyte system, mainly the liver and the spleen

streptococcal, pneumococcal and staphylococcal infections[7, 8], infectious mononucleosis[9], *Plasmodium falciparum* and *malariae* infections[10, 11], and lepromatous leprosy[12]. In experimental animals, presence of immune complexes at the level of the choroid plexus has been demonstrated during viral[6] and parasitic[13] infections.

Immune complexes formed in extravascular spaces are not cleared as rapidly as circulating immune complexes and may induce local inflammatory foci. The pathological consequences will depend on their concentration, their persistence and on the chronicity of their formation. In some clinical conditions an exchange between the extravascular and the intravascular pool of immune complexes may be observed, but this is not a general rule and a typical immune complex disease may occur in the absence of circulating immune complexes.

9.1.3 Biological activities of immune complexes

The biological properties of immune complexes are largely dependent on the presentation of antigen and/or antibody molecules in an aggregate form, and therefore at a higher density compared to the corresponding free molecules. Aggregated antigens or antibodies are bound more avidly than their isolated counterparts by cellular or humoral receptors. The biological effects of immune complexes are first determined by interreaction with these receptors (recognition step). The binding of immune complexes to the classical humoral receptor, the first component of complement and particularly its C1q constituent, can trigger the activation of the complement system and its effector mechanisms[14]. At cell surfaces, the binding of immune complexes may first occur specifically to cell receptors for antigens, possibly initiating cellular events involved in the immune response[15]; secondly, an antigen non-specific binding occurs on many cells with receptors for the Fc part of immunoglobulin molecules[16] or for complex-bound complement components[17]. The biological activities of immune complexes include activation of plasma components, mainly the complement system, and activation of cells.

9.1.3.1 *Activation of complement*

Immune complexes activate the complement system through both the classical and alternative pathways, although evidence in human beings indicates that the classical pathway is principally involved. IgG and IgM classes have this capacity, while those containing IgA, IgD and IgE do not. IgG_1 and IgG_3 are more effective in binding complement than IgG_2 and IgG_4[18]. After activation, C3 becomes bound at the site of immune complex deposition and is readily detected in tissues or on cells by fluorescent antibody techniques. The presence of bound C4 indicates involvement of activation by the classical pathway. As a result of activation of the complement system, several biological activities are generated that play a role in diseases of immune complex origin. These include:

(*a*) *Solubilization of the antigen–antibody complexes. In vitro* prepared insoluble antigen–antibody complexes become soluble following incubation in fresh serum at $37\,^\circ C$[19]. The solubilization occurs, although to a limited extent, in C2 or C4 deficient serum, but does not occur if the alternative pathway of complement is defective. This phenomenon does not seem to involve an enzymatic attack of the immune complex; following their solubilization the antigen and the antibody can be recovered without changes of their molecular weight[20]. Probably, the recruitment of some complement factors, mainly C3 and properdin factor B, into the preformed lattice allows for a deaggregation of the antibody molecules, stuck together through their Fc portion, and a partial dissociation of the antigen from the antibody. The solubilization of antigen–antibody complexes in presence of complement could have important implications *in vivo*. A reduced clearance of immune complexes from the circulation and a greater tendency of their deposition in tissues would be expected in acquired or primary complement deficiency.

(b) *C3 immune adherence.* This is a phenomenon in which leukocytes bind to C3b that is attached to membranes at the point of complement activation[14]. Leukocytes, neutrophils and macrophages of all species studied, primate erythrocytes, and platelets of the rabbit and most other non-primate mammals, except the ruminants, show this capacity. Membrane-bound C4b also induces the immune adherence of certain cells, although to a lesser extent than C3b. The immune adherence capacity of C3b is rapidly destroyed by C3b inactivator. The binding of leukocytes and non-primate platelets to C3b bound to membranes is readily measured *in vitro* and may be of great importance in localizing these cells at sites of immunological reactions *in vivo*.

(c) *Chemotaxis.* Chemotaxis of leukocytes, defined as the directional migration of cells provoked by a chemical stimulus, has been shown to be a property of activated complement components. The C567 complex as well as C5a (or possibly a degradation product of C5a) are known to possess this capacity[21]. C3a also has been found to be chemotactic for neutrophils. The effect is less marked than with C5a, and the possibility that the effect of C3a could be explained by a trace of contaminating C5a has not been entirely excluded.

(d) *Exocytosis of neutrophil granules.* Immune adherence through the C3b receptor leads to exocytosis of neutrophil granules when phagocytosis cannot occur. It has also been reported that C5a can give rise to exocytosis of cytochalasin B-treated neutrophils, thus releasing their injurious content of enzymes and basic proteins to the exterior[22].

(e) *Anaphylatoxin activity.* C3a and C5a can also stimulate mast cells to release their granules.

(f) *Lysis of cells.* Cells become lysed by action of the terminal complement components when an immune complex is formed between an antigen present on a cell and a complement-activating antibody, or when an immune-complex is brought into close opposition with the surface of certain cells (e.g. rabbit platelets, but not rabbit neutrophils). While the first condition is brought about by direct lysis, the second is a reaction of indirect or 'bystander' lysis, the terminal components (C5–C9) becoming bound to the bystander cell[23].

9.1.3.2 *Interactions with cells*

Immune complexes can activate a variety of cells by interacting with various surface receptors. Cellular activation can have several biological consequences. These reactions are discussed in this section.

(a) *Platelets*. Human platelets bear receptors for the Fc portion of immuno-globulin, and they clump and release nucleotides and vasoactive amines in response to immune complexes or aggregated immunoglobulin. IgG_1, $_2$, $_3$ and $_4$, but not the other classes of immunoglobulin, produce this response in platelets[24]. Platelets also respond to thrombin, adenosine diphosphate, collagen, prostaglandin, platelet-activating factor of basophils and mast cells, adrenalin and many other agents by clumping, and in several of these instances, by releasing their contents of vasoactive amines and the phospholipid procoagulant, platelet factor 3 (PF3). Basic proteins, somewhat analogous to the vasoactive proteins of neutrophils, are also contained within platelets. Considerable species differences exist regarding the receptors on platelets for aggregates of immunoglobulins and for C3; for example, the human platelet has receptors for the Fc portion of Ig and not C3b, while the rabbit platelet bears receptors for rabbit C3b but not Ig.

Data available concerning the role of platelets in the pathogenesis of immunopathological lesions are conflicting. In rabbit serum sickness, they appear to play a role in bringing about an increase in vascular permeability, allowing circulating immune complexes to become entrapped in the filtering membranes of the vessel walls[5]. This presumably follows their clumping within the vascular lamina and the release of vasoactive amines. In Arthus lesions and nephrotoxic nephritis, their removal prior to challenge fails to alter the development of the disease. There are conflicting data on the role of platelets in the production of disseminated intravascular coagulation by bacterial endotoxin, but it is likely that in some circumstances they are required[25].

(b) *Neutrophils*. Human neutrophils have receptors for the Fc region of IgG. Particles coated with IgG_1 and IgG_3 are phagocytosed. Attachment of erythrocytes coated with IgG antibody is followed by phagocytosis or contact-dependent lysis. Contact between neutrophils and aggregated immunoglobulins or immune complexes leads to the release of granules from the neutrophils. This process liberates proteolytic enzymes and basic peptides into the medium. These increase vascular permeability, stimulate mast cells, and generate thromboplastin, which activates the intrinsic clotting system. In human systems, IgG_1, $_2$, $_3$, $_4$ and IgA have been reported capable of such stimulation in aggregated form[24].

This process of exocytosis of neutrophil granules is probably responsible for much of the injury in acute immunological nephritis in which neutrophils participate (there is also an important neutrophil-independent mechanism) acute immunological synovitis, arthritis, and the vasculitis of the Arthus reaction. The release of superoxides, singlet oxygen, and peroxide may also play a rôle in the injurious process.

(c) *Eosinophils*. In both guinea-pigs[26] and humans[27] eosinophils have receptors for the Fc region of IgG; in the human cells these receptors are reported to be selective for IgG_1 and IgG_3. Increased reactivity has been described in the cells from patients with eosinophilic states associated with cardiac damage. Eosinophils have been shown to be cytotoxic to Schistosoma[28] and Nippostrongylus[29] when these parasites are coated with antibody. The cytotoxicity involves close contact between effector and target cells. The energy metabolism, but not protein synthesis, of the effector cell must be maintained.

(d) *Basophils and mast cells.* Although there is clear evidence that these two cell types are in many ways distinct they will be considered together in the present context. Basophils have the capacity to bind IgE antibody (and possibly to a lesser extent some IgG antibodies) cytophilically. Following the interaction of this fixed antibody with multivalent antigen the contents of the basophil granules are exocytosed. The granules contain heparin, histamine, slow-reacting substance of anaphylaxis (SRS-A), the eosinophil chemotactic factor of anaphylaxis (ECFA), and the platelet activating factor (PAF). Similar exocytosis can be produced by the reaction of the basophil with the complement fragments C3a and C5a. The receptors for these two closely related fragments are distinct, as demonstrated by the specificity of desensitization caused by each fragment.

Basophils and mast cells have assumed significance in the deposition of circulating immune complexes in acute experimental serum sickness of rabbits. An IgE-mediated anaphylactic trigger accompanies the deposition of circulating complexes and appears to be responsible for the increased vascular permeability that may be essential for the deposition of the circulating complexes in arteries and glomeruli[5].

(e) *Mononuclear phagocytes.* Cells of this lineage arise in the bone marrow, circulate as monocytes, and carry out various differentiated functions as macrophages in the pulmonary alveoli, in the lining of the hepatic and splenic sinuses, and in the peritoneal cavity and other tissue spaces. Macrophages accumulate at sites of chronic inflammation. Mononuclear phagocytes in all these sites have the same receptors for immune complexes and complement components. Human mononuclear phagocytes have receptors for the Fc region of IgG_1 and IgG_3: attachment of antibody-coated erythrocytes to these receptors is followed by phagocytosis or contact-dependent lysis[30]. Incubation of mononuclear phagocytes with complexes of IgG antibody and antigen induces secretion of hydrolytic enzymes but not cell death[31]; this is seen with complexes formed at equivalence and also in moderate antigen or antibody excess.

Erythrocytes coated with C3 are attached to macrophages but not readily engulfed. Incubation of macrophages with C3b has been reported to induce secretion of lysosomal hydrolases[32] and also of C3a, the latter possibly derived by cleavage of C3 synthesized by the macrophages. Macrophages incubated with C3b have been found to acquire the capacity to lyse tumour cells. Macrophages stimulated by lipopolysaccharide or products of activated T lymphocytes secrete collagenase, which can degrade connective tissue proteoglycans and activate the complement system.

(*f*) *Lymphocytes.* Most if not all human B cells carry receptors for IgG, Fc, C3b and C3d[33]. These Fc receptors are mainly demonstrated by their ability to bind aggregated IgG, soluble antigen–antibody complexes, or ox erythrocytes coated with rabbit antibody. The majority of B cells, in contrast to phagocytic cells and certain of the lymphocytes in the third, heterogeneous population, fail to react with indicator systems having low densities of bound IgG[34]. While the majority of human T cells are devoid of readily detectable Fc receptors, there is evidence that a fraction of antigen-stimulated T cells express receptors for IgG Fc. Another fraction of T cells has been reported to bind complexed IgM after incubation for 24 hours *in vitro*[35]. Most, if not all, unstimulated T cells are devoid of C receptors. There is evidence, however, that a fraction of antigen-stimulated T cells carries receptors for C3b, but not C3d.

Human K (killer) cells, i.e. cells capable of antibody-dependent cell-mediated cytolysis, are characterized by readily demonstrable Fc receptors in the absence of surface Ig. K cells active on IgG antibody-coated target cells carry Fc receptors of relatively high affinity, but they appear to be heterogeneous as far as complement receptors are concerned. Immune complexes have been found both to enhance and to suppress lymphocyte activation induced experimentally by immunologically specific and non-specific stimuli. Some of these differences may be explained by the particular composition and configuration of the complexes, which may determine whether the complexes react with lymphocytes through the antigenic determinants or through the Fc portion of the antibody. The activity of Fc-receptor-bearing T and B lymphocytes can be modulated via this receptor.

The effects of immune complexes on B-cell responses will depend on the stage of their differentiation. There is evidence[36] that the developing B cell acquires the Fc receptor, immunoglobulin receptor and complement receptor. In parallel with this differentiation of surface characteristics, the B cell progressively acquires responsiveness to various mitogens[37]. Its capacity to interact with immune complexes would be expected to vary during this period of receptor generation. There is considerable evidence that mature B cells can undergo inactivation following brief *in vitro* exposure to immune complexes[38]. A requirement for multivalent interaction between the immune complex and the target B cell was indicated by the finding that F(ab')$_2$ fragments of antibody formed tolerogenic complexes whereas monovalent Fab fragments did not[39]. Complexes formed between IgM and antigen can result in enhanced antibody responses *in vivo*, and this effect may be mediated through increased antigen localization[40]. At a further stage of the B-cell differentiation, when it has acquired the properties of an antibody-forming cell, it is again susceptible to alterations in its function by surface binding of multivalent antigens or immune complexes. The rate of secretion of antibody by lymphoid cells is sharply reduced after exposure to antigen[41], and it has been claimed that immune complexes bearing the antigenic determinant have a similar effect[42].

Immune complexes also appear to account for inhibition of T-cell functions in several situations. Selective inhibition of T helper-cell activity seems to be due to cell-bound antigen–antibody complexes in some model systems[43, 44]. Antigen–antibody complexes may also inhibit T-cell-mediated cytolysis. At least some of the 'serum blocking factors' found in the serum of animals and humans bearing progressively growing tumours consist of antigen–antibody complexes[45]. Inhibition by such complexes may be the result of blocking of lymphocyte receptors by antigen, with the antibody of the complexes serving mainly to cross-link the antigen. In most studies demonstrating serum-blocking factors, the nature of the effector cells in this assay has not been well characterized. It is not known whether blocking factors inhibit effector-cell activity or development of effector cells during the prolonged incubation with target cells. Blocking factors in sera from rats bearing 'enhanced' renal allografts inhibit lymphocyte cytotoxicity as tested with the microcytotoxicity test[46] but not that detected by the ^{51}Cr-release assay[47]. Other observations suggest that different effector cells are active in these two assays[48]. It is not known whether effector T cells can be inactivated via the Fc receptor of such cells.

In a model study, antibody directed against one set of antigenic specificity carried by the target cells was unable to prevent the lytic effect of T lymphocytes sensitized against another set of antigens present on the same target cells[49]. These observations suggest that blocking of lytic activity is due to masking of antigens on the target cells rather than to 'non-specific' inactivation of effector cells through the Fc receptor. The mechanism of inhibition produced by different immunoglobulin classes has not been compared. Another possible effect of immune complexes may be the activation of 'suppressor' T cells.

Finally, antigen–antibody complexes have been reported to be particularly efficient in inducing the production of anti-idiotype antibody[50]. Anti-idiotype antibody, reactive with determinants in or near the antigen-combining site of specific antibody, can also react with lymphocyte surface receptors possessing similar determinants and thus have anti-receptor activity[51]. Such antibody can react with both B and T lymphocytes[52] and its immunoglobulin class influences the outcome of the interaction: heterologous IgG anti-idiotype antibody activates T helper and B lymphocytes[53], while heterologous IgG_2 antibody has been shown to suppress specific immune responses in one model system[54]. Anti-idiotype antibody can inactivate T cells *in vivo*: graft-versus-host reactivity is specifically impaired in animals actively immunized to produce anti-idiotype antibody[55, 56].

9.1.4   Tissue injury induced by immune complexes

In vivo, the formation of immune complexes in circulation or in extracellular fluids of the host can, upon further reaction with plasma factors and cells, induce tissue injuries[5,57]. The Arthus reaction, an acute necrotizing vasculitis, is the simplest immune complex-induced lesion[58]. The lesion develops following formation of relatively large amounts of antigen–antibody complexes in extravascular spaces. A localized lesion around the vessel walls is produced if one of the reactants, either antigen or the antibody, is present in the circulation and the other injected locally. Early in the reaction, antigen and antibody diffuse toward each other, giving formation of immune complexes which can then precipitate. Following activation of complement by such immune complexes, the site of reaction becomes highly chemotactic for polymorphonuclear leukocytes (PMN). Within a few hours PMN cells infiltrate the involved tissues, which by now are undergoing necrosis. The PMNs phagocytose the antigen–antibody complexes and take them away from the site of reaction. *In vitro* studies showed that PMNs are capable of degrading rapidly the ingested complexes[59].

A more complex situation is the classical acute serum sickness, which can be induced in experimental animals or in humans by injection of foreign proteins[60,61]. The classical experimental model is constituted by the rabbit injected i.v. with a single dose of bovine serum albumin (BSA) (about 250 mg/kg)[60]. In this model, the disease develops 12–14 days after the injection, following the appearance of anti-BSA antibodies and the formation of immune complexes. Simultaneously with the presence of antigen–antibody complexes in the circulation, there is a fall in the level of serum complement and the appearance of acute inflammatory lesions in the kidney, heart, arteries, and joints, strongly reminiscent of the lesions of acute glomerumonephritis, rheumatic fever, lupus erythematosus, polyarteritis nodosa, and rheumatoid arthritis.

The study of the experimental serum sickness demonstrated soluble, circulating antigen–antibody complexes during the development of the disease, and a further localization of antigen, host IgG and host complement fractions, presumably as immunological complexes, in the site of tissue lesions. The prominent characteristics in the lesions are the increased vascular permeability, endothelial proliferation, and variable PMN infiltration. The initial step in serum sickness appears to be a systematic liberation of vasoactive substances as a result of interaction of complexes with humoral and cellular elements of the blood[5,61]. Following the resulting increased vascular permeability, complexes begin to deposit in vessel walls. The depositing complexes have a phlogogenic effect. With the combination of all antigen into complexes and its subsequent elimination from the circulation, the inflammatory lesions in all sites rapidly resolve. The circulating and fixed phagocyte cells take up and rapidly degrade most of the immune complexes formed in circulation. In acute experimental serum sickness only 0.003% of the injected antigen is deposited in the kidney in this form during the development of the glomerulonephritis, and this antigen is eliminated from the kidney with a half-life of 10 days.

The effect of complement activation has been observed in various immune complex diseases. This has been shown usually by removal of various complement components or by use of experimental animals genetically deficient in certain components. C3 and terminal components have been removed conveniently in a number of different animal species by treatment with a protein from cobra venom. The animals are rendered deficient in the components one or more days prior to the experiment. In rabbits so treated, the arteritic lesions, especially the accumulation of neutrophils, were prevented even though immune complexes were present. In Arthus reactions and nephrotoxic nephritis, neutrophils did not accumulate at the sites where immune complexes were located. Thus the attraction and/or binding of neutrophils required the biological properties of activated complement components.

However, the activation of the complement system does not appear to be always necessary for the development of lesions associated with immune complexes, particularly glomerulonephritis. Experimental conditions designed to keep small amounts of such immune complexes present in circulation for long periods of time (in order to mimic more closely the conditions likely to occur in human pathology) produce chronic progressive disease, which depends primarily on the relative amounts of antigen and antibody in the subject[62]. After one or more months of daily injections of BSA and periods of one to several weeks during which circulating antigen–antibody complexes form, rabbits develop a progressive glomerulonephritis[62]. The lesions are independent of the immunologic characteristics of the antigens. The most common and probably the earliest anatomical form of this disease is a membranous glomerulonephritis characterized by thickened glomerular capillary basement membranes with little or no endothelial proliferation[63]. Antigen, host IgG and host complement fractions are found concentrated in thickened basement membranes[62-64]. Once in this site, the immunologic reactants and the morphologically demonstrated deposits persist for long periods, as much as 1 year after cessation of antigen injection, with persistence of associated renal malfunction.

9.2 DETECTION OF IMMUNE COMPLEXES

Two main approaches have been used in order to demonstrate the occurrence of immune complexes in human diseases. These are, first, the analysis of tissue specimens and, second, the serological analysis of samples from various biological fluids.

9.2.1   Detection of immune complexes in tissues

Tissue studies by conventional histological techniques and by electron microscopy may lead to the suspicion of an involvement of immune complexes in the observed lesions on the basis of similarities with lesions induced experimentally by immune complexes. For example, typical morphological features of immune complex glomerulonephritis have been well defined through the study of animal models of this disease[57]. Moreover, immunohistochemical techniques allow a more direct demonstration of immunoglobulin deposits, associated with complement components and some identified antigens in a pattern suggestive of the presence of immune complexes[65]. Such techniques have been applied extensively to many tissues and to the demonstration of immune complex-like material within PMN leukocytes in circulation[66] or at extravascular sites of inflammation[67].

With the availability of sufficient amounts of tissue material the elution of antibodies by low pH buffers, or the destruction of a suspected antigen (e.g. DNA by the specific enzyme DNAase) allows the identification of the components of tissue-localized complexes[68, 69]. However, eluted antibodies always represent a selected fraction of the complexed molecules and the elution procedures alter some antibodies more than others, particularly IgM antibodies. The amount of immunoglobulins with an identified antibody specificity must be related to the total amount of eluted immunoglobulins in order to evaluate their relative involvement in the deposited complexes.

9.2.2   Detection of immune complexes in biological fluids

Studies on biological fluids provide evidence for the association of immune complexes with particular pathological conditions either by the direct detection of immune complexes or by demonstration of serological changes which often are associated with the presence of immune complexes[70-72].

The methods for the detection of immune complexes can be separated into two main groups. On one hand, some methods allow for selective detection of immune complexes involving one given antigen through the discrimination between free and antibody-bound antigens. They represent 'antigen-specific' methods. On the other hand, some methods have been devised in order to detect immune complexes independently of the nature of the antigen involved in the formation of these immune complexes. They represent 'antigen non-specific' methods.

9.2.2.1   Antigen-specific methods

In particular clinical conditions, it may be useful to study whether a known antigen appears in the form of immune complexes. By using a proper methodology, one can distinguish between free antigen molecules and those specifically bound to immunoglobulins. In the case of particulate antigen, morphological analysis has been applied, e.g. the electron microscopic detection of aggregated particles of hepatitis B antigen seems suggestive of their involvement in immune complexes[73]. Physico-chemical methods have been applied to this problem in combination with the detection of known antigens, e.g. neuroblastoma-specific immune complexes have been detected in the sera of patients by radioimmunocounterelectrophoresis[74]. The differentiation between free and complex-bound antigen can further be achieved by measuring the amount of antigen which is removed from a biological sample when the host immunoglobulins are specifically precipitated or absorbed, e.g. the infectivity of sera from mice infected with lactic dehydrogenase virus was shown to decrease strikingly after the specific precipitation of immunoglobulins[75]. Coprecipitation of immunoglobulins was also applied to the detection of DNA–anti-DNA complexes after a previous incubation of serum samples with radiolabelled actinomycin-D which binds as a marker to the DNA molecules[76]. An alternative approach consisted of measuring specific antibody levels before and after removal of the corresponding antigen. This has been done for the detection of DNA–anti-DNA complexes[77]. In another type of investigation the possibility of an *in vivo* formation of immune complexes involving known antigenic specificities was studied. Patients with malaria were given an injection of specific labelled anti-plasmodial antibodies. Thereafter, the solubility of these antibodies was found to be decreased in presence of polyethylene glycol in tested serum samples[78]. However, with respect to the multiplicity of antigen–antibody systems possibly involved in the *in vivo* formation of immune complexes, it is unlikely that such antigen-specific methods would be routinely used in clinical situations. Their use would probably be restricted to the assessment of the immune status in well-defined conditions.

9.2.2.2 *Antigen non-specific methods*

Antigen non-specific methods are based on the distinct properties of complexed immunoglobulin molecules as compared with free immunoglobulin molecules. The main properties which can be used are the physical changes due to the complex formation and the biological activities of immune complexes such as complement fixation or binding to cell membranes. All of these methods will detect non-specifically aggregated immunoglobulins as well as immune complexes.

(a) *Methods based on the physical properties of immune complexes*. The formation of immune complexes leads to the occurrence of new molecular structures characterized by an increased molecular size, by changes of the surface properties, solubility and electric charge as compared with the corresponding free antigens and antibodies. The extent of these changes will depend on the nature and concentration of each immunological constituent of the complex and therefore will exhibit great heterogeneity. For example, the *electric·charge* of immune complexes may differ from that of the corresponding free antibody molecules and thus complexed IgG may be found to exhibit an abnormally increased affinity for anion-exchange resins (DEAE-cellulose)[79,80] or an altered mobility by electrophoretic techniques[81]. Since this property is highly dependent on the antigen involved, it may be more useful for antigen-specific methods[81,82] than for the antigen non-specific detection of immune complexes. Surface changes characterizing immune complexes have also been related to the observed agglutination of uncoated latex particles in presence of serum containing complexed IgG[83]. However, the molecular size and solubility characteristics of immune complexes are the most widely used criteria for their detection by physical methods.

Analytical ultracentrifugation has been applied to the detection of immune complexes through the demonstration in various biological fluids of an abnormal level of some material with a relatively high sedimentation velocity. Thus, evidence which indicates the presence of immune complexes was obtained in some well-defined clinical conditions. However, the exclusive use of analytical ultracentrifugation does not allow a positive conclusion that immune complexes are present since other materials of high molecular weight may also appear in large amounts in some biological samples. Furthermore, the sensitivity of this method is low.

The use of preparative methods for separation of macromolecular aggregates, such as *sucrose gradient ultracentrifugation, gel filtration* or *selective ultrafiltration* allows for the combination of the physical analysis of samples with the characterization of various fractions by additional immunological and biological analysis. All these methods based on a separation according to molecular size are usually limited by a contamination of the macromolecular fraction by monomeric immunoglobulins or unbound complement components. Generally, the results obtained must be related to the immunoglobulin and complement levels in the tested sample. However, these preparative methods can represent an important step in the purification of immune complexes. They have been successfully applied to analytical studies of many clinical conditions, including measles[84], and leprosy[85]. They can be used in combination with added labelled markers for immune complexes, such as C1q[86,87] or antiglobulins[88]. One drawback of these techniques is that they are rather time-consuming and can hardly be used routinely for the detection of immune complexes.

Material with a decreased solubility in well-defined conditions (temperature, medium) was shown to occur frequently in serum or other biological fluid containing immune complexes. Therefore, the occurrence of an abnormal precipitation of serum proteins in a serum sample in such defined conditions may be suggestive of the presence of immune complexes. The simplest procedure is the precipitation at a cold temperature. *Cryoglobulins* may frequently represent a particular type of immune complex, but monoclonal immunoglobulins or other proteins may often be involved. Extensive

Table 9.1 Antigen non-specific methods for the detection of soluble immune complexes based on the biological properties of complexes

	Method	References
RECOGNITION OF IMMUNE COMPLEXES IN CELL-FREE SYSTEMS		
Interaction with complement		
Complement and C1q deviation tests		
Measurement of anticomplementary activity		(98, 99)
C1q deviation (using sensitized erythrocytes)	RIA	(100)
C1q inhibition assay (using IgG-coated epharose particles)	RIA	(101)
C1q latex agglutination inhibition assay		(102)
Direct measurement of C1q-immune complex interaction		
C1q agarose precipitation test		(103)
C1q-binding test	RIA	(104)
Solid-phase C1q-binding tests	RIA	(105)
	ELISA	(106)
Binding of *in vivo* complement-reacted immune complexes to conglutinin		
Solid-phase conglutinin-binding tests	RIA	(107)
	RIA/ELISA	(108, 109)
Interaction with antiglobulin: monoclonal (mRF) or polyclonal (pRF) rheumatoid factors or anti-antibodies		
mRF agarose precipitation test		(110)
Solid-phase mRF inhibition assay	RIA	(111)
pRF inhibition assay (using soluble aggregated IgG and coprecipitation with anti-IgM)	RIA	(112)
mRF inhibition assay (using IgG-coated epharose particles)	RIA	(102)
pRF latex agglutination inhibition assay		(103)
Anti-antibody inhibition assay		(113)
RECOGNITION OF IMMUNE COMPLEXES BY RECEPTORS ON CELL SURFACES		
Interaction with complement receptors on cells		
Raji cell assay	RIA	(114)
Lymphocyte complement-rosettes formation inhibition test		(115)
Interaction with Fc receptors on cells		
Platelet aggregation test		(116)
Inhibition of antibody-dependent cell-mediated cytotoxicity	RIA	(117)
Macrophage uptake inhibition test	RIA	(118)
Neutrophil inhibition test		(97)
Neutrophil-dependent red cell browning test		(97)
Detection of immunoglobulin phagocytosis by neutrophils		(119)
Lymphocyte Fc-rosettes formation inhibition test		

RIA = Radioisotope assay; ELISA = enzyme-linked immunosorbant assay. References including most recent protocols rather than first descriptions are indicated immunochemical analysis of the cryoprecipitates is required before considering cryoglobulins as possible immune complexes[89, 90].

Some media which can be used to separate serum proteins according to their physical properties can also be used to precipitate immune complexes and large serum molecules in conditions where free immunoglobulin molecules would remain soluble.

Precipitation in polyethylene glycol (PEG, MW 6000) has been applied to clinical investigation[91]. The addition to serum of PEG, an uncharged linear polymer, results in a precipitation of proteins which is proportional to the concentration of PEG. The extent of precipitation of each protein is generally proportional to its molecular size[92] so that at low concentrations of PEG, the high molecular weight proteins and immune complexes are preferentially precipitated. An abnormal increase in the protein content of PEG precipi-

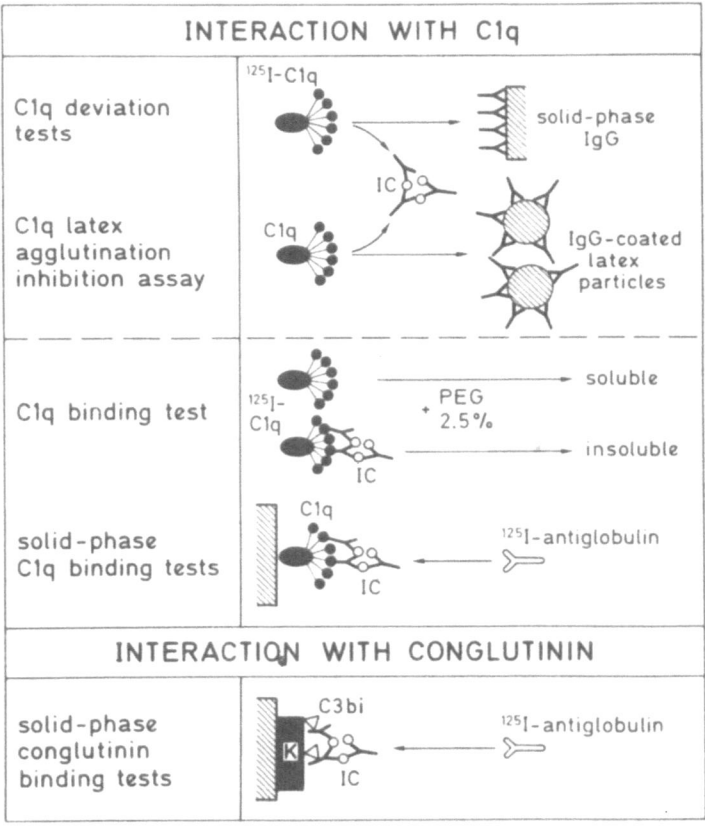

Figure 9.3 Principles and reagents of antigen non-specific methods for the detection of soluble immune complexes (IC) based on interaction with C1q or with conglutinin (K). PEG means 'polyethylene glycol'

tates was shown to be largely correlated to the level of immune complexes in some clinical conditions[93,94]. Such measurements of the total protein precipitation are influenced by the level of various serum proteins and should be considered as a rather non-specific screening test for the detection of immune complexes. More accurate information may be obtained through further analysis of the proteins precipitated at low PEG concentrations.

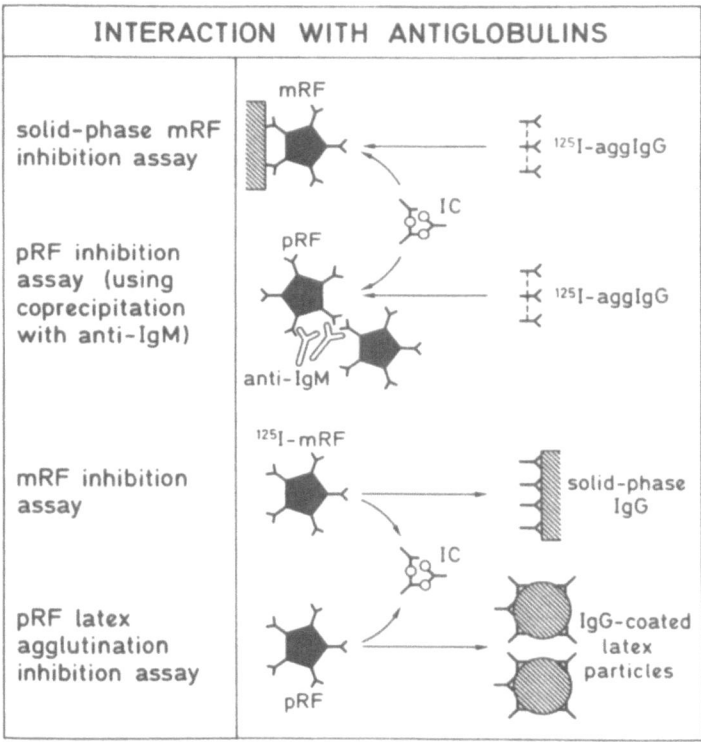

Figure 9.4 Principles and reagents of antigen non-specific methods for the detection of soluble immune complexes (IC) based on interaction with antiglobulins: monoclonal (mRF) or polyclonal (pRF) rheumatoid factors

For instance, an increase in the fraction of serum IgG which is precipitable in PEG is indicative of the presence of aggregated or complexed IgG in the tested serum sample. Furthermore, the demonstration of complement components in such PEG precipitates may suggest an *in vivo* binding of complement to macromolecular complexes. This has been particularly demonstrated for C1q[95] and C4[94]. Precipitation in PEG has also been combined with the use of added radio-labelled markers for immune complexes, such as C1q[95] or staphylococcal protein A[96].

(*b*) *Methods based on the biological properties of immune complexes.* Most detection of soluble immune complexes has been done using methods based on their biological recognition by humoral factors or by cellular receptors. More than 20 methods are now available for the detection of soluble immune complexes. The matter has recently been extensively reviewed[71]. The methods, which are summarized in Table 9.1, can be divided into four groups:

In the first group, the reaction with complement, and particularly C1q, is used to detect immune complexes. This group involves inhibition assays, such as C1q deviation assay and the C1q latex agglutination test, and direct binding assays such as C1q agarose precipitation test, the C1q binding test and the C1q solid-phase assay (Figure 9.3). These tests require the reactivity of immune complexes with complement and the inhibition assays are particularly limited by their high sensitivity to substances other than immune complexes. This interfering effect is relatively limited in the C1q binding assays. In addition, the reaction of C3bi-coated immune complexes with conglutinin has been applied to the detection of immune complexes in order to avoid the interference of substances reacting with C1q (Figure 9.3).

The second group of methods is based on the reaction of anti-immunoglobulin antibodies with immune complexes. Several types of antiglobulin have been used including monoclonal rheumatoid factor, polyclonal rheumatoid factor, anti-antibodies, and low avidity heterologous anti-

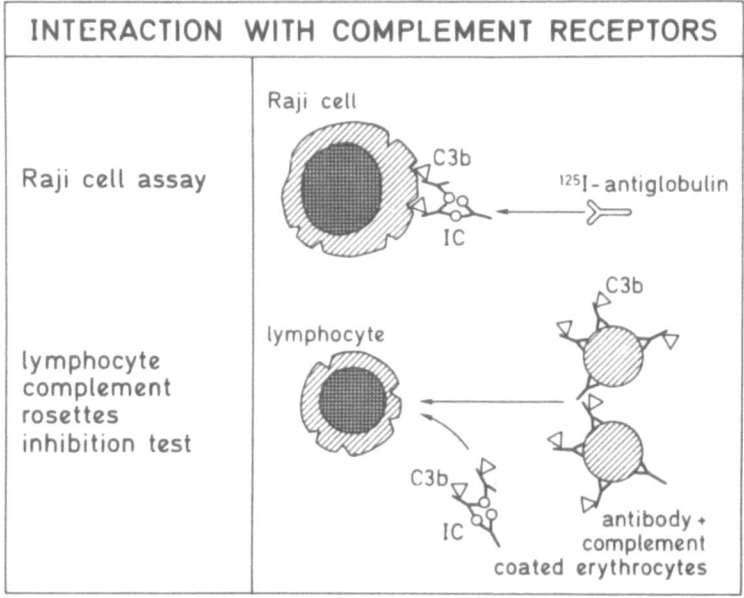

Figure 9.5 Principles and reagents of antigen non-specific methods for the detection of soluble immune complexes (IC) based on interaction with complement receptors on cells.

globulins (Figure 9.4). These tests are usually influenced by the concentration of IgG in the sample to be tested and they often suffer from interference due to the presence of rheumatoid factor in the sample.

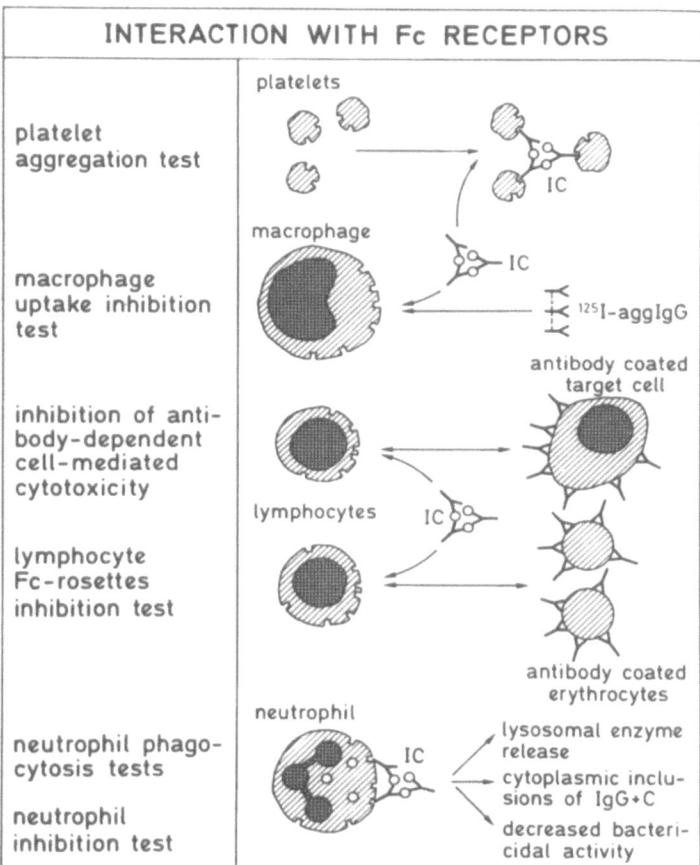

Figure 9.6 Principles and reagents of antigen non-specific methods for the detection of soluble immune complexes (IC) based on interaction with Fc receptors on various cells

The third group of methods is based on the reactivity of immune complexes with complement receptors on cells (Figure 9.5). The most familiar test in this group is the Raji cell radioassay using a lymphoblastoid cell line as a recognition unit for immune complexes. Such methods may be influenced by the presence of antilymphocyte antibodies or of antibodies to other cell membrane antigens in the samples which are analysed.

The fourth group of methods is based on the reactivity of immune complexes with Fc receptors on cells (Figure 9.6). Tests have been developed using a variety of cells including PMN leukocytes, B lymphocytes, macrophages and platelets. They are all functional assays dependent on the integrity of the cells which are used. Therefore, they may suffer from the interference of cytotoxic factors in the tested samples and they are influenced by the presence of RF in the samples. Some tests, such as the K-cell inhibition assay, are also influenced by the IgG concentration in the sample.

In view of the large number of tests available for the detection of immune complexes, one may wonder which one would be suitable for application in clinical investigation. Some answers may be provided if criteria are selected to define an ideal test system. We think that such a test should be: (a) sufficiently sensitive; (b) relatively specific but with a wide spectrum of activity for immune complexes; (c) reproducible; (d) relatively simple to allow for the standardization needed for routine laboratory procedures; (e) it should not require heat-inactivation or a particular absorption of the sample before testing.

Among the tests which are now available, six seem to fulfil most of the criteria that we have defined[97]. The six tests are: the C1q binding test, the C1q solid-phase assay, the conglutinin binding assay, the Raji cell radioassay, the monoclonal RF inhibition test and the platelet aggregation test. All six tests showed a similar range of sensitivity but the most sensitive for aggregated immunoglobulins were the Raji cell assay and the conglutinin binding assay. None of the tests requires heat-inactivation or absorption of the samples and most of them are sensitive only to immune complexes involving IgG antibodies, except for the C1q binding test which also detects IgM antibodies. However, immune complexes containing IgA or IgE antibodies cannot be detected by any other immune complexes detection method presently described.

9.2.3   Indirect evidence for the presence of immune complexes

Since most of the biological effects of immune complexes are mediated through an activation of the complement system, the involvement of complement should be regarded as an important feature, closely associated with the pathological expression of the formation of immune complexes. The analysis of complement changes can be done in serum and in extravascular fluids either by static measurements of the haemolytic activity and the protein concentration of complement components, or by evaluation of their catabolism through turnover studies or quantitation of breakdown products. In acute inflammatory states, such as in infectious diseases, the hypercatabolism of complement components can be mased by an increased synthesis and static measurements do not strictly reflect the activation of the system. Although turnover studies using labelled components have been occasionally performed, such methodology is hampered by the difficulty in avoiding functional alterations of the complement proteins during the labelling procedure. An alternative approach is the measurement of the breakdown products of C3, C4 or factor B which are released from the native molecules during the activation process. This has been achieved by immunoelectrophoresis[121] or by immunochemical quantitation, using radial immunodiffusion[122].

An important limitation of this approach is that the complement system may be activated by substances unrelated to immune complexes. Particularly, lipopolysaccharides from several bacteria can efficiently consume the complement by triggering the alternative and or the classical pathways[123-126].

9.3 ROLE OF IMMUNE COMPLEXES IN INFECTIOUS DISEASES

Immune complexes occur in many infectious diseases[127]. Evidence for the participation of such complexes in some aspects of infectious diseases is based either on immunohistochemical investigations of the tissue lesions associated with infection, or on investigations carried out on serum and other biological fluids. The relevance of such complexes appears mostly in diseases caused by infectious agents of low pathogenicity, in which the immune response of the host plays a major role in determining the pathological manifestations. With a few exceptions, immune complexes may be involved in the pathogenesis when a relatively large number of infectious agents are chronically persisting.

9.3.1 Immune complexes associated with virus infections

Most of the persistent virus infection in a wide variety of hosts are associated with virus-induced immune complex deposits and disease[6] (Table 9.2). After initiation of the infection, viruses, as self-replicating agents, provide an important supply of antigenic material which in most instances induces a corresponding immune response. After production of antiviral antibodies by the host and liberation of infectious viruses by the infected cells, immune complexes can be formed. Complement-dependent lysis of the virion can occur in some viral infections like Sindbis, herpes and measles virus infection in man[128, 129]. This lysis results in the liberation of internal viral antigens which may also be involved in the formation of immune complexes. Immune complexes are also produced at the level of virus infected cells in many virus infections caused by budding viruses like measles virus, mumps virus, and herpes virus in man. In these viral infections, viral antigens are expressed at the surface of the infected cells before virus assembly and budding through the plasma cell membrane. Antiviral antibodies reacting locally with viral antigens exposed at the surface of the infected cells cap these antigens, in a first step[130]. These antigen–antibody complexes will be partly ingested by the infected cells and partly released in the fluid phase as demonstrated in an experimental model using measles infected Hela cells and human anti-measles virus serum[3]. In this system, haemaglutinin, one of the major constituents of measles virus, was found in the complexes released in the fluid phase by the infected cells. It is possible that *in vivo*, the shedding of virus antibody complexes originally bound to the plasma membrane would be a main source of immune complexes. Virus–antibody complexes occur probably in most virus infections but are difficult to detect in acute infection, where they are present only for a short time in circulation, whereas they are frequently detected in chronic viral infection where a persistent viral replication occurs in the presence of a continuous host response. In these circumstances, complexes can be detected in the circulation and in some tissues such as kidney, skin, small vessels, choroid plexus, etc.

Table 9.2   Virus-induced immune complexes diseases

Species	Agent
Mouse	Lactic dehydrogenase virus
	Lymphocytic choriomeningitis virus
	Oncornavirus
	Coxackie B virus
	Cytomegalovirus
Mink	Aleutian mink virus
Horse	Equine infectious anaemia virus
Pig	Hog cholera virus
Man	Hepatitis B virus
	Cytomegalovirus
	Dengue virus (Dengue haemorrhagic fever)
	Epstein–Barr virus (Infectious mononucleosis, Burkitt's lymphoma and nasopharyngeal carcinoma)
	Measles virus (Subacute sclerosating panencephalitis)

9.3.1.1 *Animal models*

It has been demonstrated that immune complexes are associated with virus disease in mice infected with lactodehydrogenase (LDH) virus[131]. Mice infected at birth with lymphocytic choriomeningitis (LCM) virus survive the virus infection and produce antiviral antibodies throughout most of their life[132]. These antibodies are not protective; they will not lead to neutraliz-ation of the viruses nor to their lysis following binding of mouse complement components. But, after reacting with the virus they will generate immune complexes. Oldstone has shown using specific precipitation technique that mouse IgG and C3 are associated with infectious LCM viruses in the sera of these mice[133]. Morphological and immunopathological study of tissues of mice infected with LCM showed deposits of immune complexes with a predominance in glomeruli and choroid plexus and blood vessels. Viral antigens, IgG and C3 were present in irregular granular deposits along the capillary wall and in the mesangia of the glomeruli[6,134]. In addition, immunoglobulins eluted from kidneys of mice infected with LCM were shown to react with the three main structural proteins of LCM virus[135]. Immune complexes associated with the virus infection have also been found in mice infected with oncornavirus[136,137], polyoma[138], coxackie B[139] and cytomegalovirus[6].

9.3.1.2 *Virus-induced immune complexes diseases in man*

(a) *Hepatitis B infection.* Hepatitis B (HB) virus is a minimally cytopathic virus. The complete virus is a 43 nm virus-like particle (Dane particle) consisting of a 27 nm core containing circular double-stranded DNA and of an anti-genically distinct coat[140]. Hepatitis B virus infections occur in most human populations but with a widely different prevalence. The infections range from totally inapparent infection characterized only by the development of antibody to fulminant rapidly fatal infection resulting in complete destruction of the liver. Three antigen systems are now recognized: the HBs antigen present in the coat of the virus, HBc antigen which is part of the nucleocapsid and HBe antigen which is not yet characterized. HBs antigen is produced in great excess of virus particles (up to 10^6 excess) in the serum of patients. Hepatitis B antigens have been identified and localized in the liver cells by electron microscopy and immunofluorescence[141]. Infection with hepatitis B virus is sometimes characterized in its prodromal phase by a serum sickness syndrome which could be due to circulating immune complexes[142]. Immune complexes have been found at various stages of the disease in the circulation by the ^{125}I-C1q binding activity test and the Raji cell test, or in the form of HBs antigen–antibody complexes by immuno-electronmicroscopy[73,143,144]. There is also an association between certain cases of polyarteritis nodosa and the occurrence of immune complexes involving HBs antigen both in the serum and in the arteritis lesions[145,146]. In rare instances, glomerulonephritis is associated with presence of HBs antigen in the renal lesions[140].

Finally, it was also shown that a high proportion of patients suffering from essential mixed cryoglobulinaemia have in their cryoprecipitates either HBs antigen and/or anti-HBs antibody[147]. In some of the cryoprecipitates morphological structure corresponding to the HBs particules or to Dane particles were also detected.

(b) *Dengue haemorrhagic fever (DHF).* DHF is caused by one of the four types of Dengue virus and is an acute febrile illness associated with haemorrhagic phenomena and a shock syndrome. High mortality is observed in infants and children in south-east Asia[148]. The majority of these children display evidence of previous dengue infection. It is suggested that virus multiplication can be amplified during a second infection by the following mechanism: antibody produced on the first infection will bind but not neutralize dengue virus of another strain. The virus antibody complexes will then attach to human monocytes through their Fc receptor and the replication of the virus will be increased[148].

There is some experimental evidence that in DHF there is a massive intravascular activation of complement[148-150]. Immune complexes in sera of patients suffering from DHF have been detected using the Raji cell radioimmunoassay[144] and the C1q deviation test[100].

(c) *Epstein–Barr virus infections.* The Epstein–Barr virus (EBV) is associated with three human diseases: infectious mononucleosis (IM), Burkitt's lymphoma and nasopharyngeal carcinoma[151]. Circulating immune complexes have recently been found in the acute phase of IM[152]. In IM, autoantibodies of a wide variety of specificities and antibodies directed against haptenic structures have been described[151,153]. Several mechanisms could be responsible for appearance of autoantibodies in viral infection: (a) a mitogen effect of some viral constituent inducing polyclonal B-cell activation; (b) a release of sequestred antigens by the viral infection; (c) a virus-induced alteration of host cell membranes; (d) direct or indirect alteration of immune cells of the host. Evidently some of these mechanisms could play a role in the immune response of the host and in the generation of immune complexes. It should also be noted that immune complexes have also been found in Burkitt's lymphoma and nasopharyngeal carcinoma[154,155]. Moreover, immune complex deposits have been detected by immunofluorescence in the glomeruli of kidney biopsies of patients suffering from Burkitt's lymphoma.

(d) *Measles virus infection.* Subacute sclerosing panencephalitis (SSPE) is a progressive neurological deterioration occurring in children and adolescents. Patients with this disease have extremely high levels of antibody to measles virus in the serum and the cerebrospinal fluid. The brain tissue contains inclusion bodies and nucleocapsid material identical to measles virus. Measles virus has been isolated from their brain using the cocultivation technique and is thought to be the causing agent of SSPE[156]. Immune complexes have been found in the circulation of these patients but there is no information regarding whether or not virus or virus antigens are involved in the complex[157-159]. Some experiments suggested that in these patients a factor will block cell-mediated killing, MIF activity and lymphocyte proliferation. This factor is precipitated by antibodies against IgG and C3, which suggests that it could correspond to immune complexes[160].

9.3.2   Immune complexes associated with bacterial infections

9.3.2.1   *Infections with Gram-positive and Gram-negative cocci*

Immune complex pathology occurs frequently following streptococcal infection. Glomerulonephritis may follow streptococcal infections of either the pharynx or the skin[161, 162]. Although many strains of streptococcus elicit infection, only a few, most notably streptococcus group A, type 12, are most frequently associated with the induction of glomerulonephritis[163]. Acute poststreptococcal glomerulonephritis which has many similarities to 'one-shot' serum sickness, characteristically follows streptococcal infections, after a latent period of 7–14 days. During this period the infection resolves, titres of antibodies to a variety of streptococcal antigens increase[164] and, in the small percentage of patients who develop glomerulonephritis, there is a serum complement depression[165]. Immunopathological examination of the kidney reveals a proliferative glomerulonephritis characterized by granular deposits of IgG and C3 associated with electron dense, subepithelial deposits[7, 65, 166, 167]. Such a pattern indicates immune complex localization and strongly evocates that observed in rabbit experimental serum sickness. Materials from cell wall of the streptococcus is probably involved in such complexes[161]. In the kidney, the antigen has been demonstrated early in the course of the disease[167–169]. Within a few days after the onset, the antigen is no longer detectable, although IgG and C3 persist. Moreover, the localization of the antigen in glomeruli does not parallel the IgG and C3 deposits[5]. The finding of cryoglobulin[170], principally containing IgG, tends to support the presence of circulating complexes, as do certain of the extrarenal findings. A more complex immuno-pathogenesis has also been suggested. This includes the possibility of: (a) an *in situ* streptococcal antigen fixation and a secondary immune complex formation[171]; and (b) a cross-reaction between streptococcal components and human glomerular basement membrane antigens[161, 172]. However, the difficulty in obtaining kidney tissue from autopsy, due to the self-limited nature of acute glomerulonephritis, has not permitted a deep investigation on the glomerular-bound antibodies in order to further characterize immune complexes deposited in the kidney.

Acute immune-complex glomerulonephritis has been associated with other coccal infections, including pneumococcal otitis, staphylococcal otitis, *Staphylococcus aureus* infections of a subarachnoid–jugular shunt and *Staphylococcus epidermidis* infection of a ventriculo–jugular shunt[8, 173]. Glomerular IgG and complement deposits, similar to those observed in acute poststreptococcal glomerulonephritis, and depressed serum complement levels were found. *Staphylococcus aureus* antigens were identified in kidney from patients with immune complex nephritis and recurrent *Staphylococcus aureus* infections[174].

Patients with subacute bacterial endocarditis (SBE) may develop focal or diffuse glomerulonephritis[175]. These lesions were originally believed to be secondary to emboli originating from heart valves. Recent evidence of deposits of immunoglobulins and complement in glomeruli associated with depressed serum complement levels coupled with the rarity of bacterial isolation from glomerular lesions, suggests that renal disease in SBE represents a form of immune complex nephritis[176–178]. Streptococcal bacterial antigen has been identified in glomerular deposits and antibodies eluted from kidney were specific for the bacteria cultured from the patient's blood before death[179]. In rabbits, a typical immune complex glomerulonephritis has been induced by immunization with an infecting agent prior to the establishment of left-sided α-streptococcal endocarditis[180]. Controls receiving immunization alone, immunization and sterile endocarditis, or infective endocarditis alone did not develop diffuse glomerulonephritis. High levels of circulating immune complexes were found in 28 out of 29 patients with SBE with renal or other involvements[181]. Circulating immune complexes levels were correlated with longer duration of illness, extra-vascular manifestations of endocarditis and low levels of complement. Recently, soluble immune complexes have been detected in pleural exudates from patients with cocci and other bacterial infections[182]. The level of such complexes correlated with the depressed haemolytic complement activity and with the abnormal concentration of C3d.

9.3.2.2 Leprosy

In most infectious diseases the mechanism of tissue damage derives from combination of both microbial and host factors. However, in leprosy the infectious agent is so non-toxic (patients with early lepromatosus leprosy may have many millions of bacilli per g of skin tissue without overt clinical symptoms) that the contribution of host factors appears to be of a major importance in the determination of the lesions of the disease. The various forms of leprosy represent a wide, continuous spectrum of pathological manifestations associated with different levels of cellular and humoral immunity against the mycobacteria[183]. In the tubercoloid form, there is strong cell-mediated immunity and low antibody levels, while the reverse situation is observed in lepromatous form. The formation of immune complexes may be expected in lepromatous leprosy (LL) from the concomitant occurrence of large numbers of mycobacteria and of corresponding antibodies[184]. Indeed, there is some evidence of an involvement of immune complexes in the pathogenesis of erythema nodosom leprosum (ENL), mainly based on clinical and tissue studies[185]. Certain manifestations of ENL such as albuminuria and skin lesions, are similar to those encountered in acute serum sickness or in experimental Arthus reaction[186]. Deposits of immunoglobulin and C3, and sometimes mycobacterial antigens have been demonstrated by immunofluorescence in LL and ENL lesions[12,185,187]. Serological studies have revealed the frequent occurrence in lepromatous sera of substances which precipitate with Clq in agarose[188-190], and this has been confirmed by demonstration of an increased ^{125}I-Clq binding activity in sera from patients with ENL, with uncomplicated LL, and surprisingly in sera from patients with tuberculoid leprosy (TL)[85]. When different techniques for detection of immune complexes were applied in leprosy sera, it was found that some methods discriminated sera of patients with LL (high levels of immune complexes) from sera of patients with TL (low levels of immune complexes)[97]. In other experiments it was found that ^{125}I-C1q binding material from leprosy sera with a sedimentation rate in the range 10–25 decreased to about half of control following incubation with *M. leprae*[85]. However, antigen–antibody systems other than those involving mycobacterial antigens may be present in leprosy sera. Indeed, mixed cryoglobulins with an IgM component exhibiting anti-IgG activity were found in such sera[191]. As in other inflammatory syndromes, normal or increased levels of complement components have been reported in LL[185, 190, 192–194]. However, the finding of increased C3d level, a long-life catabolic fragment of C3, in 70% of ENL plasma provides evidence that complement is activated *in vivo* possibly by antigen–antibody complexes[85]. For a more detailed discussion, see Chapter 12.

9.3.3 Immune complexes occurring during parasitic diseases

Parasitic diseases are generally characterized by a long-term persistence of the parasite in the host. Many parasites by themselves are not highly pathogenic, and lesions associated with the disease are mostly caused by the immune response of the host against parasite antigens. Indeed, the formation of immune complexes involving antigens released from living or dying parasites is a likely major pathogenetic mechanisms. Therefore, the site of formation of such complexes would depend on the distribution of parasites and parasite antigens in the host at the time of the corresponding immune response. Even in the absence of clinically apparent renal disease, the deposition of immunoglobulins and complement in renal glomeruli is often the first sign of the association of an immune complexes disease with the parasitic infection[195]. However, it is likely that most of the immune complexes are formed in excess of antibody at the site of the localization of the parasite in tissues and one should not consider the circulation of small soluble complexes and their localization in the kidney as a prerequisite for the involvement of such immune complexes in the pathogenesis of the disease.

9.3.3.1 *Protozoal infections*

(*a*) *Malaria.* Thus most comprehensive data implicating immune complexes in the pathogenicity of malaria relate to renal lesions[196]. Several other manifestations in which immune complexes may play a role have also been studied. These include tropical splenomegaly, anaemia and autoimmunity[197]. Immunopathological studies have revealed two main types of renal involvement associated with malaria in man and experimental animals. On the one hand, glomerulonephritis very similar to that occurring during acute serum sickness is observed during the course of acute *Plasmodium falciparum* infections[10,196,198]. Granular deposits of immunoglobulins, complement and plasmodium antigens can be demonstrated in renal biopsy specimens by immunofluorescence techniques. These lesions respond very well to antimalarial therapy and urinary abnormalities usually disappear within 6 weeks. Deposits of immune complexes are not usually detectable after this length of time[196,199]. Similar findings have been reported in animal models of acute infections. On the other hand, in quartan malaria infections, chronic progressive lesions are characteristically observed. In man, deposits of immunoglobulins, complement and *P. malariae* antigens are present in the capillary walls of glomeruli[11,78,201,202] in biopsy specimens taken at the beginning of the disease but they are no longer demonstrable in the later stages of the disease.

The renal lesions are not affected following clearing of parasitaemia with anti-malaria therapy and deposits of immunoglobulins and complement persist for a long time. Immunofluorescence studies showed either typical coarse granular deposits, usually positive for IgM and/or IgG (IgG$_3$, IgG$_4$) and complement, or fine granular deposits, usually only positive for IgG, mainly IgG$_2$ subclass, without complement. A study of the antibodies eluted from renal tissue showed that they were specific for *P. malariae* in the majority of cases[203]. Owl monkeys infected with quarten malaria had lesions similar to that found in humans[204].

Until now, no reasons have been found for the development of chronic progressive renal lesions in patients with quartan malaria. However, recent experimental data suggest that specific plasmodium antigens may be involved in the immune complexes occurring in such diseases[78]. Aotus monkeys infected with quartan malaria and injected i.v. with radiolabelled anti-*P. malariae* IgG and/or normal IgG showed: (a) increased *in vivo* binding of malarial antibodies into abnormally insoluble form when precipitated by 7·5% polyethylene glycol; (b) faster disappearance of this antibody from the circulation; and (c) its increased deposition in renal glomeruli. Similar results were obtained in monkeys infected with *P. falciparum* and injected with anti-*P. falciparum* IgG but the difference when compared with controls was much less.

In patients with nephrotic syndrome and a past history of malaria infections, results similar to quartan malaria model in monkeys were found, i.e. increased binding of anti-*P. malariae* IgG with sera *in vitro*, its faster disappearance from circulation after i.v. injection, and increased deposition of IgG[78] in kidney tissue after i.v. injection. These data indicate the binding of i.v.-injected specific antibodies to soluble antigen and/or to soluble immune complexes in excess of antigen and their increased deposition at the site of kidney lesions. Decreased or normal complement components were reported in patients with renal involvement associated with *P. malariae* infections[127,195].

(b) *Trypanosomiasis*. African trypanosomiasis is characterized by sequential changes in surface antigens of the parasites during the course of the infection. This antigenic variation allows for the persistence of the infection but results also in the release of a large amount of parasite antigen during each wave of parasitaemia, which is followed by the appearance of corresponding antibodies. As in the model of chronic serum sickness, this alternation of antigen and of antibody excess is likely to favour the formation of immune complexes. Furthermore, depending on the localization of parasites, antigens may be released at the site of inoculation, in blood or in extravascular spaces. Therefore, immune complexes may be formed in various tissues as well as in circulating blood. The clinical and the histopathological picture observed in African trypanosomiasis presents some similarities with generalized immune complex disease such as systemic lupus erythematosus. Indeed, there is a disseminated vasculitis with a prevalence of lesions in the brain and in the heart. Unfortunately, very little information is available as yet on the immunopathology of these human lesions.

Strong evidence for the involvement of immune complexes in trypanosomiasis is provided by experimental infections in monkeys[205] and in mice[195]. In monkeys infected with *Trypanosoma rhodesiense*, glomerular changes are observed, with mesangial hyperplasia and with some thickening of the glomerular basement membrane. Immunofluorescence studies have shown the presence of granular deposits of IgM, C3 and properdin in glomerular lesions. The plasma level of some complement components (C3, C4, properdin) is strikingly decreased during the course of the disease, suggesting an activation of both the classical and the alternative pathway of complement.

An immune complexes pathogenesis is also associated with the development of lesions during experimental trypanosomiasis in mice. Mice sacrificed 6 weeks to 2 months after infection with *T. brucei* showed that the disease was characterized by high parasitaemia and by disseminated foci of inflammation associated with trypanosome infiltrates in various tissues. Kidney lesions were characterized by some mesangial proliferation and some thickening of the basement membranes in glomeruli. This was associated with electron-dense deposits in these basement membranes. Using immunofluorescence, deposits of IgG, IgM and C3 were found in the mesangium at the beginning of the disease, and slightly later in the capillary walls in a granular pattern. Eluates obtained from a pool of kidneys from these infected mice contained immunoglobulins specifically reacting with antigens of trypanosomes used as inoculum, but not, or poorly reacting with trypanosomes isolated from the later stages of the disease. Trypanosome antigens could be identified in glomerular lesions, using fluorescent antibodies specific for trypanosome antigens corresponding to the initial population and not to the trypanosome actually circulating at time of sacrifice[195]. These results suggest that immune complexes formed of trypanosome antigens and corresponding antibodies are localized in renal glomeruli during the course of infection. This localization may be favoured by an enhanced vascular permeability due to the release of kinins known to occur during such infections with African trypanosomiasis. Besides this finding suggesting the presence of circulating complexes, it is likely that a large amount of immune complexes is also formed locally in tissues where trypanosome infiltrates

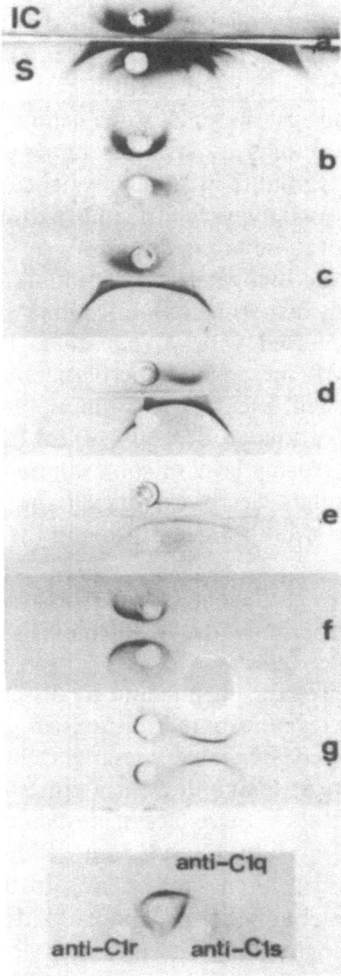

Figure 9.7 Analysis of immune complexes purified from serum of patient with kala–azar. Immunoelectrophoresis: upper well, eluate from solid-phase conglutinin; lower well, normal human serum (NHS). Trough: (a) anti-NHS; (b) anti-IgM; (c) anti-IgG; (d) anti-B1A (C3c); (e) anti-α_2d(C3d); (f) anti-Clq; (g) anti-Cls. Anode was on the right. Ouchterlony: centre well, eulate from solid-phase conglutinin

are frequently observed[206]. Inflammatory foci present between the myocardial cells were found to be associated with trypanosome antigens in identical pattern. Granular deposits of immunoglobulins were detected along the heart fibres. The major trypanosome antigens detected corresponded to trypanosomes which were no longer detectable in circulating blood but which differed from those identified in kidney lesions. Immunoglobulins eluted from these tissues were specific either for the variant trypanosome antigen detected

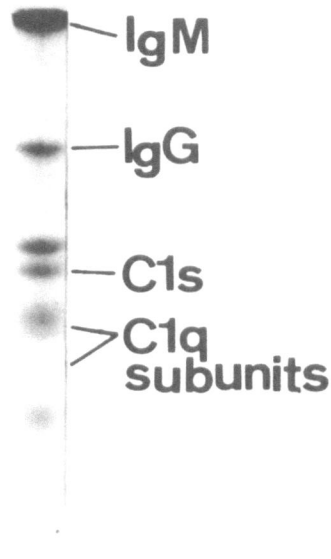

Figure 9.8 Sodium dodecylsulphate–polycyclamide gel electrophoresis (SDS–PAGE) analysis of immune complexes purified from patients with kala–azar. Sample to be analysed was diluted in 2% SDS, 0.05 M phosphate, pH 7.0, heated at 56 °C for 30 min and then applied on a 5% gel

in the lesion, or for DNA. These data suggest that there is a local formation of trypanosome–anti-trypanosome and DNA–anti-DNA complexes which persist in tissue in the presence of antibody excess. Similar mechanisms may play a role in the development of brain lesions characterizing sleeping sickness. Indeed, in some infected mice, granular deposits of immunoglobulins are seen in the choroid plexus and in perivascular areas. More recent findings strongly suggest that immune complexes formed during the course of trypanosomiasis have an important pathogenic role in the development of the lesions associated with the parasitic disease[206].

In irradiated, newborn and athymic nude mice infected with *T. brucei*, no inflammatory lesions and no deposition of IgG, IgM or trypanosomal antigens was present in tissues, although a large number of trypanosomes

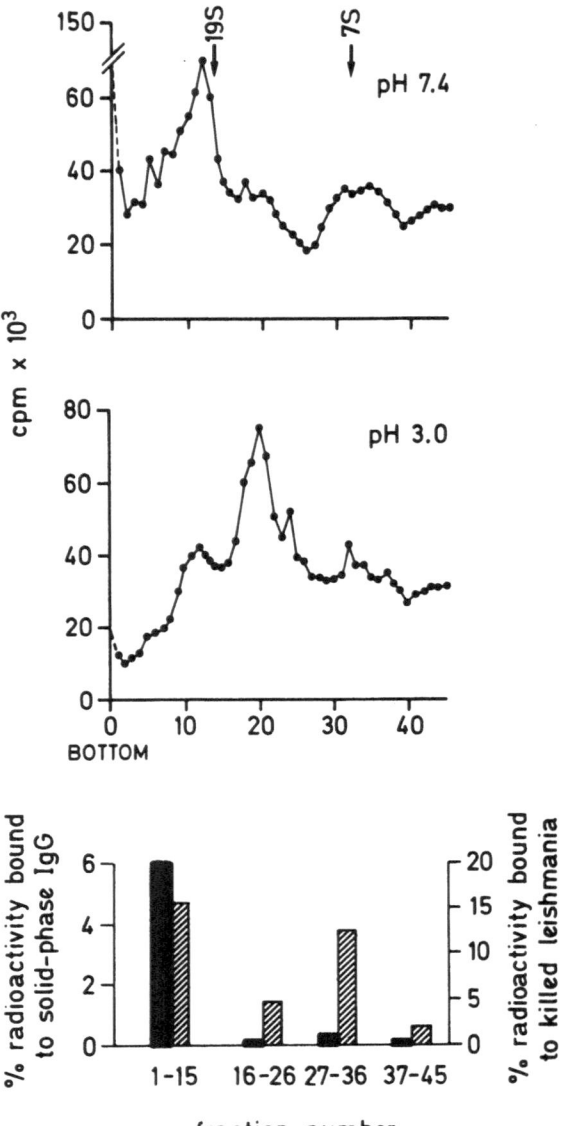

Figure 9.9 Ultracentrifugation of the immune complexes purified from serum of patient, with kala–azar. The purified complexes were labelled with ^{125}I using the lactoperoxydase method, and then applied on 10–40% sucrose density gradient either at pH 7.4 or at pH 3.0. Full line represents the radioactivity of the collected fractions. Dotted line represents the radioactivity which was found stuck to the bottom of the tube. The material fractionated at pH 3.0, pooled in four fractions, was tested for the anti-IgG (solid columns) and anti-Leishmania (hatched columns) activity. Anti-IgG activity was assessed by human IgG in solid-phase, and anti-Leishmania activity using heat killed *Leishmania tropica*

were present. The characteristic lesions could be induced in athymic nude mice by transfer of normal spleen cells or of normal T lymphocytes 1 week after the onset of the infection. The lesions were also partially induced by transfer of antibody to *T. brucei*. These data show that the immunodeficiency suppresses the development of the characteristic tissue lesions of African trypanosomiasis. Since these mice exhibit a very high parasitaemia and an infiltration of most organs with numerous parasites, it is likely that the tissues lesions observed in immunologically competent mice are not related to a direct toxicity of the parasite localized in those tissues.

(c) *Leishmaniasis.* Immune complex-like material has been reported to occur in one patient with visceral leishmaniasis (kala–azar). The C1q fixing material, with a sedimentation coefficient in the 14–24 range, was completely acid-dissociable[70]. In another case, immune complexes were detected in a 33-year-old patient affected with kala–azar. 20 ml of the serum of the patient was processed for the purification of the soluble immune complexes by freon treatment, PEG precipitation and absorption on solid-phase conglutinin[109]. Purified material contained IgM, IgG, and the complement components C3c, C3d, C1q, C1r, C1s (Figures 9.7 and 9.8). By ultracentrifugation analysis, a sedimentation coefficient greater than 21S was found for the radio-labelled purified complexes (Figure 9.9). After dissociation, anti-IgG activity was found in the fractions of about 21S sedimentation rate, and anti-leishmania activity was found in the 21 and 7S fractions.

9.3.3.2 *Helminthic infections*

(a) *Schistosomiasis.* In human schistosomiasis, the involvement of immune complexes in some aspects of the disease has been suspected. Indeed, patients with hepatosplenic schistosomiasis (*S. mansoni*) exhibit frequent urinary changes and a particular prevalence of glomerulonephritis.

Immune complexes may interfere with some of the protective immunological mechanisms and play a role in the pathogenesis of some of the lesions. IgG-dependent eosinophil-mediated damage to ^{51}Cr-labelled schistosomula *in vitro* is blocked by preincubation of effector cells with unrelated immune complexes[28]. Immunohistological findings of the involvement of immune complexes in schistosoma infections come from experimental and human infections with *S. mansoni* and *S. Japonicum*. Granular deposits containing IgG, IgM and C3 have been found in kidneys[207–209]. The presence of parasite antigens together with immunoglobulins and complement in the renal lesions was demonstrated by immunofluorescence in mice[210] and by counter-immunoelectrophoresis in baboons[203]. Soluble schistosoma antigens have been demonstrated in sera of patients and animals with *S. mansoni* infections[203,211,212]. In humans, antigens were found to occur in the circulation simultaneously with the specific antibodies lightly bound in complexes[213–215]. By ^{125}I-C1q binding activity test, circulating immune complexes have been detected in patients with *S. mansoni* infections[93]. Using three tests, ^{125}I-C1q binding activity test, conglutinin binding activity test and Raji cells – RIA, it was found that patients with the most severe hepato–splenic manifestations also displayed the highest level of circulating immune complexes. One of the major immunopathological lesions in *S. mansoni* infections is the granulomatous response to schistosoma eggs trapped in the liver, intestine and other tissues. This is a delayed hypersensitivity reaction to soluble egg antigens released from the eggs through the eggshells. Reduction in size of the granulomas after repeated exposures to egg antigens seems to be due to the blocking of antigens by antibodies. Locally formed immune complexes have been detected within the granuloma lesions[216].

(b) *Onchocerciasis*. Living *Onchocerca volvulus* is relatively harmless but the dead form initiates immunopathological mechanisms with ensuing tissue damage[127]. In generalized onchocerciasis, large numbers of microfilariae are present in the skin and other tissues. IgG and IgM specific antibodies are detectable in the sera of patients. Circulating immune complexes have been demonstrated by several techniques in the sera of patients from the Cameroons[97]. A generalized Arthus reaction, similar to a serum sickness reaction, is observed in patients treated with diethylcarbamazine. Presumably, antigens suddenly released from dying parasites form complexes with antibodies in and around blood vessels, inducing infiltration and degranulation of polymorphonuclear leukocytes. Infiltration of eosinophils in lesions is not prominent. Immune complexes occurring during the disease may contribute to the pathogenesis of lesions of the eye, leading to blindness, of the testes, leading to infertility, and also of other sites.

9.4 CONCLUSIONS

There is good evidence that immune complexes occur frequently during many viral, bacterial and parasitic infections. This evidence is based on the demonstration of immune complexes in blood and/or in tissues. The presence of soluble immune complexes has been suspected from physico–chemical analysis of serum and from the recognition of biological effects largely specific for immune complexes. The recent development of methods allowing for a quantitation of immune complexes provides a new approach for the investigation of infectious diseases. In view of the data presently available, it appears that immune complexes occur in numerous pathological conditions but their pathogenicity is variably expressed.

The main pathological manifestations of some infections are apparently directly related to the formation of immune complexes and to their localization in tissues. In these conditions, the quantitation of circulating or extravascular immune complexes and the estimation of complement catabolism may be useful in monitoring the therapy. Frequently, the formation of immune complexes may represent a secondary event during or following the course of an infection, but may account for some of the pathological manifestations, such as post-streptococcal glomerulonephritis, glomerulonephritis associated with sub-acute bacterial endocarditis and quartan malaria. Finally, immune complexes may occur in some infectious diseases without obvious direct pathological consequences. However, such complexes may sometimes interfere with important cell functions and possibly modulate the immune response of the patient in a more subtle fashion. Although circulating immune complexes can play an essential role in the development of vascular and glomerular lesions, the existence of a large extravascular pool of soluble and insoluble complexes should also be considered in relation to the frequent occurrence of inflammatory lesions in the extravascular compartment. This seems most likely in diseases such as leprosy and schistosomiasis.

The persistence and the pathogenicity of immune complexes formed in the extravascular compartment are certainly favoured by the limited clearance capacity of the mononuclear-phagocyte system in these sites.

The nature of immune complexes occurring during infectious diseases is still often unknown but it is likely that the present effort to isolate and characterize immune complexes will lead to a better definition of the antigens involved in their formation.

ACKNOWLEDGEMENTS

We wish to thank Mrs Dianne Ignoto, Mrs Martine Devouge and Mrs Jean Ringrose for their skilful secretarial services. This work has been supported by the Swiss National Foundation (Grant No. 3.847.077), the Dubois-Ferrière-Dinu Lipatti Foundation and the World Health Organization.

References

1. Lambert, P. H., Louis, J. A., Izui, S., Kobayakawa, T. (1978). Relevance of polyclonal antibody formation to the development of auto-immunity in particular relation to murine lupus. Presented at *6th International Convocation on Immunology*. June 12–15, Niagara Falls
2. Shands, J. W. (1973). Affinity of endoxin for membranes. In: *Bacterial Lipopolysaccharides*, (E. H. Hass and S. M. Wolff, eds.), pp. 189–193 (Chicago: The University of Chicago Press)
3. Perrin, L. H. and Oldstone, M. B. A. (1977). The formation and the fate of virus antigen–antibody complexes. *J. Immunol.*, **118**, 316
4. Mannik, M., Haakenstad, A. O. and Arend, W. P. (1974). The fate and detection of circulating immune complexes. In: *Progress in Immunology II* (L. Brent and J. Holborow, eds.), vol. 5, pp. 91–101 (Amsterdam: North Holland Publishing Co.)

5. Cochrane, C. G. and Koffler, D. (1973). Immune complex disease in experimental animals and man. *Adv. Immunol.*, **16**, 185

6. Oldstone, M. B. A. (1975). Virus neutralization and virus-induced immune complex disease. Virus–antibody union resulting in immunoprotection or immunologic injury – two sides of the same coin. *Prog. Med. Virol.*, **19**, 84

7. Michael, A. F., Drummond, K. N., Good, R. A. and Vernier, R. L. (1966). Acute post-streptococcal glomerulonephritis: Immune deposit disease. *J. Clin. Invest.*, **45**, 237

8. Michael, A. F., Westberg, N. G., Fish, A. J. and Vernier, R. L. (1971). Studies on chronic membranoproliferative glomerulonephritis with hypocomplementaemia. *J. Exp. Med.*, **134** (Suppl.), 208

9. Woodroffe, A. J., Row, P. G., Meadows, R. and Lawrence, J. R. (1974). Nephritis in infectious monocleosis. *Q. J. Med.*, **43**, 451

10. Futrakul, P., Boonpucknavig, V., Boonpucknavig, S., Mitrakul, C. and Bhamarapravati, N. (1974). Acute glomeronephritis complicating *Plasmodium falciparum* infection. *Clin. Pediatr.*, **13**, 281

11. Ward, P. and Kibukamusoke, J. W. (1969). Evidence for soluble immune complexes in the pathogenesis of the glomerulonephritis of quartan malaria. *Lancet*, **i**, 283

12. Shwe, T. (1972). Immune complexes in glomeruli of patients with leprosy. *Leprosy Rev.*, **42**, 282

13. Poltera, A. A. (1978). Immunopathology of cerebral trypanosomiasis in mice. Presented at the *2nd Menarini Symposium*, Immunopathology of the Central and Peripheral Nervous System. June 14–16, Milan

14. Müller-Eberhard, H. J. (1975). Complement. *Ann. Rev. Biochem.*, **44**, 697

15. Warner, N. L. (1974). Membrane immunoglobulins and antigen receptors on B and T lymphocytes. *Adv. Immunol.*, **19**, 67

16. Spiegelberg, H. L. (1974). Biological activities of immunoglobulins of different classes and subclasses. *Adv. Immunol.*, **19**, 259

17. Nussenzweig, V. (1974). Receptors for immune complexes on lympho *Adv. Immunol.*, **19**, 217

18. Augener, W., Grey, H. M., Cooper, N. R. and Müller-Eberhard, H. J. (1971). The reaction of monomeric and aggregated immunoglobulins with C1. *Immunochemistry*, **8**, 1011

19. Czop, J. and Nussenzweig, V. (1976). Studies on the mechanism of solubilization of immune precipitates by serum. *J. Exp. Med.*, **143**, 615

20. Takahashi, M., Czop, J., Ferreira, A. and Nussenzweig, V. (1976). Mechanism of solubilization of immune aggregates by complement. Implications for immunopathology. *Transpl. Rev.*, **32**, 121

21. Becker, E. L. and Henson, P. M. (1973). *In vitro* studies of immunologically induced secretion of mediators from cells and related phenomenon. *Adv. Immunol.*, **17**, 93

22. Henson, P. M. (1971). Interaction of cells with immune complexes: adherence, release of constituents, and tissue injury. *J. Exp. Med.*, **134** (Suppl.), 114

23. Thompson, R. A. and Lachmann, P. J. (1970). Reactive lysis: the complement-mediated lysis of unsensitized cells. I. The characterization of the indicator fact of and its identification as C7. *J. Exp. Med.*, **131**, 629

24. Henson, P. M. and Speigelberg, H. L. (1973). Release of serotonin from human platelet induced by aggregated immunoglobulins of different classes and subclasses. *J. Clin. Invest.*, **52**, 1282

25. Brown, D. L. (1974). Complement and coagulation. In: *Progress in Immunology II* (L. Brent and J. Holborow, eds.), vol. 1, pp. 191–200 (Amsterdam: North Holland Publishing Co.)

26. Butterworth, A. E., Sturrock, R. F. and Houba, V. (1975). Eosinophile as mediators of antibody-dependent damage to schistosomula. *Nature (Lond.)*, **256**, 727

27. Tai, P. C. and Spry, C. J. F. (1976). Studies on blood eosinophiles. I. Patients with a transient eosinophilia. *Clin. Exp. Immunol.*, **24**, 415

28. Butterworth, A. E., Sturrock, R. F., Houba, V. and Taylor, R. (1976). Schistosoma mansoni in baboons. Antibody-dependent cell-mediated damage to ^{51}Cr-labelled schistotomala. *Clin. Exp. Immunol.*, **25**, 95

29. Ogilvie, B. M. and Mackenzie, C. D. (1977). Nematode immunity with reference to strongyloidiasis. In: *Immunopathology* (P. A. Miescher, ed.), vol. 7, pp. 221–229 (Basel: Schwabe and Co.)

30. Holm, G. and Hammerström, S. (1973). Haemolytic activity of human blood monocytes lysis of human erythrocytes treated with anti-A serum. *Clin. Exp. Immunol.*, **13**, 29

31. Cardella, C. J., Davies, P. and Allison, A. C. (1974). Immune complexes induce selective release of lysosomal hydrolases from macrophages. *Nature (Lond.)*, **247**, 46

32. Schorlemmer, H. V. and Allison, A. C. (1976). Effects of activated complement components on enzyme secretion by macrophages. *Immunology*, **31**, 781

33. Shevach, E. M., Juffe, E. S. and Green, I. (1973). Receptors for complement and immunoglobulin on human or animal lymphoid cells. *Transpl. Rev.*, **16**, 3

34. Frøland, S. S. and Natwig, J. B. (1973). Identification of three different human lymphocyte populations by surface markers. *Transpl. Rev.*, **16**, 114

35. Ferrarini, M., Moretta, L., Abrile, R. and Durante, M. L. (1975). Receptors for IgG molecules on human lymphocytes forming spontaneous rosettes with sheep red cells. *Eur. J. Immunol.*, **5**, 70

36. Ryser, J. E. and Vassalli, P. (1974). Mouse bone marrow lymphocytes and their differentiation. *J. Immunol.*, **113**, 719

37. Gronowicz, E. and Continho, A. (1975). Functional analysis of B cells heterogeneity. *Transpl. Rev.*, **24**, 3

38. Feldmann, M. and Nossal, G. J. V. (1972). Tolerance, enhancement and the regulation of interactions between T cells, B cells and macrophages. *Transpl. Rev.*, **13**, 3

39. Diener, E. and Feldmann, M. (1970). Antibody-mediated suppression of the immune response *in vitro*. II. A new approach to the phenomenon of immunological tolerance. *J. Exp. Med.*, **132**, 31

40. Dennert, G. (1973). Effect of IgM on the *in vivo* and *in vitro* immune response. *Proc. Soc. Exp. Biol. Med.*, **143**, 889

41. Schrader, J. W. and Nossal, G. J. V. (1974). Effector cell blockade. A new mechanism of immune hyporeactivity induced by multivalent antigens. *J. Exp. Med.*, **139**, 1582

42. Nossal, G. J. V. and Schrader, J. W. (1975). B-lymphocyte-antigen interactions in the inhibition of tolerance or immunity. *Transpl. Rev.*, **23**, 138

43. Howard, J. G. and Mitchinson, N. A. (1974). Immunological tolerance. *Prog. Allergy*, **18**, 274

44. Kontiainen, S. and Mitchinson, N. A. (1975). Blocking antigen–antibody complexes on the T-lymphocyte surface identified with defined protein antigens. I. Lymphocyte activation during the *in vitro* response. *Immunology*, **28**, 523

45. Hellström, H. E. and Hellström, I. (1974). Lymphocyte-mediated cytotoxicity and blocking serum activity to tumor antigens. *Adv. Immunol.*, **18**, 209

46. Stuart, F. P., Fitch, F. W., Rowley, D. A. and Biesecker, J. L. (1971). Presence of both cell-mediated immunity and serum-blocking factors in rat renal allografts 'enhanced' by passive immunization. *Transplantation*, **12**, 331

47. Biesecker, J. L., Fitch, F. W., Rowley, D. A., Scollard, D. and Stuart, F. P. (1973). Cellular and humoral immunity after allogenic transplantation in the rat. II. Comparison of a ^{51}Cr-release assay and modified microcytotoxicity assay for detection of cellular immunity and blocking-serum factors. *Transplantation*, **16**, 421

48. Scollard, D. (1975). Cellular cytotoxicity assays detect different effector cell types *in vitro*. *Transplantation*, **19**, 87

49. Cerottini, J. C. and Brunner, K. T. (1974). Cell-mediated cytotoxicity allograft rejection and tumor immunity. *Adv. Immunol.*, **18**, 67

50. McKearn, T. J., Stuart, F. P. and Fitch, F. W. (1974). Anti-idiotype antibody in rat transplantation immunity. I. Production of anti-idiotype antibody in animals repeatedly immunized with allogens. *J. Immunol.*, **113**, 1876

51. Nisonoff, A. and Bangasser, S. A. (1975). Immunological suppression of idiotype specificities. *Transpl. Rev.*, **27**, 100

52. Binz, H. and Wigzell, H. (1975). Shared idiotype determinants on B and T lymphocytes reactive against the same antigenic determinants. 1. Demonstration of similar or identical idiotypes on IgG molecules on T-cells receptors with specificity for the same alloantigens. *J. Exp. Med.*, **142**, 197

53. Eichmann, K. and Rajewsky, K. (1975). Induction of T and B cell immunity by anti-idiotypic antibody. *Eur. J. Immunol.*, **5**, 661

54. Eichmann, K. (1975). Idiotype suppression. II. Amplification of a suppressor T cell with anti-idiotypic activity. *Eur. J. Immunol.*, **5**, 511

55. McKearn, T. J., Hamada, Y., Stuart, F. P. and Fitch, F. W. (1974). Anti-receptor antibody and resistance to graft-versus-host reaction. *Nature (Lond.)*, **251**, 648

56. McKearn, T. J. (1974). Anti-receptor antiserum causes specific inhibition of reactivity to rat histocompatibility antigens. *Science*, **183**, 94

57. Dixon, F. J. (1963). The role of antigen–antibody complexes in disease. *Harvey Lectures*, **58**, 21

58. Arthus, M. and Breton, M. (1903). Lesions cutanées produits par les injections de sérum de cheval chez les lapins anaphylactisé par et pour ce sérum. *C. R. Soc. Biol. (Paris)*, **55**, 147

59. Cochrane, C. G., Weigle, W. O. and Dixon, F. J. (1959). The role of polymorphonuclear leukocytes in the initiation and cessation of the Arthus vasculitis. *J. Exp. Med.*, **110**, 481

60. Dixon, F. J., Vasques, J. J., Weigle, W. O. and Cochrane, C. G. (1958). The pathogenesis of serum sickness. *A.M.A. Arch. Pathol.*, **65**, 18

61. Cochrane, C. G. and Dixon, F. J. (1976). Antigen–antibody complex induced disease. In: *Textbook of Immunopathology* (P. A. Miescher and H. J. Müller-Eberhard, eds.), vol. 1, pp. 137–156 (New York: Grune and Stratton)

62. Dixon, F. J., Feldman, J. D. and Vazques, J. J. (1961). Experimental glomerulonephritis. The pathogenesis of a laboratory model resembling the spectrum of glomerulonephritis. *J. Exp. Med.*, **113**, 899

63. Kniker, W. T. and Cochrane, C. G. (1968). Localization of circulating antigen–antibody complexes in serum sickness: the role of vasoactive and hydrodynamic forces. *J. Exp. Med.*, **127**, 119

64. Andres, G. A., Morgan, C., Hsu, K. C., Rifkind, R. A. and Seegal, B. C. (1962). Electron microscopic studies of experimental nephritis with ferritin-conjugated antibody. The basement membranes and cisternae of visceral epithelial cells in nephritic rat glomeruli. *J. Exp. Med.*, **115**, 929

65. Wilson, C. B. and Dixon, F. J. (1974). Diagnosis of immunopathological renal disease. *Kidney Int.*, **5**, 389

66. Steffelaar, J. W., De Graaff-Reitsma, C. B. and Feltkamp, T. M. (1976). Immune complex detection by immuno-fluorescence on peripheral blood polymorphonuclear leucocytes. *Clin. Exp. Immunol.*, **23**, 272

67. Britton, M. C. and Schur, P. H. (1971). The complement system in rheumatoid synovitis. II. Intracytoplasmic inclusions of immunoglobulins and complement. *Arthritis Rheum.*, **14**, 87

68. Koffler, D., Schur, P. H. and Kunkel, H. G. (1967). Immunological studies concerning the nephritis of systemic lupus erythematosus. *J. Exp. Med.*, **126**, 607

69. Lambert, P. H. and Dixon, F. J. (1968). Pathogenesis of the glomerulonephritis of NZB/W mice. *J. Exp. Med.*, **127**, 507

70. Zubler, R. H. and Lambert, P. H. (1977). Immune complexes in clinical investigation. In: *Recent Advances in Clinical Immunology* (R. A. Thompson, ed.), vol. 1, pp. 125–147 (Edinburgh: Churchill Livingstone)

71. Zubler, R. H. and Lambert, P. H. (1978). Detection of immune complexes in human diseases. *Prog. Allergy*, **24**, 1

72. Lambert, P. H. and Casali, P. (1978). Immune complexes and the rheumatic diseases. *Clinics in Rheumatic Diseases*, **4** (In press)

73. Almeida, J. D. and Wadsworth, C. (1969). Immune complexes in hepatitis. *Lancet*, **ii**, 983

74. Jose, D. G. and Seshadri, R. (1974). Circulating immune complexes in human neuroblastoma: direct assay and role in blocking specific cellular immunity. *Int. J. Cancer*, **13**, 824

75. Notkins, A. L., Mahar, S., Scheele, C. and Goffman, J. (1966). Infectious virus–antibody complex in the blood of chronically infected mice. *J. Exp. Med.*, **124**, 81

76. Izui, S., Lambert, P. H. and Miescher, P. A. (1977). Failure to detect circulating DNA–anti-DNA complexes by four radioimmunological methods in patients with systemic lupus erythematosus. *Clin. Exp. Immunol.*, **30**, 384

77. Harbeck, R. J., Bardana, E. J., Kohler, P. F. and Carr, R. I. (1973). DNA–anti-DNA complexes: their detection in systemic lupus erythematosus sera. *J. Clin. Invest.*, **52**, 789

78. Houba, V., Lambert, P. H., Voller, A. and Soyanwo, M. A. O. (1976). Clinical and experimental investigation of immune complexes in malaria. *Clin. Immunol. Immunopathol.*, **6**, 1

79. Fox, A. E., Plescia, O. J. and Mellors, R. C. (1974). Assay and characterization of polyanion–immunoglobulin complexes in sera of New Zealand Black mice. *Immunology*, **26**, 367

80. Kinkel, H. G., Müller-Eberhard, H. J., Fudenberg, H. H. and Tomasi, T. B. (1961). Gamma globulin complexes in rheumatoid arthritis and certain other conditions. *J. Clin. Invest.*, **40**, 117

81. Grubb, A. O. (1975). Demonstration of circulating IgG–lactate desydrogenase immune complexes by crossed immunoelectrophoresis. *Scand. J. Immunol.*, **4** (Suppl. 2), 53

82. Teppo, A. M., Haltia, K. and Wager, O. (1976). Immunoelectrophorectic 'tailing' of albumin due to albumin–IgG complexes. A side-effect of nitrofurantion treatment? *Scand. J. Immunol.*, **5**, 249

83. Heimer, R. and Abruzzo, J. L. (1972). A latex test for the detection of IgG aggregates and IgG–anti-IgG antibody. *Immunochemistry*, **9**, 921

84. Myllylä, G., Vaheri, A. and Penttinen, K. (1971). Detection and characterization of immune complexes by the platelet aggregation test. II. Circulating complexes. *Clin. Exp. Immunol.*, **8**, 399

85. Bjorvatn, B., Barnetson, R. S., Kronvall, G., Zubler, R. H. and Lambert, P. H. (1976). Immune complexes and complement hypercatabolism with leprosy. *Clin. Exp. Immunol.*, **26**, 388

86. Bokisch, V. A., Müller-Eberhard, H. J. and Dixon, F. J. (1974). Complement. A potential mediator of the hemorrhagic shock syndrome (dengue). *Adv. Biosci.*, **12**, 417

87. Ooi Yuet, M., Vallota, E. H. and West, C. D. (1977). Serum immune complexes in membranoproliferative and other glomerulonephritis. *Kidney Int.*, **11**, 275

88. Ludwig, F. J. and Cusumano, C. L. (1974). Detection of immune complexes using ^{125}I-goat anti (human IgG) monovalent (Fab) antibody fragments. *J. Nat. Cancer Inst.*, **52**, 1529

89. Brouet, J. C., Clauvel, J. P., Danon, F., Klein, M. and Seligmann, M. (1974). Biologic and clinical significance of cryoglobulins. *Am. J. Med.*, **57**, 775

90. Cream, J. J. (1977). Immune complexes in cryoprecipitates. *Ann. Rheum. Dis.*, **36** (Suppl. 1), 45

91. Creighton, W. D., Lambert, P. H. and Miescher, P. A. (1973). Detection of antibodies and soluble antigen–antibody complexes by precipitation with polyethylene glycol. *J. Immunol.*, **111**, 1219

92. Zubler, R. H., Perrin, L. H., Creighton, W. D. and Lambert, P. H. (1977). The use of polyethylene glycol (PEG) to concentrate immune complexes from serum or plasma samples. *Ann. Rheum. Dis.*, **36** (Suppl. 1), 23

93. Bout, D., Santoro, F., Carlier, Y., Bina, J. C. and Capron, A. (1977). Circulating immune complexes in schistosomiasis. *Immunology*, **33**, 17

94. Digeon, M., Laver, M., Riza, J. and Bach, J. F. (1977). Detection of circulating immune complexes in human sera by simplified assays with polyethylene glycol. *J. Immunol. Method*, **16**, 165

95. Zubler, R. H., Lange, G., Lambert, P. H. and Miescher, P. A. (1976). Detection of immune complexes in unheated sera by a modified ^{125}I-C1q binding test. Effect of heating on the binding of C1q by immune complexes and application of the test to systemic lupus erythematosus. *J. Immunol.*, **116**, 232

96. Hällgren, R. and Wide, L. (1976). Detection of circulating IgG aggregates and immune complexes using ^{125}I protein A from *Staphylococcus aureus*. *Ann. Rheum. Dis.*, **35**, 306

97. Lambert, P. H., Dixon, F. J., Zubler, R. H., Agnello, V., Cambiaso, C., Casali, P., Clarke, J., Cowdery, J. S., McDuffie, F. C., MacLenna, I. C. M., Masson, P., Müller-Eberhard, H. J., Pentinen, K., Smith, M., Tappeiner, G., Theofilopoulos, A. N. and Verroust, P. (1978). A collaborative study for the evaluation of eighteen methods for detecting complexes in serum. *J. Clin. Lab. Immunol.*, **1**, 1

98. Nielsen, H. and Svehag, S. E. (1976). Detection and differentiation of immune complexes and IgG aggregates by a complement consumption assay. *Acta Pathol. Microbiol. Scand., Sect. C*, **84**, 261

99. Johnson, A. H., Mowbray, J. F. and Porter, K. A. (1975). Detection of circulating immune complexes in pathological human sera. *Lancet*, **i**, 762

100. Sobel, A. T., Bokisch, V. A. and Müller-Eberhard, H. J. (1975). C1q deviation test for the detection of immune complexes, aggregates of IgG and bacterial products in human sera. *J. Exp. Med.*, **142**, 139

101. Gabriel, A. Jr. and Agnello, V. (1977). Detection of immune complexes. The use of radioimmunoassays with C1q and monoclonal factor. *J. Clin. Invest.*, **59**, 990

102. Lurhuma, A. Z., Cambiaso, C. L., Masson, P. L. and Heremans, J. F. (1976). Detection of circulating antigen–antibody complexes by their inhibitory effect on the agglutination of IgG-coated particles by rheumatoid factor or C1q. *Clin. Exp. Immunol.*, **25**, 212

103. Agnello, V., Winchester, R. J. and Kunkel, H. G. (1970). Precipitin reactions of the C1q component of complement with aggregated γ-globulin and immune complexes in gel diffusion. *Immunology*, **19**, 909

104. Zubler, R. H. and Lambert, P. H. (1976). The ^{125}I-C1q binding test for the detection of soluble immune complexes. In: In Vitro *Methods in Cell-Mediated and Tumor Immunity* Bloom and David, eds.), pp. 565–572 (New York: Academic Press)

105. Hay, F. C., Nineham, L. J. and Roitt, I. M. (1976). Routine assay for the detection of immune complexes of known immunoglobulin class using solid phase C1q. *Clin. Exp. Immunol.*, **24**, 396

106. Ahstedt, S., Hanson, L. A. and Wadsworth, C. (1976). A C1q immunoabsorbant assay compared with thin-layer gel filtration for measuring IgG aggregates. *Scand. J. Immunol.*, **5**, 293

107. Eisenberg, R. A., Theofilopoulos, A. N. and Dixon, F. J. (1977). Use of bovine conglutinin for the assay of immune complexes. *J. Immunol.*, **118**, 1428

108. Casali, P., Bosus, A., Carpentier, N. A. and Lambert, P. H. (1977). Solid-phase enzyme immunoassay or radioimmunoassay for the detection of immune complexes based on

their recognition by conglutinin: conglutinin-binding test. A comparative study with ^{125}I-labelled C1q binding and Raji cell-RIA tests. *Clin. Exp. Immunol.*, **29**, 342

109. Casali, P. and Lambert, P. H. (1978). Purification of soluble immune complexes by polymethylmethacrylate beads coated with conglutinin or C1q. Submitted for publication

110. Winchester, R. J., Kunkel, H. G. and Agnello, V. (1971). Occurrence of γ-globulin complexes in serum and joint fluid of rheumatoid arthritis patients: use of monoclonal rheumatoid factors as reagent for their demonstration. *J. Exp. Med.*, **134** (Suppl.), 286

111. Luthra, H. S., McDuffie, F. C., Hunder, G. G. and Smayoa, E. A. (1975). Immune complexes in sera and synovial fluids of patients with rheumatoid arthritis. Radioimmunoassay with monoclonal rheumatoid factor. *J. Clin. Invest.*, **56**, 458

112. Cowdery, J. S., Treadwell, P. E. and Fritz, R. B. (1975). A radioimmunoassay for human antigen–antibody complexes in clinical material. *J. Immunol.*, **114**, 50

113. Kano, K., Nishimaki, T., Palosuo, T., Loza, V. and Milgrom, F. (1978). Detection of circulating immune complexes by the inhibition of the anti-antibody. *Clin. Immunol. Immunopathol.*, **9**, 425

114. Theofilopoulos, A. N. and Dixon, F. J. (1976). Immune complexes in human sera detected by the Raji cell radioimmune assay. In: In Vitro *Methods in Cell-Mediated and Tumor Immunity* (Bloom and David, eds.), pp. 555–563 (New York: Academic Press)

115. Smith, M. D., Barrat, T. M., Hayward, A. R. and Scoothill, J. F. (1975). The inhibition of complement-dependent lymphocytes rosette formation by the sera of children with steroid-sensitive nephrotic syndrome and other renal diseases. *Clin. Exp. Immunol.*, **21**, 236

116. Myllylä, G. (1973). Aggregation of human blood platelets by immune complexes in the sedimentation pattern test. *Scand. J. Haematol.*, Suppl. 19

117. Roberts-Thompson, P. J., Hazleman, B. L., Barnett, I. G. MacLennan, I. C. M. and Mowat, A. G. (1976). Factors relating to circulating immune complexes in rheumatoid arthritis. *Ann. Rheum. Dis.*, **35**, 314

118. Mohammed, I., Thompson, B. R. and Holborow, E. J. (1977). Radiobioassay for immune complexes using macrophages. *Ann. Rheum. Dis.*, **36** (Suppl. 1), 49

119. Steffelaar, W., Ten Kate, F. J. W., Nap, M., Seaak, A. G. J., Greeff-Reitsma, C. De, Elven, E. H. van, and Feltkamp-Vroom, T. M. (1977). Immune complexes detection by immunofluorescence on polymorphonuclear leukocytes. *Clin. Exp. Immunol.*, **27**, 391

120. Morito, T., Tanimoto, K., Hashimoto, Y., Horiuchi, Y. and Juji, T. (1976). Fc-rosette inhibition by hypocomplementaemic systemic lupus erythematosus sera. *Ann. Rheum. Dis.*, **35**, 415

121. Zvaifler, N. J. (1969). Breakdown products of C3 in human synovial fluids. *J. Clin. Invest.*, **48**, 1532

122. Perrin, L. H., Lambert, P. H. and Miescher, P. A. (1975). Complement breakdown products in plasma from patients with systemic lupus erythematosus and patients with membranoproliferative or other glomerulonephritis. *J. Clin. Invest.*, **56**, 165

123. Mergenhagen, S. E., Snyderman, R. and Phillips, J. K. (1973). Activation of complement by endotoxin. In: *Bacterial Lipopolysaccharides* (E. H. Wass and S. M. Wolff, eds.), pp. 78–82 (Chicago: University of Chicago Press)

124. Loos, M. D., Bitter Suermann, D. and Dierich, M. (1974). Interaction of the first (C1), the second (C2) and the fourth (C4) component of complement with different preparations of bacterial lipopolysaccharides and with lipid A. *J. Immunol.*, **112**, 935

125. Winkelstein, J. A., Bocchini, J. A. Jr. and Schiffman, G. (1976). The role of the capsular polysaccharide in the activation of the alternative pathway by the pneumococcus. *J. Immunol.*, **116**, 367

126. Morrison, D. C. and Kline, L. F. (1977). Activation of the classical and proerdin pathways of complement by bacterial lypopolysaccharides (LPS). *J. Immunol.*, **118**, 362

127. WHO, Report of a scientific group (1977). The role of immune complexes in disease. *WHO Technical Series*, No. 606

128. Stollar, V. (1975). Immune lysis of sindbis virus. *Virology*, **66**, 620

129. Joseph, B. S., Cooper, N. R. and Oldstone, M. B. A. (1975). Immunologic injury of cultured cell infected with measles virus. I. Role of IgG antibody and the alternative complement pathway. *J. Exp. Med.*, **141**, 761

130. Joseph, B. S. and Oldstone, M. B. A. (1974). Antibody induced redistribution of measles virus antigen on the cell surface. *J. Immunol.*, **113**, 1205

131. Notkins, A. L., Mergenhagen, S. E., Rizzo, A. A., Scheele, C. and Waldmann, T. A. (1966). Elevated γ-globulin and increased antibody production in mice infected with lactic dehydrogenase virus. *J. Exp. Med.*, **123**, 347

132. Oldstone, M. B. A. and Dixon, F. J. (1969). Pathogenesis of chronic disease associated with persistent lymphocytic chroriomeningitis viral infection. I. Relationship of antibody production to disease in neonatally infected mice. *J. Exp. Med.*, **129**, 483

133. Oldstone, M. B. A. and Dixon, F. J. (1970). Persistent lymphocytic choriomeningitis viral infection. III. Virus–anti-viral antibody complexes and associated chronic disease following transplacental infection. *J. Immunol.*, **105**, 829

134. Oldstone, M. B. A. and Dixon, F. J. (1970). Pathogenesis of chronic disease associated with persistent lymphocytic choriomeningitis viral infection. Relationship of the anti-lymphocytic choriomeningitis immune response to tissue injury in chronic lymphocytic choriomeningitis disease. *J. Exp. Med.*, **131**, 1

135. Buchmeier, M. J. and Oldstone, M. B. A. (1978). Virus induced immune complex disease: identification of specific viral antigens and antibodies deposited in complexes during chronic lymphocytic choriomeningitis infection. *J. Immunol.*, **120**, 1297

136. Hirsch, M., Allison, A. and Harvey, J. (1969). Immune complexes in mice infected neonatally with Moloney leukaemogenic and murine sarcoma viruses. *Nature (Lond.)*, **223**, 739

137. Bendinelli, M. and Nardini, L. (1973). Immunodepression by Rowson–Parr virus in mice. I. Growth curves of Rowson–Parr virus and immunological relationship with Friend virus. *Infect. Immun.*, **7**, 152

138. Tonietti, G., Oldstone, M. B. A. and Dixon, F. J. (1970). The effect of induced chronic viral infections on the immunologic diseases of New Zealand mice. *J. Exp. Med.*, **132**, 89

139. Sun, S., Burch, B., Sohal, R. and Chu, K. (1967). Coxsackie B4 viral nephritis in mice and its autoimmune-like phenomena. *Proc. Soc. Exp. Biol.*, **126**, 882

140. Peterson, J. M., Dienstag, J. L. and Purcell, R. H. (1975). Immune response to hepatitis B viruses. In: *Viral Immunology and Immunopathology* (A. L. Notkins, ed.), pp. 213–237 (New York: Academic Press)

141. Edgington, T. S. and Ritt, S. J. (1971). Intrahepatic expression of serum hepatitis virus associated antigens. *J. Exp. Med.*, **134**, 871

142. Sergent, J. S., Loreskin, M. D. and Christian, C. L. (1976). Vasculitis with hepatitis B antigenemia: long-term observation in nine patients. *Medicine (Baltimore)*, **55**, 1

143. Nydegger, U. E., Lambert, P. H., Gerber, H. and Miescher, P. A. (1974). Circulating immune complexes in the serum in systemic lupus erythematosus and in carriers of hepatitis B antigen. Quantitation by binding to radiolabelled C1q. *J. Clin. Invest.*, **54**, 297

144. Theofilopoulos, A. N., Wilson, C. B. and Dixon, F. J. (1976). The Raji cell radioimmune assay for detecting immune complexes in human sera. *J. Clin. Invest.*, **57**, 169

145. Gocke, D. J., Hsu, K., Morgan, C., Bombardieri, S., Locksin, M. and Christian, C. L. (1970). Association between polyarteritis and Australia antigen. *Lancet*, **ii**, 1149

146. Trepo, C. Q., Zuckerman, A. J., Bird, R. C. and Prince, A. M. (1974). The role of circulating hepatitis B antigen–antibody complexes in the pathogenesis of vascular and hepatic manifestations in polyarteritis nodosa. *J. Clin. Pathol.*, **27**, 863

147. Levo, Y., Gorevic, P. D., Kassab, H. J., Zucker-Franklin, D. and Franklin, E. C. (1977). Association between hepatitis B virus and essential mixed cryoglobulinemia. *N. Engl. J. Med.*, **296**, 1501

148. Russel, P. K. (1971). Immunopathologic mechanism in the Dengue shock syndrome. In: *Progress in Immunology* (B. Amos, ed.), pp. 831–838 (New York: Academic Press)

149. Russel, P. K., Intavitat, A. and Kanchanapilant, S. (1969). Anti-Dengue immunoglobulins and serum B1C/a globulin levels in dengue shock syndrome. *J. Immunol.*, **102**, 412

150. Bokish, V. A., Franklin, H. T., Russel, P. K., Dixon, F. J. and Müller-Eberhard, H. J. (1973). The potential pathogenic role of complement in Dengue hemorrhagic shock syndrome. *N. Engl. J. Med.*, **289**, 996

151. Henle, W. and Henle, G. (1975). Immune responses to Epstein–Barr virus. In: *Viral Immunology and Immunopathology* (A. E. Notkins, ed.), pp. 261–273 (New York: Academic Press)

152. Wands, J. R., Perotto, J. L. and Isselbucher, K. J. (1976). Circulating immune complexes and complement sequence activation in infectious mononucleosis. *Am. J. Med.*, **60**, 269

153. McKensie, H., Parrate, D. and White, R. G. (1976). IgM and IgG antibody levels to ampicilline in patients with infectious mononucleosis. *Clin. Exp. Immunol.*, **26**, 214

154. Oldstone, M. B. A., Theofilopoulos, A. N., Gunven, P. and Klein, G. (1975). Immune complexes associated with neoplasia: presence of Epstein–Barr virus antigen–antibody complexes in Burkitt's lymphoma. *Intervirology*, **4**, 292

155. Heimer, R. and Klein, G. (1976). Circulating immune complexes in sera of patients with Burkitt's lymphoma and masopharyngal carcinoma. *Int. J. Cancer*, **18**, 310

156. Sever, J. L. and Zeman, W. (1968). Conference on measles virus and subacute sclerosing panencephalitis. *Neurology*, **18**, 1

157. Dayan, A. D. and Stokes, M. I. (1972). Immune complexes and visceral deposits of measles antigens in subacute sclerosing panencephalitis. *Br. Med. J.*, **2**, 374

158. Phillips, P. E. (1972). Immune complexes in subacute sclerosing panencephalitis. *N. Engl. J. Med.*, **286**, 949

159. Oldstone, M. B. A., Bokish, V. A., Dixon, F. J., Barbosa, L. H., Fuccillo, D. and Sever, J. L. (1975). Subacute sclerosing panencephalitis: destruction of human brain cells by antibody and complement in an autologous system. *Clin. Immunol. Immunopathol.*, **4**, 52

160. Ahmeed, A., Strong, D. M., Sell, K. W., Thurmann, G. B., Knudsen, R. C., Wistar, R. and Grace, W. R. (1974). Demonstration of a blocking factor in the plasma and spinal fluid of patients with subacute sclerosing panencephalitis. *J. Exp. Med.*, **139**, 902

161. Zabriskie, J. B. (1971). The role of streptococci in human glomerulonephritis. *J. Exp. Med.*, **134** (Suppl.), 180

162. Read, S. E. and Zabriskie, J. B. (1976). Immunological concepts in rheumatic fever pathogenesis. In: *Textbook of Immunopathology* (P. A. Miescher and H. J. Müller-Eberhard, eds.), vol. 1, pp. 471–487 (New York: Grune and Stratton)

163. Rammelkamp, C. H. Jr. (1957). Microbiological aspects of glomerulonephritis. *J. Chronic. Dis.*, **5**, 28

164. Rammelkamp, C. H. Jr. (1953). Glomerulonephritis. *Proc. Inst. Med. Chicago*, **19**, 371

165. Lange, K., Wassermann, E. and Slobody, L. B. (1960). The significance of serum complement levels for the diagnosis and prognosis of acute and subacute glomerulonephritis and lupus erythematosus. *Ann. Intern. Med.*, **53**, 636

166. Fish, A. J., Herdman, R. C., Michael, A. F., Pickering, R. J. and Good, R. A. (1970). Epidemic acute glomerulonephritis associated with type 49 streptococcal pyoderma. II. Correlative study of light, immunofluorescent and electron microscopic findings. *Am. J. Med.*, **48**, 28

167. Andres, G. A., Accinni, L., Hsu, K. C., Zabriskie, J. B. and Seegal, B. C. (1966). Electron microscopic studies of human glomerulonephritis with ferritin-conjugated antibody. Localization of antigen–antibody complexes in glomerular structures of patients with acute glomerulonephritis. *J. Exp. Med.*, **123**, 399

168. Treser, G., Sermar, M., Ty, A., Sagel, I., Franklin, M. A. and Lange, K. (1970). Partial characterization of antigenic streptococcal plasma membrane components in acute glomerulonephritis. *J. Clin. Invest.*, **49**, 762

169. Zabriskie, J. B., Utermoblen, V., Read, S. E. and Fischetti, V. A. (1973). Streptococcus-related glomerulonephritis. *Kidney Int.*, **3**, 100

170. McIntosh, R. M., Kaufman, D. B., Kulvinskas, C. and Grossman, B. J. (1970). Cryo-globulins. I. Studies on the nature, incidence, and clinical significance of serum cryoproteins in glomerulonephritis. *J. Lab. Clin. Med.*, **75**, 566

171. Wilson, C. B. and Dixon, F. J. (1976). Renal response to immunological injury. In: *The Kidney* (B. M. Brenner and R. C. Rector Jr., eds.), pp. 838–940 (Philadelphia: Saunders)

172. Markowitz, A. S. and Lange, C. F. (1964). Streptococcal-related glomerulonephritis. I. Isolation, immunochemistry and comparative chemistry of soluble fractions from type 12 nephritogenic streptococci and human glomeruli. *J. Immunol.*, **92**, 565

173. Yeh, B. P. Y., Young, H. F., Schatzki, P. F. and Bear, E. S. (1977). Immune complex disease associated with an infected ventriculojugular shunt: a curable form of glomerulonephritis. *South. Med. J.*, **70**, 1141

174. Pertschur, L. P., Vuletin, J. C., Sutton, A. L. and Velasquez, L. A. (1976). Demonstration of antigen and immune complex in glomerulonephritis due to staphylococcus aureus. *Am. J. Clin. Pathol.*, **66**, 1027

175. Glassock, R. J., Bennett, C. M., Cohen, A. H. and Zamboni, L. (1976). The glomerulopathis. In: *The Kidney* (B. M. Brenner and F. C. Rector, eds.), pp. 941–1078 (Philadelphia: Saunders)

176. Gutman, R. A., Striker, G. E., Gilliland, B. C. and Cutler, R. E. (1978). The immune complex glomerulonephritis of bacterial endocardis. *Medicine*, **51**, 1

177. Keslin, M. H., Messner, R. P. and Williams, R. C. (1973). Glomerulonephritis with subacute bacterial endocarditis. *Arch. Intern. Med.*, **132**, 578

178. Levy, R. L. and Hong, R. (1973). The immune nature of subacute bacterial endocarditis (SBE) nephritis. *Am. J. Med.*, **54**, 645

179. Perez, G. O., Rothfield, N. and Williams, R. C. (1976). Immune complex nephritis in bacterial endocarditis. *Arch. Intern. Med.*, **136**, 334

180. Arnold, S. B., Valone, J. A., Askenase, P. W., Kashgarian, M. and Freedman, L. R. (1975). Diffuse glomerulonephritis in rabbits with streptococcus viridans endocarditis. *Lab. Invest.*, **32**, 681

181. Bayer, A. S., Theofilopoulos, A. N., Eisenberg, R., Dixon, F. J. and Guze, L. B. (1976). Circulating immune complexes in infective endocarditis. *N. Engl. J. Med.*, **295**, 1200

182. Lew, P. D., Zubler, R. H., Vaudaux, P., Farquet, J. J., Waldvogel, F. A. and Lambert, P. H. (1978). Decreased heat labile opsonic activity and complement levels associated with evidence of C3 breakdown products in infected pleural effusions. *J. Clin. Invest.* (In press)

183. Godal, T. (1974). The role of immune responses to mycobacterium lepra in host defence and tissue damage in leprosy. In: *Progress in Immunology II* (L. Brent and J. Holborow, eds.), pp. 161–169 (Amsterdam: North Holland Publishing Co.)

184. Kronvall, G., Stanford, J. L. and Walsh, G. P. (1976). Studies of mycobacterial antigens with special reference to mycobacterium leprae. *Infect. Immun.*, **13**, 113

185. Wemambu, S. N. C., Turk, J. L., Waters, M. F. R. and Rees, R. J. W. (1969). Erythema-nodosum leprosum: a clinical manifestation of the Arthus phenomenon. *Lancet*, **ii**, 933

186. Waters, M. F. R. and Riddley, D. S. (1963). Necrotizing reactions in lepromatous leprosy. A clinical and histological study. *Int. J. Leprosy*, **31**, 418

187. Iveson, J. M. I., McDougall, A. C., Leatham, A. J. and Harris, A. J. (1975). Lepromatous leprosy presenting with polyarthritis myositis and immune complexes glomerulonephritis. *Br. Med. J.*, **3**, 619

188. Moran, C. J., Turk, J. L., Ryder, G. and Waters, M. F. R. (1972). Evidence for circulating immune complexes in lepromatous leprosy. *Lancet*, **ii**, 572

189. Rojas-Espinosa, O., Mendez-Navarette, I. and Estrada-Parra, S. (1972). Presence of C1q-reactive immune complexes in patients with leprosy. *Clin. Exp. Immunol.*, **12**, 215
190. Gelber, R. H., Druts, D. J., Epstein, W. V. and Fasal, P. (1974). Clinical correlates of C1q precipitating substances in the sera of patients with leprosy. *Am. J. Trop. Med. Hyg.*, **23**, 471
191. Bonomo, L. and Dammacco, F. (1971). Immune complex cryoglobulinemia in lepromatous leprosy: a pathogenic approach to some clinical features of leprosy. *Clin. Exp. Immunol.*, **9**, 175
192. Saitz, E. W., Dierks, R. E. and Shepard, C. C. (1968). Complement and second component of complement in leprosy. *Int. J. Leprosy*, **36**, 400
193. Malaviya, A. N., Pasricha, A., Pasticha, F. S. and Metha, J. S. (1972). Significance of serologic abnormalities in lepromatous leprosy. *Int. J. Leprosy*, **40**, 361
194. Petchclai, B., Chutanondh, R., Prasongsom, S., Hiranras, S. and Ramasoota, T. (1973). Complement profile in leprosy. *Am. J. Trop. Med. Hyg.*, **22**, 761
195. Lambert, P. H. and Houba, V. (1974). Immune complexes in parasitic disease. In: *Progress in Immunology II* (L. Brent and J. Holborow, eds.), pp. 57–67 (Amsterdam: North Holland Publishing Co.)
196. Berger, M., Birch, L. M. and Conte, N. F. (1967). The nephrotic syndrome secondary to acute glomerulonephritis during falciparum malaria. *Ann. Intern. Med.*, **67**, 1163
197. WHO, report of a scientific group (1975). Developments in malaria immunology. *WHO Technical Report Series*, No. 579
198. Bhamaraoravatu, N., Boonpucknavig, S., Boonpucknavig, V. and Yaemboonruang, C. (1973). Glomerular changes in acute plasmodium falciparum infection. An immunopathologic study. *Arch. Pathol.*, **69**, 289
199. Powell, K. C. and Meadows, R. (1971). The nephrotic syndrome in New Guinea. A clinical and histological spectrum. *Aust. and N. Zealand J. Med.*, **4**, 363
200. Ward, P. A. and Conran, P. B. (1969). Immunopathology of renal complications in simian malaria and human quartan malaria. *Milit. Med.*, **134**, 1228
201. Allison, A. C., Houba, V., Hendrickse, R. G., de Petris, S., Edington, G. M. and Adeniyi, A. (1969). Immune complexes in the nephrotic syndrome of African children. *Lancet*, **i**, 1232
202. Houba, V., Allison, A. C., Adeniyi, A. and Houba, J. E. (1971). Immunoglobulin classes and complement in biopsies of nigerian children with the nephrotic syndrome. *Clin. Exp. Immunol.*, **8**, 761
203. Houba, V., Koech, D. K., Sturrock, R. F., Butterworth, A. E., Kusel, J. R. and Mahmoud, A. F. (1976). Soluble antigens and antibodies in sera from baboons infected with schistosoma mansoni. *J. Immunol.*, **117**, 705
204. Voller, A., Davies, D. R. and Hutt, H. S. R. (1973). Quarton malarial infections in aotus trivirciatus with special reference to renal pathology. *Br. J. Exp. Pathol.*, **54**, 457
205. Nagle, R. B., Ward, P. A., Lindsley, H. B., Sadun, E. H., Johnson, A. J., Berkaw, R. E. and Hildebrandt, P. K. (1974). Experimental infections with African trypanosomes. VI. Glomerulonephritis involving the alternate pathway of complement activation. *Am. J. Trop. Med. Hyg.*, **23**, 15
206. Castro, B. G. F., Hochmann, A. and Lambert, P. H. (1978). The role of the host-immune response in the development of tissue lesions associated with African trypanosomiasis in mice. *Clin. Exp. Immunol.*, **33**, 12
207. Silva, L. C., Brito, T. de, Camargo, M. E., Boni, D. de, Lopez, J. D. and Gunji, J. (1970). Kidney biopsy in the hepatosplenic form of infection with schistosoma mansoni in man. *Bull. WHO*, **42**, 907
208. Andrade, Z. A., Andrade, S. G. and Sadigurska, M. (1971). Renal changes in patients with hepatosplenic schistotomiasis. *Am. J. Trop. Med. Hyg.*, **20**, 77

209. Queiroz, F. P., Brito, E., Martinelli, R. and Rocha, H. (1973). Nephrotic syndrome in patients with schistosoma mansoni infection. *Am. J. Trop. Med. Hyg.*, **22**, 622

210. Natali, P. G. and Cioli, D. (1976). Immune complex nephritis in schistosoma mansoni infected mice. *Eur. J. Immunol.*, **6**, 359

211. Berggren, W. L. and Weller, T. H. (1967). Immunoelectrophoretic demonstration of specific circulating antigen in animals infected with schistosoma mansoni. *Am. J. Trop. Med. Hyg.*, **16**, 606

212. Gold, R., Rosen, F. S. and Weller, T. H. (1969). A specific circulating antigen in hamsters infected with schistosoma mansoni. Detection of antigen in serum and urine, and correlation between antigenic concentration and worm burden. *Am. J. Trop. Med. Hyg.*, **18**, 545

213. Madwar, M. A. and Voller, A. (1975). Circulating soluble antigens and antibody in schistosomiasis. *Br. Med. J.*, **1**, 435

214. Smith, M. D., Verroust, P. J., Morel-Maroger, L. M., Pasticier, A. and Couland, J. P. (1975). Circulating immune complexes in schistosomiasis. *Br. Med. J.*, **2**, 274

215. Phillips, T. M. and Draper, C. C. (1975). Circulating immune complexes in schistosomiasis. *Br. Med. J.*, **2**, 476

216. Houba, V., Butterworth, A. E., Sturrock, R. F. (1977). Eosinophils and the immune response. In: *Immunopathology* (P. A. Miescher, ed.), vol. 7, pp. 233–243 (Basel: Schwabe)

10
Infection in the Compromised Host

E. H. NAUTA

10.1	INTRODUCTION	344
10.2	DEFENCE DISTURBANCES	350
10.3	PREDISPOSING FACTORS	355
10.4	RELATIONSHIP BETWEEN THE UNDERLYING DISEASE AND REDUCED RESISTANCE	357
10.5	THE RELATIONSHIP BETWEEN DEFECTIVE RESISTANCE AND THE TYPE OF INFECTION	360
	10.5.1 *Bacterial infections*	360
	10.5.2 *Non-bacterial infections*	361
	10.5.2.1 *Fungal infections*	361
	10.5.2.2 *Protozoal infections*	361
	10.5.2.3 *Viral infections*	362
10.6	CLINICAL PICTURES OF INFECTIONS SEEN IN VARIOUS UNDERLYING DISEASES	362
	10.6.1 *Acute leukaemia in adults*	362
	10.6.2 *Clinical pictures*	364
	10.6.2.1 *The teeth*	367
	10.6.2.2 *Urinary tract infections*	367
	10.6.2.3 *Septicaemia*	368
	10.6.2.4 *Hepatitis B*	368
	10.6.3 *Infections in Hodgkin's disease and other lymphoproliferative disorders*	368
	10.6.4 *Infections in acute lymphatic leukaemia*	369
	10.6.5 *Multiple myeloma and Waldenström's disease*	369

10.6.6   *Infections after splenectomy*   370
10.6.7   *Infections after organ transplantation*   370

10.7   DIAGNOSIS AND TREATMENT OF INFECTIONS   370

10.8   ADDITIONAL THERAPY   374
10.8.1   *Granulocyte transfusion*   374
10.8.2   *Isolation and decontamination*   376
         10.8.2.1   *Reverse isolation*   376
         10.8.2.2   *Decontamination*   376
10.8.3   *Reinforcement of body defences*   377

10.1   INTRODUCTION

Man lives in an environment populated by micro-organisms. He is continually in contact with his own rich flora of bacteria, fungi, and any other parasites on the internal and external surfaces of his body and with the microflora in the world around him. An idea of approximately how many bacteria there are in the flora of an individual is given by the following

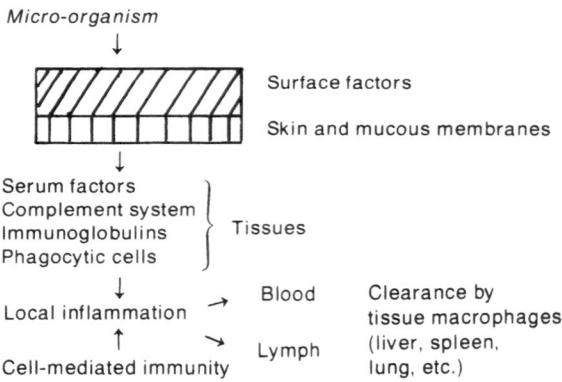

Figure 10.1   Schematic representation of defence against micro-organisms

numbers. The surface of the skin and mucous membranes carry about 10^{14} bacteria, the skin accounting for approximately 10^{12}, comprising staphylococci, micrococci, and corynebacteria; the entire digestive tract carries about 10^{14} bacteria, 10^{10} of them residing in the mouth. The proximal part of the small intestine has 10^2 to 10^3 bacteria per ml and the concentration in the rectum reaches 10^{12} bacteria per g of faeces. The mucous membranes of the urinary tract and the lower respiratory tract are sterile.

For defence against these (potentially pathogenic) micro-organisms, the human body has several mechanisms at its disposal. Every congenital or acquired weakness in the links of this chain of mechanisms means an increased chance of infection. A patient with one or more disturbances in this defence system is described as 'compromised'. Conversely, every infection (disease) can be seen as reflecting a defect in the defence system. In the developed countries of the world pathogenic micro-organisms play a smaller role in infections (for example in epidemics) than reduced resistance with respect to the normal microflora of the host[1].

Table 10.1   Host resistance to infection

Body surfaces

Skin – horn layer, desquamation, skin microflora, pH (fatty acids, lactic acid), lysozyme

Mucous membranes – epithelial layer, adhesion factors, bacterial interference

Gastro-intestinal tract – salivation, swallowing, peristalsis, defaecation, lysozyme in saliva, gastric acidity, deconjugated bile salts, fatty acids, O_2, eH, pH

Respiratory tract – mucous production, ciliary motion, coughing

Urinary tract – urination

Vagina – acidity

Cellular and humoral factors at body surfaces – complement, lysozyme, lactoferrin, transferrin, interferon, glycoproteins

Phagocytic cells: granulocytes and macrophages

Immune system: secretory IgA, IgG, IgM, cell-mediated immunity (T lymphocytes and macrophages)

'Second line of defence' (tissues)

Serum factors – complement, lysozyme, lactoferrin, transferrin, β-lysin, interferon, glycoproteins

Phagocytic cells

Immune system – cell-mediated immunity, immunoglobulins (B lymphocytes and plasma cells)

General influences

Nutritional, endocrine, and metabolic factors

Age and genetic factors

The defence against micro-organisms (Figure 10.1) consists of an intact barrier formed by the skin and mucous membranes together with a number of additional factors, phagocytic cells, and an immune system consisting of B and T lymphocytes collaborating with macrophages. To cause an infection, micro-organisms must break through the skin or mucous membrane barrier and an infection may be defined as the combined responses of the host to micro-organisms or other parasites which have penetrated the body and multiplied there (Table 10.1).

The mucous membranes are more vulnerable than the skin and are therefore the most important port of entry for micro-organisms. Besides their purely mechanical resistance, the skin and mucous membranes have several other defence mechanisms. The skin possesses a protective horn layer in which desquamation effects the removal of an appreciable number of bacteria, and the low pH created by fatty acids produced by *Propriono-bacterium acnes* and sebaceous glands and by the lactic acid production of sweat glands impedes colonization by micro-organisms. Sweat also contains lysozyme, which kills some Gram-positive bacteria. Mucous membranes have less mechanical protection (lacking the horn layer and being only one cell-layer thick) but possess humoral and cellular defence mechanisms.

In the digestive tract bacteria are removed mechanically by saliva, swallowing, peristalsis, and defecation. Lysozyme with an anti-bacterial action is present in saliva, nasal secretions, and tears. Because of its very low pH, gastric acid is bactericidal, and as a result the stomach is the only part of the digestive tract which is virtually free of viable bacteria. The rest of the tract has what is called colonization resistance, i.e. the local (mainly anaerobic) bacteria prevent colonization by other micro-organisms because of bacterial competition[2-4].

Colonization resistance arises from such things as the utilization of nutrients by the bacteria, oxygen tension, pH, and the blocking of receptor sites on the mucous membranes. Furthermore biliary acids formed by bacteria and volatile fatty acids produced by anaerobic bacteria prevent colonization as well as lowering of the eH and the production of bacteriocins. In addition to this bacterial competition, there is considerable microbial synergism, which can also play an important role in infections[4].

In the respiratory tract mucus production, ciliary movements and coughing contribute to the defence against micro-organisms so effectively that normally no micro-organisms are present below the glottis. In the upper part of the tract the microflora of the host prevent colonization by bacterial interaction, and the nose offers barriers to large particles in the form of hairs, the turbulence of air currents, and a ciliary movement which directs the flow of mucous containing the micro-organisms towards the pharynx. The nasal secretions contain lysozyme and secretory IgA which hampers adherence of micro-organisms. The bronchi and bronchioli also have mucus and a ciliary epithelium. However, small particles can penetrate the deeper parts of the respiratory tract. The alveoli lack cilia and in this region micro-organisms are eliminated by phagocytosis.

The urinary tract is sterile except for the distal part of the urethra, where micturition impedes colonization, possibly in combination with a lower pH, secretory IgA, and the bactericidal effect of prostatic fluid. In the vagina the normal bacterial flora, which is composed mainly of lactobacilli producing lactic acid, keeps the pH low, which inhibits colonization by other bacteria. Besides these factors, humoral and cellular mechanisms[5] play a role on the surface of mucous membranes[6-9]. The non-immunological humoral factors include complement, lysozyme, lactoferrin, transferrin, interferon and virus-inhibiting glycoproteins.

Cellular resistance is provided by phagocytosis, performed by granulocytes and macrophages.

The immunological defence at the level of the mucous membranes is carried out by immunoglobulins (secretory IgA, IgM, and IgG) synthesized by the B lymphocytes, as well as by cell-mediated immunity brought about by T lymphocytes together with macrophages[5]. Bacteria activate the immune response on the surface of these mucous membranes. In the mucosa there are B lymphocytes, plasma cells and T lymphocytes. Immunoglobulins at this site are partially derived from the circulation and partially from local production. Lymphokines are also formed locally. Together with complement factors, immunoglobulins can opsonize, neutralize, or lyse micro-organisms; furthermore both exotoxins and endotoxins can be neutralized and the attachment of micro-organisms to mucosa by immunoglobulins impeded. In the pathogenicity of a large number of bacterial species, for instance the enteropathogenic *Escherichia coli*, attachment to the mucosa plays an important role, since infection cannot occur without it.

On the mucosa there is an interaction between micro-organisms and the host. Some bacteria have surface factors promoting adhesion, for instance the pili of *Neisseria gonorrhoeae* and the M protein of *Streptococcus pyogenes* group A. Furthermore, the mucosa of the host has specific bacterial receptors and exerts a positive or negative attraction[10] leading to a specific attachment to certain areas of the skin and mucosa by certain endogenous flora, for instance in the upper respiratory tract, the digestive tract, and the vagina[11].

Thus, we find many staphylococci on the skin, many streptococci in the mouth, Gram-negative flora and anaerobic bacteria in the digestive tract, and lactobacilli in the vagina, with the host living in a stable symbiotic equilibrium with the normal microflora. This was recognized as early as 1905 by Metchnikoff. This equilibrium is achieved by an interaction between the host and the microflora and between the species composing the microflora.

The skin, mucous membranes, and their various surface factors form the first line of defence. Normally, there are no micro-organisms in the tissues and micro-organisms must penetrate the barrier formed by the skin and mucosa before an infection can develop. If they succeed in doing so, they proliferate locally in the tissue and induce an inflammatory reaction. Mediators of inflammation then give rise locally to an enhanced permeability of the blood vessels permitting the passage of phagocytic cells and serum factors. The serum factors important for defence include immunoglobulins and non-immunological factors such as complement, lysozyme, transferrin, lactoferrin, and β-lysine. Lysozyme produced by monocytes, macrophages and granulocytes can split the glycopeptide in the cell wall of

Gram-positive bacteria, which leads to osmotic lysis of the bacteria. Lacto-ferrin and transferrin interfere with the bacterial iron metabolism. β-lysine released from blood platelets during coagulation is bactericidal for most of the Gram-positive bacteria[12-18]. Specific immunoglobulins and complement have an opsonizing action and this promotes phagocytosis and intra-cellular killing.

Micro-organisms (e.g. *Streptococcus pneumoniae* and *Haemophilus in-fluenzae*) with a thick polysaccharide capsule, which hampers phagocytosis, can only be opsonized by specific antibodies and complement. Specific anti-bodies in combination with complement can also have a bacteriolytic effect on Gram-negative bacteria, and cross-reacting antibodies can sometimes play an important role as well. The importance of leukokinen (Tuftsin), the active peptide which is synthesized in the spleen, is a matter of controversy[19]. A humoral factor with an important role in viral infections is interferon.

With the mediation of such humoral factors, phagocytosis is performed by two types of cell–granulocytes and macrophages[13,20]. Under the influ-ence of chemotactic stimuli, migration of granulocytes and monocytes occurs[21,22], and products of micro-organisms, activated complement (C3a and C5a), factors deriving from leukocytes and lymphokines[23,24] are important for chemotaxis. In addition, humoral mechanisms can induce granulocytosis and monocytosis via increased synthesis[25].

Opsonization is necessary for efficient phagocytosis, because the mem-brane of phagocytic cells bears receptors for the Fc fragment of IgG (sub-classes 1 and 3) and for the complement factor C3. Opsonization can also be brought about by the combination of IgM and complement. Neutrophil granulocytes have special importance as far as micro-organisms which are pathogenic extracellularly (i.e. outside the phagocytosing cells) are con-cerned. Recently, it became known that eosinophil granulocytes too can eliminate extracellular micro-organisms. An important part in the defence against extracellular parasites is also played by specific antibodies.

Adhesion of a micro-organism to a granulocyte or macrophage is followed by ingestion and the formation of a phagolysosome by fusion of a phago-some and a lysosome; this in turn is followed by degranulation of the lyso-somes, and intracellular killing and digestion of the micro-organism by lysosomal enzymes, and by the myeloperoxidase system by which super-oxide, singlet oxygen, hydrogen peroxide, and an activated halide are formed[13,20,26-28]. These processes are energy-dependent, the energy stored in ATP being delivered by glycolysis. The granulocyte has a short life and usually dies after phagocytosis. The macrophage lives much longer, and after phagocytosis remnants of micro-organisms (residual bodies) are often found in it.

If phagocytosis is inadequate, the invading micro-organisms can continue to proliferate and the inflammation can either spread locally or be dis-seminated via the lymph or blood and cause infections at distant sites.

Granulocytes and macrophages in the liver (Küpffer cells), spleen, lymph nodes and other tissues can clear micro-organisms from the circulation.

There is also another kind of cellular resistance called cell-mediated immunity (CMI), which is regulated by T lymphocytes in collaboration with macrophages. CMI is very important in infections caused by (facultative) intracellular micro-organisms such as mycobacteria, Salmonella spp., Listeria and Brucella spp., viruses, fungi, and protozoa. After renewed contact with an antigen, sensitized T lymphocytes form lymphokines which are thought to activate macrophages to a higher degree of phagocytosis and intracellular killing. At present, several lymphokines are known, but their function in vivo is not fully understood. Transfer factor is a dialysable extract derived from sensitized T lymphocytes which has been claimed to be able to restore the specific cellular immunity[24,29-35].

In the defence against viruses there are some additional factors. Extracellular virus can be neutralized by specific antibodies (present in the circulation and on the surface of mucous membranes), secretory IgA, interferon, and non-specific virus-inhibiting glycoproteins. Neutralization prevents the adsorption to mucosa of, for instance, enteroviruses and respiratory viruses. A virus-infected cell can only be killed by T cells, sometimes in association with macrophages, which secondarily can lead to the death of the virus. This mechanism requires further elucidation[36]. As soon as the virus penetrates a cell and begins to proliferate, the synthesis of interferon occurs. Interferon stimulates the production of an anti-viral protein that prevents virus replication. This is an important defence mechanism, one which begins to operate before cellular and humoral immunity develop. Interferon is species-specific and not virus-specific. Its synthesis can be provoked in animals by endotoxin and by synthetic interferon inducers (e.g. anion polymers and polynucleotides), but these inducers are too toxic for use in man. However, interferon produced by cells in vitro can be administered to patients[35].

The immune defence system is obviously extremely important in the ability of the body to throw off an infection. If an individual comes into contact with a new micro-organism, it takes about 5-10 days before an adequate specific reaction of the humoral and cellular immunity system occurs. A secondary response to a recurrent infection or a vaccination occurs within 2-3 days. Sometimes, micro-organisms are not completely eliminated and remain latent intracellulary (e.g. Mycobacterium tuberculosis, Salmonella spp. and herpes viruses).

Nutrition, endocrine and metabolic factors, age and genetic predisposition have an important influence on the defence mechanisms, particularly antibody formation and phagocytosis. These factors are of particular significance for individuals in the less developed countries, for post-operative patients, and for the elderly[15,16,21,37-44].

It is evident from the foregoing that there is a high degree of interaction between the various defence mechanisms. Cellular and humoral immunity are closely related and seldom function separately[30,45].

10.2 DEFENCE DISTURBANCES

Disturbances in the resistance of the host can affect one or more of the defence mechanisms of the skin and mucosa; surface factors, phagocytosis, and cellular or humoral immunity. Malignant diseases, cytotoxic drugs, immunosuppressive drugs, corticosteroids, radiotherapy, antibiotics and other medicaments take effect at various levels and often enhance each other's attack on the host's defence.

Factors which can disturb the anatomical barrier of the skin and mucous membranes (Table 10.2) include mechanical damage (e.g. surgery, trauma, burns, decubitis, tumour necrosis, skin diseases, skin infections, intra-vascular and urinary catheters, and intubation) and interference with cell division leading to mucosal ulceration (e.g. cytotoxic drugs, irradiation and corticosteroids). Since various parts of the skin and mucous membranes bear a specific and constant microflora, the site of the lesion often deter-mines which particular micro-organism will cause the infection[46-48].

Table 10.2   Disturbed defence of skin and mucous membranes

Surface factors
Alteration of endogenous microflora by antibiotics, disinfectants, colonization by micro-organisms, gastrectomy

Depression of immunoglobulins, cell-mediated immunity, phagocytosis, or interferon production due to underlying disease, cytotoxics, corticosteroids, X-irradiation

Interference with mechanical elimination of micro-organisms
Foreign bodies, obstruction, ileus, aspiration

Disturbed cell division
Ulceration due to cytostatics, corticosteroids, X-irradiation, graft-versus-host reaction

Mechanical injury
Trauma, burns, surgical or diagnostic procedures, supportive care (catheter, intubation), decubitis, infections, tumour necrosis, endoscopy

---

Changes in surface factors may be brought about by a reduction of humoral and cellular factors and by changes in the flora by the administration of antibiotics or corticosteroids, disinfection of skin or mucosa, and coloniz-ation in the hospital environment via food or contact with persons or objects. Achlorhydria can promote colonization by certain bacteria in the digestive tract[49-51].

Reduction of humoral factors on mucous membranes, for instance IgA, IgM, IgG, the complement system and lysozyme, can reduce the adhesion of micro-organisms to mucosa, the inactivation of exo- and endotoxins, and the neutralization of micro-organisms[21,52]. Interference with the mechanical elimination of bacteria, caused by obstruction, aspiration, foreign bodies, ileus and the like, can play a role in the local growth of micro-organisms. Prostheses (artificial heart valves, ventriculo-atrial or ventriculo-peritoneal drains, orthopaedic prostheses etc.) can lead to locally reduced resistance. After even a very slight and clinically undetected bacteraemia an infection may develop. Lastly, injections and infusions of fluids or blood components can be contaminated, and this forms a particularly serious threat to patients with lowered resistance. Many diseases and therapies can lead to disturbances in the reaction to chemotactic factors, to the adhesion and migration of phagocytic cells, and to opsonization, ingestion and intracellular killing[16,20,21,50,53].

A shortage of phagocytic cells can be caused by underlying disease, cytotoxic therapy, irradiation, corticosteroids and so on. Disturbances in the functioning of these cells can be congenital or acquired. Functional disorders of these cells may depend on the presence of immunoglobulins, complement and other humoral factors, but metabolic factors are also important for energy-dependent processes such as chemotaxis, migration, ingestion and intracellular killing. Disorders of sugar metabolism, for instance in uncontrolled diabetes mellitus[16,21,54] acidosis or phosphate deficiency, disturb the energy regulation that is dependent on glycolysis. It has been reported that under a prolonged parental nutrition a decrease in the phosphate level may develop which, in turn, lowers the ATP level[55,56]. Haemodialysis also leads to a disturbance of the phagocytosis performed by granulocytes[57]. Lowering of the transferrin level also increases the susceptibility of the patient to infections[15,16]. A good nutritional state is also of great importance in the resistance to infections, particularly with respect to opsonization, phagocytosis, and intracellular killing[16,37,40,42-44].

In haematological malignant processes such as acute or chronic lymphatic leukaemia, in paraproteinaemia, where there has been immunosuppression for organ transplantation and in treatment with cytotoxic drugs, corticosteroids, irradiation, or the administration of anti-lymphocyte globulin, a disturbance occurs in the functioning of B and T lymphocytes[16,20,21,30,53,58-61]. In acute forms of leukaemia it is known that the immature cells function defectively, but it is not known whether the functioning of the mature cells is completely normal. Corticosteroids lead to reduced stickiness, a weakened reaction of granulocytes to chemotactic stimuli, and monocytopenia, and interfere with cell-mediated immunity[16,21,22,53,62-69].

Most of the micro-organisms which cause clinical infections belong to the endogenous microflora of the host, and the treatment of infections or suspected infections with antimicrobial drugs causes marked changes in this microflora. It selects insensitive strains, promotes the growth of fungi, and reduces the patient's resistance to colonization by exogenous micro-organisms. Furthermore, during hospitalization the hospital environment will contribute to colonization of the patient by a selected, unusual, and antibiotic-resistant flora via hospital personnel, other patients, instruments and other objects, food, infusions, diagnostic and therapeutic procedures, medicaments etc.[49,50,70-77].

As this review indicates, the diversity of the patients who are compromised is extremely wide. Very many of the developments in both diagnostic and therapeutic fields can lead to altered resistance. The rest of this chapter will be devoted to a resumé of the infections occurring in the 'compromised host' *sensu strictu*, which are characterized by the frequent occurrence of infections caused in many cases by micro-organisms which are seldom associated with infection in individuals with intact resistance (e.g. opportunistic infections). These infections usually occur after the successful treatment of other infections caused by known pathogenic micro-organisms, and are called super-infections. They are now more frequent than in the past because therapy may prolong the life of a patient with a serious underlying disease while it does not cure the disease. Not only are such super-infections often very difficult to cure because of the antibiotic resistance of the micro-organism and the often limited therapeutic range of the available antimicrobial drugs (e.g. gentamicin, pentamidin, amphotericin B), but in addition it is often very difficult to arrive at the diagnosis.

As a result of reduced immunological resistance or inadequate phago-cytosis, latent infections (herpes simplex, varicella-zoster, cytomegalo-virus, *Salmonella* spp., *Mycobacterium tuberculosis*) and hidden foci of infection (in the teeth, sinuses, respiratory passages, tonsils, prostate, or urinary tract) or micro-organisms which may be found to colonize on mucosal surfaces (e.g. *Candida* spp., *Pneumocystis carinii*, *Aspergillus* spp., and *Toxoplasma gondii*) may produce manifest infections. The greatly reduced or virtually absent inflammatory reaction in such patients often means that the signs of infection are minimal, and the problems associated with the identification of the micro-organism involved (isolation from the patient, preparation for microscopy, culture, sensitivity determination, and serology) make it difficult to track down an infection, and it is in these very patients that infections may run a serious course and treatment should be started as early as possible. Only close daily observation, interrogation and examination make it possible to diagnose such an infection promptly and attention must be paid to even very small indications.

The group of patients with whom we are concerned consists mainly of individuals with myeloproliferative and lymphoproliferative diseases, solid tumours and organ transplants. Brief reference will also be made to infection problems associated with burns, splenectomies, acquired forms of hypogammaglobulinaemia, Kahler's disease, and Waldenström's disease. There is available a large body of literature on infections in patients with malignant haematological conditions, solid tumours and organ transplants[71, 76, 78–92]. Infection remains the most important cause of morbidity and mortality in cases of malignant haematological processes in spite of the progress made in the field of anti-microbial agents[71, 82, 86].

In those patients with a markedly diminished resistance even small indications such as accelerated respiration, coughing or cyanosis should raise suspicion of an infection of the respiratory tract. Signs of a developing pneumonia can be minor at both physical examination and radiological investigation. Micturition complaints are often absent in cases of urinary tract infections, and at examination the signs of pharyngitis, rectal lesions, pneumonia, acute abdomen, or neck stiffness may be minimal. Nevertheless, pharyngitis and rectal lesions can be ports of entry for sepsis. It is also important to keep in mind that in patients with granulocytopenia there may be few or no granulocytes in the area of the inflammation, which means that there will be little cell infiltration and ultimately little pus will be produced. Furthermore, few granulocytes will be seen when preparations of sputum, CSF, urine or wound exudates etc. are examined.

Fever remains the most important sign of an infection and must be taken very seriously[93]. In acute myeloid leukaemia about 60% of fever episodes are based on an infection. Since almost every infection is accompanied by fever, an elevated temperature must always be regarded as a symptom of infection unless this possibility can be ruled out. On the other hand it is incorrect to institute anti-bacterial therapy solely because of temperature elevation. Even a drop in temperature under antibiotic therapy does not constitute proof that an infection is present[71, 82, 86, 90, 94–97].

As already mentioned, it is always necessary to seek predisposing factors. Despite the occurrence of many unusual infections, most infections are caused by a relatively small group of micro-organisms such as Gram-negative bacteria, *Staphylococcus aureus*, *Candida albicans*, varicella-zoster virus, herpes simplex virus, and hepatitis B virus[76, 86, 98].

For the prevention of infection, anti-microbial drugs do not provide a solution. They select insensitive micro-organisms and increase the susceptibility of the patient to colonization by exogenous micro-organisms. Micro-organisms will always remain on the skin and mucosa, and even after attempts to 'decontaminate' patients completely in strict isolation and with a sterile diet it usually proves impossible to eliminate all bacteria[99]. Prophylaxis of these infections should be directed primarily towards the best possible maintenance of the normal natural defence mechanisms of the body and the elimination of those factors which may compromise the patient. We should therefore attempt to keep the endogenous flora of the patient as normal as possible; the use of antibiotics should be restricted[82]. An attempt should be made to limit exogenous colonization by avoiding hospitalization whenever possible, and to reduce exposure by isolation[100, 102]. Invasive diagnostic and therapeutic procedures (e.g. in-dwelling catheters, hyperalimentation) should be avoided as much as possible. In this respect it seems useful to apply the techniques developed to reduce the chance of endogenous infections by strict isolation with partial decontamination to eliminate potentially pathogenic micro-organisms selectively[82, 83, 99, 103, 104]. (See Table 10.3.) Repeated bacteriological investigations of the isolated patient can provide evidence which will indicate that the patient is a carrier of, or has been colonized by, certain micro-organisms such as *Candida albicans* in the digestive tract or *Staphylococcus aureus* in the nose or on the skin, which can then be controlled if necessary. It may be important to treat a hidden focus found in the sinuses, teeth, prostrate, etc. Patients who have had tuberculosis should be treated prophylactically with isoniazide. In some cases the resistance may be increased by active or passive immunization. The value of administering the more experimental drugs which stimulate the defence system specifically or non-specifically is still uncertain (see below).

Despite the many preventive measures available, it may nevertheless be necessary to institute anti-microbial therapy and reference has already been made to the importance of the early diagnosis of an infection. For this purpose, careful monitoring of the patient is imperative, and use can be made of such modern techniques as echography, organ scanning, electron-microscopical investigation for virus diagnosis and so on. In some centres

Table 10.3   Prevention of infections by maintenance of defence mechanisms

Preservation of endogenous microflora
Limitation of hospitalization
Surveillance of hospital environment
Isolation
Strict antibiotic policy

Preservation of intact skin and mucous membranes

Bacteriological inventory of the isolated patient
Treatment of asymptomatic infections
Treatment of carrier state of certain micro-organisms

Selective or total decontamination of skin and mucous membranes

Reinforcement of body defences
Treatment of underlying and concurrent disease(s)
Elimination of obstructions
Optimal nutrition (calories, protein, vitamins, minerals)
Granulocyte transfusions
Lithium therapy
Passive immunization (varicella-zoster, hepatitis B, measles)
Active immunization (influenza, herpes zoster, cytomegalovirus, hepatitis B, *Pseudomonas* spp., *Haemophilus influenzae, Streptococcus pneumoniae*)
Stimulation of T lymphocytes and/or monocytes by: microbial antigens, levamisole, transfer factor, thymosin, immune RNA, administration of interferon

use is made of the Limulus test by which the presence of endotoxin of Gram-negative bacteria in the blood and CSF can be demonstrated. The reliability of this test is still uncertain because false–positive results are often obtained in blood samples. For the CSF this test is reliable. The nitroblue tetra-zolium reduction (NBT) test seems to be of limited value[105]. Counter-electrophoresis and enzyme immunoassays for the rapid demonstration of bacterial antigens seem to be very promising methods[106–109].

If an infection is suspected on the basis of a high fever, anamnestic data, the results of physical and radiological examination etc. antibiotic therapy must be instituted and directed against micro-organisms whose presence is suggested by the localization and the laboratory data. The initial antibiotic therapy will almost always have to be directed at Gram-negative bacteria (such as *Pseudomona* and *Klebsiella* spp.) and will consist of two bactericidal drugs which must be given parenterally in high doses. If these drugs do not produce good results, the possibility must be considered either that resistant bacteria are present or that the infection is due to fungi, viruses or protozoa. This is especially so when the patient has been previously treated for an infection.

Additional therapy is sometimes required in the form of transfusions of granulocytes. The value of this treatment is fairly well established, but the exact indication for its use is not yet entirely clear. This subject will be discussed below. Attention should also be given to such general measures as optimal nutrition, treatment of endocrine disorders, elimination of obstruc-tions, and bacterial checks on the apparatus in use, food, water, infusion fluids, blood components and personnel.

For the rapid institution of treatment in patients with reduced resistance, it is important to be aware of certain patterns of infection which may develop. These patterns are dependent on the underlying disease as well as the therapy applied and on the type of disturbance of the resistance associ-ated with it, such as disruption of the continuity of the skin or mucosa, granulocytopenia, monocytopenia and immunosuppression. It is also import-ant to take into account the stage of the disease because more intensive chemotherapy and more frequent administration of anti-microbial drugs applied when the disease process has become more extensive will lead to a further reduction of the resistance and the patient will develop very abnormal flora[71,76,82,86,98].

10.3 PREDISPOSING FACTORS

It is extremely difficult to distinguish the influence of the various pre-disposing factors which are outlined below. The natural history of the relationship between infection and malignant disease is appreciably altered by treatment with various cytotoxic drugs, antibiotics, supportive care and improved culture techniques[30,58,71,76,78,82,86,89].

(1) Granulocytopenia remains the dominant factor in patients with malignant disease, particularly in acute leukaemia in adults. When the number of granulocytes falls below 1000 per mm^3, the incidence of infection increases. Furthermore, the frequency and severity of infection are correlated with the duration and the severity of the granulocytopenia[82,83,87,96,97]. Of all cases of septicaemia, 75% are associated with counts of less than 500 granulocytes per mm^3, and this percentage rises sharply when there are fewer than 100 per mm^3. In cases of granulocytopenia and defective granulocyte function we find mainly infections caused by extracellular pathogenic micro-organisms, such as the Gram-positive and Gram-negative bacteria and *Candida albicans*.

(2) When the synthesis of immunoglobulins is disturbed we can expect disturbed opsonization, a reduction in the neutralization of toxins and blocking of attachment of micro-organisms such as *Salmonella* spp. to the mucous membranes, as well as defective bacteriolysis of Gram-negative bacteria and diminished virus neutralization. In this situation it is mainly bacterial infection which develop and in IgG deficiency respiratory tract infections are common.

(3) When the cell-mediated immunity is disturbed, as is found particularly in lymphoproliferative diseases and in immunosuppression for organ transplantation, the proportion of infections with facultative and obligatory intracellular micro-organisms increases. These micro-organisms live or proliferate within the macrophages and are resistant to intracellular killing and can only be successfully attacked by macrophages in collaboration with specific sensitized T lymphocytes. They include *Salmonella*, *Candida*, *Listeria* and *Cryptococcus*, and strictly intracellular micro-organisms such as *Mycobacteria*, *Histoplasma*, *Coccidioides*, *Brucella*, *Pasteurella tularensis*, *Toxoplasma gondii* and viruses. It is possible that a number of these strictly intracellular parasites can persist for a long time in the macrophages and in granulomas under an equilibrium which becomes established between the parasite and the host. Examples of this are infections by virus (e.g. herpes simplex virus, varicella-zoster virus, cytomegalo virus and hepatitis B virus) and by bacteria (e.g. *Brucella* or *Mycobacteria*). Chronic infections can also occur, for instance with hepatitis B virus, and slow virus infections are also known (e.g. the progressive multi-focal leuko-encephalopathy).

(4) Additional factors that primarily disturb the integrity of the skin and mucosa may also play an important role, such as diagnostic and surgical procedures, burns, catheterization, contaminated intravenously administered fluids or blood components and other forms of supportive care, ulceration, obstruction, ischaemia, etc.[46-48].

(5) While the original infection is usually caused by the normal colonizing host flora, e.g. *Staphylococcus aureus* and *E. coli*, antibiotic therapy alters the flora and predisposes to an infection that will be caused by resistant or

opportunistic micro-organisms, whose acquisition is promoted by hospital environments.

10.4 RELATIONSHIP BETWEEN THE UNDERLYING DISEASE AND REDUCED RESISTANCE

Disturbances of resistance are largely dependent on the underlying disease, the type and stage of the disease, and on the treatment. Of increasing importance are the classifications of certain diseases which until recently were seen as one entity. For instance, the lymphoproliferative diseases are subdivided on the basis of immunological and cytochemical characteristics into T, B, and Null cell malignancies, which leads to a better understanding of the disorders[110,111] (see Table 10.4).

(1) In adult patients with acute leukaemia, the main predisposing factor is the combination of granulocytopenia and defective functioning of these cells. During an admission, these patients have fewer than 100 granulocytes per mm³ for about half of the time. An important factor in recovery from serious infections is the capacity of the granulocytopenic patient to react to the infection with an increase in the production of granulocytes. In the absence of this, the prognosis is very poor[82,102].

Monocytopenia often develops in these patients. Functional disorders of cells in leukaemia have also been described, e.g. disturbances of migration, chemotaxis, phagocytosis, and intracellular killing; whether this also holds for the mature cells is not entirely certain[112]. An important additional factor in these patients is the occurrence of mucosal ulceration under cytotoxic drug therapy and interruption of the continuity of the skin caused by supportive care and diagnostic procedures. In a later stage of the disease, the prolonged and intensive chemotherapy may often lead to a distinct disturbance of immunity, although humoral immunity is often relatively well preserved. While bacterial infections are mainly encountered in the early stage of acute leukaemia, infections caused by intracellular parasites such as yeasts, viruses and protozoa may occur later. Furthermore, in the late stages, because of prior antibiotic treatment, infections due to highly resistant bacteria occur, and hepatitis B infections occur frequently because of transfusions of blood products[58,71,76,82,86,98,112].

(2) Children with acute lymphatic leukaemia have few infections in the early stages of the disease, partly due to the fact that the chemotherapy directed against lymphoblasts (vincristine, prednisone) is less intensive, which results in a less severe granulocytopenia. Diminished resistance in these cases of acute lymphatic leukaemia is based on disturbed cellular immunity. In later stages of the disease granulocytopenia develops.

(3) Patients with Hodgkin's disease and other lymphoproliferative diseases also have few infections in the early stages. In these diseases the

Table 10.4 Acquired disturbances of phagocytosis and immunity in certain diseases

	Opsonization	Chemotaxis	Migration	Ingestion	Intracellular killing	Granulocytopaenia	Monocytopaenia	B lymphocytes	T lymphocytes
Haematological diseases:									
AML				+		+			
ALL					++				++
CLL				+	++				++
Lymphoproliferation		+					.		
Paraproteinaemia	+	++			+			+	
Splenectomy				+					
Fe prive an.					+				
Immunological diseases:									
Rheumatoid arthritis		+		++					
SLE	++		.	++					
Lowered C3	++	+							
Immunological complex diseases	+			+					
Metabolic diseases:									
Diabetes mellitus		++	++	++					
Hypophosphataemia		++	++	++	+				
Burns		+			+				
Corticosteroids							+	+	+
Cytostatic drugs				+		+	+	+	+

predominant feature is a disturbance of the cell-mediated immunity, which is attributable to the disease itself, and the number or functioning of the T lymphocytes is reduced. Therapy further reduces resistance and the diminished cell-mediated immunity leads to infections with (facultative) intracellular parasites.

Lymphoproliferative diseases may promote infection of, for instance, respiratory or urinary passages by obstruction. In the stage of the disease in which granulocytopenia occurs, there may be infections resembling those seen in adult patients with acute leukaemia and granulocytopenia; however, due to the disturbed cell-mediated immunity more of them are caused by fungi, protozoa, *Listeria, Salmonella, Mycobacterium tuberculosis* and viruses[58,60,85,113-118].

(4) Chronic myeloid leukaemia is rarely complicated by infections. A blast crisis may give rise to the same situation as in acute leukaemia in adults, in which the diminished resistance is due mainly to granulocytopenia and ulceration of mucosa. This disease can, in addition, lead to obstruction of the respiratory, urinary, and biliary tracts etc. Periods of fever in these patients are not only caused by infections but can also be due to the disease process itself[58].

(5) Chronic lymphatic leukaemia is associated with infections resembling those seen in other lymphoproliferative disorders. The disease originates in the T lymphocytes and leads to a defective cell-mediated immunity. Initially, there are few infections, some of which are caused by varicella-zoster virus. In the later stages, immunoglobulin synthesis may decline and this leads to more infections, especially by micro-organisms in which opsonization is important. In the stage of the disease requiring cytotoxic drug therapy, the clinical picture of the infections is analogous with that seen in the later stages of lymphoma[58].

(6) In multiple myeloma and Waldenström's disease the B lymphocytes do not function normally and antibody production is decreased; this increases the frequency of infections, predominantly those caused by bacteria for whose elimination opsonization is important. There is usually hypo- or a-gammaglobulinaemia of one or more of the immunoglobulins. IgG deficiency in these diseases leads particularly to respiratory tract infections. Under intensive cytotoxic drug therapy, granulocytopenia can also occur, which leads to infections of the type described in acute leukaemia[58,59,88,119,120].

(7) Patients with solid tumours develop infections related mainly to local lesions in the affected organ caused by the tumour itself, and to obstruction, mucosal lesions, and granulocytopenia. In tumours of the digestive tract and of the genital tract in women there are more anaerobe infections. Iatrogenic procedures and surgical treatment can also play an important role in these conditions.

(8) In patients with organ transplants, infections are very important and are responsible for an appreciable percentage of the mortality. Many bacterial infections are related not only to granulocytopenia but also to the transplanted organ. In patients given a bone-marrow transplant the number of infections is unusually high due to the frequent occurrence of a graft-versus-host reaction. Furthermore, in all patients who have undergone an organ transplantation the prolonged and intensive immunosuppressive therapy which they have usually undergone leads to a severe disturbance of cell-mediated immunity.

(9) Infections after splenectomy are frequent because the spleen serves as a mechanical sieve for circulating micro-organisms and, furthermore, until the age of 2 years it is the site of the primary response for IgG synthesis. The latter observation explains why so many children develop bacterial infections after splenectomy, for in them the spleen is essential for the phagocytosis of blood-borne bacteria. The predominant infections after splenectomy are those caused by bacteria in which opsonization is important[121]. Adults also frequently develop bacterial infections after splenectomy[19,122-127].

(10) Burns are important in giving rise to problems of infection. Predisposing factors include not only the loss of the skin barrier but also a disturbed granulocyte function in the form of a diminished reaction to chemotactic stimuli and a reduced level of intracellular killing[128-131]. In addition, contact with the hospital environment, and the use of antibiotics both locally and generally are of great importance. In burn patients the administration of antibiotics must be strictly limited and reserved for cases of septicaemia[132].

(11) The predisposition of immunologically determined diseases must also be considered. Thus in rheumatoid arthritis disturbed chemotaxis and phagocytosis has been described, perhaps due to the presence of rheumatoid-factor complexes which affect granulocyte mobility and the ingestion of particles[21]. Again in systemic lupus erythematosus, disturbed ingestion in diseases with reduced levels of complement, such as SLE and glomerulonephritis, decreased chemotaxis and opsonization have also been described[21,52,133]. Hypergammaglobulinaemia E disturbs chemotaxis[21].

10.5   THE RELATIONSHIP BETWEEN DEFECTIVE RESISTANCE AND THE TYPE OF INFECTION

10.5.1   Bacterial infections

As already noted the factors of importance in the development of bacterial infections include a disturbance of the mechanical protection provided by the skin and mucous membranes, and also surface factors, defective phagocytosis by granulocytes and monocytes and disorders of the humoral immunity and complement system (see above and Table 10.5)[30,134].

10.5.2 Non-bacterial infections

10.5.2.1 Fungal infections

As far as *Candida, Aspergillus*, and *Mucormycetes* are concerned the most important factors in infections with these fungi are loss of the integrity of the skin or mucous membranes or of phagocytosis. For other infections, such as those caused by *Cryptococcus, Histoplasma*, and *Coccidioides*, cell-mediated immunity plays the most important role. (See Chapter 2, for a more detailed discussion.)

The normal bacterial flora of the skin and mucosa probably also provides protection against colonization by fungi and the occurrence of fungal infections is also promoted by ulceration, foreign bodies (catheters), obstruction, and the use of antibiotics and corticosteroids[14,30,33,79,135–141].

10.5.2.2 Protozoal infections

The disturbed cell-mediated immunity is of special importance here. The factors promoting such infections are colonization from the environment and reactivation of latent infections. The only really important infections in this category are those caused by *Toxoplasma gondii* and *Pneumocystis carinii*[30,79,142–144]. Malaria can also be reactivated under immunosuppressive therapy, and one case of amoeba-encephalomeningitis has been described in a patient with Hodgkin's disease. *Giarda lamblia* infections may occur in IgA-deficient individuals and one case has been described in a patient with Hodgkin's disease. A number of cases of disseminated infection

Table 10.5 Relation of predisposing factors to type of infection

Type of infection		Disturbance of
Bacterial		Integrity of skin and mucous membranes
		Surface factors and endogenous microflora
		Phagocytosis and opsonization
Non-bacterial		
Fungal	*Candida*	Microflora
	Aspergillus	Skin and mucous membranes
	Mucor	Phagocytosis and opsonization
	Cryptococcus	
	Histoplasma	Cell-mediated immunity
	Coccidioides	
Protozoal		Cell-mediated immunity
Viral		Immunoglobulins
		Cell-mediated immunity

with Strongyloides have been reported in patients with a lymphoproliferative disease or leukaemia, all of whom were treated with prednisone and came from an endemic region. (For a detailed discussion, see Chapter 3.)

10.5.2.3 Viral infections

A shortage of immunoglobulins means insufficient neutralization of extra-cellular virus and loss of inhibition of the attachment of viruses to mucous membranes. Cell-mediated immunity is necessary for the control of intra-cellular virus. When this form of immunity is severely disturbed, dis-seminated virus infections can occur, for instance of varicella-zoster and herpes simplex. The former can also be reactivated in irradiated areas[58,79,117,118,145–148]. (See Chapter 13.)

10.6 CLINICAL PICTURES OF INFECTIONS SEEN IN VARIOUS UNDERLYING DISEASES

10.6.1 Acute leukaemia in adults

In patients with acute leukaemia, bacterial infections are frequent. Accord-ing to the literature, the micro-organisms responsible for these bacterial infections are largely dependent on the hospital environment. Most of the publications on this subject come from large centres to which patients had been referred from other hospitals. In the first hospital to which these patients were admitted mention is made of different pathogenic micro-organisms, i.e. the 'more ordinary' bacteria, from those later reported by the larger centres[75,90]. Thus, due to the use of broad-spectrum antibiotics, the composition of the flora changes and with it the bacteriological pattern of the infections.

This is also seen when the situation is reviewed historically: in the 1960s infections caused by Gram-positive cocci such as *Staphylococcus aureus* and *Streptococci* had the highest incidence, whereas after that mainly Gram-negative infections were reported. In some hospitals, while *Pseudomonas* infections predominated in recent years, at the present time, with the introduction of carbenicillin and gentamicin, *Klebsiella*, Enterobacteria of the genus *Serratia* and multi-resistant *E. coli* strains are the most preva-lent[70,71,75,76,80,82,86,98,149,150]. Furthermore, in recent years there has been an increase in infections caused by higher bacteria (*Nocardia* spp.), fungi, protozoa and viruses. The pattern of these infections has been strongly influenced by antibiotic administration and colonization in the hospital environment[14,49–51,70,74,77,79,98]. In the future, non-bacterial infections will probably play an even greater role.

Adult patients with acute leukaemia show particular patterns of infection. The main sites of these infections are the lower respiratory tract and the digestive tract with anorectal, pharyngeal and oesophageal lesions. Infections in these patients can also originate in the skin, particularly in the axillary and inguinal regions, and also as a result of the introduction of catheters and other iatrogenic procedures. Urinary tract infections do not, however, seem to occur much more frequently than in other patients (Table 10.6).

The predominant micro-organisms playing a role in large hospitals are Gram-negative bacteria (*E. coli*, *Pseudomonas aeruginosa*, and *Klebsiella pneumoniae*), *Staphylococcus aureus* and non-bacterial pathogens such as *Candida*, *Aspergillus*, and *Mucor* spp. There are few reports of infections caused by anaerobic bacteria.

Table 10.6   Clinical pictures of infection in acute myeloid leukaemia and lymphoproliferative disorders

Acute myeloid leukaemia	
Site	*Micro-organisms*
Lower respiratory tract	*Escherichia coli*
Digestive tract:	
Pharyngitis	*Klebsiella* spp.
Oesophagitis	*Pseudomonas* spp.
Anorectal lesions	*Staphylococcus aureus*
Skin infections	*Candida* spp.
Septicaemia	*Aspergillus* spp.
Hepatitis B	*Mucor* spp.

Lymphoproliferative disorders	
Site	*Micro-organisms*
In early stage: herpes zoster	HZV virus
post-stenotic infections	
In later stage: as in AML	also:
also:	*Listeria monocytogenes*
Meningoencephalitis	*Cryptococcus neoformans*
Disseminated herpes zoster	*Nocardia asteroides*
	Salmonella spp.
	Pneumocystis carinii
	Toxoplasma gondii
	Cytomegalovirus

Septicaemia can arise from infections in any of the above-mentioned sites and is seen mainly in patients with severe granulocytopenia (fewer than 100 granulocytes per mm^3). It is in this range of granulocyte numbers that the most severe and most widespread infections are seen. Because the inflammatory reaction of the granulocytes and monocytes is so weak, it is often very difficult to diagnose an infection in these patients and to find its focus[71,76,82,86,98]. It can usually be localized as a pneumonia or gastro-intestinal ulceration, and sometimes in the skin. Smaller lesions (e.g. in the anorectal, pharyngeal or oesophageal regions) can also give access to a pathogen.

Sepsis due to more than one micro-organism has quite frequently been described in the literature[71,81,82].

Fungal infections increase in frequency with increasing duration of the disease. The diagnosis is invariably very difficult to make and is very often not reached before the death of the patient. According to studies done in the USA, post mortem investigations have shown severe fungal infections in 13–21% of cases[14,79,82,86]. Infections due to viruses in acute leukaemia include not only those due to hepatitis B virus seen after multiple trans-fusions but also those of herpes simplex type I leading to stomatitis and oesophagitis[79,145].

10.6.2 Clinical pictures

(1) Pulmonary infections have the highest incidence in these patients and are the most frequently fatal of all the forms of infection. Because of the weak inflammatory reaction, there are generally few signs or symptoms in the early phase, and the physical, diagnostic, and radiological investigations reveal no abnormalities. Sputum production may be minimal, and the sputum is not usually purulent. As previously noted Gram preparations of sputum show very few granulocytes, which makes diagnosis extremely difficult, because any bacteria present might have originated from an oropharyngeal contamination. For the preparation and culture of sputum, according to Mulder, it is important to wash the material[151]. Contamination can also occur from Gram-negative rods which can start to colonize the upper respiratory passages after contact with the hospital environment or in association with antibiotic therapy.

To establish the diagnosis it is thus often necessary to perform a trans-tracheal aspiration, and, if no material is obtained, transtracheal selective bronchial brushing or a lung puncture or biopsy may be necessary to find the causative micro-organisms. It is often difficult to reach a decision on the merits of a lung biopsy, because the patient is usually extremely ill. Further-more, because thrombocytopenia is usually present, a thrombocyte trans-fusion is necessary prior to this procedure. Such aggressive diagnostic procedures are mainly required for the diagnosis of non-bacterial infec-tions[106,139,142,144,152,153]

In cases of pneumonia, the micro-organisms most commonly found are Gram-negative rods (*E. coli*, *Pseudomonas aeruginosa*, and *Klebsiella pneumoniae*) and *Staphylococcus aureus*. There are few reports of pneumonia caused by *Streptococcus pneumoniae*. The mortality due to Gram-negative bacillary pneumonias is extremely high, even with the administration of the newer antibiotics and granulocyte transfusions, and it still amounts to about 40% of the cases[86,98]. Early diagnosis and treatment of these respiratory infections in individuals with acute leukaemia is therefore very important in these cases. After the successful treatment of bacterial infections, these patients tend to develop pneumonia induced by *Candida albicans*, *Aspergillus* or *Mucor* spp. The sputum is virtually always negative and under the microscope any micro-organisms which are seen are best visualized in KOH preparations. However, the possibility of a false-positive result due to contamination from the upper respiratory tract must be kept in mind. The diagnosis is seldom reached before death, and can usually only be made by lung biopsy. In patients with a pulmonary infection and negative sputum in whom the pneumonia does not respond to anti-bacterial therapy, the possibility of a fungal pathogen must be considered. (In cases of fungal infection blood cultures are usually negative.) Under these conditions, there should be no hesitation about applying aggressive diagnostic procedures without delay. Treatment can only be expected to be successful if it is started promptly and directed specifically to the responsible parasite. Since the possible causes of pneumonia are numerous, it is essential to have a specific diagnosis for specific therapy. It is impossible to treat patients for all of the possible pathogens. In addition, some forms of therapy are toxic. Because the administration of empirical therapy for one of the possible pathogens generally means a loss of time, the use of aggressive diagnostic methods is justified.

In general, the radiographic picture is not very helpful in the diagnosis of a pneumonia. However, an aspergillus infection can also be manifested as an aspergilloma or as tram-rail-like lesions or as multiple lung emboli, and *Pneumocystis carinii* can lead to bilateral infiltrative anomalies arising from the hilus. If, finally, it is not possible to use aggressive diagnostic methods and there is strong suspicion of a fungal infection, therapy with amphothericin B must be instituted, sometimes in combination with 5-fluorocytosine[14,106,137,154–161], and usually also with a therapy directed against Gram-negative micro-organisms. Another useful antifungal agent is miconazole[158,160,162]. Lung infiltrates can, however, also be due to an infection with *Pneumocystis carinii*, which is extremely difficult to diagnose. This parasite is seldom to be found in the sputum and is sometimes present in material obtained by selective transtracheal bronchial brushing, but a lung puncture or biopsy is usually necessary[106,113,142,144,152,153]. Visualization of the parasite requires staining with metanamine silver. Serological diagnosis is not reliable for *Pneumocystis carinii*. Pentamidine isostenate can be used for treatment, but must be started early. Currently, cotrimoxasole is used in high dosage or in combination with sulfonamide and pyrimethamine; together with this therapy citrovorum factor is necessary[79,142,144,163,234]. This kind of infection is seen mainly in children with acute leukaemia when the corticosteroid dosage is reduced.

Reactivation of lung tuberculosis or infection with cytomegalovirus is seldom seen in patients with acute leukaemia (but when this does occur, it is often found in combination with *Pneumocystis carinii*, Gram-negative bacteria, *Cryptococcus neoformans*, or *Toxoplasma gondii*).

(2) Infections of the upper respiratory tract (sinusitis, otitis media) are not very frequent in acute leukaemia. Sinusitis can be caused by *Staphylococcus aureus*, Gram-negative bacteria, viruses, and occasionally by *Mucor* spp.

(3) Infections arising in the digestive tract start most frequently at three sites – anorectal, pharyngeal and oesophageal. Infections starting from anorectal lesions such as fissures and haemorrhoids are the most frequent. These lesions can easily be missed at physical examination, because, due to the granulocytopenia, the inflammatory reaction is weak and true abscesses seldom develop. In most cases, however, defecation is painful.

Whenever an infection is suspected, the patient must be examined minutely and frequently, including the anal region. When granulocytopenia is present, even small lesions can probably lead to bacteraemia during defaecation. This region is one of the most important portals via which Gram negative rods reach the bloodstream. Sometimes a larger, and in a few cases a very extensive, inflammation develops, with the production of a watery secretion containing many micro-organisms (Gram-negative rods and a mixed anaerobic flora) with few granulocytes.

Mucosal lesions in the oropharynx can be associated with the use of cytotoxic drugs and corticosteroids, or may be caused by viral infections. Prior hospitalization and administration of antibiotics can also promote the colonization of the oropharynx by Gram-negative bacteria and by yeasts. The patient develops fever, a sore throat, difficulty in swallowing, and sometimes rigors. Again in these cases, few signs of inflammation are found at examination. The throat is red but there is no exudate and no glands are palpable in the neck. The Gram preparation and the culture of a throat smear show many kinds of micro-organisms, which makes it very difficult to identify the pathogen. The possible pathogens are Gram-negative rods, *Staphylococcus aureus*, and yeasts. A candida infection of the oropharynx usually leads to ulceration and bleeding. Herpes simplex stomatitis is often accompanied by a candida superinfection. Despite the weak inflammatory reaction, bacteraemia or candidaemia can originate from this site.

It is now becoming increasingly recognized that in adult patients with acute leukaemia the incidence of oesophagitis is high and at autopsy, oesophagitis is found in about one-third of the cases, usually with candida infection[14,79,164]. Candida oseophagitis may be preceded by pharyngitis, but can also occur alone. The pathological changes are usually seen in the lower third of the oesophagus, and are ascribed to cytotoxic therapy and the regurgitation of gastric acid. The patient usually has a burning pain retrosternally and dysphagia. In most cases there are distinct radiographic abnormalities, but the various pathogens do not lead to a specific radiological picture and a definite diagnosis can only be made in a biopsy specimen, obtained by oesophagoscopy. Not only *Candida* but also Herpes simplex type I and Gram-negative rods may be found in the biopsy. Because the candida infection is usually rather superficial, this type of pharyngitis can be adequately treated by local therapy in the form of a fungostatic drug such as nystatin, pimaricin or miconazole given in a lozenge, to be sucked in the mouth. (If there are lesions in the mouth the best form of treatment is the administration of a cream to which amphotericin B has been added.) In severe cases of candida oesophagitis, parenteral therapy with amphotericin B is required.

The oesophagus is an important access route for disseminated candida infections throughout the body (e.g. the eyes, liver, spleen, skin, kidneys), and when such an infection is suspected the patient must be closely observed for signs of localization in one or other organ. In suspected dissemination, fundoscopy is of great value, because the typical abnormalities of candida endophthalmitis can be found. Blood cultures are nearly always negative. However, positive blood culture does not always mean that a disseminated candida infection is present, because it can be due to a transient candidaemia arising from an infected intravascular catheter. Therefore, when a blood culture is positive all catheters must be removed and a careful watch kept for signs of an organ localization, with repeated blood cultures, urine cultures, fundoscopy, thorax X-rays, and, if necessary, oesophagoscopy. The diagnostic usefulness of serology for *Candida* is not yet established (but see also chapter 2)[106,108,109,137,165].

10.6.2.1 *The teeth*

During granulocytopenia, slumbering oral infections such as gingivitis, paradontosis, root granuloma, and root abscesses can be reactivated. In these patients it is therefore important to investigate and treat the teeth in a favourable period when there is no granulocytopenia nor thrombocytopenia.

10.6.2.2 *Urinary tract infections*

These infections are not very frequent in patients with acute leukaemia, but, as might be expected, occur more frequently when there are predispositions such as catheterization, instrumentation, prostate hypertrophy or other forms of obstruction. In this group of patients the use of indwelling catheters should only be considered on very strict indications. In general, patients with urinary tract infections seldom complain of symptoms related to the urinary tract because of the weak inflammatory reaction which is usually present. Since there are only a few cells or none at all in the urine during granulocytopenia, the urine must be checked for micro-organisms in a Gram preparation and quantitative cultures made. The urinary tract is seldom the source of sepsis in the absence of an obstruction. If *Candida* spp. are found in the urine of a patient who does not have or has not had a catheter, the possibility of disseminated candidiasis must be considered after exclusion of the possibility that a urine sample has been contaminated, for instance from the vulva. Some cytotoxic drugs can cause chemical cystitis because of the mucosal ulceration produced.

10.6.2.3 *Septicaemia*

In adults with acute leukaemia, septicaemia develops in about one-third of the cases. At present, mainly Gram-negative micro-organisms are found[70,71,75,82,86,166-169] and less frequently *Staphylococcus aureus*, and *Candida*. It is not unusual to find more than one micro-organism. Anaerobic micro-organisms are relatively rare, being seen more frequently in association with solid tumours of the digestive tract and in the female genital tract. In cases of septicaemia it is essential to find the focus or portal of entry. In bacteraemias every organ must be considered, but the focus is most often a pneumonia, an anorectal lesion, or pharyngitis. Vein and bladder catheters predispose to sepsis. Candida septicaemia almost always originates in the oesophagus or some other part of the digestive tract or is associated with catheterization. The possibility of a secondary localization in an organ must always be kept in mind (bone, lungs, brain, liver, skin, eyes, etc.)[14,70,137,167,170].

10.6.2.4 *Hepatitis B*

Hepatitis B occurs frequently in adults with acute leukaemia, since it is correlated with the numerous transfusions these patients require. This infection is to some degree dependent on the standards maintained by the blood bank. Besides an acute form of hepatitis, a chronic aggressive hepatitis frequently occurs in carriers of the HBS antigen. Other causes of hepatitis may also be found, such as cytomegalovirus[86,145].

10.6.3 Infections in Hodgkin's disease and other lymphoproliferative disorders

The first stage of this disease is characterized by few infections[76,82,84,86] (as discussed on page 357). Herpes zoster infections, particularly in irradiated regions, are seen most frequently, for these patients have a reduced resistance to the herpes zoster-varicella virus[58,114,117,118,146,171]. Patients who have not had chicken pox invariably contract a herpes zoster infection if exposed. The incubation period is 15–30 days. When there is a known contact, a non-immune patient can be given specific zoster immunoglobulin prophylactically.

Obstruction (reversible with radiation therapy) can also lead to infection. In lymphoproliferative disorders the fever which may be present can sometimes be based on the underlying disease and not on an infection. In therapy-resistant forms of Hodgkin's disease and in recurrences in which granulocytopenia develops, infections which may occur resemble those seen in acute leukaemia. Due to the defective cell-mediated immunity there is an increase in the incidence of infections with facultative and obligatory intracellular micro-organisms as already outlined.

Unusual micro-organisms which can cause infections include *Listeria monocytogenes* (with bacteraemia, pneumonia and encephalomeningitis), *Cryptococcus neoformans* (sometimes in a disseminated form, and also causing meningitis), *Nocardia asteroides* (pneumonia, subcutaneous infections and encephalomeningitis), and *Salmonella* spp. There are also infections caused by cytomegalovirus, *Pneumocystis carinii*, and sometimes *Toxoplasma gondii*. Occasionally, reactivation of tuberculosis occurs. The differential diagnosis of lung infiltrates is particularly difficult in these patients (Gram-negative bacteria, *Listeria* and *Cryptococcus*, Cytomegalovirus, *Pneumocystis carinii*, and *Toxoplasma gondii*) and usually requires aggressive diagnostic procedures (see page 365). The possibility of meningoencephalitis caused by bacteria and fungi must always be kept in mind.

When humoral immunity is also considerably reduced, infections caused by encapsulated micro-organisms such as *Haemophilus influenzae* and *Streptococcus pneumonia* may be seen[1,127,134]. Recent reports in the literature indicate that splenectomy in patients with a lymphoproliferative affection also leads to the more frequent occurrence of bacterial infections[118,125].

10.6.4 Infections in acute lymphatic leukaemia

As discussed above (see page 357) patients with this disease, especially children, develop infections less often than those with non-lymphatic leukaemia. However, when chemotherapy is intensified because of recurrence or failure to achieve a remission, infections similar to those seen in adults with acute myeloid leukaemia occur. In later phases of the disease more than 50% of the patients die from a disseminated viral infection.

10.6.5 Multiple myeloma and Waldenström's disease

In the past, infections caused by *Streptococcus pneumoniae* and *Haemophilus* spp. were commonly seen in these diseases, whereas at present, because of antibiotic therapy, there are more infections with Gram-negative rods and *Staphylococcus aureus*. In the later stages of these diseases under the influence of intensive chemotherapy, the opportunistic infections increase in frequency[58,59,88,119].

10.6.6   Infections after splenectomy

Children aged 2 years or younger have a high risk of serious infections (meningitis and sepsis) after splenectomy (see page 360). In recent years there have also been more reports of infections caused by *Streptococcus pneumoniae* and *Haemophilus* spp. in adults, as in patients with Hodgkin's disease[121,122,124,126,127]. In the splenectomized patient who runs a fever it is of great importance to start antibiotic therapy against *Streptococcus pneumoniae* and *Haemophilus influenzae* immediately after the sampling of blood (and if necessary the cerebrospinal fluid (CSF)) for culture.

10.6.7   Infections after organ transplantation

In patients who have had organ transplants the development of granulocytopenia is followed by infections resembling those seen in adults with acute leukaemia and granulocytopenia, except that the disturbed cellular immunity in the former also results in more infections caused by fungi, protozoa, *Listeria* and *Salmonella* spp., *Mycobacterium tuberculosis*, and cytomegalovirus. (Legionnaire's disease has been described after a transplant[172]). Kidney recipients show predominantly urinary tract infections; liver recipients often develop liver abscesses via the portal vein and/or biliary tracts, frequently in association with bacteraemia, and many heart recipients develop pneumonia[53,58,85,91,113,116,135,136,137–141,143,146,148,172–181].

10.7   DIAGNOSIS AND TREATMENT OF INFECTIONS

As has been stressed the signs of an infection in patients with a malignant haematological condition or in those who are under immunosuppression therapy are usually limited and non-specific, because of the weak inflammatory reaction, particularly during granulocytopenia. It is important to be aware of the types of infection which can occur in the various underlying diseases, the stage of the disease, and what predisposing factors are present[71,76,81–84,86,87,89–91,95,96,98].

The main sign of infection is again fever and, according to the literature, 60% of patients with a myelo- or lymphoproliferative disease have a confirmed infection while 20% probably have no infection. Other causes of fever include a reaction to transfusion of blood components, treatment with cytotoxic or other drugs, bleeding, local thrombophlebitis or phlebothrombosis related to intravascular catheters, contaminated infusions, or the underlying disease itself (e.g. lymphoproliferative disorders, chronic myeloid leukaemia).

A detailed history must always be taken, and attention should also be paid to such relatively minor complaints as dyspnoea, cough, sore throat, difficulty in swallowing, retrosternal pain, gastric complaints, pain on defaecation, trouble with micturition, headache, and so on. As already stated physical examination should be extremely thorough, with special attention to sites where infections are frequently seen, such as the pharynx, lungs, anorectal region, skin (particularly axillary and inguinal areas). Examination for any neck stiffness must never be omitted. Consideration must also be given to intravenous catheters, bladder catheters, and signs of obstruction. Urine should be investigated bacteriologically and radiographs should be made of the thorax from two directions. Because of the absence of distinct inflammatory reactions, the site of an infection is often not found with certainty at this examination, and extensive bacteriological investigation is necessary (see Table 10.7).

Table 10.7 Diagnosis of infection

Attention to minor signs and symptoms
Analysis to identify causes of fever
Knowledge of types of infections
Investigation of predisposing factors
Detailed history and thorough physical examination
Repeated chest X-rays
Microscopial preparations of suspected sites
Collection of material for cultures and serology

If necessary: more extensive diagnostic investigations

Lung biopsy, oesophagoscopy, fundoscopy, organ-scanning, echography, counter-electrophoresis for bacterial antigens
CSF puncture
Cryptococcus antigen in CSF and serum
Candida serology, antigen in serum
Rapid diagnosis of viral infections by the use of immunofluorescence studies, immunoperoxidase tests, radio-immunoassay, counter-immunoelectrophoresis, electron microscopy

Before antibiotic therapy is instituted, material must be collected for at least two blood cultures (including anaerobic cultures) and for cultures of sputum, urine, pharyngeal, nasal, and rectal secretions, and also samples from suspected sites, and sometimes also samples of CSF. Samples of the serum of the patient must be stored for serological investigation at various times during the course of the disease. Since even the first results on cultures are not available before at least 24 h, microscopical preparations should also be made, where possible, to provide a basis for the choice of the initial antibiotic therapy. When the investigations do not provide the necessary information, it will often be necessary to treat the patient provisionally. The choice of therapy is difficult, because bouts of fever are not always caused by an infection, and broad-spectrum antibiotic therapy may lead to marked changes in the microbial flora of the patient and predispose to colonization by resistant flora as well as to other infections due to opportunistic micro-organisms.

These super-infections are always extremely difficult to treat and their occurrence in later stages is unavoidable in most of the patients. On the other hand, an untreated infection can rapidly become serious and the chance of recovery is much less when antibiotic therapy is started late. Thus when a rise in temperature cannot be explained by a non-infectious cause and severe granulocytopenia is present, the institution of antibiotic therapy is in general obligatory. However, the physician must also terminate such therapy if no infection can be demonstrated within a few days (usually four).

Initial therapy started after specimens have been taken for cultures usually consists of a combination of penicillin or cephalosporin and an aminoglycoside. For a first infection, a simpler combination (e.g. Ampicillin and Kanamycin) will generally suffice. For subsequent infections and after a stay in hospital, the therapy should in general consist of a combination of a carbenicillin or a cephalosporin and Gentamicin, Amikacin, Tobramycin or some other aminoglycoside antibiotic. Sometimes the bacteriological data will make it possible for a more specific choice of antibiotics to be made; for instance, in cases of colonization by *Klebsiella* species, a cephalosporin combined with an aminoglycoside could be used, and for a *Pseudomonas* infection a combination of carbenicillin and an aminoglycoside should be given[82, 86, 95, 96, 182-185].

Because of the granulocytopenia, preference should be given to bactericidal antibiotics, which should be given parenterally in high doses and preferably in synergistic combinations. The dosage of Gentamicin, Tobramycin or Amikacin can best be chosen on the basis of a nomogram[186-188], which improves the prediction of the concentration reached in the body. When possible, it is advisable to determine the serum concentrations of these antibiotics.

Such treatment is adequate for most of the Gram-negative rods including *Pseudomonas* spp., for Gram-positive micro-organisms including *Staphylococcus aureus*, and for most anaerobes such as *Bacteroides* spp., when carbenicillin is used. For most micro-organisms the combination of carbenicillin and Gentamicin is synergistic, but they must be administered separately.

After the institution of antibiotic therapy, the patient must be thoroughly examined daily and radiographs of the chest must be made at regular intervals until the focus of the infection is found and the micro-organism identified. If blood cultures are positive, the search for the source must be continued, the more so because local therapy can be of essential importance (for instance in cases with an abscess, empyema, obstruction, a catheter etc.). It is not unusual to find the source of the infection after a few days, for instance in the lung (pneumonia), anorectal lesions, or septic arthritis.

When the *in vitro* sensitivity of the isolated micro-organism is known, the preliminary antibiotic therapy must be changed if necessary. The choice must be made from among bactericidal antibiotics with the narrowest spectrum possible. If the patient does not show improvement on this treatment, even when a positive culture has demonstrated a micro-organism sensitive to the chosen antibiotic, another cause must be sought. If cultures are negative and no focus is found but the condition of the patient improves and the temperature becomes normal, the antibiotic therapy can generally be withdrawn 5 days after the temperature is normal. If the cultures are negative but the condition of the patient does not improve, a non-bacterial cause must be considered, e.g. a fungal, viral, or protozoal infection. In some cases a resistant bacterium may be involved and a third antibiotic can be added to the therapy (e.g. a cephalosporin, carbenicillin, clindamycin, or metronidazole).

Long continuation of antibiotic therapy after reasonable exclusion of an infection has very distinct drawbacks, not only because toxicity of these drugs can occur but also because of the possibility that a resistant microbial flora will develop and lead to another infection. According to Green[102], the chance of a super-infection of this kind is 12% after 6 days of therapy, 25% after up to 12 days, and 50% with more than 12 days of treatment. In general, once reasonable exclusion of an infection has been reached, antibiotic therapy can be withdrawn within 4 days. After that, a thorough investigation of the patient must be undertaken. If appropriate, antifungal therapy may be considered[96].

When the cultures are negative but an infection originating from an anorectal lesion or a lesion elsewhere in the digestive tract is suspected, a drug against anaerobic micro-organisms may be given, for instance metronidazole. If the blood cultures remain positive or a patient with a known infection with a known micro-organism having a known *in vitro* sensitivity does not improve under adequate bactericidal therapy and shows a persistent severe granulocytopenia, granulocyte transfusion should be considered. It seems probable that benefit can only be expected from such a transfusion when there are fewer than 100 granulocytes per mm³ (see under *Additional therapy*, page 374). (It is known that Gentamicin is not effective as monotherapy for *Pseudomonas* in the presence of severe granulocytopenia[70,182], probably because of the limited therapeutic index and the low concentration reached in the body.) As already mentioned on page 372 better results can be expected with Gentamicin using a dosage nomogram. As noted good results are obtainable with the combination of Gentamicin (Tobramycin or Amicacin) and a carbenicillin, or a carbenicillin alone.

A more extensive diagnostic investigation may be required to detect the pathogenic micro-organism, e.g. a fungus or protozoa (see Table 10.5). In cases with lung infiltrates it is often necessary to use more aggressive diagnostic methods, as discussed on page 371, because the sputum is often negative for non-bacterial micro-organisms and may have become contaminated via the oropharynx during sampling, which makes the culture results unreliable. For infections originating from the digestive tract, the pharynx, oesophagus and anus must be examined and the faeces investigated for the presence of *Candida*, *Salmonella*, and *Lamblia*.

When a disseminated infection is suspected, the organ of its origin must be sought; in this respect fundoscopy, urine investigation for *Candida*, repeated chest X-rays, gallium-67 scanning, computed tomographic scanning and echography are useful. If meningoencephalitis is suspected, a spinal puncture to collect a sample of CSF must be performed without delay. In active infections *Cryptococcus* antigen may be found in the CSF[117] (see also page 368) or blood[14, 139]. Counter-electrophoresis makes it possible to demonstrate bacterial antigens, which is important for rapid diagnosis in cases with septicaemia[107, 137, 165].

The diagnosis of virus infections remains difficult, but it is important to store (in the refrigerator) a number of serum samples from each patient in order to be able to identify any rising titres due to infection with a specific agent. Several serum samples should be obtained in the acute phase and 2–3 weeks after the onset of a clinical picture suggesting infection. Virus cultures take considerable time, but rapid diagnosis of blister and other fluids, including CSF, is possible with electron microscopy, in cases of a few viruses. Inclusion bodies in cells collected from oral swabs may be seen in herpes simplex. Cytomegalovirus pneumonia can be diagnosed in sections and cultures of lung biopsy material and sometimes from surface sputum. Furthermore, in cases of hepatitis the hepatitis virus and core antigens may be found in the serum.

Rapid diagnosis is now also possible with the use of immunofluorescence studies, immunoperoxidase tests, radioimmunoassay, and counter-immuno-electrophoresis[145, 189, 190]. Some progress has been made in the treatment of viral infections, especially of herpes viruses with drugs such as adenine arabinoside[145, 191–193], and in some cases interferon has been used[194].

10.8 ADDITIONAL THERAPY

10.8.1 Granulocyte transfusion

Although new antibiotics have greatly improved the treatment of infections in patients with granulocytopenia, an infection with or without septicaemia may sometimes persist during this treatment if the granulocytopenia is severe. In animal models it has been shown conclusively that granulocyte transfusions are effective in such situations, but it is less certain whether this holds for humans. Many factors influence the results of this type of therapy. Recently, indications of effectiveness have been obtained in randomized studies, but they have all been done in very small groups of patients. Some of these patients improve on antibiotic therapy alone, others show fever but no infection, and some show spontaneous bone marrow recovery. The effect of granulocyte transfusions in these studies varies widely.

For these transfusions, use may be made of the granulocytes of healthy donors or of patients with chronic granulocytic leukaemia collected by filtration leukophoresis, continuous-flow centrifugation, or by the buffy coat method. It has been shown that these granulocytes retain most of their functions *in vitro* and *in vivo* (e.g. chemokinesis, phagocytosis, and killing)[69,195]. Granulocyte function is not influenced by pre-treatment of the donor with corticosteroids[64,69,195].

A daily transfusion of more than 10^{10} granulocytes is required. This increases the number of granulocytes in the patient only by several hundred per mm^3. These daily transfusions must be continued until improvement is obtained, and according to the literature for at least 4 days. Studies which have been done have not made it clear at what level of the patient's granulocytes transfusion is most beneficial. Some authors consider less than 1000 per mm^3 to be an indication for granulocyte transfusion, others less than 500 per mm^3. Still others recommend transfusion of granulocytes only when an infection or septicaemia does not respond to adequate antibiotic therapy. There is a distinct improvement in patients in whom the granulocytopenia persists under transfusion when this treatment is continued[82,83,87,195–201].

An absolute indication for granulocyte transfusion is persistently positive blood cultures or failure of infections to improve under adequate bactericidal antibiotic therapy with persisting severe granulocytopenia. This situation occurs when the granulocyte level stays below 100 per mm^3 [82,83,87]. In addition to the precise indication for granulocyte transfusion, many other questions remain to be answered, e.g. the number of cells to be transfused each time, and the optimal timing and frequency of transfusions. A number of centres advocate prophylactic transfusions when granulocytopenia is present, but this does not seem appropriate and moreover may be impossible because of the number of donors required. Routine transfusion seems neither feasible nor desirable[195,202]. Furthermore, complications can accompany both the collection and administration of granulocytes. During filtration leukophoresis, complement activation may occur in the donor and lead to granulocytopenia due to margination of granulocytes, e.g. in the lungs, and this may be accompanied by pulmonary diffusion disturbances and elevated lung resistance[57,195,203,204], as has been described in haemodialysis patients. Problems which can occur in the recipient include the induction of HLA antibodies, which may complicate further transfusion. In addition, the formation of leukocyte antibodies can be induced[195].

The donor must in any case belong to the same ABO blood group as the patient, because some erythrocytes will unavoidably be transfused at the same time. Leukocyte cross-matching should also be done. When erythrocytes must be transfused, it is important to make the transfused material

extremely leukocyte-poor by filtration through a cotton-wool filter[205].
Thrombocyte preparations can be made leukocyte-poor by prolonged
centrifugation[206]. In a few cases a graft-versus-host reaction has been
induced by granulocyte transfusion. To avoid this, the granulocyte material
can be irradiated with 1500 rad before transfusion[207].

10.8.2 Isolation and decontamination

As was stated at the beginning of this chapter, the origin of micro-organisms
leading to an infection can be exogenous or endogenous. In general, an
exogenous micro-organism that causes an infection will first colonize the
patient and then (temporarily) belong to his endogenous microflora.
Various conditions promote this colonization, as discussed on page 345.
Most of the infections occurring in these patients are endogenous in origin
(mainly from the digestive tract). An important place must always be
assigned to preventive measures to avoid infection. The exogenous acquisition of micro-organisms can be prevented by adequate isolation, and the
endogenous source can be eliminated by decontamination of the skin and
the mucous membranes of the oropharynx, digestive tract, nose, and
genitalia.

10.8.2.1 *Reverse isolation*

A number of possibilities are available for reverse isolation, i.e. nursing in a
single room, an ultra-clean room, a 'life-island', or a laminar air-flow room.
The ordinary room is almost worthless for reverse isolation; the ultra-clean
room does not prohibit colonization but does delay it. Use of a 'life-island'
does not completely guarantee non-colonization either, because the isolators
frequently become contaminated; in addition, they are difficult to operate
and create many psychological problems for the patient. Only the laminar
air-flow isolator is satisfactory both bacteriologically and psychologically.

10.8.2.2 *Decontamination*

For decontamination of the skin and orifices, antiseptics can be used. For
intestinal decontamination, use is made of poorly absorbed antibiotics
against aerobic and anaerobic intestinal flora in combination with antifungal drugs. During the decontamination procedure, the patient should be
nursed in a laminar air-flow isolator and should be given sterile food.
  Regimes for total decontamination of the digestive tract usually consist of
treatment with Gentamicin or neomycin combined with a cephalosporin or
vancomycin with nystatin or amphotericin B by mouth. The mouth and
oropharynx (important for respiratory tract infections) and genitalia can be
treated with a cream containing antibiotics and fungotoxic drugs. Such

regimes make it possible to obtain a considerable reduction in the percentage of infections, particularly of serious infections, in patients with lowered resistance[99, 208].

Partial intestinal decontamination is intended solely to eliminate the potentially pathogenic aerobic flora and maintain the anaerobic flora which provide colonization resistance, so that the patient does not acquire exogenous micro-organisms too rapidly[83, 103]. Partial decontamination can be effected by a combination of neomycin (or kanamycin) and polymyxin (or colistin) and nalidixic acid with amphotericin B (or miconazole). Selective decontamination seems very promising from preliminary results, and just as effective, and less liable to lead to vulnerability than total decontamination. Moreover, it is less difficult to carry out and less of a burden for both the patient and the medical personnel.

In controlled studies, patients given strict reverse isolation and decontamination developed only half as many infections as those in control groups and only one-fourth as many serious infections. Furthermore, the mortality from infections dropped appreciably and septicaemia was rare[99]. Decontamination without isolation gave widely differing results in various studies. This form of prophylaxis must be discarded, because of the patients' extreme sensitivity to colonization by micro-organisms resistant to this regime.

Little data are available on the effect of adequate reverse isolation alone. This raises the question of whether the combination of strict reverse isolation and sterile food might not be effective for the prevention of infections. The short-term effect would probably be limited, because most of the early infections are endogenous, but this approach offers the great advantage of avoiding the acquisition of bacteria from the environment which is extremely important for the group of patients with reduced resistance, since the responsible micro-organisms of later infections are probably acquired in the hospital. A second advantage of isolation for this group of patients is that it makes it possible to protect the hospital environment against contamination with the antibiotics they take, as well as against their microflora. This problem has, as yet, received little attention.

10.8.3 Reinforcement of body defences

Some measures can be taken to restore or increase the resistance of the body defences (Table 10.3), such as treatment of the underlying and concurrent disease(s), elimination of obstructions, optimal nutrition, and granulocyte transfusions etc., if indicated. Passive immunization is possible with hyperimmune gammaglobulin immediately after contact with hepatitis B[154, 209], varicella-zoster or measles virus.

Active immunization may be considered for *Streptococcus pneumoniae*[210–213], *Haemophilus influenzae*[214], *Pseudomonas aeruginosa*[215–217], influenza, hepatitis B[145], cytomegalovirus[115] or varicella-zoster virus[218].

The value of the administration of more experimental drugs which stimulate the T lymphocytes and/or monocytes by microbial antigens (e.g. BCG), the use of levamisole[219-222], transfer factor[31,32,34,35,223], thymosine[224], immune RNA[230], and interferon[44,194,209,227] are still in the experimental stages[35]. Lithium can stimulate the production of granulocytes[225,226] and requires further trials.

References

1. Drutz, D. J. (1976). Immunity and infection. In: *Basic and Clinical Immunology* (H. H. Fudenberg, D. P. Stites, J. L. Caldwell and J. V. Wells, eds.) (Canada: Lange)
2. van der Waaij, D., Berghuis-de Vries, J. M. and Lekkerkerk-van der Wees, J. E. C. (1971). Colonization resistance of the digestive tract in conventional and antibiotic-treated mice. *J. Hyg.*, **69**, 405
3. van der Waaij, D. and Berghuis-de Vries, J. M. (1974). *J. Hyg.*, **72**, 379
4. Sommers, H. M. (1975). The indigenous microbiota of the human host. In: *The Biologic and Clinical Basis of Infectious Diseases* (G. P. Youmans, P. Y. Paterson and H. M. Sommers, eds.) (Philadelphia: W. B. Saunders Company)
5. Hauptman, S. P. and Tomasi, T. B. (1976). The secretory immune system. In: *Basic and Clinical Immunology* (H. H. Fudenberg, D. P. Stites, J. L. Caldwell and J. V. Wells, eds.) (Canada: Lange)
6. McClelland, D. B. L. Immunity to infection in the gastrointestinal tract. In: *Immunology of the Gastrointestinal Tract* (P. Asquith, ed.) (Edinburgh: Churchill Livingstone)
7. Waldman, R. H. and Ganguly, R. (1974). Immunity to infections on secretory surfaces. *J. Infec. Dis.*, **130**, 419
8. Waldman, R. H. and Ganguly, R. (1976). Role of immune mechanisms on secretory surfaces in prevention of infections. In: *Infection and the Compromised Host* (J. C. Allen, ed.) (Baltimore: Williams & Wilkins Company)
9. Walker, W. A. and Isselbacher, K. J. (1977). Intestinal antibodies. *N. Eng. J. Med.*, **297**, 767
10. *The Lancet* (1977). Bacterial adhesiveness and the gut. *Lancet*, **i**, 1293
11. Rowlands, D. T. and Daniele, R. P. (1975). Surface receptors in the immuno response. *N. Engl. J. Med.*, **293**, 26
12. Donaldson, D. M. (1973). B-Lysin and host resistance. In: *'Non-Specific' Factors Influencing Host Resistance*, p. 316 (Basel: Karger)
13. Klebanoff, S. J. (1975). Antimicrobial mechanisms in neutrophilic polymorphonuclear leukocytes. *Sem. Hematol.*, **12**, 117
14. Krick, J. A. and Remington, J. S. (1976). Opportunistic invasive fungal infections in patients with leukemia and lymphoma. *Clin. Haematol.*, **5**, 249
15. Payne, S. M. and Finkelstein, R. A. (1978). The critical role of iron in host–bacterial interactions. *J. Clin. Invest.*, **21**, 1428
16. Quie, P. G. (1975). Pathology of bactericidal power of neutrophils. *Sem. Hematol.*, **12**, 143
17. Weinberg, E. D. (1974). Iron and susceptibility to infectious disease. *Science*, **184**, 952
18. Weinberg, E. D. (1975). Nutritional immunity. Host's attempt to withhold iron from microbial invaders. *J. Am. Med. Ass.*, **231**, 39
19. Spirer, Z., Zakuth, V., Diamant, S., Mondorf, W., Stefanescu, T., Stabinsky Y. and Fridkon, M. (1977). Decreased tuftsin concentrations in patients who have undergone splenectomy. *Br. Med. J.*, **2**, 1574
20. Stossel, T. P. (1975). Phagocytosis: recognition and ingestion. *Sem. Hematol.*, **12**, 83

21. Miller, M. E. (1975). Pathology of chemotaxis and random mobility. *Sem. Hematol.*, **12**, 59
22. Senn, H. J. and Jungi, W. F. (1975). Neutrophil migration in health and disease. *Sem. Hematol.*, **12**, 27
23. Keller, H. U., Hess, M. W. and Cottier, H. (1975). Physiology of chemotaxis and random mobility. *Sem. Hematol.*, **12**, 47
24. Leading article (1978). Lymphokines: an increasing repertoire. *Br. Med. J.*, **1**, 62
25. van Waarde, D., Hulsink-Hesselink, E. and van Furth, R. (1976). A serum factor including monocytosis during an acute inflammatory reaction caused by newborn calf serum. *Cell Tis. Kinet.*, **9**, 51
26. Babior, B. M. (1978). Oxygen-dependent microbial killing by phagocytes. *N. Engl. J. Med.*, **298**, 659–712
27. Dannenberg, A. M. (1975). Macrophages in inflammation and infection. *N. Engl. J. Med.*, **293**, 489
28. van Furth, R. and van Zwet, T. L. (1973). *In vitro* determination of phagocytosis and intracellular killing by polymorphonuclear phagocytes. In: *Handbook of Experimental Immunology*, 2nd edition (D. M. Weir, ed.) (Oxford: Blackwell Scientific Publications Ltd.)
29. Gershon, L. D. and Remington, J. S. (1974). Resistance against *Cryptococcus* conferred by intracellular bacteria and protozoa. *J. Infect. Dis.*, **123**, 22
30. Neu, H. C. (1976). The role of cellular and humoral factors in infections. *Clin. Haematol.*, **5**, 449
31. Polmar, S. H. (1973). Transfer-factor therapy of immunodeficiencies. *N. Engl. J. Med.*, **289**, 1420
32. Potter, H., Rosenfeld, S. and Dressler, D. (1974). Transfer-factor. *Ann. Intern. Med.*, **81**, 838
33. Solomkin, J. S., Mills, E. L., Giebink, G. S., Nelson, R. D., Simmons, R. L. and Quie, P. G. (1978). Phagocytosis of *Candida albicans* by human leukocytes: opsonic requirements. *J. Infect. Dis.*, **137**, 30
34. Wybran, J., Levin, A. S., Spitler, L. E. and Fudenberg, H. (1973). Rosette-forming cells, immunologic deficiency diseases and transfer factor. *N. Engl. J. Med.*, **288**, 710
35. Wybran, J. (1976). Experimental aspects of immunotherapy. In: *Basic and Clinical Immunology* (H. H. Fudenberg, D. P. Stites, J. L. Caldwell and J. V. Wells, eds.) (Canada: Lange)
36. Merigan, T. C. (1974). Host defenses against viral disease. *N. Engl. J. Med.*, **290**, 323
37. Golden, M. H. N., Golden, B. E., Harland, P. S. E. G. and Jackson, A. A. (1978). Zinc and immunocompetence in protein-energy malnutrition. *Lancet*, **i**, 1226
38. Kay, M. M. B. (1976). Aging and the decline of immune responsiveness. In: *Basic and Clinical Immunology* (H. H. Fudenberg, D. P. Stites, J. L. Caldwell and J. V. Wells, eds.) (Canada: Lange)
39. Leading article (1969). Genetics and infection. *Br. Med. J.*, **2**, 317
40. Seth, V. and Chandra, R. K. (1972). Opsonic activity, phagocytosis and bactericidal capacity of polymorphs in undernutrition. *Arch. Dis. Child.*, **47**, 282
41. Caldwell, J. L. (1976). Genetic regulation of immune responses. In: *Basic and Clinical Immunology* (H. H. Fudenberg, D. P. Stites, J. L. Caldwell and J. V. Wells, eds.) (Canada: Lange)
42. Dionigi, R., Zonta, A., Dominioni, L., Gnes, F. and Ballabio, A. (1977). The effects of total parenteral nutrition on immunodepression due to malnutrition. *Ann. Surg.*, **185**, 467
43. Douglas, S. D. and Schopfer, K. (1974). Phagocyte function in protein-calorie malnutrition. *J. Clin. Exp. Immunol.*, **17**, 121
44. Good, R. A., Fernandes, G., Yunis, E. J., Cooper, W. C., Jose, D. C., Kramer, T. R. and Hansen, M. A. (1976). Nutritional deficiency, immunologic function, and disease. *Am. J. Pathol.*, **84**, 599

45. Marchalonis, J. J. (1976). Cell cooperation in immune response. In: *Basic and Clinical Immunology* (H. H. Fudenberg, D. P. Stites, J. L. Caldwell and J. V. Wells, eds.) (Canada: Lange)

46. Garibaldi, R. A., Burke, J. P., Dickman, M. L. and Smith, C. B. (1974). Factors predisposing to bacteriuria during indwelling urethral catheterization. *N. Engl. J. Med.*, **291**, 215

47. Montgomerie, J. Z. and Edwards, J. E. (1978). Association of infection due to *Candida albicans* with intravenous hyperalimentation. *J. Infect. Dis.*, **137**, 197

48. Ryan, J. A., Abel, R. M., Abbott, W. M., Hopkins, C. C., Chesney, T. M., Colley, R., Phillips, K. and Fischer, J. E. (1974). Catheter complications in total parenteral nutrition. *N. Engl. J. Med.*, **290**, 757

49. Pollack, M., Nieman, R. E., Reinhardt, J. A., Charache, P., Jett, M. P. and Hardy, P. H. (1972). Factors influencing colonization and antibiotic-resistance patterns of Gram-negative bacteria in hospital patients. *Lancet*, **ii**, 668

50. Seelig, M. S. (1966). The role of antibiotics in the pathogenesis of *Candida* infections. *Am. J. Med.*, **40**, 887

51. Valenti, W. M., Trudell, R. G. and Bentley, D. W. (1978). Factors predisposing to oropharyngeal colonization with Gram-negative bacilli in the aged. *N. Engl. J. Med.*, **298**, 1108

52. Newman, S. L., Vogler, L. B., Feigin, R. D. and Johnston, R. B. (1978). Recurrent septicaemia associated with congenital deficiency of C_2 and partial deficiency of factor B and the alternative complement pathway. *N. Engl. J. Med.*, **299**, 290

53. Cline, M. J. (1974). Drugs and phagocytes. *N. Engl. J. Med.*, **291**, 1187

54. Bagdade, J. D., Root, T. K. and Bulger, R. J. (1974). Impaired leukocyte function in patients with poorly controlled diabetes. *Diabetes*, **23**, 9

55. Craddock, P. R., Yamata, Y., van Santen, L., Gilberstadt, S., Silvis, S. and Jacob, H. S. (1974). Acquired phagocytic dysfunction. *N. Engl. J. Med.*, **290**, 1403

56. *The Lancet* (1977). Hypophosphatemia. *Lancet*, **ii**, 122

57. Chervenick, P. A. (1977). Dialysis, neutropenia, lung dysfunction and complement. *N. Engl. J. Med.*, **296**, 810

58. Hersh, E. M., Whitecar, J. P., McCredie, K. B., Bodey, G. P. and Freireich, E. J. (1971). Chemotherapy, immunocompetence, immunosuppression and prognosis in acute leukemia. *N. Engl. J. Med.*, **285**, 1211

59. Paglieroni, T. and MacKenzie, M. R. (1977). Studies on the pathogenesis of an immune defect in multiple myeloma. *J. Clin. Invest.*, **59**, 1120

60. Siegal, F. P. (1976). Inhibition of T-cell rosette formation by Hodgkin-disease serum. *N. Engl. J. Med.*, **295**, 1314

61. Tattersall, M. H. N. (1975). Aggressive cancer treatment and its role in predisposing to infection. *Eur. J. Cancer*, **11 (suppl.)**, 9

62. Dale, D. C., Fauci, A. S. and Wolff, S. M. (1974). Alternate-day Prednisone. Leukocyte kinetics and susceptibility to infections. *N. Engl. J. Med.*, **291**, 1154

63. Fauci, A. S. and Dale, D. C. (1974). The effect of *in vitro* hydrocortisone on subpopulation of human lymphocytes. *J. Clin. Invest.*, **53**, 240

64. Glasser, L., Huestis, D. W. and Jones, J. F. (1977). Functional capabilities of steroid-recruited neutrophils harvested for clinical transfusion. *N. Engl. J. Med.*, **297**, 1033

65. MacGregor, R. R. (1977). Granulocyte adherence changes induced by hemodialysis, endotoxin, epinephrine and glucocorticoids. *Ann. Intern. Med.*, **86**, 35

66. Rosenthal, S. and Balow, J. E. (1975). Mechanisms of glucocorticosteroids suppression of cell-mediated immunity. In: *Mononuclear Phagocytes in Immunity, Infection and Pathology* (R. van Furth, ed.) (Oxford: Blackwell Scientific Publications)

67. Stevenson, R. D. (1977). Mechanism of anti-inflammatory action of glucocorticosteroids. *Lancet*, **i**, 225

68. van Zwet, T. L., Thompson, J. and van Furth, R. (1975). Effect of glucocorticosteroids on the phagocytosis and intracellular killing by peritoneal macrophages. *Infect. Immun.*, **12**, 699

69. Steigbigel, R. T., Baum, J., MacPherson, J. L. and Nusbacher, J. (1978). Granulocyte bactericidal capacity and chemotaxis as affected by continuous-flow centrifugation and filtration leukapheresis steroid administration, and storage. *Blood*, **52**, 197

70. Bodey, G. P. and Rodriguez, V. (1973). Advances in the management of *Pseudomonas aeruginosa* infections in cancer patients. *Eur. J. Cancer*, **9**, 435

71. Bodey, G. P., Rodriguez, V., Chang, H. Y. and Narboni, G. (1978). Fever and infection in leukemic patients. *Cancer*, **41**, 1610

72. Casewell, M. W. and Phillips, I. (1978). Epidemiological patterns of *Klebsiella* colonization and infection in an intensive care ward. *J. Hygi. (Cambridge)*, **80**, 295

73. Curie, K., Speller, D. C. E., Simpson, R. A., Stephens, M. and Cooke, D. I. (1978). A hospital epidemic caused by a Gentamicin-resistant *Klebsiella* aerogenes. *J. Hygi. (Cambridge)*, **80**, 115

74. *The Lancet* (1966). *Pseudomonas aeruginosa*. *Lancet*, **i**, 1139

75. McGowan, J. E., Barnes, M. W. and Finland, M. (1975). Bacteremia at Boston City Hospital: occurrence and mortality during 12 selected years (1935–72), with special reference to hospital-acquired cases. *J. Infect. Dis.*, **132**, 316

76. Schimpff, S. C. (1975). Diagnosis of infection in patients with cancer. *Eur. J. Cancer*, **11** (suppl.)

77. Shooter, R. A. (1971). Bowel colonization of hospital patients by *Pseudomonas aeruginosa* and *Escherichia coli*. *Proc. R. Soc. Med.*, **64**, 989

78. Allen, J. C. (1976). Infection complicating neoplastic disease and cytotoxic therapy. In: *Infection and the Compromised Host* (J. C. Allen, ed.) (Baltimore: Williams & Wilkins)

79. Armstrong, D., Chmel, H., Singer, C., Tapper, M. and Rosen, P. P. (1975). Non-bacterial infections associated with neoplastic disease. *Eur. J. Cancer*, **11**, suppl. 79

80. Bouza, E., Burgaleta, C. and Golde, D. W. (1978). Infections in hairy-cell leukemia. *Blood*, **51**, 851

81. Chang, H. Y., Rodriguez, V., Narboni, G., Bodey, G. P. and Freireich, E. J. (1975). Causes of death in adults with acute leukemia. *Medicine*, **55**, 256

82. The EORTC International Antimicrobial Therapy Project Group (1978). Three antibiotic regimes in the treatment of infection in febrile granulocytopenic patients with cancer. *J. Infect. Dis.*, **137**, 14

83. Guiot, H. F. L. and van der Meer, J. W. M. (1978). Infections in granulocytopenia. The efficacy of partial antibiotic decontamination. *Proc. Courchevet*

84. Infectious Complications in Haematological Diseases (1976). *Clinics in Haematology* (G. P. Bodey, ed.), vol. 5, no. 2 (London: W. B. Saunders Company Ltd.)

85. Levin, M. J. and Zaia, J. A. (1977). Immunosuppression and infection progress. *N. Engl. J. Med.*, **296**, 1406

86. Levine, A. S., Schimpff, S. C., Graw, R. G. and Young, R. C. (1974). Haematologic malignancies and other marrow failure states: progress in the management of complicating infections. *Sem. Hematol.*, **11**, 141

87. van der Meer, J. W. M., Alleman, M. and Boekhout, M. Infectious episodes in severely granulocytopenic patients. (Submitted for publication)

88. Meyers, B. R., Hirschman, S. Z. and Axelrod, J. A. (1972). Current patterns of infection in multiple myeloma. *Am. J. Med.*, **52**, 97

89. Nauta, E. H. and van Furth, R. (1975). Infection in immunodepressed patients. *Infection*, **3**, 202

90. Sickles, E. A., Greene, W. H. and Wiernik, P. H. (1975). Clinical presentation of infection in granulocytopenic patients. *Arch. Intern. Med.*, **135**, 715

91. Simmons, R. L., Balfour, H. H., Lopez, C., Mauer, S. M., Kjellstrand, C. M., Buselmeier,

T. J. and Najarian, J. S. (1975). Infection in immunosuppressed transplant recipients. *Surg. Clin. N. Am.*, **55**, 1419

92. Snow, R. M. and Dismukes, W. E. (1975). Cryptococcal meningitis. *Arch. Intern. Med.*, **135**, 1155

93. Dinarello, C. A. and Wolff, S. M. (1978). Pathogenesis of fever in man. *N. Engl. J. Med.*, **298**, 607

94. Goodall, P. T. and Vosti, K. L. (1975). Fever in acute myelogenous leukemia. *Arch. Intern. Med.*, **135**, 1197

95. Gurwith, M. J., Brunton, J. L., Lank, B. A., Ronald, A. R., Harding, G. K. M. and McCullough, D. W. (1978). Granulocytopenia in hospitalized patients. *Am. J. Med.*, **64**, 127

96. Rodriguez, V. and Bodey, G. P. (1976). Antibacterial therapy–special considerations in neutropenic patients. *Clin. Haematol.*, **5**, 347

97. Bodey, G. P., Buckley, M., Sathe, Y. S. and Freireich, E. J. (1966). Quantitative relationships between circulating leucocytes and infection in patients with acute leukemia. *Ann. Intern. Med.*, **64**, 328

98. Valdivieso, M. (1976). Bacterial infection in haematological diseases. *Clin. Haematol.*, **5**, 229

99. Levine, A. S. (1976). Protected environment–prophylactic antibiotic programmes; clinical studies. *Clin. Haematol.*, **5**, 409

100. Ayliffe, G. A. J. (1975). Antibiotic policies. *J. Antimicrobial Chemother.*, **1**, 255

101. Cartwright, R. Y. (1978). Use of antibiotics. *Br. Med. J.*, **2**, 108

102. Greene, W. H., Schimpff, S. C., Young, V. M. *et al.* (1973). Emperic carbenicillin, gentamicin, and cephalothin therapy for presumed infection. *Ann. Intern. Med.*, **78**, 825

103. Guiot, H. F. L. and van Furth, R. (1977). Partial antibiotic decontamination. *Br. Med. J.*, **1**, 800

104. Schimpff, S. C., Greene, W. H., Young, V. M., Fortner, C. L., Jepsen, L., Nancy, C., Block, J. and Wiernik, P. H. (1975). Infection prevention in acute non-lymphocytic leukemia. *Ann. Intern. Med.*, **82**, 351

105. Steigbigel, R. T., Johnson, P. K. and Remington, J. S. (1974). The nitroblue tetrazolium reduction test versus conventional hematology in the diagnosis of bacterial infection. *N. Engl. J. Med.*, **290**, 235

106. Aisner, J., Schimpff, S. C. and Wiernik, P. H. (1977). Treatment of invasive *Aspergillosis*: relation of early diagnosis and treatment to response. *Ann. Intern. Med.*, **86**, 539

107. Miller, G. G., Witwer, M. W., Braude, A. I. and Davis, C. E. (1974). Rapid identification of *Candida albicans* septicemia in man by gas–liquid chromatography. *J. Clin. Invest.*, **54**, 1235

108. Sommers, H. M. (1975). Laboratory diagnosis of bacterial and fungal infections. In: *The Biologic and Clinical Basis of Infectious Diseases* (G. P. Youmans, P. Y. Paterson, H. M. Sommers, eds.) (Philadelphia: W. B. Saunders Company)

109. Warren, R. C., Bartlett, A., Bidwell, D. E., Richardson, M. D., Voller, A. and White, L. O. (1977). Diagnosis of invasive *Candidosis* by enzyme immunoassay of serum antigen. *Br. Med. J.*, **1**, 1183

110. *The Lancet* (1977). Enzyme markers in leukemia. *Lancet*, **ii**, 539

111. Murphy, S. B. and Mauer, A. M. (1977). Terminal transferase and lymphoblastic neoplasms. *N. Engl. J. Med.*, **297**, 502

112. DiBella, N. J. and Brown, G. L. (1978). Immunologic dysfunction in the myeloproliferative disorders. *Cancer*, **42**, 149

113. Abdallah, P. S., Mark, J. B. D. and Merigan, T. C. (1976). Diagnosis of cytomegalovirus pneumonia in compromised hosts. *Am. J. Med.*, **61**, 326

114. Hillinger, S. M. and Herzig, G. P. (1978). Impaired cell-mediated immunity in Hodgkin's disease mediated by suppressor lymphocytes and monocytes. *J. Clin. Invest.*, **21**, 1620

115. Leading article (1977). Cytomegalovirus in immune compromised hosts. *Br. Med. J.*, **1**, 1048

116. *The Lancet* (1977). Cytomegalovirus in adults. *Lancet*, **ii**, 541

117. Ruckdeschel, J. C., Schimpff, S. C., Smyth, A. C. and Mardiney, M. R. (1977). Herpes zoster and impaired cell-associated immunity to the varicella-zoster virus in patients with Hodgkin's disease. *Am. J. Med.*, **62**, 77

118. Weitzman, S. A., Aisenberg, A. C., Siber, G. R. and Smith, D. H. (1977). Impaired humoral immunity in treated Hodgkin's disease. *N. Engl. J. Med.*, **297**, 245

119. MacGregor, R. R., Negendank, W. G. and Schreiber, A. D. (1978). Impaired granulocyte adherence in multiple myeloma: relationship to complement system, granulocyte delivery, and infection. *Blood*, **51**, 591

120. Siegal, F. P., Siegal, M. and Good, R. A. (1978). Role of helper, suppressor and B-cell defects in the pathogenesis of the hypogammaglobulinemias. *N. Engl. J. Med.*, **299**, 172

121. Drachman, R. H. (1976). Splenic and reticuloendothelial function and infection. In: *Infection and the Compromised Host* (J. C. Allen, ed.) (Baltimore: Williams & Wilkins Company)

122. Chilcote, R. R., Baehner, R. L. and Hammond, D. (1976). Septicemia and meningitis in children splenectomized for Hodgkin's disease. *N. Engl. J. Med.*, **295**, 789

123. Constantoulakis, M., Trichopoulos, D., Avgoustaki, O. and Economidou, J. (1978). Serum immunoglobulin concentrations before and after splenectomy in patients with homozygous B-thalassaemia. *J. Clin. Pathol.*, **31**, 546

124. Ertel, I. J., Boles, E. T. and Newton, W. A. (1977). Infections after splenectomy. *N. Engl. J. Med.*, **296**, 1174

125. Infections in 92 splenectomized patients with Hodgkin's disease: a clinical review. (1975). *Am. J. Med.*, **59**, 695

126. Likhite, V. V. (1976). Immunological impairment and susceptibility to infection after splenectomy. *J. Am. Med. Assoc.*, **236**, 1376

127. Weitzman, S. A. and Aisenberg, A. C. (1977). Fulminant sepsis after the successful treatment of Hodgkin's disease. *Am. J. Med.*, **62**, 47

128. Alexander, J. W. and Fisher, M. W. (1970). Immunological determinants of *Pseudomonas* infections of man accompanying severe burn injury. *J. Trauma*, **10**, 565

129. Bjornson, A. B., Altemeier, W. A. and Bjornson, H. S. (1977). Changes in humoral components of host defense following burn trauma. *Ann. Surg.*, **186**, 88

130. Grogan, J. B. and Miller, R. C. (1973). Impaired function of polymorphonuclear leukocytes in patients with burns and other trauma. *Surg. Gynecol. Obstet.*, **137**, 784

131. Neilan, B. A., Taddeine, L. and Strate, R. G. (1977). T lymphocyte rosette formation after major burns. *J. Am. Med. Assoc.*, **238**, 493

132. Burke, J. F., Quinby, W. C., Bondoc, C. C., Sheehy, E. M. and Morenho, H. C. (1977). The contribution of a bacterially isolated environment to the prevention of infection in seriously burned patients. *Ann. Surg.*, **186**, 377

133. Perez, H. D., Lipton, M. and Goldstein, I. M. (1978). A specific inhibitor of complement (C5)-derived chemotactic activity in serum from patients with systemic lupus erythematosus. *J. Clin. Invest.*, **21**, 29

134. Drutz, D. J. and Graybill, J. R. (1976). Infectious diseases. In: *Basic and Clinical Immunology* (H. H. Fudenberg, D. P. Stites, J. L. Caldwell and J. V. Wells, eds.) (Canada: Lange)

135. Kaplan, M. H., Rosen, P. P. and Armstrong, D. (1977). Cryptococcosis in a cancer hospital. *Cancer*, **39**, 2265

136. Davies, S. F., Khan, M. and Sarosi, G. A. (1978). Disseminated histoplasmosis in immunologically suppressed patients. *Am. J. Med.*, **64**, 94

137. Edwards, J. E., Lehrer, R. I., Stiehm, E. R., Fischer, T. J. and Young, L. S. (1978).

Severe candidal infections. Clinical perspective, immune defense mechanisms, and current concepts of therapy. *Ann. Intern. Med.*, **89**, 91

138. Gallis, H. A., Berman, R. A., Cate, T. R., Hamilton, J. D., Gunnels, J. C. and Stickel, D. L. (1975). Fungal infection following renal transplantation. *Arch. Intern Med.*, **135**, 1163

139. Fisher, B. D. and Armstrong, D. (1977). Cryptococcal interstitial pneumonia. *N. Engl. J. Med.*, **297**, 1440

140. Schröter, G. P. J. and Weil, R. (1977). Listeria monocytogenes. Infection after renal transplantation. *Arch. Intern. Med.*, **137**, 1395

141. Schröter, G. P. J., Hoelscher, M., Putnam, C., Porter, K. A. and Starzl, T. E. (1977). Fungus infections after liver transplantation. *Ann. Surg.*, **186**, 115

142. Editorial (1976). Treatment of *Pneumocystis carinii* pneumonitis. *N. Engl. J. Med.*, **295**, 726

143. Gleason, T. H. and Hamlin, W. B. (1974). Disseminated toxoplasmosis in the compromised host. *Arch. Intern. Med.*, **134**, 1059

144. Hughes, W. T. (1977). *Pneumocystis carinii* pneumonia. *N. Engl. J. Med.*, **297**, 1381

145. Feldman, S. and Cox, F. (1976). Viral infections and haematological malignancies. *Clin. Haematol.*, **5**, 311

146. Rand, K. H. *et al.* (1977). Cellular immunity and herpes virus infections in cardiac-transplant patients. *N. Engl. J. Med.*, **296**, 1372

147. Pollard, R. B., Rand, K. H., Arvin, A. M. and Merigan, T. C. (1978). Cell-mediated immunity to Cytomegalovirus infection in normal subjects and cardiac transplant patients. *J. Infect. Dis.*, **137**, 541

148. Thomas, E. D. *et al.* (1975). Bone-marrow transplantation. *N. Engl. J. Med.*, **292**, 832

149. Finland, M. (1970). Changing ecology of bacterial infections as related to antibacterial therapy. *J. Infect. Dis.*, **122**, 419

150. Willemze, R., Hartgrink-Groeneveld, C. A., Speck, B. and Eernisse, J. G. (1975). Treatment of acute myelogenous leukemia in adults. *Neth. J. Med.*, **18**, 17

151. Mulder, J. (1938). *Acta Med. Scand.*, **97**, 165

152. Feldman, N. T. (1975). An assessment of transbronchial lung biopsy. *N. Engl. J. Med.*, **293**, 299

153. Greenman, R. L., Goodall, P. T. and King, D. (1975). Lung biopsy in immuno-compromised hosts. *Am. J. Med.*, **59**, 488

154. Bennett, J. E. (1974). Chemotherapy of systemic mycoses. *N. Engl. J. Med.*, **290**, 30

155. Bennett, J. E. (1977). Flucytosine. Diagnosis and treatment. Drugs five years later. *Ann. Intern. Med.*, **86**, 319

156. Cartwright, R. Y. (1975). Antifungal drugs. *J. Antimicrobial Chemother.*, **1**, 141

157. Eilard, T., Beskow, D., Norrby, R., Wåhlén, P. and Alestig, K. (1976). Combined treatment with amphotericin B and flucytosine in severe fungal infections. *J. Antimicrobial Chemother.*, **2**, 239

158. Miconazole (1977). New possibilities in the treatment of systemic mycoses. Reports on the experimental and clinical evaluation of miconazole. *R. Soc. Med.*, **70**, suppl. 1

159. Montgomerie, J. Z., Edwards, J. E. and Guze, L. B. (1975). Synergism of Amphotericin B and 5-fluorocytosine for *Candida* species. *J. Infect. Dis.*, **132**, 82

160. Sawyer, P. R., Brogden, R. N., Pinder, R. M., Speight, T. M. and Avery, G. S. (1975). Miconazole: a review of its antifungal activity and the therapeutic efficacy. *Drugs*, **9**, 406

161. Utz, J. P. *et al.* (1975). Therapy of *Cryptococcosis* with combination of flucytosine and Amphotericin B. *J. Infect. Dis.*, **132**, 368

162. Leading article (1977). Miconazole: a new antimycotic drug. *Br. Med. J.*, **2**, 347

163. *The Lancet* (1975). *Pneumocystis carinii* pneumonitis. *Lancet*, **ii**, 1023

164. Kodsi, B. E., Wickremesinghe, P. C., Kozinn, P. J., Iswara, K. and Goldberg, P. K. (1976). *Candida* esophagitis. *Gastroenterology*, **71**, 715

165. Everett, E. D., LaForce, F. M. and Eickhoff, Th. E. (1975). Serologic studies in suspected visceral Candidiasis. *Arch. Intern. Med.*, **135**, 1075

166. McCabe, W. R. (1974). Gram-negative bacteremia. *Adv. Intern. Med.*, **19**, 135

167. Teplitz, C. (1965) Pathogenesis of *Pseudomonas vasculitis* and septic legions. *Arch. Pathol.*, **80**, 297

168. Young, L. S., Martin, W. J., Meyer, R., Weinstein, R. J. and Anderson, E. T. (1977). Gram-negative rod bacteremia: microbiologic, immunologic, and therapeutic considerations. *Ann. Intern. Med.*, **86**, 456

169. Zinner, S. H. and McCabe, W. R. (1975). Gram-negative rod bacteremia in cancer patients. A review with emphasis of the antibody response. *Eur. J. Cancer*, **11**, 39

170. Fishman, L. S., Griffin, J. R., Sapico, F. L. and Hecht, R. (1972). Hematogenous *Candida* endophthalmitis – a complication of Candidemia. *N. Engl. J. Med.*, **286**, 675

171. Arvin, A. M., Pollard, R. B., Rasmussen, L. E. and Merigan, T. C. (1978). Selective impairment of lymphocyte reactivity to varicella-zoster virus antigen among untreated patients with lymphoma. *J. Infect. Dis.*, **137**, 531

172. Bock, B. V., Edelstein, P. H., Snyder, K. M., Hatayama, C. M., Lewis, R. P., Finegold, S. M., Kirby, B. D., George, W. L., Owens, M. L., Haley, C. E. and Meyer, R. D. (1978). Legionnaires' disease in renal-transplant recipients. *Lancet*, **i**, 410

173. Anderson, R. J., Schafer, L. A., Olin, D. B. and Eickhoff, T. C. (1973). Infectious risk factors in the immunosuppressed host. *Am. J. Med.*, **54**, 453

174. Ascher, N. L., Simmons, R. L., Marker, S. and Najarian, J. S. (1978). Listeria infection in transplant patients. *Arch. Surg.*, **113**, 90

175. Calne, R. Y. and Williams, R. (1977). Orthotopic liver transplantation: the first 60 patients. *Br. Med. J.*, **1**, 471

176. Kauffman, C. A., Israel, K. S., Smith, J. W., White, A. C., Schwarz, J. and Brooks, G. F. (1978). Histoplasmosis in immunosuppressed patients. *Am. J. Med.*, **64**, 923

177. Leading article (1978). Fatal Cytomegalovirus infection after renal transplantation. *Br. Med. J.*, **1**, 1506

178. Mason, J. W., Stinson, E. B., Hunt, S. A., Schroeder, J. S. and Rider, A. K. (1976). Infections after cardiac transplantation: relation to rejection therapy. *Ann. Intern. Med.*, **85**, 69

179. Rand, K. H., Pollard, R. B. and Merigan, T. C. (1978). Increased pulmonary superinfections in cardiac-transplant patients undergoing primary Cytomegalovirus infection. *N. Engl. J. Med.*, **298**, 951

180. Stinson, E. B., Bieber, C. P., Griepp, R. B., Clark, D. A., Shumway, N. E. and Remington, J. S. (1971). Infectious complications after cardiac transplantation in man. *Ann. Intern. Med.*, **74**, 22

181. Suwansirikul, S., Rao, N., Dowling, J. N. and Ho, M. (1977). Primary and secondary Cytomegalovirus infection. *Arch. Intern. Med.*, **137**, 1026

182. Lumish, R. M. and Norden, C. W. (1976). Therapy of neutropenic rats infected with *Pseudomonas aeruginosa*. *J. Infect. Dis.*, **133**, 538

183. Parry, M. F. and Neu, H. C. (1978). A comparative study of ticarcillin plus tobramycin versus carbenicillin plus gentamicin for the treatment of serious infections due to Gram-negative bacilli. *Am. J. Med.*, **64**, 961

184. Reynolds, H. Y., Levine, A. S., Wood, R. E., Zierdt, C. H., Dale, D. C. and Pennington, J. E. (1975). *Pseudomonas aeruginosa* infections: persisting problems and current research to find new therapies. *Ann. Intern. Med.*, **82**, 819

185. Smith, C. R., Baughman, K. L., Edwards, C. Q., Rogers, J. F. and Lietman, P. S. (1977). Controlled comparison of Amikacin and Gentamicin. *N. Engl. J. Med.*, **296**, 349

186. Hull, J. H. and Sarubbi, F. A. (1976). Gentamicin serum concentrations: pharmacokinetic predictions. *Ann. Intern. Med.*, **85**, 183

187. Reeves, D. S. (1977). Prescription of aminoglycosides by nomogram. *J. Antimicrobial Chemother.*, **3**, 533

188. Wilkinson, P. M., Gorst, D. W., Tooth, J. A. and Delamore, I. W. (1977). The management of fever in blood dyscrasias: results of a prospective controlled trial of a prescribing aid for Gentamicin. *J. Antimicrobial Chemother.*, **3**, 297

189. Atanasiu, P. (1977). Laboratory techniques for rapid diagnosis of viral infections: a memorandum. *Bull. WHO*, **55**, 33

190. Editorial notes (1978). Rapid diagnosis of viral infections. *Ann. Intern. Med.*, **88**, 708

191. Merigan, T. C. (1976). Efficacy of adenine arabinoside in herpes zoster. *N. Engl. J. Med.*, **294**, 1233

192. Stuart-Harris, C. (1975). Prospects for antiviral chemotherapy. *J. Antimicrobial Chemother.*, **1**, 133

193. Withley, H. J., Ch'ien, L. T., Dolin, R., Galasso, G. J. and Alford, C. A. (1976). Adenine arabinoside therapy of herpes zoster in the immunosuppressed. *N. Engl. J. Med.*, **294**, 1193

194. *The Lancet* (1978). Interferon treatment of herpes zoster. *Lancet*, **ii**, 84

195. McCullough, J. (1978). Leukapheresis and granulocyte transfusion. *Arch. Pathol. Lab. Med.*, **102**, 53

196. Alavi, J. B., Root, R. K., Djerassi, I., Evans, A. E., Gluckman, S. J., MacGregor, R. R., Guerry, D., Schreiber, A. D., Shaw, J. M., Koch, P. and Cooper, R. A. (1977). Clinical trial of granulocyte transfusions for infection in acute leukemia. *N. Engl. J. Med.*, **296**, 607

197. Clift, R. A., Sanders, J. E., Thomas, E. D., Williams, B. and Buckner, C. D. (1978). Granulocyte transfusions for the prevention of infection in patients receiving bone-marrow transplants. *N. Engl. J. Med.*, **298**, 1052

198. Herzig, R. H., Herzig, G. P., Graw, R. G., Bull, M. I. and Ray, K. H. (1977). Successful granulocyte transfusion therapy for Gram-negative septicemia. *N. Engl. J. Med.*, **296**, 701

199. *The Lancet* (1975). Granulocyte transfusions. *Lancet*, **i**, 377

200. McCredie, K. B. and Hester, J. P. (1976). White blood cell transfusions in the management of infections in neutropenic patients. *Clin. Haematol.*, **5**, 379

201. Schiffer, C. A. (1977). Principles of granulocyte transfusion therapy. *Med. Clin. N. Am.*, **61**, 1119

202. Broggs, D. R. (1976). Neutrophils in the blood bank. *N. Engl. J. Med.*, **295**, 726

203. Hammerschmidt, D. E., Craddock, P. R., McCullough, J., Kronenberg, R. S., Dalmasso, A. P. and Jacob, H. S. (1978). Complement activation and pulmonary leukostasis during nylon fiber filtration leukapheresis. *Blood*, **51**, 721

204. O'Flaherty, J. T., Craddock, P. R. and Jacob, H. S. (1978). Effect of intravascular complement activation on granulocyte adhesiveness and distribution. *Blood*, **51**, 731

205. Diepenhorst, P. *et al.* (1972). *Vox Sang.*, **23**, 308

206. Eernisse, J. G. and Brand, A. (1977). *Br. J. Haematol.*, **35**, 674

207. Ford, J. M., Cullen, M. H., Lucey, J. J., Tobias, J. S. and Lister, T. A. (1976). Folate graft-versus-host disease following transfusion of granulocytes from normal donors. *Lancet*, **ii**, 1167

208. Dietrich, M., Gaus, W., Vossen, J., van der Waaij, D. and Wendt, F. (1977). Protective isolation and antimicrobial decontamination in patients with high susceptibility to infection. *Infection*, **5**, 107

209. Grady, G. F., Lee, V. A. *et al.* (1975). Hepatitis B immune globulin – prevention of hepatitis from accidental exposure among medical personnel. *N. Engl. J. Med.*, **293**, 1067

210. Austrian, R. (1977). Pneumococcal infection and Pneumococcal vaccine. *N. Engl. J. Med.*, **297**, 938

211. *The Lancet* (1978), Pneumococcal vaccines. *Lancet*, **i**, 131

212. Riley, I. D., Andrews, M., Howard, R., Tarr, P. I., Pfeiffer, M., Challands, P. and

Jennison, G. (1977). Immunisation with a polyvalent Pneumococcal vaccine. *Lancet*, **i**, 1338

213. Smit, P., Oberholzer, D., Hayden-Smith, S., Koornhof, H. J. and Hilleman, M. R. (1977). Protective efficacy of Pneumococcal polysaccharide vaccines. *J. Am. Med. Assoc.*, **238**, 2613

214. Makele, P. H. *et al.* (1977). Polysaccharide vaccines of group A *Neisseria meningitidis* and *Haemophilus influenzae* type b: field trial in Finland. *J. Infect. Dis. (suppl.)*, **136**, 43

215. Alexander, J. W. and Fisher, M. W. (1974). Immunization against *Pseudomonas* in infection after thermal injury. *J. Infect. Dis.*, **130**, 152

216. *The Lancet* (1975). Pseudomonas vaccines. *Lancet*, **ii**, 168

217. Young, L. S., Meyer, R. D. and Armstrong, D. (1973). *Pseudomonas aeruginosa* vaccine in cancer patients. *Ann. Int. Med.*, **79**, 518

218. Commentory: Varicella-zoster virus vaccine. (1977). *J. Am. Med. Assoc.*, **238**, 1731

219. *The Lancet* (1975). Levamisole. *Lancet*, **i**, 151

220. Ramot, B., Biniaminov, M., Shoham, C. and Rosenthal, E. (1976). Effect of levamisole on E-rosette-forming cells *in vivo* and *in vitro* in Hodgkin's disease. *N. Engl. J. Med.*, **294**, 809

221. Russell, A. S., Brisson, E. and Grace, M. (1978). A double-blind, controlled trail of levamisole in the treatment of recurrent herpes' labialis. *J. Infect. Dis.*, **137**, 597

222. Symoens, J. and Rosenthal, M. (1977). Levamisole in the modulation of the immune response: the current experimental and clinic state. *J. Reticuloendothelial Soc.*, **21**, 175

223. Lawrence, H. S. (1972). Immunotherapy with transfer factor. *N. Engl. J. Med.*, **287**, 1092

224. Wara, D. W., Goldstein, A. L., Doyle, N. E. and Ammann, A. J. (1975). Thymosin activity in patients with cellular immunodeficiency. *N. Engl. J. Med.*, **292**, 70

225. Rothstein, G., Clarkson, D. R., Larsen, W., Grosser, B. I. and Athens, J. W. (1978). Effect of lithium on neutrophil mass and production. *N. Engl. J. Med.*, **298**, 178

226. Stein, S., Hanson, G. H., Koethe, S. and Hansen, R. (1978). Lithium-induced granulocytosis. *Ann. Intern. Med.*, **88**, 809

227. Hirsch, M. S. (1978). Interferon – its hour come at last? *N. Engl. J. Med.*, **298**, 1022

228. *The Lancet* (1977). Therapy-linked leukemia. *Lancet*, **i**, 519

229. Prince, A. M., Szmuness, W., Mann, M. K., Vyas, G. N., Grady, G. F., Shapiro, F. L., Suki, W. N., Friedman, E. A. and Stenzel, K. H. (1975). Hepatitis B 'immune' globuline, effectiveness in prevention of dialysis-associated hepatitis. *N. Engl. J. Med.*, **293**, 1063

230. Sell, S. and Mendelsohn, J. (1978). Transfer of specific immunity with RNA. *Arch. Pathol. Lab. Med.*, **102**, 217

231. Weiner, M. H. and Yount, W. J. (1976). Mannan antigenemia in the diagnosis of invasive *Candida* infections. *J. Clin. Invest.*, **58**, 1045

232. Bohnhoff, M., Miller, L. P. and Martin, W. R. (1964). *J. Exp. Med.*, **120**, 805

233. Hamilton, J. D. and Elliott, D. M. (1975). Combined activity of amphotericin B and 5-fluorcytosine against *Cryptococcus* neoformans *in vitro* and *in vivo* in mice. *J. Infect. Dis.*, **131**, 129

234. Hughes, W. T., Kuhn, S., Chaudhary, S., Feldman, S., Verzosa, M., Aur, R. J. A., Pratt, C. and George, S. L. (1977). Successful chemoprophylaxis for *Pneumocystis carinii* pneumonitis. *N. Engl. J. Med.*, **297**, 1419

11
Autoimmunity in Infectious Disease

L. E. GLYNN

11.1   INTRODUCTION   390

11.2   THE IMMUNOLOGICAL RESPONSE   390
    11.2.1   *Carriers and haptens*   391
    11.2.2   *Acquisition of natural tolerance*   393

11.3   ENHANCEMENT OF IMMUNE RESPONSE BY
      MICRO-ORGANISMS   393
    11.3.1   *Freund's adjuvant*   394
    11.3.2   *Other chemical substances*   394

11.4   VIRUSES AND AUTOIMMUNE DISEASES   395

11.5   CROSS-REACTIVITY OF ANTIGENS OF PARASITE
      AND HOST   396
    11.5.1   *Chemical characteristics of bacterial antigens*   396
    11.5.2   *Dominant determinants in mammalian tissues*   399
            11.5.2.1   *Nature of cellular antigens in cross-reactivity*   399
    11.5.3   *Autoimmune reactions and tissue injury*   400
            11.5.3.1   *Types of response*   400
    11.5.4   *Intracellular antigens*   402

11.6   EXAMPLES OF AUTOIMMUNITY ASSOCIATED
      WITH SPECIFIC MICROBIAL INFECTIONS   402
    11.6.1   *Syphilis*   402
    11.6.2   *Streptococci*   402

11.6.2.1	*Rheumatic fever*	403
	(a) *Cross-reacting antigens in streptococci*	404
	(b) *Nature of cross-reacting material in*	
	human myocardium	407
11.6.2.2	*Acute glomerulonephritis*	409
11.6.3	*Mycobacteria*	410
11.6.4	Escherichia coli	411
11.6.5	Yersinia	411
11.6.6	Erysipelothrix rhusiopathiae	412
11.6.7	*Viruses*	413

11.1 INTRODUCTION

The appearance of an autoimmune reaction whether manifested by the development of antibodies or cells sensitized to host antigens implies a breakdown in those mechanisms normally responsible for the immunological tolerance to such autochthonous substances. In order adequately to consider the means by which infection may influence and overcome immunological tolerance it is necessary firstly to consider those theoretical pathways that may circumvent the tolerant state and secondly how infectious disease can act upon them. The student of infectious diseases concerned particularly with their clinical features will also want to know how and to what extent autoimmunity is responsible for the clinical manifestations associated with any particular infection.

11.2 THE IMMUNOLOGICAL RESPONSE

The immunological process is complex and involves the participation of several cell types acting in ordered sequence. Antigens, whether exogenous or endogenous are usually processed by macrophages[1] which then present the antigen to a T lymphocyte. that is a lymphocyte whose structure and function has been modified by a temporary sojourn in the thymus. Those T lymphocytes naturally endowed with receptors capable of reacting with the antigen so presented co-operate in some not yet completely understood fashion with B lymphocytes, that is lymphocytes that have matured without thymus influence[2,3]. These lymphocytes are plasma cell precursors and when influenced by appropriately activated T lymphocytes mature into immunoglobulin secreting cells, the immunoglobulin possessing specificity for determinants on the antigen originally concerned. It has become apparent in recent years that immunological tolerance can result from interference with the function of either T or B lymphocytes both of which, with few exceptions, are required for a humoral immune response[4]. T cells are more easily rendered tolerant than B cells, that is they require a smaller dose of antigen, and this tolerance appears more rapidly and is sustained for much longer periods than that of B cells in the same animal. Natural tolerance to most autochthonous antigens is of the T-cell variety since they are mostly circulating in very small quantities. B-cell tolerance is mainly to materials such as the common serum proteins which are normally present in relatively high concentration. An autoimmune reaction to antigens of the former category therefore only needs to overcome the tolerance of the T cells. Help from T cells[5,6] can be either specific, i.e. will only co-operate with B cells reacting to antigens with similar specificity, or non-specific, i.e. capable of co-operation with B cells of quite unrelated specificity[7,8,9].

For an infection to induce an autoimmune reaction it would only be necessary therefore for T cells to be activated either specifically or non-specifically. Little is known of non-specific activation by infecting agents but it is possible that some of the autoimmune manifestations associated with mycobacterial infections are mediated in this way.

Specific T-cell activation is probably the basis of what is probably the commonest cause of infection-induced autoimmunity, namely that due to cross-reacting antigens. Such cross-reacting antigens are common in some families of micro-organisms, e.g. the Enterobacteriaceae[10] and the strepto-cocci[11]. The mechanism is best understood by a more detailed consideration of the immunological response.

11.2.1 Carriers and haptens

The majority of naturally occurring antigens are complex and consist of two functionally distinct components: a carrier, usually protein in nature and responsible for the immunogenicity of the molecule, i.e. its capacity to induce an immune response, and a haptenic moiety, frequently non-protein in nature, not immunogenic on its own, but responsible for the specificity of the antibodies or sensitized cells which constitute the immune response[12]. Cross-reactive antigens need only resemble each other in their haptenic components. An autochthonous antigen does not induce an immune response, not because the B cells are unable to synthesize the appropriate globulin, but because the T cells are tolerant to the carrier component of the molecule. Should a foreign antigen be introduced, i.e. one whose carrier component is foreign and therefore capable of reacting with a host T cell, an immune response will occur with anti-hapten specificity even if the hapten is identical to one occurring in host tissue; the resulting antibody will react with the corresponding host antigen.

It may not always be necessary for the haptenic component of a complex antigen to be covalently bound to its carrier protein. Non-antigenic plant polysaccharides, for example, can be induced to stimulate a specific immune response if injected adsorbed on to the surface of some micro-organisms, notably streptococci[13]. It is therefore conceivable that in a like fashion an infecting agent could render specifically immunogenic any host haptens present in the vicinity.

Although immunological tolerance to a complex molecule is more commonly regarded as involving the immunogenic carrier protein, there is now convincing evidence that tolerance can also develop to haptenic determinants such as those, for example, which are provided by the sugar residues on some glycoproteins or polysaccharides. Thus, although exogenous polysaccharides such as plant gums are readily made antigenic by adsorption on to streptococci, endogenous polysaccharides such as hyaluronic acid are not.

It would appear, therefore, that in the presence of the free hapten, such as may be presumed to exist with hyaluronic acid, tolerance cannot be overcome even when the carrier protein itself is foreign[14]. The work of Coulson and Stevens[15] has clearly shown such a blocking effect of free hapten against specific antibody production. In their experiments, antibodies against dextran were produced in guinea-pigs injected with *Leuconostoc mesenteroides*, but free dextran given before the beginning of the immunizing schedule successfully prevented antibody formation. The mechanism of this variety of tolerance has not yet been established but its mode of induction is strongly suggestive of B-cell tolerance. Such hapten mediated suppression of the responsiveness of B cells presumably only operates where hapten is present in significant quantities and as far as auto-haptens are concerned would only involve haptenic material readily available in the tissue fluids. Haptenic material present within cells and only released on cellular injury, would not be expected to act in this manner. This no doubt accounts for the old observation of Asherson and Dumonde[16] that rabbits, although incapable of mounting an immune response to extracts of rabbit liver, readily produce such autoreactive antibodies if immunization of the rabbit is carried out with similar extracts of rat liver.

The specific immunosuppressive effect of circulating haptenic determinants is quite remarkable and particularly well illustrated in rabbits immunized with human blood group A substance. Although this is a poor antigen when administered alone, excellent responses are obtained when the material is injected adsorbed on to β-haemolytic streptococci. Rabbits, however, can be divided into two groups according to the presence or absence of rabbit A-like substance and it is only in the A negative group that specific antibodies capable of agglutinating group A red cells are produced[17]. The ability of an infecting organism to induce an autoimmune response to autochthonous haptenic material by simple adsorption on to the organismal surface is therefore largely restricted to substances not normally present in tissue fluids.

11.2.2 Acquisition of natural tolerance

All hypotheses concerning the acquisition of natural tolerance require the presence of the antigen in a form accessible to the immunological apparatus. Sequestered antigens, i.e. those that are either intracellular or for other reasons segregated from contact with peripatetic lymphocytes are therefore usually capable of inducing an autoimmune response should they for any reason be released from their sequestered position, either by cell damage or by changes in permeability permitting access of lymphocytes. Both these processes may well occur in consequence of microbial invasion and undoubtedly contribute to the autoimmune reactions frequently associated with virus infections especially of the central nervous system.

Since many foreign proteins are homologous with many self proteins it is evident that the difference between a tolerated 'self' antigen and its immunogenic foreign homologue is frequently extremely slight. It is, therefore, not surprising that even mild treatment of 'self' antigens may occasionally be sufficient to induce enough change in a self protein to render it autoantigenic. For example, heat aggregation or alkaline denaturation of immunoglobulin G has been shown to render this protein auto-antigenic in many species[18,19]. Moreover, although 'self' proteins are tolerated in their intact state many show autoimmune capacity when fragments of their peptide chains have been removed by proteolytic activity. Once again the immunoglobulins are conspicuous in this respect; rabbits, for example, frequently showing auto-antibodies to the Fab fragments of their immunoglobulins whilst being entirely unreactive to the intact molecules[20,21]. Inflammatory reactions to microbial infections frequently result in local release of lysosomal enzymes capable of hydrolysing proteins in such a manner as to yield autoantigenic fragments[117] and such fragments of immunoglobulins have indeed been found in the contents of abscesses[22].

It is important to appreciate that the antibodies formed to an altered or fragmented autoantigen may react with the unaltered antigen despite the immunological tolerance of the host to the unaltered form. For example, classical rheumatoid factor is presumably induced by denatured IgG, but not by the native form. Nevertheless that factor binds with equal affinity to both the native and denatured forms of the molecule[118,119]. An autoantibody to an altered protein that showed no reaction with its native counterpart is, however, unlikely to be of any pathogenic significance in the absence of any sustained supply of the altered protein.

11.3 ENHANCEMENT OF IMMUNE RESPONSE BY MICRO-ORGANISMS

Micro-organisms and their products have been extensively used to enhance the immune response to other antigens either administered simultaneously mixed with the antigen or given alone before or after the antigen. Amongst the many organisms used for this purpose the mycobacteria are outstanding, but similar adjuvant properties are also shown by *Bordetella pertussis*, and by the lipopolysaccharides of many Gram-negative organisms[23].

11.3.1 Freund's adjuvant

Of the many adjuvants now available, that introduced by Freund is most widely used experimentally, not only for its ability to increase the level of an antibody response, but more especially because it appears to be able in certain situations to facilitate the breakdown of tolerance to antigens administered with it. Thus almost without exception the experimental production of autoimmune encephalitis, adrenalitis, thyroiditis and orchitis makes use of this effect of Freund's adjuvant; without it the experiment is either a failure or requires extremely prolonged and repeated immunization.

It now seems probable that this function of Freund's complete adjuvant depends upon the ability of the acid fast bacilli to stimulate T lymphocytes to co-operate non-specifically with B cells[24]. Consequently any antigen whose inability to excite an immune response in a particular recipient is due to tolerance confined to T cells, may induce a response if given as an emulsion with Freund's complete adjuvant. This interpretation of the mode of action of this adjuvant is supported by the work of Smith and Bridges[25] which showed that success or failure to break tolerance is largely dependent upon the degree of tolerance to be overcome. In their experiments with rabbits made tolerant to bovine serum albumin, tolerance during the early stages was virtually absolute and resistant to the most potent stimuli; later, between the phase of high tolerance and the return of susceptibility, there is a stage of relative tolerance during which an immune response is only obtainable to a strong antigenic stimulus. During this phase the influence of Freund's adjuvant was clearly demonstrable. In modern parlance the phase of high tolerance involves the B cells as well as T cells and it is consequently resistant even to the adjuvant; the phase of relative tolerance involves only the T cells and is therefore capable of avoidance by their non-specific activation. The state of heightened immunological reactivity long recognized in patients with clinical tuberculosis is, no doubt, at least in part, attributable to this ability of tubercle bacilli to lead to non-specific activation of T cells.

11.3.2 Other chemical substances

Amongst the metabolites of many micro-organisms are several substances capable of being incorporated into body proteins[26]. Amongst such substances are D-amino acids or unusual amino acid homologues, for example, azetidine and pipecolic acid, the three- and five-carbon homologue respectively of proline. Should such components be incorporated into a tissue protein, and there is evidence that this does occur, e.g. with collagen being synthesized in the presence of azetidine, the product may well be sufficiently foreign to excite an immunological reaction against itself[27].

11.4 VIRUSES AND AUTOIMMUNE DISEASES

Viruses with their obligate intracellular parasitism and their correspondingly unique metabolism are peculiarly endowed with potential for the genesis of autoimmune reactions[28]. Firstly, when they enter a cell some enzymatic attack on the surface membrane could sufficiently modify some of the surface antigens as to render then autoantigenic. Since, moreover, such antigens are of necessity on the cell surface, antibodies to them could be particularly cytotoxic. Secondly, when virus particles leave a cell they frequently carry with them cell wall antigens incorporated into their own surface glycoproteins. Such incorporated antigens may well endow the virus particle with the capacity to excite antibodies capable of reacting with such cell surface antigens of the host. Finally, as a result of the transcription and translation of viral nucleic acids within the host cells neo-antigens may appear upon these cells capable of inducing an apparently autoimmune reaction to the cells so affected.

It is not, however, exclusively by their effect on antigen production that viruses may be significantly involved in the development of autoimmunity. Several viruses show a distinct predilection for infecting lymphocytes, i.e. the cells directly involved in the immune response[29]. It would not be surprising, therefore, if such affected cells occasionally manifested signs of impaired recognition of self with the resulting elaboration of a variety of autoantibodies. The human disease systemic lupus erythematosus is strongly suspected of arising on such a basis although direct evidence of viral involvement is still lacking[30, 31]. The remarkably similar disease in NZB mice and their NZB–NZW hybrids rests upon a much firmer virological basis[32] although even here the relative importance of the virus and the genetic make up of the host still remain to be clarified.

The alteration of lymphocytes by viral infection so as to interfere with their ability to distinguish 'self' from non-'self' antigens implies some lasting change in constitution possibly associated with permanent residence of the virus in the affected cell. Inability of a virus to replicate in lymphocytes from a given patient when similar cells from a normal individual readily support such replication has been taken as evidence not only of a viral aetiology of the disease from which the patient is suffering but as indicating persistence of intracellular virus. Thus Denman[33] has found that lymphocytes from patients recovered from a cold sore or suffering from infectious mononucleosis fail to replicate herpes simplex virus whereas vesicular stomatitis virus replicate normally. A similar finding with lymphocytes from patients with polyarteritis, systemic lupus and dermatomyositis suggests that here too the interference with replication is indicative of some persistent viral agent within the lymphoid cells and by inference responsible for the auto-immune phenomena underlying the pathogenesis of these diseases.

The consistent failure to demonstrate viruses by objective methods in the many diseases in which they are strongly suspected of playing an aetiological role has led to the view that perhaps only a fragment of the viral nucleic acid is retained within the cell.

11.5 CROSS-REACTIVITY OF ANTIGENS OF PARASITE AND HOST

Finally in this enumeration of the possible mechanisms by which infection can lead to the development of autoimmune disease we come to the question of cross-reactivity between the antigens of the parasite and those of the host, and this is, at least numerically, probably the most important cause of autoimmunization. Such cross-reactivity is readily identified by a variety of techniques the most commonly employed using a labelled antibody to the organism concerned and appropriately sectioned tissues containing the suspected cross-reactive antigens. The site of such antigens is then revealed by its ability to bind labelled antibody. Essential controls for such a demon-stration involve the ability of both the organisms alone and tissue extract alone to remove the antibodies from the antiserum. One of the earliest observations of such cross-reactivity by this method was that of Kaplan and Meyeserian[34] (1962) who demonstrated it between β-haemolytic strepto-cocci and an antigen in the sub-sarcolemmal region of human and several other mammalian cardiac muscle fibres. Other immunological methods commonly employed to detect and/or confirm the immunological nature of such cross-reactions include complement fixation, precipitation and the agglutination of red cells coated with suitable extracts of the organism or the putative antigen.

11.5.1 Chemical characteristics of bacterial antigens

The two major, but closely related problems of cross-reacting antigens are the identification in chemical terms of the substances responsible in the tissues and in the micro-organisms involved. A truly enormous volume of material has now accumulated on the subject of microbial antigens and their distribution within the structure of the organism itself: capsule, cell wall, cytoplasmic membrane or cytoplasm, and differences of opinion frequently expressed because of the difficulties in obtaining organismal fractions in an adequate state of purity. A notable example was the identifi-cation of the material in streptococci that cross-reacts with something in the sub-sarcolemmal region of mammalian myocardial fibres: Kaplan and

Suchy[35] maintained that the antigen was intimately associated with the M proteins and Zabriskie and Freimer[36] proposed that it was a component of the cytoplasmic membrane quite distinct from M protein.

Of the capsular polysaccharides, most is known chemically of those derived from pneumococci. With the exception of some relationship to the carbohydrate moiety of the ABH blood group substances shown by Type XIV pneumococcal polysaccharide, there is little evidence that these pneumococcal products play any part in cross-reactions of autoimmunological significance.

Because of the accepted aetiological relationship between β-haemolytic streptococci and both rheumatic fever and glomerulo nephritis, a major effort has been directed towards the identification of the antigenic structure of these organisms; and this structure may with various modifications be accepted as the standard for most bacteria. At least six distinct components have now been recognized, an outer layer of hyaluronic acid, then a layer of polysaccharide specific for each of the streptococcal groups. The individual types are distinguishable by specific proteins, the M proteins, and these in turn are supported by the rigid structure of the cell wall. This is a highly complex structure which can be regarded as a single macromolecule known as murein in which three distinct molecular structures are incorporated: (1) A complex polysaccharide chain in which the repeating unit is a disaccharide unit consisting of N-acetylglucosamine and N-acetylmuramic acid. (2) To the lactic acid side chain on C3, which is a feature of muramic acid, is attached a tetrapeptide of L-analyl-D-glutamyl-L-lysyl-D-alanine and adjacent chains in the same or adjacent planes are linked by bridges of pentaglycine, extending from the free amino group of lysine in one tetrapeptide to the carboxyl group of the D-alanine in another. (3) In all Grampositive organisms a teichoic acid, i.e. another polymer this time consisting of alternating residues of phosphoric acid and glycerol, or phosphoric acid and ribitol[37,38], is joined to the polysaccharide chain by phosphodiester linkage to the hydroxyl on C6 of the muramic acid. Deep to the cell wall lies the cytoplasmic membrane, a highly complex structure, complex since it incorporates the innumerable enzymes required for the synthesis of all the cell wall components including the group and type specific components as well as the hyaluronate capsule.

This basic structure of murein offers endless possibilities for antigenic variation in diverse bacterial species. Thus in the tetrapeptide, lysine can be replaced by one of many diaminoacids, e.g. diaminopimelic acid, and various peptides can replace the bridging pentaglycine. In the teichoic acid moiety an amino acid is usually joined to C2 of the glycerol or ribitol but this can be replaced by N-acetylglucosamine, or gentobiose or other residues.

Although it has been customary to depict the antigenic composition of bacterial cell walls in concentric layers, it is more probable, in view of the ready accessibility of most of these antigens to their specific antibodies, that they exist in the form of a mosaic. Under the electron microscope the dense wall is covered by a fimbriated material of fuzzy appearance which is readily removed by trypsin. This, according to Fox[39] 'provides a three-dimensional reticulum with interstices exposing most of the cell wall antigens to enzymatic degradation or binding by specific antisera'.

Gram-negative organisms are usually characterized by a complex lipopolysaccharide which lies outside the murein component of the cell wall. These lipopolysaccharides are the somatic O antigens of this class of organisms and are of considerable importance immunologically not only because of their antigenic specificity but because of their capacity to act as adjuvants and to stimulate the transformation of B cells[40,41]. The great diversity of their antigenic specificity is related to the wide range of monosaccharides involved. The complexity of these antigens reaches its maximum in the Enterobactericaceae where they have been analysed into three layers: the outermost is composed of long side chains made up of a repeating branched tetrasaccharide of abequose, mannose, rhamnose and galactose; these side chains are attached to another linear polysaccharide of which the repeating unit consists of N-acetylglucosamine, glucose, galactose, glucose, galactose; this in turn is attached to another polysaccharide of which the repeat unit consists of two heptose molecules and an octulosonic acid. The lipid component, which is believed to be attached to the latter, is itself composed of glucosamine, phosphate and acetyl residues and β-hydroxymyristic acid.

The variations on this theme appear endless and account both for the extraordinary diversity of antigenic types in this family and the opportunity to induce antibodies cross-reacting with host determinants.

In many micro-organisms the dominant antigens have carbohydrate determinants and it is natural to assume that cross-reactivity with mammalian tissues would be mediated through similar determinants on those tissues. There is, however, little convincing supporting evidence. The outstanding exception is that presented by Goldstein[42,43] of a cross-reaction between the C-polysaccharide of *Streptococcus pyogenes* and material extracted from heart valves. The basis of this cross-reactivity was attributed by these authors to the presence of N-acetyl glucosamine as the dominant determinant in streptococcal group A polysaccharide and its presence also in the polysaccharides of the connective tissues of the heart valves. Kasp-Grochowska *et al.*[44] were unable to confirm these results and could find no evidence of cross-reactivity between streptococcal antigens and extracellular antigens of connective tissue. Some at least of the findings of Goldstein *et al.* could be attributed to non-immunological precipitation of collagen present in the extracts, and others to cross-reactivity between antigens in streptococci and those present in the mycobacteria used by them in the adjuvant for the raising of antisera to bovine heart valve extracts.

On theoretical grounds it is extremely unlikely that cross-reactions with connective tissue antigens would be stimulated by any micro-organisms, since the basis of such cross-reactivity resides in the presence of non-tolerant B cells. The presence of antigenic determinants readily available in the connective tissues would most probably lead to tolerance by the B cells and hence remove the very basis of the cross-reactivity. A typical example of such a potential connective tissue antigen is hyaluronic acid. Despite the presence of the identical polysaccharide in the capsule of streptococci no antibodies to it have been found. Nor can this be attribted to any lack of covalent linkage between the capsular material and streptococcal protein, since a similar failure to induce antibodies to hyaluronic acid has been reported despite covalent linkage between the polysaccharide and a carrier protein[14].

11.5.2 Dominant determinants in mammalian tissues

That cross-reactivity between microbial and mammalian antigens is mainly dependent upon the non-tolerance of the B-cell population to the determinants concerned, is supported by the observation that almost without exception the mammalian antigens involved are cell-bound and usually intracellular in distribution, i.e. they are unlikely to have been available for the natural induction of B-cell tolerance.

11.5.2.1 Nature of cellular antigens in cross-reactivity

The nature of the cellular antigens involved in cross-reactivity are exciting increasing attention. Since pathogenicity of the resulting antibodies must depend upon their ability to reach the cross-reacting antigens involved, much effort is now being concentrated upon the chemistry and architecture of cell membranes. Here almost all classes of chemical compound are represented, including polysaccharide, protein and lipid[45], all of which are also represented in the structure of micro-organisms. As an example of cross-reactivity involving proteins the type specific M protein of β-haemolytic streptococci has been especially well studied but with mainly negative results. Thus although the early papers of Kaplan et al.[46] associated the cross-reactivity between some strains of group A streptococci and myocardium with the M antigen, recent experiments with purified M protein clearly show the absence of such cross-reactivity. Thus antibodies raised in rabbits to purified M antigen failed to show any reaction with myocardium by the fluorescein labelled antibody method, and the anti-myocardial antibodies present in patients with rheumatic fever could not be removed by absorption with M protein[47].

An extremely important cross-reactivity between Type I M protein and the HLA antigens on human lymphocyte cell membranes was claimed by Hirota and Terasaki[48] based on the removal of HLA antibodies by absorption with Type I M protein. A similar suggestion of cross-reactivity derives from the observation of Pellegrino *et al.*[49] that lymphocytes from patients with anti-MI antibodies are stimulated to DNA synthesis by the presence of MI protein and that this is inhibited by any anti-HLA serum independent of HLA type. Unfortunately the results of Fox and Peterson[50] are at complete variance with these and the question of any relationship between M protein and HLA antigens remains an open one. There are nevertheless some older observations based on the rejection time of skin grafts by animals after streptococcal infections that do suggest an immunological relationship between these organisms and transplantation antigens[51,52].

11.5.3   Autoimmune reactions and tissue injury

The presence of autoimmune reactions whether mediated by humoral antibodies or specifically sensitized cells is only of pathogenic interest if it can be shown that such reactions are responsible for tissue injury. Four types of immunologically mediated damage were distinguished by Coombs and Gell[53], and all four are potentially capable of acting in those autoimmune situations arising in association with infectious disease.

11.5.3.1   *Types of response*

Type I hypersensitivity is the variety originally known as anaphylactic and is mediated by IgE, which by virtue of its characteristic binding to the surface of mast cells leads to the release of histamine, serotonin, heparin and probably other pharmacologically active substances when such sensitized mast cells are brought into contact with the antigen to which the IgE is reactive. There is little evidence at present that this type of autoimmune reaction contributes to the pathogenesis of infectious disease.

Type II reactions are those in which an antigen–antibody reaction takes place on a cell surface either because circulating antibody is present specific for a cell surface antigen or occasionally because cell-bound antibody reacts with some circulating antigen. Where the complex so formed is capable of activating complement, cell lysis results with consequent inflammatory response to the damaged cells. Where such a cross-reaction occurs to a natural component of the cell surface the reaction may be justifiably regarded as autoimmune, but a similar situation can arise as a result of material released from an infecting agent passively coating some host cells which would thus become susceptible to lysis in the presence of antibody and complement[54,55]. Such a reaction is essentially hetero-immune and is sometimes referred to as 'passive immune kill'.

Type III hypersensitivity is the variety mediated by the deposition of immune complexes. Insoluble complexes, i.e. those formed in the presence of excess of antibody, are readily removable by the reticuloendothelial system and are therefore usually innocuous unless formed locally as in the experimental induction of an Arthus reaction. It is the soluble complexes, formed in an excess of antigen, which are potentially more dangerous since they are likely to be deposited at various sites where for one reason or another vascular permeability is increased. The injurious effects of such deposits are associated with their capacity to activate complement which in turn releases chemotactic factors for polymorphonuclear cells and other pharmacologically active materials. The interaction between the complexes and platelets also contributes to local tissue injury associated with these complexes. As a mechanism for the mediation of autoimmune damage associated with infectious disease, type III reactions appear to be of major importance[56, 57].

Type IV reactions are those mediated by sensitized lymphocytes and typified by the tuberculin reaction. In contrast to the other types of hypersensitivity they are slow in onset, usually requiring 24–48 hours for maximum development, are transferable by cells but not by serum, and are characterized histologically by perivascular infiltrations of lymphocytes and macrophages. Tissue injury associated with these reactions is brought about by the release of a variety of active substances designated lymphokines from the sensitized lymphocytes[58, 59] and of potent tissue destroying enzymes from the macrophages[60].

Although type IV reactions probably play a significant role in those autoimmune reactions arising in consequence of infectious disease, even less is known of the mechanism by which they arise than is the case with cross-reacting humoral immunity. Since the cells involved belong to the T series of lymphocytes it would appear that the breakdown of tolerance implied in the development of such autoimmune reactions must differ fundamentally from that which leads to a humoral response. It is now becoming evident, however, that T cells belong to several different subsets distinguishable by different surface markers and these subsets subserve distinct functions[61]. Thus the effector cell of the type IV reaction may well differ fundamentally from the initially sensitized T cell and its susceptibility to tolerance induction may more closely resemble that of a B cell than a T cell. If this be so then non-specific activation of the first-order sensitized T cell may account as readily for cross-reactive type IV reactions as for any of the humorally mediated responses.

A fifth type of hypersensitivity reaction has recently been recognized in which an antibody directed towards a determinant on a cell surface may result, not in cell injury but in functional hyperactivity[62]. The antibody most typical of this type of reaction is the long-acting thyroid stimulator (LATS) now widely regarded as the agent responsible for hyperthyroidism of primary toxic goitre. Whether or not infectious agents are ever responsible for stimulating this type of autoimmune response is at present unknown.

11.5.4 Intracellular antigens

Although for reasons of immunological tolerance cross-reactivity between mammalian and organismal antigens is most probable with intracellular materials, the non-pathogenicity of such antibodies must not be taken for granted. Antibodies might be carried into cells by wandering lymphocytes (emperipolesis) and intracellular antigens are of course released either as part of their normal physiological function or as a consequence of cellular injury or death. Such a release of antigen could then result in an antigen–antibody interaction damaging to neighbouring cells, with consequent release of more antigen, or to the release of antigen into the circulation with the resulting formation of immune complexes with all the inherent potentiality for systemic lesions which these entail. An immune response to a microbial antigen that cross-reacts with an intracellular antigen of the host is not therefore to be regarded as an entirely innocuous phenomenon.

11.6 EXAMPLES OF AUTOIMMUNITY ASSOCIATED WITH SPECIFIC MICROBIAL INFECTIONS

11.6.1 Syphilis

Although the Wassermann reaction as originally described[63] made use of tissue heavily infected with *Treponema pallidum* and was therefore regarded as involving a heterogenous antigen belonging to this causative organism, subsequent observations clearly indicated that the antigen involved derived from host tissue and not from the infective agent[64]. The material cardiolipin, so called because of its ready availability from cardiac muscle, is a diphosphatidyl glycerol and occurs especially in the inner membrane of the mitochondria. Although it possesses immunological activity, as shown by its role in the Wassermann reaction, antibodies to it do not react with intact mitochondria thus indicating a non-accessible situation within the membrane.

Since cardiolipins capable of reacting with WR-positive sera are extractable from most mammalian hearts, including human ones, the Wassermann reaction must be regarded as an autoimmune reaction. In view, however, of the inaccessible state of the cardiolipin *in vivo* its pathogenic significance is probably negligible.

11.6.2 Streptococci

Of all the organisms associated with the development of autoimmunity the best studied are streptococci. Not only are these organisms themselves a centre of major investigation but of even greater interest is the mechanism by which the autoimmune reactions are engendered. The reason for this unusual interest is of course the long-suspected relationship between a previous streptococcal infection and two important disease entities, rheumatic fever and acute glomerulonephritis.

11.6.2.1 *Rheumatic fever*

The streptococcal aetiology of rheumatic fever rests upon three main sources of evidence, epidemiological, serological and prophylactic. One of the first recognized features of the disease was its tendency to appear some 1–3 weeks after a febrile sore throat; and with the development of clinical bacteriology it was soon established that β-haemolytic streptococci of group A could be isolated with high frequency from the throat during this prodromal phase.

The opportunity provided by the Second World War of studying epidemics of streptococcal sore throat amongst young adults living under overcrowded conditions in service camps enabled Coburn and Young[65] to carry out their now classical studies on the relationship of rheumatic fever to previous streptococcal infection. This study and the subsequent work of Rammelkamp *et al.*[66] not only established the aetiological relationship of the streptococcus to the disease, but indicated that many of the factors predisposing to rheumatic fever such as poverty, overcrowding, latitude and season operate mainly through their influence on the incidence of streptococcal infections.

The incidence of rheumatic fever following a known streptococcal infection of the upper respiratory tract varies from 0.3% in sporadic cases to 3.0% in epidemics. This tenfold variation is apparently related to the greater severity of the primary disease in its epidemic form[67].

The serological evidence of a recent streptococcal infection is based on a high or rising titre of antibodies to one or more of the 20 or so antigens known to be released by the growing organisms. The antibody most commonly determined is the antistreptolysin-O, mainly because of its ease of measurement. By this means it has been shown that acute rheumatic fever is associated with such an infection in some 80% of cases. If, however, antibodies are determined against three or more of the organismal antigens the evidence of recent infection approaches an incidence of 100%[68].

Once it was established that streptococci were the causative agents of rheumatic fever attempts at prophylaxis immediately followed the introduction of reliable antibacterial drugs such as the sulfonamides and penicillin. The success of such prophylaxis[69], especially in reducing the incidence of relapses in patients recovered from a previous attack, provided the final confirmation of the relationship established on serological and epidemiological grounds.

That rheumatic fever is not the result of direct infection of the affected tissues, namely heart or joints, has been clearly established by many investigators, notably Watson[70]. Moreover the quiescent interval between the throat infection and the symptoms of rheumatic fever are contrary to what would be expected from direct bacterial involvement. The same criticism may be offered of any hypothesis incriminating a direct toxic effect upon the affected tissues of materials released by the organisms.

Finally the advent of potent antibiotics has shown that the critical events leading to a subsequent attack of rheumatic fever occur within the first 5 days of the throat infection[71]. It is the rising titre of antibodies against the various streptococcal products that occurs during this period which draws attention to the possible importance of immunological processes in the pathogenesis.

An immunological pathogenesis, however, could be entirely associated with exogenous antigens and in patients with rheumatic fever this is indeed suggested by the significantly higher titres of various streptococcal antigens found as compared to titres from patients with uncomplicated streptococcal infection[72, 73]. An immunological pathogenesis of the kind envisaged would most probably be mediated by the deposition of immune complexes and although superficially similar lesions can be induced in rabbits by injection of large amounts of foreign serum[74], human serum sickness bears little similarity to rheumatic fever. Furthermore if the lesions are a non-specific response to the deposition of immune complexes why is the disease exclusively related to infection with streptococci?

It is therefore evident that if the disease is mediated by an immune response it must be to something peculiar to streptococci. It had already been suggested by Brockman et al.[75] when they reported a high incidence of complement-fixing antibodies to an extract of human heart in the sera of children with rheumatic fever, that mammalian cardiac tissue contained material capable of acting as an autoantigen. It was natural, therefore, to consider the possibility that the peculiarity of the streptococci lay in their ability to enhance in some way the potential antigenicity of certain auto-antigens. That streptococci are capable of converting haptenic substances to complete antigens had already been shown by Glynn and Holborow[13]; and Kaplan[76] subsequently reported that if streptococci are grown in a medium including an extract of beef heart, then antibodies to a cardiac antigen appeared in the serum of rabbits immunized with these organisms. Further work by Kaplan and his colleagues[77] and by Gery and Davis[78] showed the presence of organ specific, but not species specific, antigen(s) in the heart of several mammalian species and it is probably this antigen present in beef heart broth that is absorbed by the streptococci and is responsible for the appearance of anti-heart antibodies in the immunized animals.

(a) Cross-reacting antigens in streptococci. Organisms other than streptococci are, however, also capable of absorbing haptenic material and rendering it antigenic although much less effectively than streptococci[13]. It was Kaplan and Meyeserian[34] who first showed the unique feature of some strains of these organisms in that, even when grown in cultures entirely free from materials of animal origin, they could still induce the formation of antibodies specific for antigens in myocardium and in some smooth muscle fibres (Figure 11.1). This important finding was rapidly confirmed by other workers[36, 79].

Although the first studies of this apparently cross-reacting antigen in streptococci was restricted to a type 5 strain[34] it soon became established that it was also present in many others and probably in the majority of types of group A streptococci. Thus Nakhla and Glynn[80] reported it present in nine of 10 types examined but absent in other Gram-positive cocci with the exception of a single strain of group G.

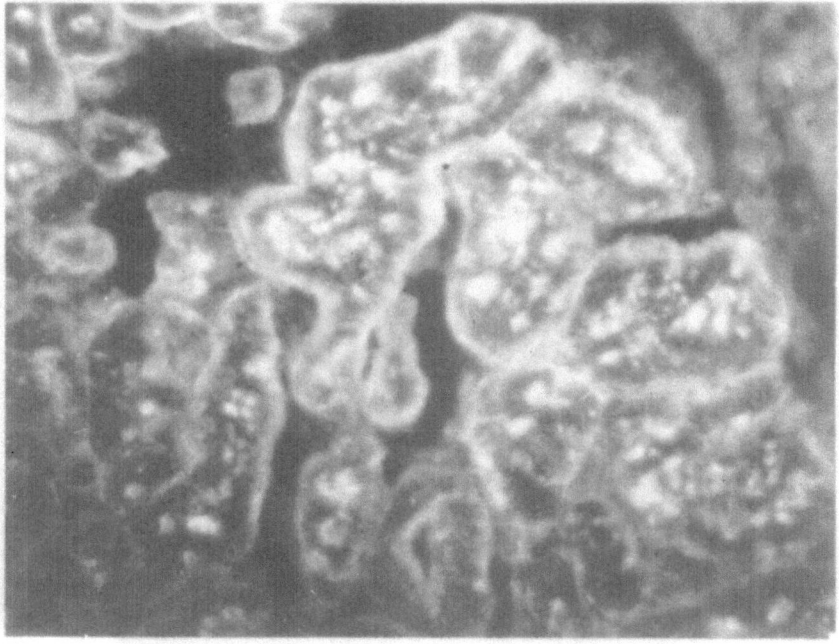

Figure 11.1 Section of human myocardium treated with a rabbit antigroup A streptococcal antiserum followed by fluorescein conjugated goat–anti-rabbit immunoglobulin antiserum. Note the specific staining of the sub-sarcolemmal region. × 368

The pathogenic significance of these cross-reacting antimyocardial antibodies is difficult to assess. Although claims have been made that animals immunized with appropriate strains of streptococci develop in addition to the cross-reacting antibodies myocardial lesions consisting of foci of muscle cell necrosis, none of the lesions resembles those of rheumatic fever. Moreover, many patients with upper respiratory tract infections with streptococci develop these antibodies without showing any subsequent signs of cardiac involvement. Finally, passive transfer of the antibodies has no demonstrable effect upon the target organ. It is evident, therefore, that although these antibodies are a feature of the 'post-streptococcal' state their pathogenic significance is still *sub judice*. Zabriskie[81], however, has adduced evidence that their pathogenic activity is largely a function of concentration and that the titre in rheumatic fever is significantly higher than in non-complicated cases of streptococcal infection.

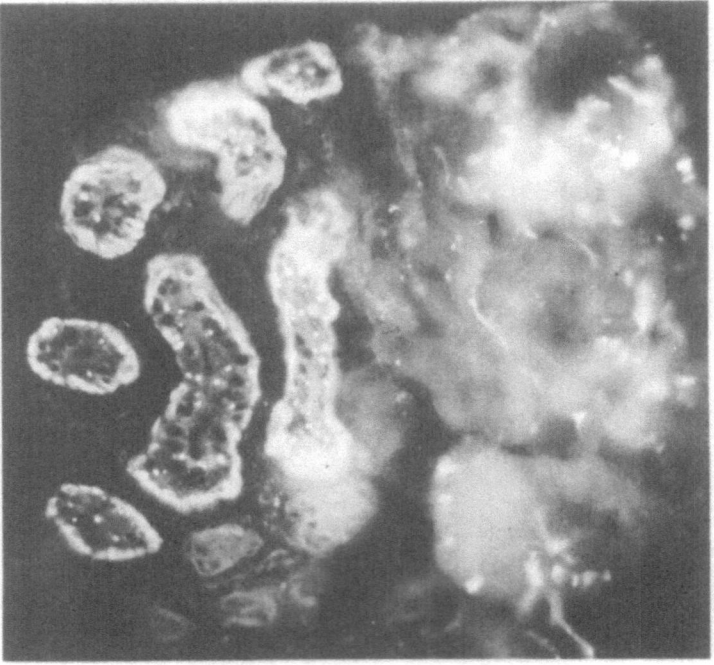

Figure 11.2 Section of human skin treated as in Figure 11.1 and showing cross-reaction with the myoepithelial cells of the sweat glands. × 368

Rheumatic fever is a disease by no means confined to the myocardium, and lesions, especially in severe cases, are found in the heart valves, joints, blood vessels, skin, subcutaneous tissues and, in the related condition of chorea, in the central nervous system. If the myocardial lesions are mediated by cross-reacting antibodies then it is probable that many of these other lesions are similarly mediated. In a detailed study of this problem Kingston and Glynn[82], by means of the fluorescein labelled antibody method, found that several sera raised in rabbits against various strains of β-haemolytic streptococci showed unequivocal cross-reactions with fibroblasts, both in the heart valves and in the dermis, with endothelium covering the heart valves, with various skin appendages especially the cells of the sheaths of the hair follicles and with the myoepithelial cells of the sweat glands. Positive reactions were also given by the epithelium of the interlobular bile ducts, Küpffer cells and the mesangium of the renal glomeruli. The reaction of some of these antisera with central nervous tissue was especially interesting. Some cells in the cortical white matter subsequently identified as fibrous astrocytes were selectively stained, and virtually identical staining was obtained with serum from a patient with severe chorea. Moreover, this reaction with chorea serum was completely removed by absorption with the strain of streptococci that induced the anti-astrocyte response in the rabbit[83] (Figures 11.2–4).

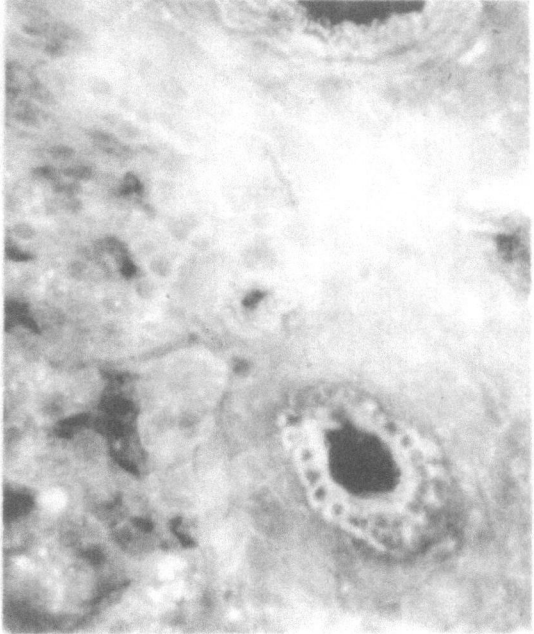

Figure 11.3   Section of human liver treated as in Figure 11.1 and showing cross-reaction with cytoplasma of bile ductule epithelial cells

(b) *Nature of cross-reacting material in human myocardium.* This extraordinary range of cross-reactivity taken at its face value implies a remarkable range of similar antigens in the streptococcus itself. This seems extremely unlikely, but some light is thrown on this problem by the work of Kasp-Grochowska and Glynn[84] on the chemical nature of the material in human myocardium that cross-reacts with anti-streptococcal sera. This material was identified as an ethanolamine plasmalogen, and antibodies to it gave a myocardial staining pattern identical to that obtained with positive anti-streptococcal antisera. Despite the fact that these antibodies are more readily removed by absorption with streptococci than with the plasmalogen itself, there is no chemical evidence for the presence of plasmalogen as such in streptococci[85]. The most probable cross-reactive material in these organisms is the polyglycerophosphate component of the teichoic acid. Although neither α- nor β-glycerophosphates were able to inhibit the agglutination of red cells coated with cardiac plasmalogen by antiplasmalogen antiserum it is possible that greater success would have been achieved with a polymer of one or other of these glycerophosphates.

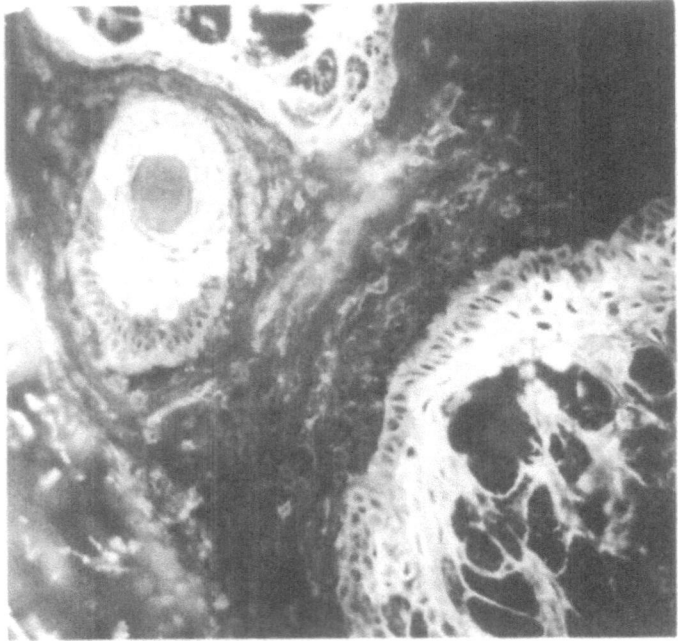

Figure 11.4 Human skin treated as in Figure 11.1 and showing staining of epithelial components of hair follicles as well as dermal fibrocytes. × 208

Although plasmalogen does participate without doubt in several of the immunological tests used by Kasp-Grochowska and Glynn, they have suggested an alternative hypothesis for its role in the genesis of the cross-reactions between streptococci and tissue antigens, namely that it participates in the formation of complexes between the organisms and tissue derived materials which complexes are responsible for initiating the autoimmune responses.

Plasmalogen is potentially an excellent complexing agent owing to its content of highly unsaturated fatty acids. In the plasmalogen isolated by Kasp-Grochowska and Glynn argentation chromatography of the methyl esters of the fatty acids revealed a high content of polyunsaturated fatty acids with four or more double bonds. Fluorescence studies of these fatty acids confirmed the presence of highly unsaturated materials which readily undergo peroxidation and the excitation and emission maxima coincided with the figures given by Fletcher, Dillard and Tappel[86] for peroxidizing tissues that contain unsaturated fatty acids with 2–4 double bonds.

That streptococci can initiate such peroxidation has indeed been indicated by Malke[87], who showed that some of the so-called bacteriocine-like activity of group A streptococci was the result of peroxide production. Thus locally increased peroxide could initiate oxidation of unsaturated fatty acids yielding carbonyl groups capable of cross-linking through amino groups with glyco-proteins, proteins or lipids. Such cross-linking could result in complexes of streptococcal and tissue antigens capable of inducing the formation of auto-antibodies. Since the cross-reacting autoantibodies associated with strepto-coccal infections are removable by either the tissue involved or the streptococcus it would appear that the antibodies involved must have a complex reactive site involving determinants on both the organism and the tissue. Antibodies of such complexity are, however, not unknown; note, for example, removal of antibodies to AB blood group in group O sera, by absorption with either A or B substance[88]. A similarly complex immune response embracing two determinants has been suggested to explain the greater cell-mediated cytotoxicity against some virus-infected cells when both the target cells and aggressor cells are syngeneic, the inference being that the effective determinant is a complex of viral and transplantation antigen.

This hypothesis of a plasmalogen-linked complex of antigen from the organism and that from the tissue would also account for the well-corroborated observation of Lyampert[89], that some cross-reacting anti-myocardial antibodies induced by streptococci can only be absorbed by organisms of the same M type. In such circumstances the complex antigen presumably involves both cardiac antigen and type specific protein.

The hypothesis is reminiscent of that put forward by Cavelti[90,91] to account for the cardiac lesions he obtained when rats were injected with an emulsion of rat heart and killed group A haemolytic streptococci. Although this work was not confirmed, it could well be, because the *in vitro* circumstances necessary for the required interactions as outlined above were at the time unknown and success was, therefore, entirely dependent upon the chance provision of the appropriate conditions.

11.6.2.2 *Acute glomerulonephritis*

The relationship of streptococcal infection to acute glomerulonephritis is strikingly different from its relationship to rheumatic fever in three important respects. Firstly, whereas no particular type of group A streptococcus is associated with rheumatic fever, the ability to induce glomerulitis appears to be restricted to a few so-called nephritogenic types, notably types 5 and 12. Secondly, whereas all cases of rheumatic fever are regarded as secondary to a streptococcol infection a significantly large proportion of cases of glomerulonephritis are unrelated to such infection. Nevertheless, post-streptococcal glomerulonephritis is a well-recognized entity. Thirdly, rheumatic fever is not a complication of any streptococcal infection but appears to be restricted to infections of the upper respiratory tract. Acute glomerulonephritis shows no such restriction and has been known, for example, to occur with considerable frequency as a consequence of strepto-coccal impetigo[120-122].

Of the two generally accepted methods by which an immune reaction can induce glomerular lesions, namely the deposition of immune complexes and the specific reaction of an autoantibody to a glomerular component, the evidence in post-streptococcal nephritis strongly favours the former. Although there have been claims to have demonstrated specific antigens in nephritogence strains of streptococci which cross-react with glomerular basement membrane[92] the lesions do not resemble those of Goodpasture's syndrome, and the immunoglobulin deposits in the affected glomeruli do not lie on the membrane but on its epithelial side.

If, indeed, post-streptococcal nephritis results from the deposition of immune complexes involving streptococcal but not tissue antigens[93] it should no longer be regarded as an autoimmune manifestation. On the other hand, if this is so, it is difficult to account for the restriction of the disease to infection with only a few strains of streptococci.

11.6.3 Mycobacteria

The adjuvant activity of acid fast micro-organisms employed so successfully in Freund's complete adjuvant for the experimental production of auto-immune diseases has drawn attention to the possibility that infection with these organisms might be complicated by autoimmune reactions which could contribute to the clinical features associated with such infections. An investigation of this possibility was made[94] in rabbits infected with *Myco-bacterium tuberculosis* or with *Pasteurella pseudo-tuberculosis*. Although studies were restricted to humoral antibodies, positive evidence of an auto-immune response was obtained in four out of 21 rabbits infected with *M. tuberculosis* and in five of the 21 rabbits infected with *P. pseudotuberculosis*. The antibodies were directed against a variety of antigens present in the liver, spleen, kidneys, heart, lung and lymph nodes and showed a moderate degree of interspecies cross-reactivity, but no organ specificity. The results were explained most simply by the assumption that at least five antigens were involved, with up to three of these in any one organ.

Ultra centrifugal fractionation of saline homogenates of the liver of the rabbits showed that the antigens were chiefly localized in the microsomal and supernatant fractions with none in the nuclei and very little in the mitochondria. Although it was not possible to incriminate the antibodies directly in the genesis of any of the lesions in the infected animals, their ability to induce cytopathic changes in the corresponding cells in tissue culture implies the presence of some, at least, of the antigens upon the cell surface. Consequently participation of these antibodies in the pathology associated with these infections remains a distinct possibility.

Of the other naturally occurring infections with mycobacteria, leprosy has received most attention. From the intracellular habitat and prolonged persistence of the organisms it might be inferred that autoimmune manifestation would be a conspicuous feature of the disease. With the possible exception of the lepromin test[95] there is little evidence of autoimmunity associated with leprosy and it now seems doubtful whether a positive lepromin test is indicative of such a reaction[96].

11.6.4 *Escherichia coli*

In 1959 Broberger and Perlmann[97] reported their finding of an antibody in children with ulcerative colitis that reacted with a phenol extract of fetal human colon. Subsequently, Perlmann[98] and his colleagues in 1965 showed that these sera also reacted with a lipopolysaccharide extracted from the colon of germ-free rats and that the reaction was inhibited by polysaccharide extracted from certain strains of *E. coli*, notably strain 014.

Asherson and Holborow[10] found that rabbits immunized with *E. coli* 0.86, developed antibodies capable of reacting with mucus-secreting cells of the rabbit colon and to a much less extent with similar cells in the small intestine and even more rarely with stomach. There is, however, little evidence that these cross-reacting antibodies are pathogenic and although they are common in children with ulcerative colitis they are only rarely found in adults. Unfortunately, little is known of cell-mediated immunity to cross-reactive antigens in colitis. This may well be of greater significance than humoral antibodies in the pathogenesis of ulcerative colitis, since lymphocytes capable of killing colon cells in culture have been found in that disease[99].

11.6.5 *Yersinia*

Although infection with organisms of this genus are uncommon in this country, they are extremely common in other parts of Europe, especially Scandinavia. The species *Yersinia enterocolitica* is widespread in that country and appears to be a common cause of acute enteritis[100,101]. A small but significant proportion of cases develop a mono- or polyarthritis shortly after the subsidence of the initial intestinal symptoms, and although in the majority of these patients the arthritis subsides in a few weeks, in others especially those with severe joint symptoms, the arthritis may last for several months or even a year.

Attempts to identify the cause of the arthritis have excluded the presence of living organisms by means of cultures and of dead organisms by staining with fluorescent antibodies[102]. This is in marked contrast to the findings of Greenwood and Whittle[103] in patients with arthritis complicating meningococcal infection, where either the living organisms or antigen was readily identified. Larsen, therefore, favours an autoimmune basis for the on-going arthritis that complicates Yersinia infections which apparently occur almost exclusively in the genetically predisposed. The incidence of the HLA antigen B27 in yersinial arthritis namely 43/49 (88%)[104,105] supports this view. Similar genetic findings have also been reported in the reactive arthritis associated with infections with Salmonella and Shigella[106]. There is at present no evidence that the presence of the gene for HLA-B27 predisposes to infection with any of these organisms but only with the subsequent development of reactive arthritis. In the series reported by Aho and his colleagues[104], it can be calculated that persons possessing HLA-B27 have 50 times more chance of developing such an arthritis than those without this gene. Its mode of action is still purely speculative but it may well be involved with factors predisposing to autoimmunization, especially perhaps in Scandinavia where elevated yersinia antibodies have been found in patients with such putative autoimmune diseases as thrombocytopaenia, haemolytic anaemia, chronic liver disease, glomerulonephritis and thyroiditis.

It is of some interest that the association of the HLA-B27 gene with reactive arthritis to known infective agents is restricted to Gram-negative micro-organisms. Rheumatic fever and the reactive arthritis seen occasionally in pneumococcal infections show no such association with this genetic marker. Can it be that the endotoxin characteristic of Gram-negative organisms is an essential requirement for this genetic association?

11.6.6 *Erysipelothrix rhusiopathiae*

Although this organism is rarely responsible for any serious infection in man it is a cause of major losses amongst weanling pigs. The disease is typically septicaemic with a marked tendency to involve the joints. Its main interest to immunopathologists is that the arthritis shows a strong tendency to persist after recovery has occurred from the other systemic manifestations of the disease, and that the chronically affected joints are frequently sterile[107,108]; attempts to identify residual antigens in these joints are usually unsuccessful. There is, therefore, some reason to suppose that the persistent arthritis, which closely resembles rheumatoid arthritis pathologically, might be dependent upon the development of an autoimmune reaction during the course of the initial infection[109].

11.6.7 Viruses

The mechanisms by which viruses might induce autoimmune reactions have already been discussed and it should therefore not appear surprising that many viral infections are associated with the appearance of autoantibodies. Thus autohaemolytic anaemia, possibly of the cold type, is a well-recognized complication of infectious mononucleosis[110] and rheumatoid factor has been reported with an incidence of 14%[111] in that disease.

In the prodromal period of viral hepatitis, vasculitis and arthritis are the result of local deposition of complexes of viral surface antigen and antibody. These are not, therefore, examples of autoimmunity. In the stage of chronic hepatitis which may follow an initial viral hepatitis, there is, however, increasing evidence that autoimmunization to hepatocyte membrane antigens contributes to the persistence of the lesions[112,113,114].

The importance of viral infections in the possible pathogenesis of chronic inflammatory disease probably depends upon two features especially peculiar to viruses: firstly, the ability of many viruses to persist indefinitely in the infected host and secondly, the necessary interaction between virus and cell membrane both when entering and leaving the infected cell. This may effect immunologically significant changes in the cell surface antigens. Some of these may be dependent upon the major histocompatibility locus, such as the H-2 associated antigens of mice, and could account for the well-defined genetic restriction of some forms of murine viral disease. Thus, Zinkernagel and Doherty[115,116] have suggested that the killing of virus-infected cells by T cells could be due to such viral alteration of histocompatibility antigens. There is not yet, however, any evidence of such an HLA restriction to killing by T cells in man, but it would help to explain some of the remarkable examples now coming to light of genetic restriction of human disease, e.g. ankylosing spondylitis and HLA-B27.

References

1. Unanue, E. R. (1972). The regulatory role of macrophages in antigenic stimulation. *Adv. Immunol.*, **15**, 45
2. Claman, H. N., Chaperon, E. A. and Triplett, R. F. (1966). Immunocompetence of transferred thymus-marrow cell combinations. *J. Immunol.*, **97**, 928
3. Miller, J. and Mitchell, C. G. (1968).
4. Weigle, W. O. (1973). Immunological unresponsiveness. *Adv. Immunol.*, **16**, 61
5. Mitchison, N. A. (1969). In: *Immunological Tolerance* (M. Landy and W. Braun, eds.), p. 149 (New York: Academic Press)
6. Rajewsky, K. V., Schirrmacher, V., Nase, S. and Jerne, N. K. (1969). The requirement of more than one antigenic determinant for immunogenicity. *J. Exp. Med.*, **129**, 1131
7. Hartmann, K. H. (1971). Induction of hemolysin response *in vitro*. II. Influence of thymus-derived cells during the development of antibody-producing cells. *J. Exp. Med.*, **133**, 1325
8. Hunter, P., Munro, A. and McConnell, I. (1972). Properties of educated T cells for rosette formation and co-operation with B cells. *Nature (New Biol.)*, **236**, 52

9. Waldmann, H. and Munro, A. (1973). T-cell dependent mediator in the immune response. *Nature (Lond.)*, **243**, 356

10. Asherson, G. L. and Holborow, E. J. (1966). Autoantibody production in rabbits. VII. Autoantibodies to gut produced by the injection of bacteria. *Immunology*, **10**, 161

11. Kingston, D. and Glynn, L. E. (1976). Anti-streptococcal antibodies reacting with brain tissue. I. Immunofluorescent studies. *Br. J. Exp. Pathol.*, **57**, 114

12. Landsteiner, K. (1919). Über die Bedeutung der Proteinkomponente bei den Präzipitin-reaktionen der Azoproteins. *Biochem. Z.*, **93**, 106

13. Glynn, L. E. and Holborow, E. J. (1952). The production of complete antigens from polysaccharide haptens by streptococci and other organisms. *J. Pathol. Bacteriol.*, **64**, 775

14. Humphrey, J. H. (1943). Antigenic properties of hyaluronic acid. *Biochem. J.*, **37**, 460

15. Coulson, E. J. and Stevens, H. (1961). Some observations on the immunochemistry of dextrans. *J. Immunol.*, **86**, 241

16. Asherson, G. L. and Dumonde, D. C. (1962). Characterization of auto-antibodies produced in the rabbit by the injection of rat liver. *Br. J. Exp. Pathol.*, **43**, 12

17. Glynn, L. E., Holborow, E. J. and Johnson, G. D. (1956). The influence of the A-like substance of rabbits on their immune response to human group A substance. *J. Immunol.*, **76**, 357

18. McCluskey, R. T., Miller, F. and Benacerraf, B. (1962). Sensitization to denatured autologous gamma-globulin. *J. Exp. Med.*, **115**, 253

19. Williams, R. C. and Kunkel, H. G. (1963). Antibodies to rabbit γ-globulin after immuniz-ation with various preparations of autologous γ-globulin. *Proc. Soc. Exp. Biol. Med.*, *N.Y.*, **112**, 554

20. Mandy, W. J. and Lewis, F. B. (1966). Homoreactant: A new serum factor in normal rabbits. *Nature (Lond.)*, **212**, 791

21. Mandy, W. J. (1967). A new serum factor in normal rabbits. III. Specificity for antigenic determinants uncovered by papain or pepsin digestion. *J. Immunol.*, **99**, 815

22. Waller, M. (1974). IgG hydrolysis in abscesses. II. Hydrolysis of Ripley IgG by enzymes from abscess leucocytes. *Immunology*, **26**, 735

23. Whitehouse, M. W. (1978). The chemical nature of adjuvants. In: *Immunochemistry*, An advanced textbook (L. E. Glynn and M. W. Steward, eds.), p. 571 (Chichester: John Wiley and Sons)

24. Allison, A. C., Denman, A. M. and Barnes, R. D. (1971). Co-operating and controlling functions of thymus-derived lymphocytes in relation to autoimmunity. *Lancet*, **ii**, 135

25. Smith, R. T. and Bridges, R. A. (1958). Immunological unresponsiveness in rabbits produced by neonatal injection of defined antigens. *J. Exp. Med.*, **108**, 227

26. Natori, Y., Trowbridge, H. O., Toreson, W. E. and Tarver, H. (1961). Studies on ethionine. V. Sex differences in incorporation *in vivo* of ethionine into rat proteins. *J. Biol. Chem.*, **236**, 2821

27. Brown, P. C. and Glynn, L. E. (1973). The antigenicity of sequential polypeptides. II. The antigenicity of some sequential polymers including several related to collagen. *Immunology*, **25**, 251

28. Symposium (1971). Viruses and autoimmune disease. *Am. J. Clin. Pathol.*, **56**, 259

29. Wheelock, E. F. and Toy, S. T. (1974). Participation of lymphocytes in viral infections. *Adv. Immunol.*, **16**, 123

30. Lewis, R. M., Tannenberg, W., Smith, C. and Schwartz, R. S. (1974). C–type viruses in systemic lupus erythematosus. *Nature (Lond.)*, **252**, 78

31. Mellors, R. C. and Mellors, J. W. (1976). Antigen related to mammalian type C-RNA viral p-30 proteins is located in renal glomeruli in human systemic lupus erythematosus. *Proc. Natl. Acad. Sci. (Wash.)*, **73**, 233

32. Mellors, R. C., Shirai, T. and Aoki, T. (1971). Wild type Gross leukaemia virus and the pathogenesis of the glomerulonephritis of New Zealand mice. *J. Exp. Med.*, **133**, 113

33. Denman, A. M., Appleford, D. J., Imrie, R. C., Kinsley, M. J., Pelton, B. K. and Schnitzer, T. (1977). Viral replication in lymphocytes and the pathogenesis of connective tissue diseases. In: *Experimental Models of Chronic Inflammatory Diseases* (L. E. Glynn and H. D. Schlumberger, eds.), p. 77 (Berlin: Springer-Verlag)

34. Kaplan, M. H. and Meyeserian, M. (1962). An immunological cross-reaction between group A streptococcal cells and human heart tissue. *Lancet*, i, 706

35. Kaplan, M. H. and Suchy, M. L. (1964). Immunologic relation of streptococcal and tissue antigens. II. Cross-reaction of antisera to mammalian heart tissue with a cell wall constituent of certain strains of group A streptococcus. *J. Exp. Med.*, **119**, 643

36. Zabriskie, J. B. and Freimer, E. H. (1966). An immunological relationship between the group A streptococcus and mammalian muscle. *J. Exp. Med.*, **124**, 661

37. Martin, H. H. (1966). Biochemistry of bacterial cell walls. *Annu. Rev. Biochem.*, **35**, 457

38. Horecker, B. L. (1966). Biosynthesis of bacterial polysaccharides. *Annu. Rev. Microbiol.*, **20**, 253

39. Fox, E. N. (1974). M proteins of group A streptococci. *Bacteriol. Rev.*, **38**, 57

40. Munoz, J. (1964). Effect of bacteria and bacterial products on antibody response. *Adv. Immunol.*, **4**, 397

41. Fournie, G. J., Lambert, P. H. and Miescher, P. A. (1974). Release of DNA in circulating blood and induction of anti-DNA antibodies after injection of bacterial lipopolysaccharides. *J. Exp. Med.*, **140**, 1189

42. Goldstein, I., Halpern, B. and Robert, L. (1967). Immunological relationship between streptococcus A polysaccharide and the structural glycoproteins of heart valve. *Nature (Lond.)*, **213**, 44

43. Goldstein, I. Rebeyrotte, P., Parlebas, J. I. and Halpern, B. (1968). Isolation from heart valves of glycopeptides which share immunological properties with streptococcus haemolyticus group A polysaccharides. *Nature (Lond.)*, **219**, 866

44. Kasp-Grochowska, E., Kingston, D. and Glynn, L. E. (1972a). Immunology of bovine heart valves. I. Cross-reaction with the C-polysaccharide of streptococcus pyogenes. *Ann. Rheum. Dis.*, **31**, 282. (1972b). Immunology of bovine heart valves. II. Reaction with connective tissue components. *Ibid.*, p. 290

45. Gomperts, B. D. (1977). *The Plasma Membrane: Models for Structure and Function* (London: Academic Press)

46. Kaplan, M. H. *et al.* (1962). *J. Immunol.*, **80**, 254

47. Fox, E. N. and Grossman, B. J. (1969). Antigenicity of the M proteins of group A haemolytic streptococci. IV. The absence of antigenic determinants common to mammalian heart muscle. *J. Immunol.*, **102**, 970

48. Hirota, A. A. and Terasaki, P. I. (1970). Cross-reaction between human transplantation antigens and streptococcal M proteins. II. *Science*, **168**, 1095

49. Pellegrino, M. A., Ferrone, S., Safford, J. W., Hirata, A. A., Terasaki, P. J. and Reisfeld, R. A. (1970). Stimulation of lymphocyte transformation by streptococcal type M1 protein. Relationship to HL-A antigens. *J. Immunol.*, **109**, 97

50. Fox, E. N. and Peterson, R. D. A. (1970). Streptococcus M protein vaccines, rheumatic fever and human histocompatibility antigens. *J. Immunol.*, **105**, 103

51. Rapaport, F. T. and Chase, R. M. Jr. (1964). Homograft sensitivity induction by group A streptococci. *Science*, **145**, 407

52. Rapaport, F. T., Chase, R. M. and Soloway, A. C. (1966). Transplantation antigen activity of bacterial cells in different animal species and intracellular localization. *Ann. N.Y. Acad. Sci.*, **129**, 102

53. Coombs, R. R. A. and Gell, P. G. H. (1963). Classification of allergic reactions responsible for clinical hypersensitivity and disease. In: *Clinical Aspects of Immunology* (P. G. H. Gell and R. R. A. Coombs, eds.) (Oxford: Blackwell Scientific Publications)

54. Assoku, R., Penhale, W. and Buxton, A. (1970). An immunological basis for the anaemia

of acute Salmonella gallinarum infection of chicken. I. Haematological changes and their association with *in vivo* modification of the erythrocytes. *Clin. Exp. Immunol.*, **7**, 865

55. Assoku, R. and Penhale, W. (1970). An immunological basis for the anaemia of acute Salmonella gallinarum infection of chicken. II. The relationship of the immune response to the development of the haemolytic anaemia. *Clin. Exp. Immunol.*, **7**, 875

56. Cochrane, C. G. and Koffler, D. (1973). Immune complex disease in experimental animals and man. *Advan. Immunol.*, **16**, 185

57. Henson, P. M. (1977). Immune complex diseases: cellular mediators and the pathogenesis of inflammatory tissue injury produced by immune complexes. In: *Experimental Models of Chronic Inflammatory Diseases* (L. E. Glynn and H. D. Schlumberger, eds.), p. 94 (Berlin: Springer-Verlag)

58. Dumonde, D. C., Wolstencroft, R. A., Panayi, G. S., Matthew, M., Morley, J. and Howson, W. T. (1969). Lymphokines. Non-antibody mediators of cellular immunity generated by lymphocyte activation. *Nature (Lond.)*, **224**, 38

59. Bloom, B. R. (1971). *In vitro* approaches to the mechanism of cell-mediated immune reaction. *Adv. Immunol.*, **13**, 101

60. Allison, A. C. and Davies, P. (1975). Increased biochemical and biological activities of mononuclear phagocytes exposed to various stimuli with special reference to secretion of lysosomal enzymes. In: *Mononuclear Phagocytes* (R. van Furth, ed.) (Oxford: Blackwell Scientific Publications)

61. Good, R. A. (1976). Immunodeficiency in developmental perspective. In: *Textbook of Immunopathology* (P. A. Miescher and H. G. Müller-Eberhard, eds.), p. 555 (New York: Grune and Stratton)

62. Roitt, I. M. (1972). *Essential Immunology* (Oxford: Blackwell Scientific Publications)

63. Wassermann, A., Neisser, A. and Bruch, C. (1906). Eine serodiagnostische Reaktion bei Syphilis. *Dtsch. Med. Wochenschr.*, **32**, 745

64. Landsteiner, K., Müller, R. and Pötzl, O. (1907). Über Komplementbindungsreaktionen mit dem serum von Dourinetieren. *Wien. Klin. Wochenschr.*, **20**, 1421

65. Coburn, A. F. and Young, D. C. (1949). *Epidemiology of Haemolytic Streptococcus* (Baltimore: Williams and Wilkins)

66. Rammelkamp, C. H., Denny, F. W. and Wannamaker, L. W. (1952). Studies on the epidemiology of rheumatic fever. In: *Rheumatic Fever* (L. Thomas, ed.), p. 72 (Minneapolis: University of Minnesota Press)

67. Stollerman, G. H. (1954). The epidemiology of primary and secondary rheumatic fever. In: *The Streptococcus, Rheumatic Fever and Glomerulonephritis* (J. W. Uhr, ed.), p. 311 (Baltimore: Williams and Wilkins)

68. McCarthy, M. (1952). The immune response in rheumatic fever. In: *Rheumatic Fever* (L. Thomas, ed.), p. 136 (Baltimore: Williams and Wilkins)

69. Kohn, K. H., Milzer, A. and MacLean, H. (1950). Oral penicillin prophylaxis of recurrences of rheumatic fever. *J. Am. Med. Assoc.*, **142**, 20

70. Watson, R. F., Hirst, G. K. and Lancefield, R. C. (1961). Bacteriologic studies of cardiac tissues obtained at autopsy from eleven patients dying with rheumatic fever. *Arthritis Rheum.*, **4**, 74

71. Denny, F. W. Jr., Wannamaker, L. W., Brink, W. R., Rammelkamp, C. H. Jr. and Custer, E. A. (1950). Prevention of rheumatic fever: treatment of the preceding infection. *J. Am. Med. Assoc.*, **143**, 151

72. Rantz, L. A., Maroney, M. and Di Capro, J. M. (1950). Antibody response after haemolytic streptococcal respiratory infection in childhood. *J. Clin. Invest.*, **29**, 840

73. Rantz, L. A., Maroney, M. and Di Capro, J. M. (1952). Infection and reinfection by haemolytic streptococci in early childhood. In: *Rheumatic Fever* (L. Thomas, ed.), p. 90 (Baltimore: Williams and Wilkins)

74. Rich, A. F. and Gregory, J. E. (1943). Experimental evidence that lesions with basic

characteristics of rheumatic carditis can result from anaphylactic hypersensitivity. *Bull. John Hopkins Hosp.*, **73**, 289

75. Brockman, H., Brill, J. and Frendzell, J. (1937). Komplementablenkung mit Organextracten von Rheumatikern BBF-Reaktion bei sogennanten akuten Gelenksrheumatismus. *Klin. Wochenschr.*, **16**, 502

76. Kaplan, M. H. (1958). Immunologic studies of heart tissue. *J. Immunol.*, **80**, 254

77. Kaplan, M. H. and Craig, J. M. (1963). Immunologic studies of heart tissue. VI. Cardiac lesions in rabbits associated with autoantibodies to heart induced by immunization with heterologous heart. *J. Immunol.*, **90**, 725

78. Gery, I. and Davies, A. M. (1961). Organ specificity of the heart. I. Animal immunization with heterologous heart. *J. Immunol.*, **87**, 351. II. Immunization of rabbits with homologous heart. *Ibid.*, **87**, 357

79. Nakhla, L. S. (1966). MD thesis (University of London)

80. Nakhla, L. S. and Glynn, L. E. (1967). Studies on the antigen in β-haemolytic streptococci that cross-reacts with an antigen in human myocardium. *Immunology*, **13**, 209

81. Zabriskie, J. B., Hsu, K. C. and Seegal, B. C. (1970). Heart reactive antibody associated with rheumatic fever; characterization and diagnostic significance. *Clin. Exp. Immunol.*, **7**, 147

82. Kingston, D. and Glynn, L. E. (1971). A cross-reaction between Str. pyogenes and human fibroblasts, endothelial cells and astrocytes. *Immunology*, **21**, 1003

83. Kingston, D. and Glynn, L. E. (1976). Anti-streptococcal antibodies reacting with brain tissue. I. Immunofluorescence studies. *Br. J. Exp. Pathol.*, **57**, 114

84. Kasp-Grochowska, E. and Glynn, L. E. (1977). The role of plasmalogen in the cross-reaction between group A streptococcus and human myocardium. *Br. J. Exp. Pathol.*, **58**, 359

85. Goldfine, H. and Hagen, P. O. (1972). Bacterial plasmalogens. In: *Ether lipids: Chemistry and Biology*, p. 329 (New York: Academic Press)

86. Fletcher, B. L., Dillard, C. J. and Tappel, A. L. (1973). Measurement of fluorescent lipid peroxidation products in biological systems and tissues. *Analyt. Biochem.*, **52**, 1

87. Malke, H., Starke, R., Jacob, H. E. and Köhler, W. (1974). Bacteriocine-like activity of group A streptococci due to the production of peroxide. *J. Med. Microbiol.*, **7**, 367

88. Morgan, W. T. J. and Watkins, W. M. (1956). The product of the human blood group A and B genes in individuals belonging to group AB. *Nature (Lond.)*, **177**, 521

89. Lyampert, J. M., Vvedenskaya, O. I. and Danilova, T. A. (1966). Study on streptococcus. Group A antigens common with heart tissue elements. *Immunology*, **11**, 313

90. Cavelti, P. A. (1947a). Studies on the pathogenesis of rheumatic fever. I. Experimental production of autoantibodies to heart and skeletal muscle and connective tissue. *Arch. Pathol.*, **44**, 1

91. Cavelti, P. A. (1947b). Studies on the pathogenesis of rheumatic fever. II. Cardiac lesions produced in rats by means of autoantibodies to heart and connective tissue. *Arch. Pathol.*, **44**, 13

92. Markowitz, A. S. and Lange, C. F. (1964). Streptococcal related glomerulonephritis. I. Isolation, immunochemistry and comparative chemistry of soluble fractions from type 12 nephritogenic streptococci and human glomeruli. *J. Immunol.*, **92**, 565

93. Andres, G. A., Accinni, L., Hsu, K. C., Zabriskie, J. B. and Seegal, B. C. (1966). Electron microscopic studies of human glomerulonephritis with ferritin conjugated antibody–localization of antigen–antibody complexes in glomerular structures of patients with acute glomerulonephritis. *J. Exp. Med.*, **123**, 399

94. Thewaini Ali, A. J. and Oakley, C. L. (1967). Autoantibodies in experimental chronic infective disease. *J. Pathol. Bacteriol.*, **93**, 413

95. Rees, R. J. W. (1964). The significance of the lepromin reaction in man. *Progr. Allergy*, **8**, 224

96. Turk, J. L. and Bryceson, A. D. M. (1971). Immunological phenomena in leprosy and related diseases. *Adv. Immunol.*, **13**, 209

97. Broberger, O. and Perlmann, P. (1959). Autoantibodies in human ulcerative colitis. *J. Exp. Med.*, **110**, 657

98. Perlmann, P., Hammarstrom, S., Lagerkrantz, R. and Gustafsson, B. E. (1965). Antigen from colon of germ-free rats and antibodies in human ulcerative colitis. *Ann. N.Y. Acad. Sci.*, **124**, 377

99. Perlmann, P. and Broberger, O. (1963). *In vitro* studies of ulcerative colitis. II. Cytotoxic action of white blood cells from patients on human fetal colon cells. *J. Exp. Med.*, **117**, 717

100. Ahvonen, P. (1972). Human yersiniosis in Finland. I. Bacteriology and serology. *Ann. Clin. Res.*, **4**, 40. II. Clinical features. *Ibid.*, **4**, 49

101. Larsen, J. H. (1972). Human yersiniosis in Denmark. *Scand. J. Immunol.*, **1**, 412

102. Larsen, J. H. (1976). Yersinia enterocolitica infections and arthritis. In: *Infection and Immunology in the Rheumatic Diseases* (D. C. Dumonde, ed.), p. 133 (Oxford: Blackwell Scientific Publications)

103. Greenwood, B. M. and Whittle, H. C. (1976). The pathogenesis of meningococcal arthritis. In: *Infection and Immunology in the Rheumatic Diseases* (D. C. Dumonde, ed.), p. 119 (Oxford: Blackwell Scientific Publications)

104. Aho, K., Ahuonen, P., Lassus, A., Sievers, K. and Tiilikainen, A. (1973). HL-A27 antigen and reactive arthritis. *Lancet*, **ii**, 157

105. Aho, K., Ahuonen, P., Lassus, A., Sievers, K., and Tiilikainen, A. (1974). HL-A27 in reactive arthritis. A study of yersinia arthritis and Reiter's disease. *Arthritis Rheum.*, **17**, 25

106. Aho, K., Ahuonen, P., Lassus, A., Sievers, K. and Tiilikainen, A. (1976). Yersinia arthritis and related diseases: clinical and immunogenetic implications. In: *Infection and Immunology in the Rheumatic Diseases* (D. C. Dumonde, ed.), p. 341 (Oxford: Blackwell Scientific Publications)

107. Ajmal, M. (1969). Erysipelothrix rhusiopathiae and spontaneous arthritis in pigs. *Res. Vet. Sci.*, **10**, 579

108. Ajmal, M. (1971). Experimental erysipelothrix arthritis. I. *Res. Vet. Sci.*, **12**, 403; II. *Res. Vet. Sci.*, **12**, 412

109. Glynn, L. E. (1977). Erysipelothrix arthritis in rabbits. In: *Experimental Models of Chronic Inflammatory Disease* (L. E. Glynn and H. D. Schlumberger, eds.), p. 238 (Berlin: Springer-Verlag)

110. Dacie, J. V. (1962). *The Haemolytic Anaemias, Congenital and Acquired.* II. The Autoimmune Anaemias (London: Churchill)

111. Carter, R. L. (1966). Antibody formation in infectious mononucleosis. II. Other 19S antibodies and false-positive serology. *Br. J. Haematol.*, **12**, 268

112. Miller, J., Smith, M. G. M., Mitchell, C. G., Reed, W. D., Eddleston, A. L. W. F. and Williams, R. (1972). Cell-mediated immunity to a human liver-specific antigen in patients with active chronic hepatitis and primary biliary cirrhosis. *Lancet*, **ii**, 296

113. Smith, M. G. M., Golding, P. L., Eddleston, A. L. W. F., Mitchell, C. G., Kemp, A. and Williams, R. (1972). Cell-mediated immune responses in chronic liver disease. *Br. Med. J.*, **1**, 527

114. Paronetto, F. and Vernace, S. J. (1975). Immunological studies in patients with chronic active hepatitis. Cytotoxic activity of lymphocytes to autochthonous liver cells grown in tissue culture. *Clin. Exp. Immunol.*, **19**, 99

115. Zinkernagel, R. and Doherty, P. (1974). Immunological surveillance against altered self components by sensitized T lymphocytes in lymphocytic choriomeningitis. *Nature (Lond.)*, **251**, 547

116. Zinkernagel, R. and Doherty, P. (1974). Restriction of *in vitro* T-cell-mediated cytotoxicity in choriomeningitis within a syngeneic or semiallogenic system. *Nature (Lond.)*, **248**, 701

117. Waller, M. and Curry, N. (1970). The demonstration of plasma agglutinators in human sera. *Vox. Sang. (Basel)*, **19**, 34
118. Gaarder, P. I. and Natvig, J. B. (1974). The reaction of rheumatoid Anti-Gm antibodies with native and aggregated Gm-negative IgG. *Scand. J. Immunol.*, **3**, 559
119. Dissanayake, S., Hay, F. C. and Roitt, I. M. (1977). The binding constants of IgM rheumatoid factors and their univalents fragments for native and aggregated human IgG. *Immunology*, **32**, 309
120. Updyke, E. L., Moore, M. S. and Conroy, E. (1955). Provisional new type of group A streptococcus associated with nephritis. *Science*, **121**, 171
121. Dillon, H. C., Reeves, M. S. and Maxted, W. R. (1968). Acute glomerulonephritis following skin infection due to streptococci of M-type 2. *Lancet*, **i**, 543
122. Hall, W. D., Blumberg, R. W. and Moody, M. D. (1973). Studies in children with impetigo. Bacteriology serology and incidence of glomerulonephritis. *Am. J. Dis. Child.*, **125**, 800

12
Immunology of Chronic Infections

J. L. TURK

12.1   INTRODUCTION   422

12.2   MECHANISMS OF SURVIVAL OF MICRO-
ORGANISMS   423
     12.2.1   *Antigenic variation*   423
     12.2.2   *Intracellular residence*   424
     12.2.3   *Failure of cellular immunity*   424

12.3   IMMUNOLOGICAL SPECTRA IN CHRONIC
INFECTIONS   426

12.4   GENETIC SUSCEPTIBILITY   427

12.5   MYCOBACTERIAL INFECTIONS   427
     12.5.1   *Leprosy*   427
         12.5.1.1   *The clinical spectrum*   427
         12.5.1.2   *The nature of granuloma formation*   429
         12.5.1.3   *Immunological parameters*   429
             (a)   *The Lepromin test*   429
             (b)   In vitro *parameters of cellular immunity*   430
             (c)   *Evidence for non-specific defect*   431
             (d)   *Immunoglobulins, complement and
humoral antibodies*   431
         12.5.1.4   *Reaction states in leprosy*   432
             (a)   *Reversal reactions*   432
             (b)   *Erythema nodosum leprosum (ENL)*   432
         12.5.1.5   *Animal models*   433
     12.5.2   *Tuberculosis*   434

12.6   SYPHILIS   436

12.7   PARASITIC INFECTIONS   440
       12.7.1   *Leishmaniasis*   440
       12.7.2   *Trypanosomiasis*   444

12.8   HELMINTHIC INFECTIONS   446
       12.8.1   *Onchocerciasis*   446
       12.8.2   *Schistosomiasis*   446

12.9   FUNGAL INFECTIONS   447
       12.9.1   *Systemic mycoses*   447
       12.9.2   Candida albicans   448

12.10 SUMMARY   449

12.1   INTRODUCTION

Chronic infection can occur with a wide range of micro-organisms. Although all the organisms that cause acute infectious diseases can cause infections with some degree of chronicity, there are a number of groups of micro-organisms that especially produce chronic infections. There are many reasons why infections show chronicity. Chronic infections usually result from the infecting organism developing qualities which protect it from the defence mechanisms of the host while at the same time not producing factors that are directly lethal to the host. In addition there a number of infections by organisms of low toxicity in which host resistance may be poor. Poor host resistance may be as much the result of a low degree of antigenicity as of a weakness in the immunological recognition mechanisms of the host. Thus there are two prerequisites for chronic infections. The first is an ability of the infectious agent to avoid host defence mechanisms, and the second is for it to be of low toxicity so that the host can survive a prolonged state of parasitism by large numbers of live micro-organisms.

Another feature of chronic infections is that the organism *per se* is frequently not the cause of the pathological processes associated with that disease, for many of the organisms that cause such infections do not secrete exotoxins, nor do they carry endotoxins as part of their cell walls. Pathological processes in these infections are frequently the result of hypersensitivity mechanisms and the immunological processes underlying these hypersensitivity mechanisms are usually separate from those underlying host resistance. This may be because they are directed against different antigens in the organism or, as in many cases, because host resistance depends solely on cell-mediated immune mechanisms, whereas the hypersensitivity reaction may be an antibody-induced phenomenon. In infection with a micro-organism of unvarying antigenicity, one may observe at the same time proliferation of the organism due to a specific failure of cellular immunity, and hypersensitivity reactions due to the interaction between antigens derived from the host and high levels of humoral antibody directed against these antigens.

An additional factor in the development of chronic infections is the role of antibiotics and chemotherapeutic agents. In many situations a failure of host resistance may persist under a cover of excess antigen. In these circumstances reduction of the antigenic load may result in the release of host resistance mechanisms and a return of immunity, or even the development of powerful hypersensitivity reactions. A further situation where therapy may influence the clinical picture occurs when sudden massive killing of the micro-organism results in a flood of soluble antigen into the circulation. This may result in acute serum-sickness-like symptoms due to massive immune complex deposition, or to a state of endotoxaemia as in the Jarisch–Herxheimer reaction.

This chapter will first discuss the mechanisms of survival of infecting organisms in the immunized host. It will then go on to discuss a number of chronic infectious diseases in some detail, highlighting particularly the role of immunological mechanisms in the production of pathological lesions. It is hoped that as a result, some insight will be developed into the immunological basis of the spectrum of clinical features that may occur.

12.2 MECHANISMS OF SURVIVAL OF MICRO-ORGANISMS

12.2.1 Antigenic variation

As host resistance is mainly dependent on immunological mechanisms, the most powerful tool at the disposal of the organism is its ability to vary its antigenic structure. Individual antigens are controlled by individual genes and only one antigen controlled by a gene at a particular locus can be expressed at a time. However, there is a potential to express a number of different antigenic types corresponding to the genes present at that locus. Under adverse conditions the organism may be induced to switch antigens. Such changes may occur as the result of the presence of specific antibody in the environment. While this kind of switch could be due to mutation or recombination, evidence is accumulating which suggests that antigenic variation could be due to a switch in gene activity.

Antigenic variation of this type is a particular feature of parasitic infections and has been studied extensively in malaria, trypanosomiasis, schistosomiasis and hookworm infection. Trypanosomes for instance change their surface antigen by secreting a coat composed of a different glycoprotein. In other situations these organisms can bind host serum proteins to their surface which give the organism additional protection from antibodies. In many situations antigenic variation is induced by residence in a partially immune host.

12.2.2 Intracellular residence

A feature common to many of the organisms which cause chronic infectious diseases is that they are obligate or facultative intracellular parasites and such organisms appear to be effectively protected from the action of circulating humoral antibody. Among these facultative intracellular organisms are Mycobacteria and parasites such as *Leishmania* spp. which are found mainly within macrophages. Viruses can only replicate in an intracellular environment and thus spend a considerable part of their life-cycle in an environment where they appear to be inaccessible to the action of antibody. Such organisms appear to need cell-mediated immunity for their elimination. Other organisms which do not appear to be eliminated by antibody and need cell-mediated immunity as part of host resistance include *Treponema pallidum* and fungi and on this basis it is likely that they also spend some part of their life-cycle intracellularly. Organisms needing cell-mediated immunity for their control can readily cause infections as a result of specific failure of host resistance despite the presence of a high level of circulating antibody, and under such circumstances there is rapid proliferation of the organism. Frequently there is a release of soluble antigen, resulting in the development of clinical features such as arthritis, glomerulonephritis and cutaneous vasculitis, which indicate immune complex deposition. (See Chapter 9 for a detailed discussion.)

12.2.3 Failure of cellular immunity

As will be discussed later, a number of chronic infectious agents cause disease states in which host resistance may be poor or absent. The lepromatous form of leprosy and the kala-azar form of leishmaniasis are only two examples of a more general phenomenon which includes the systemic mycoses and helminthic infections such as onchocerciasis. In other diseases such as syphilis, low host resistance may be a necessary but transient phase of the disease in the majority of individuals infected. A low resistance state may in other conditions, form one pole of a spectrum of clinical manifestations and variations in host resistance either upwards or downward may result in a change in both clinical and histopathological features of the disease.

There are a number of theoretical ways in which host resistance may be lost. These may be determined and understood best from experimental models of immunological tolerance, immunological enhancement and suppressor cells. Immunological tolerance differs from the other two models in that it presupposes the depression of a clone of effector cells (T lymphocytes) by a high concentration of antigen which persists over a period of time. Although the classical model of immunological tolerance is the inhibition of allograft rejection by the introduction of antigen in late fetal or early neonatal life, there is evidence that partial depression of clonal proliferation and the immune response can result from the introduction of antigen in the requisite dosage in later life. Reduction of the antigenic load could result in a return of cell-mediated immune function and a change in the clinical and histopathological status of the individual. Such a reduction in a chronic infection could be the result of chemotherapy or treatment with antibiotic drugs.

Both the blocking antibody of the immunological enhancement phenomenon and suppressor cells, whether T lymphocytes or B lymphocytes, can modulate cell-mediated immune mechanisms. Such homeostatic control can work on the central level by preventing the proliferative response of T cells to antigen, or interfere with the reaction of effector cells with antigen in the periphery. In many immune responses studied it is likely that antigen stimulates both effector cells and suppressor elements at the same time. An upset in this fine balance in one direction can result in further suppression and complete immunological unresponsiveness, whereas an upset in the other direction will result in an increase in host resistance or the development of increased hypersensitivity reactions. In certain chronic infectious diseases there is a degree of parallelism between host resistance and the manifestation of delayed hypersensitivity. However a number of examples are being found in which there is a dissociation between strong host resistance and hypersensitivity states associated with strong delayed hypersensitivity. In these situations it is likely that host resistance is directed towards one group of antigens, whereas cell-mediated hypersensitivity reactions are directed against another group in the same organism.

The reason why some individuals develop what is primarily a low resistance form of disease and others develop a high resistance form is poorly understood. Decreased host resistance similar to that induced by an upset in immune regulation could be due to the inhibitory effect of specific humoral antibody or immune complexes formed between such antibody and soluble antigen released from the organism into the circulation. Such a process is equivalent to the immunological enhancement of tumour growth and has been referred to as immune facilitation[1]. Although the antibody which reacts with cell-mediated immunity in immunological enhancement is described as IgG_2, that in the immunological facilitation phenomenon is an IgG_1 homocytotropic antibody. This would indicate that, depending on the situation, there could be competition for the antigenic site of the infecting organism involving antibodies with a wide variation of class. It may be that the important factor is not the class of the antibody but its affinity, the stronger affinity depending on the stereochemical fit between antibody and antigen. The stronger the bond, the greater the inhibition of cellular immunity and host resistance.

Other factors that can affect host resistance are the state of nutrition of the individual (see Chapters 1 and 6) and the role of intercurrent infections. There is no doubt that protein calorie malnutrition can under certain circumstances affect the ability of the individual to develop certain parameters of cell-mediated immunity. Thus the ability to develop tuberculin sensitivity is retarded in children with malnutrition[2]. In addition there is considerable evidence of the ability of one infection to interfere with the response to another infection. Among the earliest observations was that of von Pirquet[3] who observed a reduced state of tuberculin hypersensitivity in children with measles. Tuberculin insensitivity may appear 1 to 3 weeks before the development of the rash and can persist for an average of 18 days. Moreover the addition of live measles virus to lymphocytes in culture will suppress their response to tuberculin. Malaria is another disease in which impairment of the immune response has been well documented. Children with acute *Plasmodium falciparum* infection have been shown to have a diminished antibody response to tetanus and to *Salmonella typhi* vaccine. A similar failure has been found in trypanosomiasis, in which there is also an impairment of cell-mediated immunity as judged by skin tests with tuberculin and with *Candida* antigen, as well as skin sensitization with dinitrochlorobenzene (DNCB)[4].

12.3 IMMUNOLOGICAL SPECTRA IN CHRONIC INFECTIONS

Evidence of an immunological basis for the spectrum of clinical manifestations is accumulating in a number of chronic infectious diseases. These include:

(1) *Bacterial* – leprosy, tuberculosis, syphilis.
(2) *Fungal* – blastomycosis, histoplasmosis, candidiasis.
(3) *Protozoal* – leishmaniasis, trypanosomiasis (Chagas' disease).

Two types of spectrum may be defined; in the first, which might be called a 'horizontal' spectrum, there may be movement in either direction from a high resistance pole to a low resistance pole, as exemplified by the pattern of disease found in leprosy. The other, which might be called a 'vertical' spectrum, is a progression from low resistance to high resistance as seen in the pattern of clinical events in syphilis where there is initially low resistance to the infecting organism followed by a higher state of resistance sufficient to allow a balance between immune mechanisms and the infecting organism, but insufficient to eliminate the organism completely. Such a balance is, however, unstable, and in a proportion of patients it can be so disturbed as to result in tertiary manifestations of the disease.

12.4 GENETIC SUSCEPTIBILITY

Not everyone exposed to organisms causing chronic infection is actually infected, and not everybody infected develops clinical symptoms. Furthermore, as discussed above, one individual may develop a high resistance form of the disease, whereas another may show manifestations indicative of a low state of host resistance. In addition to the state of nutrition of the individual and the presence or absence of intercurrent infection, it is likely that genetic factors may also play a considerable role in determining the path that an infection may take.

In leprosy, for instance, it has been postulated that the disease develops in individuals who have a natural weakness to develop cell-mediated immunity to mycobacterial antigens[5]. This hypothesis was put forward as a result of a study in which tuberculin-negative children with a family history of leprosy were vaccinated with vole tuberculosis vaccine and it was found that only 18% converted to tuberculin positivity, as opposed to a 90% conversion rate in children from families without leprosy. Further evidence for genetic control of susceptibility to *M. leprae* is obtained from a study of twins with leprosy[6] which showed that of 62 monozygotic pairs 37 (59.7%) were concordant for leprosy and 32 were also concordant for the type of leprosy. Differences in the intensity of contact with infectious cases and differences in the general state of health were the most likely cause of only one twin being affected in the other pairs. More recently evidence has begun to accumulate which indicates that genetic control of host response to *M. leprae* is HLA-linked[7]. In these studies siblings with the same type of leprosy were found to have a significant excess of identical HLA haplotypes. However, siblings affected with different types of leprosy shared a haplotype less often than expected. This was taken to indicate that both susceptibility to and the type of leprosy are controlled by at least two HLA-controlled genes.

12.5 MYCOBACTERIAL INFECTIONS

12.5.1 Leprosy

12.5.1.1 *The clinical spectrum*

The spectrum of leprosy has been particularly well defined[8-10] and the five-group system of classification (Table 12.1) is now used by all immunologists working in this field. This is based on (i) the cytology of cells of the mononuclear phagocyte system (whether histiocyte or epithelioid), (ii) the bacterial density in lesions in untreated patients, and (iii) the degree of lymphocytic infiltration. The groups are no more than arbitrary points in a spectrum and, in the very early stages of the disease, a patient may not develop sufficiently definite characteristics to be placed accurately on the spectrum. Such

Table 12.1 Summary of the clinical, histological, bacteriological and immunological findings of the five groups of the leprosy spectrum

	TT	BT	BB	BL	LL
Skin lesions					
Numbers	1 to 3	Very few to moderate	Moderate	Moderate to many	Very many
Symmetry	Very symmetrical	Asymmetrical	Asymmetrical	Slightly asymmetrical	Symmetrical
Anaesthesia	Very marked	Marked	Marked to moderate	Slight to nil	Nil
Nerve enlargement					
Cutaneous sensory	Common	May occur	0	0	0
Peripheral nerves*	0 or 1	Common; asymmetrical	Common; asymmetrical	Moderately asymmetrical	Symmetrical
Skin histology					
Granuloma cell	Epithelioid	Epithelioid	Epithelioid	Histiocyte	Foamy histiocyte
Lymphocytes	+++	+++	+	± or ++	±
Dermal nerves	Destroyed	Mostly destroyed	Some visible	Visible	Easily visible
Bacilli numbers (routine examination)	0	0, + or ++	+, ++ or +++	++++	+++++
Lymph nodes					
Paracortical infiltrate	Nil, immunoblasts	Sarcoid-like	Diffuse epithelioid	Diffuse histiocytes	Massive infiltrate foamy histiocytes Virchow cells
Germinal centres	Normal	Normal	Normal	Some hypertrophy	Gross hypertrophy
Reactions					
Lepromin test	+++	++	± or 0	0	0
ENL	0	0	0	Rare	Very common
Reversal (Lepra)	?	Common	Very common	Very common	(Rare)†

* Nerves of predilection, i.e. ulnar, median, lateral popliteal, facial, great auricular, and posterior tibial
† Lepra reactions are occasionally seen in treated LL patients who have developed from borderline (BT, BB or BL) in the absence of treatment

patients are considered to have 'indeterminate' leprosy and may later develop a more typical form of the disease or recover spontaneously. The only stable points on the spectrum are at the polar tuberculoid (TT) – high resistance – and lepromatous polar (LLp) – low resistance – poles. Thus an untreated patient with borderline tuberculoid (BT) may downgrade or lose resistance and move across the spectrum to borderline (BB), borderline lepromatous (BL) or even lepromatous subpolar (LLs). Similarly a patient with BL on effective treatment may develop a reversal or 'upgrading' reaction and move to BB or BT as he develops immunity against the organism. Having swung across the spectrum in this way, he may lose resistance again if treatment is stopped prematurely and swing back to his original position on the spectrum. The most unstable point is BB, and a patient rarely stays at this point for long, moving rapidly to BT or BL.

12.5.1.2   *The nature of granuloma formation*

The granuloma in the skin of lepromatous patients consists of large undifferentiated macrophages similar to those seen in experimental animals at the site of injection of a non-antigenic colloidal material such as aluminium hydroxide[11], where there is a conspicuous absence of lymphocytes and other inflammatory cells. The macrophages may be packed with globi of *M. leprae* in untreated patients and these cells change gradually into epithelioid cells as the spectrum is crossed through borderline to tuberculoid. This is associated with an increased infiltration with lymphocytes and a gradual decrease in the bacterial load. The epithelioid cell appearance is a measure of the activation of macrophages and is associated with increased ability to eliminate intracellular organisms. Such macrophage activation has been obtained in cultures of blood-derived macrophages from patients with tuberculoid leprosy when they are exposed to *M. leprae in vitro*, in the presence of lymphocytes. Under similar conditions no activation was observed in cultures of macrophages from patients with lepromatous leprosy[12].

12.5.1.3   *Immunological parameters*

(a) *Lepromin test*. The Mitsuda lepromin test is a nodular granulomatous reaction which occurs between 2 and 4 weeks after the intradermal injection of a crude preparation of *M. leprae* derived from autoclaved infected human tissue. This reaction is positive only in the high resistance (TT and BT) forms of the disease. Its main value is to detect the inability of patients at the lepromatous end of the spectrum to react to the injection of *M. leprae* with an epithelioid cell granuloma, and therefore is a marker of a specific absence of cell-mediated immunity to this organism. The reaction cannot be used as an indication of contact with *M. leprae* as non-infected individuals have been found to develop a positive reaction to the antigen.

A 48-hour typical delayed hypersensitivity reaction, which is known as the Fernandez reaction, also occurs after the injection of lepromin. Most leprologists find that there is a better correlation between the 4-week Mitsuda reaction and host resistance, and that the reaction remains negative in LL patients even after many years of treatment when the bacterial load has fallen to undetectable levels. Many attempts have been made to produce a more purified lepromin and, now that it has been discovered that *M. leprae* will grow in the armadillo, a purified standardized reagent will shortly be readily available.

(b) In vitro *parameters of cellular immunity*. The nature of the immunological changes that occur in leprosy has been studied *in vitro* by Myrvang et al.[13], who found that circulating lymphocytes of patients with lepromatous leprosy failed to be transformed by whole *M. leprae* (lymphocyte transformation test – LTT). There was a similar failure of *M. leprae* to inhibit the migration of leukocytes from capillary tubes *in vitro*. This defect decreases across the leprosy spectrum and patients at the tuberculoid end of the spectrum show strong reactivity in both these tests. Although LL lymphocytes are not transformed by *M. leprae*, in many cases they can be induced to transform by *M. tuberculosis*. Initially it appeared that there was a strong correlation between the specific LTT with *M. leprae* and cellular immunity. A subsequent report suggests that the correlation is not necessarily with the ability of the host to eliminate the infecting organism but with the strength of the allergic reaction shown by the patient[14]. LTT responses may frequently be stronger in actively inflamed BT than in TT. Moreover the response in the LTT test may vary depending on the nature of this antigenic preparation[15]. Thus borderline patients with active nerve damage may show stronger response using sonicated antigen than whole bacilli. Patients with predominantly cutaneous lesions, however, react better to whole bacilli than to the sonicated preparation. There have been variable reports of the LTT response of leprosy patients using non-specific mitogens such as phytohaemagglutinin (PHA), and, in untreated lepromatous patients, there may be a serum factor that non-specifically depresses the response to PHA and in the mixed leukocyte reaction[16,17]. This non-specific lymphocyte-depressing factor can be shown to decrease with time on treatment.

A significant proportion of new arrivals in a leprosy endemic area, who had initially been shown to be unresponsive to *M. leprae* in the LTT, were found to develop positive reactivity after contact with leprosy patients[18], and, in a study of families of known lepromatous patients, it was found that contacts without any evidence of clinical disease had a lower proportion of positive responses to *M. leprae* than contacts of patients with tuberculoid disease. This lack of correlation between LTT and disease might be considered as further suggestive evidence that the LTT test is not a reaction with the antigens that are primarily associated with host resistance.

(c) *Evidence for a non-specific defect in cell-mediated immunity in leprosy patients.* There are a number of reports indicating that there may be a non-specific defect in T-cell function in lepromatous leprosy. These range from an inability to be sensitized with DNCB[19] to a decrease in the proportion of T- and an increase in the proportion of B-lymphocytes in the peripheral blood[20-22], and wide replacement of the paracortical areas of lymph nodes by macrophages packed with *M. leprae*[23].

However, there are enough indications that the basic defect is a specific one and that non-specific deficiencies in cellular immunity develop secondary to a primary defect in the ability to eliminate *M. leprae*. In the first place, there is no clear parallel between failure to be sensitized to picryl chloride and failure to show tuberculin sensitivity, and the incidence of the failure of sensitization is lower among patients who have received treatment for leprosy over 18 months[24]. Secondly, despite an inability to sensitize 50% of lepromatous patients with DNCB, there is no difficulty in sensitizing them to develop delayed hypersensitivity to keyhole limpet haemocyanin[25]. However, the most striking evidence for the specificity of the primary lesion is that there is no increased incidence of other infections or tumours in leprosy patients, which indicates that immunological surveillance mechanisms are otherwise unimpaired. In addition the failure of lymphocytes to react *in vivo* by transformation also appears to be specific to *M. leprae*[13].

In patients with tuberculoid leprosy where there is a high degree of host resistance to *M. leprae*, there may occasionally also be a failure of ability to be sensitized to picryl chloride[24]. Tuberculoid patients may also be found to show a significantly decreased incidence of tuberculin positivity as compared with a control population. However, a significant delay in skin allograft rejection has been demonstrated in lepromatous and, to a lesser degree, in tuberculoid patients[26]. These defects may in part be explained by the presence of a non-specific lymphocyte depressing factor in the sera of all lepromatous and, at a lower titre, in some tuberculoid patients.

(d) *Immunoglobulins, complement and humoral antibodies.* High levels of IgG are consistently found in the sera of untreated lepromatous patients. High levels of IgA and IgM have also been described but appear to be more variable. High levels of both C2 and C3 (β_1 /β_1 globulin) are also recorded. (For review, see reference 27.)

Sera from all patients with lepromatous leprosy have antibodies which react strongly with culture filtrates of *M. tuberculosis*. These antibodies are not found in TT although low levels are found in BT[28]. Such antibodies cross-react with antigens from other mycobacteria. In a similar study[29] precipitins against *M. kansasii* and *M. smegmatis* were found in the sera of lepromatous patients and in half of patients with 'tuberculoid' lesions that were bacillary-positive (probably BB and BT). However, precipitins were not found in the sera of bacillary-negative tuberculoid patients (probably TT).

Numerous reports describe the detection of antibodies to autoantigens in lepromatous patients. Wager[30], from a review of the literature, gives the following incidences: antinuclear factor 30%; LE cells 8%; rheumatoid factors 50%; thyroglobulin autoantibodies 40%; cryoglobulin 95% and biologically false positive tests for syphilis 70%. The incidence of autoantibodies has marked geographical variation and the presence of autoantibodies may be related to the length of disease, lack of regularity of treatment and incidence of reactional states; however, so far there has been no published evidence of correlation with any of these factors. High levels of precipitating antimycobacterial antibodies in lepromatous leprosy are paralleled by marked plasma cell proliferation and germinal centre formation in peripheral lymph nodes, despite replacement of T-cell areas by macrophages filled with mycobacteria[23,31].

12.5.1.4 Reaction states in leprosy

(a) *Reversal reactions*. These reactions occur in borderline leprosy (BT, BB and BL) and occasionally in LLs, usually developing within the first year of the onset of therapy. Skin lesions become red and swollen. Some patients become mildly febrile and there is frequently severe peripheral nerve involvement. This type of reaction is often associated with a movement across the clinical spectrum towards tuberculoid, from which it would appear that the patient is regaining cell-mediated immunity as the bacterial load is being reduced by therapy. These changes can be monitored histologically in the skin and in lymph node biopsies. In the lepromatous state the paracortical areas of lymph nodes are replaced by macrophages full of bacilli and are depleted of lymphocytes, presumably T cells, while B-cell areas often show greatly increased activity. In reversal reactions lymphocytes can be seen to begin to appear in the paracortical areas round the postcapillary venules. This is suggestive of a return of T-cell activity[31]. In addition there is evidence of increase in LTT activity to *M. leprae*[14].

It would thus appear that reversal reactions are caused by a rapid increase in cell-mediated immunity against *M. leprae*. This is associated with the decrease in antigenic load that follows the onset of therapy and with it the patient regains or increases the capacity to produce hypersensitivity reactions at the site of residual bacterial deposition. Therefore the sites of this reaction are those where *M. leprae* particularly accumulate in borderline leprosy, i.e. the skin and peripheral nerves. Histological appearance of these reactions is consistent with their being due to delayed hypersensitivity.

(b) *Erythema nodosum leprosum (ENL)*. This occurs in patients at or near the lepromatous end of the spectrum where cell-mediated immunity against *M. leprae* is very low or absent. However, these patients have high levels of circulating antimycobacterial antibodies.

Although ENL may rarely occur in untreated patients, it usually develops for the first time during the first 12 months of treatment with sulphones. In the skin, the lesions of ENL generally occur as repeated crops of painful erythematous papules. In severe episodes, they may become haemorrhagic, pustular and necrotic. Histologically there is an intense perivascular poly-morphonuclear leukocytic infiltration reminiscent of that seen in the Arthus reaction in experimental animals. Significant, often severe, vasculitis may also be detected. The vessels affected are generally deep in the dermis and frequently show necrotic changes. In some cases the lesions are more superficial and are associated with capillary necrosis, and fragmented (dead) bacilli are present[32].

In biopsies of ENL lesions in 38 lepromatous patients, immunoglobulins and β_{1C}/β_{1A} globulin were detected in areas of polymorph infiltration in 20 of them[33]. No such deposits were found in the lesions from 13 patients with lepromatous leprosy who did not have ENL. The deposits seen were granular in form and did not correspond to the areas of bacillary infiltration. Deposits were sometimes demonstrated within the walls of blood vessels in the deep dermis.

ENL lesions may also occur in other tissues in lepromatous leprosy which contain accumulations of *M. leprae*. These present as neuritis (in particular of the ulnar and median nerves), lymphadenitis, orchitis and iridocyclitis. Arthritis is a less frequent complication[34]. In addition there may be systemic upset with fever and significant proteinuria, and there may be evidence of immune complex deposition in the kidney[35]. These obser-vations suggest that patients with ENL may develop illness due to circulating immune complexes as well as Arthus-like reactions locally, but at present there is little evidence to confirm this. The demonstration of circulating complexes in diseases other than in systemic lupus erythematosus has been found particularly elusive. So far there have only been isolated findings of C1q precipitable material in the serum of patients with lepromatous leprosy. Results using this technique are, however, variable and do not necessarily correlate with systemic disorders. Moreover C1q can be precipi-tated by many other substances in the serum as well as specific immune complexes. These include aggregates of γ-globulin, biological polyanions including polysaccharides, and circulating immunoglobulin–anti-immuno-globulin complexes including cryoglobulins.

12.5.1.5   *Animal models*

It has not yet been possible to grow *M. leprae in vitro*. The earliest successful studies on the transmission of *M. leprae* to experimental animals were in mice, when in 1960 Shepard[36] produced a limited proliferation of the organism in their footpads. However Rees and his colleagues[37] were able to overcome the resistance in mice by injecting *M. leprae* into the footpads and ears of mice which had been thymectomized at the age of 6 weeks, given total body irradiation of 900 rad and transfused with syngeneic bone marrow. After 9 months these mice showed a histological appearance similar to that seen in lepromatous leprosy and some developed nodular swelling of their footpads. Thus a disease similar to lepromatous leprosy can be produced in mice whose immunological activity, and especially cell-mediated immunity, has been depleted enough to accept and retain allogenic skin grafts. The development of lepromatous leprosy could be prevented by serial injection of syngeneic lymphocytes. However, when the lymphocyte injections were withheld until lepromatous leprosy had developed, the mice were found to regain cell-mediated immunity[38]. This reversal reaction was associated with a move across the spectrum to a borderline (BT) position. Histologically there was evidence of increased lymphocytic infiltration of the infected tissue with degeneration of bacilli both in the skin and in Schwann cells of peripheral nerves.

More recently a new animal model has been introduced into leprosy research following the demonstration that infection of the nine-banded armadillo with *M. leprae* can result in the development of advanced disseminated leprosy within 15 months[39]. Further studies indicated that the disease was produced in 40% or more of animals injected with the organism. Moreover lepromatous tissue from the armadillo may contain more than 100 times more organisms than an equivalent amount of human lepromatous tissue. The armadillo therefore can become an important source of organisms and antigens for research purposes, as well as providing a natural model for investigating the disease.

12.5.2 Tuberculosis

Despite the large amount of literature on this condition, an immunological spectrum similar to that for leprosy has only recently been defined[40]. Four points on the spectrum have been defined equivalent to TT, BT, BL and LL. These are described as follows:

RR – reactive: micronodular localized tuberculosis
RI – reactive intermediate: nodular or micronodular localized tuberculosis with cavitation; unilateral or bilateral lymphadenopathy; tubercular serositis
UI – unreactive intermediate: nodular or micronodular chronic diffuse tuberculosis with cavitation and fibrosis; tubercular lymphadenopathy complicated by fistula formation
UU– unreactive: acute miliary tuberculosis.

The definition of localized micronodular tuberculosis was based on the size and discrete quality of the lesions on X-ray and their limitation to one or two segments of the lung. Nodular lesions were larger in size but still localized in their distribution. The lesions of nodular or micronodular chronic diffuse tuberculosis were characterized by one or more cavities and a prolonged course of disease and relative resistance to therapy.

The cell-mediated immune reactivity of the patients was assessed by tuberculin skin testing in which three types of reactivity were found:

(a) Typical delayed hypersensitivity reaction present at 24 hours, peaking at 48 hours with strong induration and persisting up to 72 and 96 hours;

(b) Early reactions with rapid development persisting until 24 hours, chiefly with erythema and oedema gradually decreasing and disappearing at 48 hours;

(c) Biphasic reactions with an early phase visible from 3 to 24 hours with erythema and oedema, gradually decreasing at 48 hours.

In addition cell-mediated immune reactivity was assessed by the leukocyte migration inhibition test (LMT) using tuberculin as antigen. Typical delayed hypersensitivity reactions were found in 100% of patients with RR, 30% with RI and 5% with UI. UU patients showed no response to tuberculin. Reactivity as assessed by LMT followed a similar pattern (Table 12.2). The

Table 12.2 The spectrum of human tuberculosis, as defined on the basis of clinical, bacteriological, histological and immunological data[40]

	Reactive (RR)	Reactive intermediate (RI)	Unreactive intermediate (UI)	Unreactive (UU)
Skin test to PPD:				
Typical delayed reaction (%)	100	30	5	—
Early reaction (%)	—	13	15	—
Mixed reaction (%)	—	57	80	—
Leukocyte migration inhibition	+++	++−	±−−	−−−
Humoral anti-PPD antibodies (%)	5	70	98	100
Mycobacteria:				
In sputum	−−−	−−−	++−	+++
In the tissue	−−−	+−−	+++	+++
Immunologic change in lymph node:				
Germinal centres and plasma cells	−−+	−−+	+++	−−+
Paracortical area	+++	++−	+−−	−−−
Response to antimycobacterial treatment (%)	100	90	33	0

presence of mycobacteria in the sputum and tissues was inversely proportional to cell-mediated immunity as assessed by these parameters. Humoral antibody levels were also inversely proportional to the parameters of cell-mediated immunity. The ability to respond to antimycobacterial therapy paralleled the strength of cell-mediated immune reactivity. These recent studies indicate that host resistance in this disease is likely to be genetically controlled in the same way as in leprosy, and it will be of interest to find out whether a similar linkage with HLA haplotypes exists.

12.6 SYPHILIS

Treponema pallidum is another organism that causes a chronic infection with a wide range of clinical manifestations (Table 12.3). However, as noted, whereas in the case of leprosy and tuberculosis, patients can move from side to side across a spectrum depending on the strength of host resistance, in syphilis there is a predictable progression from low resistance to high resistance during the course of disease. Initially resistance is low, so that the organism rapidly spreads throughout the tissues. This is followed by a gradual increase in resistance sufficient to control the spread of the organism without actually eliminating it completely. This balance is, however, unstable and in a proportion of individuals it can be so disturbed as to result in the tertiary manifestations of the disease. These may take on either a high resistance tuberculoid form (gummatous) or a low resistance form (cerebral).

T. pallidum can enter cells in the same way as mycobacteria, and thus escape the action of circulating antibody[41]. Antibody alone confers only partial resistance in experimental models[42,43]. Moreover diffuse spread of the organism can be obtained in models in which cell-mediated immunity is reduced and antibody production remains normal[44]. In addition *T. pallidum* appears to have a natural ability to suppress the immune response of the host. When injected into newborn rabbits, the organism produces a runt-like syndrome associated with depletion of splenic lymphoid tissue[45].

Infection with *T. pallidum* runs a progressive and relentless course in many infected patients. This has been traditionally divided into four phases: primary, secondary, latent and tertiary disease. The organism spreads rapidly throughout the body before the primary lesion has developed, and both the primary and secondary forms of the disease are characterized by a low state of host resistance. During the later phases of the secondary form of the disease when the skin lesions may be papular rather than macular, resistance begins to improve and the patients begin to strike a balance with the organism which is all but eliminated. Then at a later date something happens, resistance fails, and the patient goes into the tertiary form of the disease. This may take the form of localized gummatous lesions or the more diffuse proliferation of the organism characteristic of the neurological forms of the disease. It has been known for many years that whereas positive delayed hypersensitivity tests with treponemal antigens were found in late secondary and latent syphilis, they were almost universally negative in primary and early secondary syphilis[46,47]. Moreover in cerebrospinal syphilis the reaction is negative in 50% of patients, whereas in the other tertiary forms of the disease it is positive in 95% of patients[46].

Table 12.3 Syphilis

		T-cell function				B-cell function		
		LTT						
		T. pallidum						
	Luetin skin test	UK	Ethiopia	PHA	Presence of T. pallidum	Antibody	Immune complexes	Vasculitis
Primary								
sero − ve	−	−	−	++				
sero + ve		+	−	+±	++	+		+
Secondary								
macular	−	−	−	+++	+++	+++		?
papular	++	+	−	+±	++	++	++	−
Latent	+ or −	+	±	++	−	+		−
Tertiary								
gumma	+++		+		+	+		++
neurosyphilis	±				+++	+++		++

Lymphocyte transformation and proliferation of lymphocytes cultured with specific antigen *in vitro* (LTT) has been used to investigate further the spectrum of cellular immunity in syphilis[48,49]. These studies were made in England and in Ethiopia, where the course of the disease was somewhat different in that the secondary lesions were more of the papular type, and it was possible also to collect a series of patients with a cardiovascular tertiary form of the disease. In England, patients with sero-negative primary syphilis were universally negative in the LTT. Half the patients with sero-positive primary syphilis reacted to *T. pallidum* whereas cells from most patients with macular secondary syphilis were unresponsive. After 4 to 8 days of antibiotic therapy, patients even in the macular secondary stage of the disease showed a dramatic increase in lymphocyte reactivity. A similar increased skin-test reactivity to *T. pallidum* has also been described by Noguchi in patients with secondary syphilis following treatment[46]. In Ethiopian patients with early syphilis, regardless of clinical type, there was a complete failure of responsiveness to *T. pallidum*. This absence of reactivity in the LTT was found in forms of the disease in which many patients in the UK were positive, e.g. sero-positive primary syphilis. Strong reactivity was found, however, in patients with latent and cardiovascular syphilis. Increased reactivity was found in only half the patients with early syphilis following treatment.

The consistent absence of specific reactivity in certain forms of early syphilis would therefore appear to be due to positive immunosuppression. There is accumulated evidence that this is to some extent non-specific. Thus it can be shown that there is a parallel depression of lymphocyte responsiveness to phytohaemagglutinin (PHA) and tuberculin (PPD). In addition a factor can be demonstrated in the plasma of these patients which inhibits the response of lymphocytes from normal individuals to PHA and PPD[51,52]. This factor could be related to the release of anti-lymphocytic factors by *T. pallidum* or the presence of antigen–antibody complexes, which if formed in antibody excess can specifically inhibit lymphocyte transformation to the homologous antigen, and if complexed with IgM antibody can non-specifically depress stimulation by mitogen. These inhibitory plasma factors may, however, be evidence of a deeper upset in immunological control mechanisms caused by the presence of excessive amounts of antigen in the tissues, and may parallel the presence of a population of immunologically specific suppressor cells. (A similar phenomenon has been described in leprosy. It has been found that patients with borderline leprosy do not respond to *M. leprae* in the LT test[15] and that plasma from these patients inhibits lymphocyte responsiveness to PHA. Some of these patients develop 'reversal reactions' in which their lesions become inflamed, probably as a result of delayed hypersensitivity. During the 'reaction' the patient's lymphocytes become reactive to *M. leprae* in the LT test and their plasma loses its inhibitory capacity.)

Evidence is now beginning to accumulate which suggests that the lymphocyte transformation reaction correlates in both leprosy and syphilis with delayed hypersensitivity. However, the correlation between these two reactions and protective immunity is not as strong as might be expected. Patients with tuberculoid (TT) leprosy in whom protective immunity is highest do not show such strong lymphocyte reactivity to *M. leprae* as those with BT leprosy in whom protective immunity is weaker. Patients in England with syphilitic re-infection clearly lack protective immunity. However, they frequently show strong reactivity to *T. pallidum* in the LTT. It would also appear from a number of studies that the clinical appearance of the lesion is related to delayed hypersensitivity rather than to immunity. The gummatous form of the disease is particularly associated with strong hypersensitivity reactions.

Immune complex disease as well as cellular hypersensitivity can also contribute to the clinical manifestations of syphilis. Antibodies against *T. pallidum* occur early in the disease; during the time when the primary lesion is present the antibodies are initially IgM but later are IgG. The contribution of immune complexes to the clinical manifestations of the early (secondary macular) stages of the disease are suggested by the occasional occurrence of iridocyclitis, arthritis and proteinuria. In addition there may be a fully developed nephrotic syndrome with electron-microscopic evidence of immune complex deposition on the glomerular basement membrane.

It is clear from a number of studies that patients who are infected with *T. pallidum* do not necessarily go through the whole spectrum of the disease. It is well documented for instance, that only one-third of patients who have passed into the latent stage will develop tertiary stigmata. In a number of these it used to be considered that one-third developed neurosyphilis, one-third gummatous disease and one-third cardiovascular disease[53, 54]. However, in a recent survey in Ethiopia the only tertiary form of the disease discovered was the cardiovascular form. In addition it is clear that not all patients will develop papular lesions in the secondary form of the disease. Thus the clinical manifestations that develop will depend firstly on the strength of protective immunity, which if developed sufficiently can terminate the infection at any stage. Secondly the clinical manifestations developed will depend on the relative strengths of both cellular and humoral hypersensitivity reactions. Thus the clinical manifestations of secondary disease may be relatively weak or inapparent. Moreover two-thirds of patients passing into the latent stage of the disease, in which the patient reaches a balance between protective immunity and the infecting organism, fail to pass into the tertiary phase of the disease. It could be that tertiary stigmata only develop if this balance between the host and the infecting organism is upset by external events. This could be the result of a temporary depression of protective immunity that might develop as a result of, for example, malnutrition or intercurrent infection.

12.7 PARASITIC INFECTIONS

12.7.1 Leishmaniasis

A further group of diseases, in which a clinical spectrum related to the immunological response of the host exists, consists of those due to infection with protozoa of the genus *Leishmania*. *Leishmania* are obligatory intracellular parasites of macrophages of the skin and viscera of vertebrates. They are primarily parasites of small rodents and are transmitted by sandflies (usually of the genus *Phlebotomus*). The clinical pattern of the disease varies depending on the infecting species of the *Leishmania* (Table 12.4). *Leishmania* spp. are flagellates but they retain the promastigote form only in the insect host and in culture media. When infecting man and other vertebrates they take on the 'amastigote' form. *Leishmania* spp. can be identified on the basis of morphological and ultrastructural appearances, characteristics in culture, DNA and enzyme analysis, serological tests, host and vector specificity, reactions to drugs and epidemiological findings.

Three of the principal diseases of man caused by *Leishmania* spp. are cutaneous leishmaniasis caused by *L. tropica*, mucocutaneous leishmaniasis (espundia) caused by *L. braziliensis* and visceral leishmaniasis (kala-azar) caused by *L. donovani*. These diseases present with distinct clinical features. Cutaneous leishmaniasis caused by *L. tropica* presents as a spectral disease like leprosy with two polar forms, the features of which depend upon the response of the host to the parasite. The forms are diffuse cutaneous leishmaniasis and lupoid or recidiva leishmaniasis[27] (Table 12.5).

Oriental sore, which is the common form taken by the infection, falls somewhat between these two rarer extremes. In oriental sore a nodule appears in the skin some weeks after the inoculation of *L. tropica* by a sandfly. After 2–8 months it ulcerates and becomes crusted. Healing gradually takes place over the next few months, leaving in the end a characteristic depressed mottled scar. Oriental sore is a self-healing disease which is followed by permanent immunity to re-infection and is accompanied by strong delayed hypersensitivity to leishmanial antigen. Positive lymphocyte transformation in the presence of specific leishmanial antigen can be demonstrated, as also can the production of lymphokine in the supernatant from sensitized lymphocytes incubated with specific antigen. Only a low level of antibody can be detected in the serum.

In lupoid or recidiva leishmaniasis which is also caused by *L. tropica*, the lesion never quite heals or sometimes heals and then relapses. Classically, there is a typical scar around whose borders small nodules recrudesce, ulcerate and heal, so that the lesion gradually spreads but no metastases develop. Histologically the lesion shows an intense cellular reaction forming a tuberculoid granuloma, and parasites are scanty or absent. Marked delayed hypersensitivity, often with an earlier Arthus component, may be found.

Diffuse cutaneous leishmaniasis (DCL) is rare and is found mainly in

Table 12.4 Summary of immunopathological features of leishmanial infections in man[70]

Disease	Aetiologic agent	Self-cure	Cutaneous lesion		Lesions of			Delayed cutaneous hypersensitivity to leishmanial antigens		Humoral anti-bodies	Immunity to re-infection
			Nodular	Ulcerous	Mucosa	Cartilage	Viscera	During infection	After cure		
Kala-azar (visceral) leishmaniasis	L. donovani	−	+	−	−	−	++++	−	++	++++	+
Kala-azar (Mediterranean infantile)	L. infantum	−	+	−	−	−	++++	−	++	++++	+
Post-kala-azar-dermal leishmanoid (Indian)	L. donovani	−	++++	−	−	−	−	±	++	++	+
Oriental sore (cutaneous leishmaniasis)	L. tropica (major, minor)	+	+	++++	−	−	−	++	++++	+	+
Diffuse cutaneous leishmaniasis	L. tropica (Ethiopia)	−	++++	−	−	−	−	−	±	+	+
Diffuse cutaneous leishmaniasis	L. pifanoi (Venezuela)	−	++++	−	+	−	−	−	−	+	++
Leishmaniasis recidiva	L. tropica	−	+	+	−	−	−	+++	±	±	++
Chicleros ulcer	L. mexicana	+	++	+++	−	++	−	++	++++	++	++
'Uta'	L. peruviana	+	++	+++	−	−	−	++	++++	++	+
Leishmaniasis tegumentaria americana	L. braziliensis	+	++	+++	−	−	−	++	++++	+	+
'Espundia' (mucocutaneous leishmaniasis)	L. braziliensis	−	++	+++	+++	+++	−	++	+++++	++	+

Ethiopia where it is caused by *L. tropica*, and in Venezuela where it is caused by *L. pifanoi*. The initial lesion may be a macule, papule or nodule which rarely ulcerates. The lesion does not heal but spreads locally and metastasises to other areas of the skin. The histological appearance is of heavily parasitized macrophages and lymphocytes and epithelioid cells are typically absent. Delayed hypersensitivity to leishmanial antigen is notably absent. Strains of *L. tropica* isolated from DCL and oriental sore in Ethiopia appear to be identical using serological techniques. The presence of high levels of circulating antibody and absent delayed hypersensitivity in two conditions where self-healing does not occur (DCL and kala–azar) has suggested that healing depends on cell-mediated immunity and that antibodies in leishmaniasis may not be protective.

Table 12.5   Features of polar forms of cutaneous leishmaniasis[27]

Features	Diffuse cutaneous leishmaniasis	Lupoid or recidiva leishmaniasis
Clinical	Disseminated nodules	Local scar with peripheral spread
Histology	Parasitized macrophages (MM)*	Tubercles (TT)†
Delayed hypersensitivity to leishmanin	Negative	Positive, with occasional Arthus
Antibodies	Variable	Not studied
Immunoglobulins	Normal	Not studied
Response to treatment	Poor, relapses	Variable, improved by steroids

*MM – macrophage
**TT – tuberculoid

Espundia is a form of infection with *L. braziliensis* in which metastatic lesions involve the nasopharyngeal mucosa causing intense local tissue necrosis. These lesions develop months or years after the initial primary infection despite the evidence of both cell-mediated immunity and humoral antibody production. The ability of the *Leishmania* parasites to resist killing by activated macrophages in the presence of both cellular and humoral allergy would appear to indicate further factors in host resistance to this parasite. This phenomenon may be related to the observation that the fate of *Leishmania* in activated macrophages would seem to depend on a particular host–parasite combination[55]. Thus *Leishmania* spp. that can elicit infections in a given host may develop the ability to resist the effects of activated macrophages of that host. For example, activated guinea-pig macrophages derived from a *Leishmania*-immune animal do not destroy *L. enriettii* (the species that infects guinea-pigs) *in vitro*, while this parasite is killed by activated mouse cells. *L. enriettii* readily infects guinea-pigs but fails to infect mice. *L. tropica* on the other hand, infects mice and is not destroyed by the activated cells of that host. Other factors that need to be taken into account when assessing the mechanism of host resistance to *Leishmania* spp. include the observation that pretreatment of experimental animals with cyclophosphamide, which decreases antibody production without any observable effect on delayed hypersensitivity, will increase the intensity of the local lesion and also increase the incidence of formation of metastases[56]. This suggests that more attention should be paid to the role of antibody in host resistance to this organism. It may be that control of this infection is due to a synergism between cell-mediated immunity and antibody production, and that a decrease in either function can result in an increased incidence of widespread metastatic lesions. The course of *Leishmania* infection can also be affected by intercurrent infection with another parasite, for example, the plasmodium of malaria. Chronic infection of hamsters with plasmodia caused the development of a larger leishmanial skin lesion than would have been found in animals without malaria[57].

Infection with *L. donovani* usually results in kala–azar, in which there is gross parasitization of systemic macrophages in the spleen, liver, blood and bone marrow. The skin is rarely involved. The Leishmanin test is negative and humoral antibodies are high. The condition lies at the low host resistance end of the spectrum similar to DCL and cases usually terminate fatally without treatment. After treatment the extremely high antibody levels fall and cell-mediated immunity may return as indicated by delayed hypersensitivity to Leishmanin. This shift across the spectrum towards the tuberculoid pole is accompanied by the development of immunity to re-infection. In some patients a purely cutaneous relapse may occur following visceral leishmaniasis. This condition is known as post-kala–azar-dermal-leishmanoid and the wide variation in skin-test response and histological pattern could indicate that patients might be lying at a number of points in the leishmaniasis spectrum. A histological spectrum analogous to that proposed by Ridley and Jopling[9] for leprosy has been devised by Bryceson for the spectrum of leishmaniasis[58]. In this classification the letter M has been substituted for the letter L of the leprosy spectrum. The letter M has been used to indicate the degree of macrophage, as opposed to lymphocytic, infiltration of the lesion. The pole of the spectrum, equivalent to LL in leprosy, is referred to as MM and in this group are found the more severe cases of DCL which are characterized by intense dermal infiltration with macrophages, often vacuolated and full of parasites, and an absence of small lymphocytes. Less severe cases of DCL may show the macrophage intermediate (MI) or intermediate (II) pattern. The full spectrum is as follows:

MM – macrophage
MI – macrophage intermediate
II   – intermediate
IT   – intermediate tuberculoid
TT – tuberculoid

Table 12.6   The histological spectrum in leishmaniasis[27]

Designation		Histological features	
(MM)	Macrophage	Thin intact epidermis, clear subepidermal zone. Dermal infiltration with macrophages, often vaccuolated, full of parasites; histiocytes, many vessels containing monocytes, absence of lymphocytes	
(MI)	Macrophage intermediate	MM together with scanty lymphocytes scattered throughout or grouped deeply beneath the lesion	DCL* before treatment
(II)	Intermediate	Epidermis thickened, intact early, may ulcerate later. No clear zone. Lymphocytes intimately mixed with large fleshy histiocytes, moderate numbers of parasites or MM areas alongside IT or TT areas	
(IT)	Intermediate tuberculoid	Epidermis ulcerated; where intact shows re-duplication of the layers, nuclear damage and hyperkeratosis. Lymphocytes predominate, early arrangement into tubercles around clumps of epithelioid cells, parasites scanty	Oriental sore and DCL in relapse
(TT)	Tuberculoid	Epidermis ulcerated. Tubercle formation, often with giant cells. Parasites rare or invisible	Lupoid leishmaniasis.
(TF)	Tuberculoid fibrosis	Tubercles being destroyed by fibrosis. Re-epithelialization	All types healing
(F)	Fibrosis		
(R)	Resolving	Patchy perivascular infiltration with lymphocytes and histiocytes. Absence of tubercle formation and of parasites	DCL healing without immunological shift

* Diffuse cutaneous leishmaniasis

TF   – tuberculoid fibrosis
F   – fibrosis
R   – resolving.

Diffuse cutaneous leishmaniasis before treatment ranges between MM and II. Oriental sore and DCL in relapse lie between MI and TF. Lupoid leishmaniasis is found in the TT–TF range. The spectrum as such runs between MM and TT, the points TF, F and R are added to provide points during healing (Table 12.6).

12.7.2   Trypanosomiasis

Chagas' disease, due to infection with *Trypanosoma cruzi*, has a number of features suggesting that it is a further example of a disease with a vertical spectrum. The acute form of the disease occurs mainly in children. The condition consists of intermittent fever, associated oedema and inflammation of the face, and trypanosomes may be found in the blood. Death may occur within 2 to 4 weeks and the mortality is in the region of 10%[59]. In this form of the disease there may be an acute myocarditis in which the muscle fibres are separated by a diffuse infiltration with mononuclear cells. Immunological activity is suggested by the diffuse lymph node enlargement and splenomegaly. While trypanosomes may be demonstrated in large numbers in the blood in the first weeks of infection, after 6–10 weeks it is difficult to demonstrate them by direct microscopy. Despite the high parasitaemia, circulating precipitins may be demonstrated. The children then pass into the asymptomatic or latent stage of the disease, which usually lasts from 10 to 20 years before entering the third or chronic stage. Patients at this stage frequently do not give a history of an acute episode and may be well into middle-age before presenting with the typical cardiac manifestations. This would indicate that the acute illness may take on a relatively mild form. In the chronic form of the disease there is diffuse fibrosis of the myocardium and infiltration with lymphocytes, macrophages and plasma cells. Polymorphs and eosinophils may also be present. The condition is progressive and the pathological changes lead to early myocardial failure. In the chronic form the parasite is not found in the circulation and may be difficult to demonstrate even in the cardiac lesions.

Thus there is a continuous progression through an acute illness in which there is marked proliferation of parasites to a state of balance between the organism and host resistance. As indicated this balance may last for 10–20 years until disturbed in some way, resulting in the development of the chronic cardiac condition. The relative roles of humoral antibody and cell-mediated immunity in host resistance have not been worked out. Specific precipitins are formed during the phase of proliferation of organisms[59] and there is evidence in vitro for the development of cell-mediated immunity in mice infected with T. cruzi.

Kumar et al.[60] have described three types of cardiac lesions in mice infected with T. cruzi. These subdivisions were made according to the survival times of the mice. The description 'acute' myocarditis was given to those which survived for less than 50 days after infection, 'subacute' for 50–84 days, and 'chronic' for 84–154 days. This subdivision was based on the disappearance of parasitaemia 70 days after inoculation. Kumar et al.[61] showed that treatment with cyclophosphamide during infection reduced the survival time of mice which developed the chronic form of the disease, and, in another study[62], γ-radiation and cyclophosphamide, given during the latent phase of chronic Chagas' disease in mice, were shown to induce a fresh acute phase with outbreaks of high parasitaemia and a high mortality rate. This would indicate that the balance between the organism and immunity which gives rise to the latent period in this disease is very fine and can be easily disturbed. The mechanism for such a disturbance in human disease is not known but it may again include factors such as malnutrition or intercurrent infection.

12.8   HELMINTHIC INFECTIONS

12.8.1   Onchocerciasis

Onchocerciasis is an example of a helminthic infection in which there is evidence for a spectrum of clinical patterns, possibly dependent on the response of the host to infection. Clinically the disease is characterized by skin changes with subcutaneous nodules containing adult worms, and by ocular lesions, usually of the anterior segment of the eye, which often lead to blindness. Numerous microfilariae are found in the dermis and characteristically these are found without any evidence of inflammatory tissue reaction. In contrast to the more common generalized form, a localized form of the disease may be found. This condition, referred to as 'sowda' (arabic – black) is manifested as a thickened area of hyperpigmentation localized in distribution to one lower extremity. This may be associated with papular eruption and swelling of the regional lymph node. Microfilariae of *Onchocerca volvulus* are difficult to find histologically or to demonstrate using the standard skin-snip technique. These observations have suggested that the more common generalized form of the disease is a low resistance form analogous to lepromatous leprosy and diffuse cutaneous leishmaniasis, whereas the rarer sowda type is a high resistance form analogous to tuberculoid leprosy or lupoid leishmaniasis. In a study of 84 patients with generalized onchocerciasis and 20 patients with sowda, Bartlett *et al.*[63] found that they could demonstrate delayed hypersensitivity to onchocercal antigens only in patients with sowda. Patients with the more common generalized form of the disease produced negative delayed hypersensitivity to this antigen, although giving strong delayed hypersensitivity to a non-cross-reacting helminthic antigen derived from the hookworm *Necator americanus*. This would indicate that generalized onchocerciasis is associated with a specific defect in cell-mediated immunity. Despite differences in cellular immunity in the two forms of this disease, no differences have been detected in antibody production. Antibody levels against onchocercal antigens are high in both forms, and immediate weal and flare reactions to these antigens indicate a parallel increase in IgE. The role of these antibodies and immune complex formation in producing the typical ocular lesions that lead to blindness in this condition is as yet poorly understood. However, the inflammatory reaction which occurs is generally around dead microfilariae and consists of a perivascular lymphocytic infiltration associated with vascular changes and could be due to immune complex deposition.

12.8.2   Schistosomiasis

Schistosomiasis is a chronic infection with trematode helminths which enter the body in the larval form through the skin. Unlike onchocerciasis, the disease that develops is not the result of any failure of immunological reaction, but occurs as a result of a heightened immune response. The pathological lesions which develop are the result of granuloma development around and in relation to ova deposited in the tissues by adult worms. The presence of these granulomas leads to pipe-stem fibrosis of the liver and fibrosis followed by calcification in the bladder, as well as in other sites in the body. Histologically these granulomas consist of epithelioid cells, lymphocytes and plasma cells surrounding the ova, which are referred to as pseudo-tubercles. The ova themselves are surrounded by a rim of fibrinoid material (Hoeppli phenomenon) which is thought to represent antigen–antibody complexes. The immunological basis of granuloma development in this disease has been reviewed by Warren[64]. Schistosome ova were injected intravenously into mice so that they would be deposited in the lungs. If the mice were previously sensitized by an intraperitoneal injection of ova, the granulomas formed more rapidly and were much larger than those in controls. Sensitivity could be transferred with lymphocytes and granuloma formation was correlated with delayed hypersensitivity, lymphocyte transformation and macrophage migration inhibition to schistosome antigens. Suppression of granuloma formation could be produced by a number of immunosuppressive and cytotoxic agents, and by neonatal thymectomy. This would indicate that the lesions depended on intact T-cell function. However, immunological studies of the fibrinoid material deposited round the ova has also demonstrated the presence of antigen–antibody complexes containing soluble schistosome antigens. In *Schistosoma mansoni* infection, the infiltrate is mainly mononuclear and the soluble egg antigen is a powerful T-cell stimulator, which suggests that cell-mediated immunity plays the major role in the formation of this type of granuloma. However in *Schistosoma japonicum* infection, more polymorphonuclear leukocytes are found, which indicates that antigen–antibody complexes may be playing a more important role.

There are a number of reports of glomerular lesions in schistosomiasis. Immunofluorescence and electron microscopy have demonstrated deposits of immunoglobulin and complement in the glomerular capillary walls, particularly in relation to proliferating mesangial cells. So far, schistosome antigen has not been demonstrated in these diseases. However, there is every reason to believe that kidney disease in patients with schistosomiasis is of immunological origin. (See also Chapter 9, page 329.)

12.9 FUNGAL INFECTIONS

12.9.1 Systemic mycoses

A spectrum of clinical appearances may also be found in the chronic systemic mycoses, such as South American blastomycosis[65] and histoplasmosis. In the generalized form of these diseases the lesions are usually systemic, but in South American blastomycosis there is also a diffuse cutaneous form of the disease. In the localized cutaneous form of South American blastomycosis, there is delayed hypersensitivity to paracoccidioidin, low levels of complement-fixing antibodies to the polysaccharide antigen of *Paracoccidiomyces brasiliensis* and a good response to treatment with sulphonamides. The diffuse cutaneous or systemic forms of the disease are associated with negative skin reactivity to paracoccidioidin and high levels of complement-fixing antibodies, even detectable precipitins, against polysaccharide antigens derived from the infecting organism. The low resistance forms respond poorly to treatment and relapses occur even after treatment with amphotericin B. Delayed hypersensitivity to tuberculin, trichophytin and candidin, as well as the ability to be sensitized with DNCB, may also be depressed in some patients[66]. There may also be impaired lymphocyte transformation with PHA[67]. However, there is no indication of increased susceptibility of these patients to other infections, indicating that the primary defect in host resistance is specific.

12.9.2 *Candida albicans*

Candida albicans is a normal skin commensal. Under normal conditions it is not pathogenic, although most people develop a state of delayed hypersensitivity to it. Failure to develop delayed hypersensitivity and cellular immunity results in the condition of chronic mucocutaneous candidiasis (CMCC). This condition affects the mouth, skin and nails, persists for many years and relapses frequently despite therapy. Intractable infection with *C. albicans* occurs in advanced Hodgkin's disease and in patients on high doses of systemic corticosteroids, as well as in babies with congenital thymic deficiency. In all of these there is a demonstrable non-specific failure of T-cell function, as shown by the inability of lymphocytes to be transformed by PHA, and reduced ability to be sensitized with DNCB. However, in a number of children, some with a family history of the condition, others with endocrine deficiencies, there may be a different immunological defect. Such children have a normal PHA response and both antigen recognition and lymphocyte proliferation in the presence of specific antigen are normal. Despite this, they fail to show contact sensitivity when sensitized with DNCB. The defect has been localized not to the immune response, but to an inability of lymphocytes to produce migration inhibitory factor and other pharmacological mediators of delayed hypersensitivity[68,69]. In a further group there may be a specific failure of lymphocytes to respond to *Candida* antigens despite normal reactivity *in vitro* of lymphocytes to other antigens and normal ability to be sensitized with DNCB. Despite a slightly depressed response to PHA, this may be considered to be a specific deficiency in the immune response similar to that in lepromatous leprosy.

One other situation that has been described as giving rise to CMCC is that of a patient with a lymphocytotoxic serum factor which inhibited both the normal immune response *in vitro* to *Candida* antigens and the mixed lymphocyte response with lymphocytes from unaffected individuals.

In most patients with CMCC, despite the varying defects in cell-mediated immunity described above, there is generally a high level of precipitating antibody to *Candida* antigens, indicating the need for normal T-cell function in the control of infection with this organism. This description of the defects that might underlie CMCC illustrates the various mechanisms that can reduce host resistance to such organisms. (See Chapter 2 for a discussion of fungal infections.)

12.10 SUMMARY

Variable clinical patterns of disease occur in patients with chronic infections depending on the strength and nature of the immune response of the host. Pathological lesions dependent on enhanced cell-mediated immunity and delayed hypersensitivity characterize tuberculoid leprosy, syphilitic gummas and schistosome granulomas. In many patients rapid dissemination of the infecting organism is due to a failure of the specific immune response against that organism. Specific immunodeficiency can be found in a wide range of bacterial, fungal, protozoal and helminthic diseases. These include lepromatous leprosy, secondary syphilis, mucocutaneous candidiasis, diffuse cutaneous leishmaniasis, kala-azar and onchocerciasis. Such failures of host resistance could be due to a fundamental disturbance in the immunological regulatory mechanism as a result of an upset in the balance between suppressor and effector cells. It could also be related to the extremely high antigenic load carried by the host during these infections. Other clinical aspects, such as cutaneous vasculitis, arthritis and glomerulonephritis may be due to the deposition of immune complexes containing antibody and soluble antigen, especially at the vascular basement membrane. Such immune complexes are frequently formed in patients with low host resistance associated with a failure of cellular immunity, e.g. erythema nodosum leprosum. High circulating antibody levels in patients with low host resistance illustrate the frequent dissociation of cellular immunity and antibody production in these infections.

References

1. Voisin, G. (1971). Immunological facilitation, a broadening of the concept of the enhancement phenomenon. *Prog. Allergy*, **15**, 328
2. Harland, P. S. E. G. (1965). Tuberculin reactions in malnourished children. *Lancet*, **ii**, 719
3. Von Pirquet, C. (1908). Das verhalten der kutanen Tuberkulin reaction wahrend der Masern. *Dtsch. Med. Wochenschr.*, **34**, 1297
4. Greenwood, B. M. (1974). Immunosuppression in malaria and trypanosomiasis. In: Ciba Foundation Symposium 25 *Parasites in the Immunized Host: Mechanisms of Survival*, p. 137 (Amsterdam: Associated Scientific Publishers)

5. Jamison, D. G. and Vollum, R. L. (1968). Tuberculous conversion in leprous families in Northern Nigeria. *Lancet*, **ii**, 1271

6. Chakravarti, M. R. and Vogel, F. (1973). A twin study in leprosy. *Top. Human Genet.*, **1**, 1

7. De Vries, R. R. P., Fat, R. F. M. L. A., Nijenhuis, L. E. and van Rood, J. J. (1976). HLA-linked genetic control of host response to *Mycobacterium leprae*. *Lancet*, **ii**, 1328

8. Ridley, D. S. and Jopling, W. H. (1962). A classification of leprosy for research purposes. *Lepr. Rev.*, **33**, 119

9. Ridley, D. S. and Jopling, W. H. (1966). Classification of leprosy according to immunity. A five group system. *Int. J. Lepr.*, **34**, 255

10. Ridley, D. S. (1974). Histological classification and the immunological spectrum of leprosy. *Bull. WHO*, **51**, 451

11. Gaafar, S. M. and Turk, J. L. (1970). Granuloma formation in lymph nodes. *J. Pathol.*, **100**, 9

12. Godal, T., Rees, R. J. W. and Lamvik, J. O. (1971). Lymphocyte mediated modification of blood derived macrophage function *in vitro*: inhibition of growth of intracellular mycobacteria with lymphokines. *Clin. Exp. Immunol.*, **8**, 625

13. Myrvang, B., Godal, T., Ridley, D. S., Froland, S. S. and Song, Y. K. (1973). Immune responsiveness to *Mycobacterium leprae* and other mycobacterial antigens throughout the clinical and histopathological spectrum of leprosy. *Clin. Exp. Immunol.*, **14**, 541

14. Bjune, G., Barnetson, R. St. C., Ridley, D. S. and Kronvall, G. (1976). Lymphocyte transformation test in leprosy, correlation of the response with inflammation of lesions. *Clin. Exp. Immunol.*, **25**, 85

15. Barnetson, R. St. C., Bjune, G., Pearson, M. M. H. and Kronvall, G. (1976). Antigenic heterogeneity in patients with reactions in borderline leprosy. *Br. Med. J.*, **4**, 435

16. Bullock, W. E. and Fasal, P. (1971). Studies of immune mechanisms in leprosy. *J. Immunol.*, **106**, 888

17. Nelson, D. S., Penrose, J. M., Waters, M. F. R., Pearson, J. M. H. and Nelson, M. (1975). Depressive effect of serum from patients with leprosy on mixed lymphocyte reactions, influence of anti-leprosy treatment. *Clin. Exp. Immunol.*, **22**, 385

18. Godal, T. and Negassi, K. (1973). Subclinical infection in leprosy. *Br. Med. J.*, **3**, 557

19. Waldorf, D. S., Sheagren, J. N., Trautman, J. R. and Block, J. B. (1966). Impaired delayed hypersensitivity in patients with lepromatous leprosy. *Lancet*, **ii**, 773

20. Dwyer, J. M., Bullock, W. E. and Fields, J. P. (1973). Disturbance of the blood T : B ratio in lepromatous leprosy. *N. Engl. J. Med.*, **288**, 1036

21. Gajl-Peczalska, K. J., Lim, S. D., Jacobson, R. R. and Good, R. A. (1973). B-lymphocytes in lepromatous leprosy. *N. Engl. J. Med.*, **288**, 1033

22. Nath, I., Curtis, J., Bhutani, L. K. and Talwar, G. P. (1974). Reduction of a subpopulation of T-lymphocytes in lepromatous leprosy. *Clin. Exp. Immunol.*, **18**, 81

23. Turk, J. L. and Waters, M. F. R. (1968). Immunological basis for depression of cellular immunity and the delayed allergic response in patients with lepromatous leprosy. *Lancet*, **ii**, 436

24. Bullock, W. E. (1968). Studies of immune mechanisms in leprosy. *N. Engl. J. Med.*, **278**, 298

25. Turk, J. L. and Waters, M. F. R. (1969). Cell-mediated immunity in patients with leprosy. *Lancet*, **ii**, 243

26. Han, S. H., Weiser, R. S. and Kau, S. T. (1971). Prolonged survival of skin allografts in leprosy patients. *Int. J. Lepr.*, **39**, 1

27. Turk, J. L. and Bryceson, A. D. M. (1971). Immunological phenomena in leprosy and related diseases. *Adv. Immunol.*, **13**, 209

28. Rees, R. J. W., Chatterjee, K. R., Pepys, J. and Tee, R. D. (1965). Some immunologic aspects of leprosy. *Am. Rev. Respir. Dis.*, **92**, 139

29. Norlin, M., Navalkar, R. G., Ouchterlong, O. and Lind, A. (1966). Characterization of

leprosy sera with various mycobacterial antigens using double diffusion in gel analysis III. *Acta Pathol. Microbiol. Scand.*, **67**, 555

30. Wager, O. (1969). Immunological aspects of leprosy with special reference to autoimmune disease. *Bull. WHO*, **41**, 793

31. Turk, J. L. and Waters, M. F. R. (1971). Immunological significance of changes in lymph nodes across the leprosy spectrum. *Clin. Exp. Immunol.*, **8**, 363

32. Fernandez, J. M. M. (1936). Bacteriologia de la reaccion leprosa. Investigacion del *Mycobacterium leprae* en las lesiones cutaneas de reaccion leprosa. *Rev. Bras. Leprol.*, **4**, 9

33. Wemambu, S. N. C., Turk, J. L., Waters, M. F. R. and Rees, R. J. W. (1969). Erythema nodosum leprosum: A clinical manifestation of the Arthus phenomenon. *Lancet*, **ii**, 933

34. Karat, A. B. A., Karat, S., Job, C. K. and Furness, M. A. (1967). Acute exudative arthritis in leprosy. Rheumatoid arthritis-like syndrome in association with erythema nodosum leprosum. *Br. Med. J.*, **3**, 770

35. Drutz, D. J. and Gutman, R. A. (1973). Renal manifestations of leprosy: Glomerulonephritis a complication of erythema nodosum leprosum. *Am. J. Trop. Med. Hyg.*, **22**, 496

36. Shepard, C. C. (1960). The experimental disease that follows the injection of human leprosy bacilli into foot-pads of mice. *J. Exp. Med.*, **112**, 445

37. Rees, R. J. W., Waters, M. F. R., Weddell, A. G. M. and Palmer, E. (1967). Experimental lepromatous leprosy. *Nature (Lond.)*, **215**, 599

38. Rees, R. J. W. and Weddell, A. G. M. (1968). Experimental models for studying leprosy. *Ann. N.Y. Acad. Sci.*, **154**, 214

39. Storrs, E. E., Walsh, G. P., Burchfield, H. P. and Binford, C. H. (1974). Leprosy in the armadillo: new model for biochemical research. *Science*, **183**, 851

40. Lenzini, L., Rotolli, P. and Rotolli, L. (1977). The spectrum of human tuberculosis. *Clin. Exp. Immunol.*, **27**, 230

41. Sykes, J. A. and Miller, J. N. (1971). Intracellular location of *Treponema pallidum* (Nichols strain) in the rabbit testis. *Infect. Immunol.*, **4**, 307

42. Bishop, N. H. and Miller, J. N. (1976). Humoral immunity in experimental syphilis. I. The demonstration of resistance conferred by passive immunization. *J. Immunol.*, **117**, 191

43. Weiser, R. S., Erickson, D., Perine, P. L. and Pearsall, N. (1976). Immunity to syphilis: Passive transfer in rabbits using serial doses of immune serum. *Infect. Immun.*, **13**, 1402

44. Metzger, M. (1976). In: *The Biology of the Parasitic Spirochaetes* (R. C. Johnson, ed.), p. 317 (New York: Academic Press)

45. Festenstein, H., Abrahams, C. and Bokkenheuser, V. (1967). Runting syndrome in neonatal rabbits infected with *Treponema pallidum*. *Clin. Exp. Immunol.*, **2**, 311

46. Noguchi, H. (1911). A cutaneous reaction in syphilis. *J. Exp. Med.*, **14**, 557

47. Michelson, H. E. (1932). The superficial lymph glands in early syphilis. *Arch. Dermatol. Syphil.*, **25**, 457

48. Friedmann, P. S. and Turk, J. L. (1975). A spectrum of lymphocyte responsiveness in human syphilis. *Clin. Exp. Immunol.*, **21**, 59

49. Friedmann, P. S. and Turk, J. L. (1978). The role of cell-mediated immune mechanisms in syphilis in Ethiopia. (Submitted for publication)

50. Planner, H. (1929). In: *Handbuch der Haut- und Geschlechtskrankheiten* (J. Jadassohn, ed.), p. 468 (Berlin: Springer)

51. Levene, G. M., Turk, J. L., Wright, D. J. M. and Grimble, A. G. S. (1969). Reduced lymphocyte transformation due to a plasma factor in patients with active syphilis. *Lancet*, **ii**, 246

52. From, E., Thestrup-Pedersen, K. and Thulin, H. (1976). Reactivity of lymphocytes from patients with syphilis towards *T. pallidum* antigen in the leucocyte migration and lymphocyte transformation tests. *Br. J. Vener. Dis.*, **56**, 224

53. Gjestland, T. (1955). The Oslo study of untreated syphilis – An epidemiologic investigation of the natural course of untreated syphilis based on a restudy of the Boeck–Bruusgaard material. *Acta Derm. Venereol.*, **35** (Suppl.), 34

54. Olansky, S., Schuman, S. H. and Peters, J. J. (1956). Untreated syphilis in the male negro. X. Twenty years of clinical observation of untreated and presumably non-syphilitic groups. *J. Chronic Dis.*, **4**, 77

55. Mauel, J., Behin, R., Biroum-Noerjasin and Doyle, J. J. (1974). Survival and death of *Leishmania* in macrophages. In: Ciba Foundation Symposium 25, *Parasites in the Immunized Host*, p. 225 (Amsterdam: Associated Scientific Publishers)

56. Belehu, A., Poulter, L. W. and Turk, J. L. (1976). Modification of cutaneous leishmaniasis in the guinea-pig by cyclophosphamide. *Clin. Exp. Immunol.*, **24**, 125

57. Belehu, A., Poulter, L. W. and Turk, J. L. (1976). Influence of rodent malaria on the course of *Leishmania enriettii* infection of hamsters. *Infect. Immun.*, **14**, 457

58. Bryceson, A. D. M. (1969). Diffuse cutaneous leishmaniasis in Ethiopia. *Trans. R. Soc. Trop. Med. Hyg.*, **63**, 708

59. Laranja, F. S., Dias, E., Nebrega, G. and Miranda, A. (1956). Chagas's disease. A clinical, epidemiological and pathologic study. *Circulation*, **14**, 1035

60. Kumar, R., Kline, I. K. and Abelmann, W. H. (1969). Experimental *Trypanosoma cruzi* myocarditis: relative effects upon the right and left ventricle. *Am. J. Pathol.*, **57**, 31

61. Kumar, R., Kline, I. K. and Abelmann, W. H. (1970). Immunosuppression in experimental acute and subacute Chagasic myocarditis. *Am. J. Trop. Med. Hyg.*, **19**, 932

62. Brener, Z. and Chiari, E. (1971). The effects of some immunosuppressive agents in experimental chronic Chagas's disease. *Trans. R. Soc. Trop. Med. Hyg.*, **65**, 629

63. Bartlett, A., Turk, J., Ngu, J., Mackenzie, C. D., Fuglsang, H. and Anderson, J. (1978). Variation in delayed hypersensitivity in onchocerciasis. *Trans. R. Soc. Trop. Hyg.*, **72**, 372

64. Warren, K. S. (1976). Immunopathology due to cell-mediated (type Ir) reactions. In: *Immunology of Parasitic Infections* (S. Cohen and E. Sadun, eds.), p. 448 (Oxford: Blackwell Scientific Publications)

65. Da Silva Lacaz, C. (1967). *Compendio de Micologia Medica*, p. 212 (Sau Paulo: Sarvier)

66. Mendes, E. and Raphael, A. (1971). Impaired delayed hypersensitivity in patients with South American blastomycosis. *J. Allergy*, **47**, 14

67. Mendes, N. F., Musatti, C. C., Leao, R. C., Mendes, E. and Naspitz, C. K. (1971). Lymphocyte cultures and skin allograft survival in patients with South American blastomycosis. *J. Allergy*, **48**, 40

68. Chilgren, R. A., Meuwissen, H. J., Quie, P. G., Good, R. A. and Hong, R. (1969). The cellular immune defect in chronic mucocutaneous candidiasis. *Lancet*, **i**, 1286

69. Valdimarsson, H., Holt, L., Riches, H. R. C. and Hobbs, J. R. (1970). Lymphocyte abnormalities in chronic mucocutaneous candidiasis. *Lancet*, **i**, 1259

70. Belehu, A. (1975). Experimental studies of experimental cutaneous leishmaniasis in rodents – modification by cyclophosphamide and malaria. (University of London: Ph.D. thesis)

13

Immunology of Persistent and Recurrent Viral Infections

C. J. GIBBS, Jr, G. J. NEMO
and A. R. DIWAN

13.1 INTRODUCTION   455

13.2 DEFINITION OF PERSISTENT RECURRENT
      INFECTIONS   457

13.3 PATTERNS OF DISEASES ASSOCIATED WITH
      PERSISTENT AND RECURRENT INFECTIONS   457

13.4 MECHANISMS OF VIRAL PERSISTENCE   458

13.5 DNA VIRUSES WHICH CAUSE PERSISTENT
      RECURRENT INFECTIONS IN HUMANS   458
      13.5.1 *Hepatitis B*   458
              13.5.1.1 *Replication of hepatitis B virus* 459
              13.5.1.2 *Disease pattern associated with HBV infection* 459
              13.5.1.3 *Immune response in HBV infections* 459
              13.5.1.4 *Humoral antibody responses in HBV*
                        infection   460
              13.5.1.5 *Cellular immune response*   460
              13.5.1.6 *Other immunological factors*   461
              13.5.1.7 *Occurrence of different specificity of HBs–Ag*
                        and anti-HBs–Ag in humans and experi-
                        mental animals   461

		13.5.1.8	Occurrence of defective Dane particles in sera of HBs–Ag carriers	462
		13.5.1.9	Hepatitis A	462
		13.5.1.10	Non-A non-B hepatitis	462
	13.5.2	Herpes simplex virus type 1 and type 2 infections		462
		13.5.2.1	Humoral immune response	463
		13.5.2.2	Cell-mediated immunity	463
		13.5.2.3	Role of Fc receptors in HSV infection	464
		13.5.2.4	Herpes infection and histocompatibility antigens of the HLA system	465
	13.5.3	Epstein–Barr virus (EBV)		465
		13.5.3.1	Humoral immunity to EBV in infectious mononucleosis	465
		13.5.3.2	Cell-mediated immunity to EBV in infectious mononucleosis	466
		13.5.3.3	Immunodeficiency and EBV	466
		13.5.3.4	Endogenous reactivation of EBV infections	467
	13.5.4	Cytomegalovirus		467
		13.5.4.1	Humoral immunity	467
		13.5.4.2	Cell-mediated immunity	467
		13.5.4.3	Cytomegalovirus and Guillain–Barré syndrome	468
	13.5.5	Varicella–zoster virus		468
		13.5.5.1	Humoral immune response	469
		13.5.5.2	Herpes zoster	469
		13.5.5.3	Cell-mediated immunity	469
		13.5.5.4	Interferon production	470
	13.5.6	Adenoviruses		470
	13.5.7	Papovaviruses		471
		13.5.7.1	Papovaviruses and progressive multifocal leukoencephalopathy	471
13.6	RNA VIRUSES WHICH CAUSE PERSISTENT RECURRENT INFECTIONS IN HUMANS			472
	13.6.1	Subacute sclerosing panencephalitis (measles virus)		472
		13.6.1.1	Humoral immunity in SSPE	472
		13.6.1.2	Cellular immunity in SSPE	474
	13.6.2	Chronic progressive panencephalitis (rubella)		476
		13.6.2.1	Congenital rubella	477
		13.6.2.2	Humoral immunity in congenital rubella	477
		13.6.2.3	Cellular immunity in congenital rubella	478
	13.6.3	Foamy viruses		479

13.7 UNCONVENTIONAL VIRUSES WHICH CAUSE
PERSISTENT INFECTIONS IN HUMANS 480

13.8 SUMMARY AND CONCLUSIONS 482

13.1 INTRODUCTION

The development and widespread use of live attenuated and killed viral vaccines has reduced the incidence of epidemics due to acute viral diseases and has shifted the focus of attention to the role of viruses in chronic, persistent and recurrent viral infections. Chronic progressive diseases may be caused by conventional viruses as in measles and rubella, or by unconventional slow viruses as in kuru and Creutzfeldt–Jakob disease (CJD). These agents may persist in the host for periods of months or years causing little or no clinical signs or pathological changes. Technical advances in the study of virus–cell interactions at the cellular and molecular levels have served to enhance our understanding of the host–parasite relationship in persistently infected cells.

As early as 1951 von Magnus[1] demonstrated that undiluted passage of influenza virus resulted in the production of incomplete virus particles. When preparations of incomplete virions were inoculated into mice, the survivors developed long-term resistance to acute disease when challenged with preparations of complete virus. Since von Magnus's discovery, advances in biochemical and biophysical techniques have provided the methodology to segregate these virus populations successfully. Incomplete particles are now referred to as defective-interfering or DI particles. They are generated spontaneously during undiluted passages of animal viruses in culture, and are classified as deletion mutants with the following general properties: (i) structurally they are composed of normal viral proteins and a deleted viral genome, (ii) functionally they are unable to reproduce in the absence of their non-defective helper virus, and (iii) as a consequence of their dependence they interfere specifically with the intracellular replication of the helper virus. The importance of defective viral particles in the establishment and maintenance of certain persistent infections has been proposed[2] and demonstrated[3]. Recent advances in virus genetics has led to the development of temperature sensitive 'TS' mutants. The role of these mutants in the establishment and maintenance of persistently infected cell cultures has been delineated by several workers[4–7]. With the discovery of RNA-dependent DNA polymerase or reverse transcriptase[8,9], integration of viral nucleic acid into the cellular genome has become a workable hypothesis in explaining viral persistence of members of the retrovirus group. Furthermore, several reports with transfection experiments have suggested that a similar mechanism may operate with other RNA viruses such as respiratory syncytial virus, measles, Sindbis and tick-borne encephalitis[10,11] viruses, even though no reverse transcriptase or DNA polymerase activity has been shown to be associated with these agents.

All the aforementioned advances have contributed significantly to our understanding of viral persistence *in vitro*. In studies *in vivo* an additional element is added, the contribution of the immune response to viral persistence within the intact animal. Immunology has made rapid progress and contributed significantly to our understanding of both humoral and cell-mediated immune responses to viral infection. Over the years immunology has dealt mainly with the humoral response and techniques were developed primarily to detect and measure the presence of antibodies. This technology was useful in diagnostic and seroepidemiological studies of viral infections that occur naturally, and in studies to quantitate antibody responses following vaccination. Studies of the various types of immunoglobulin and their evolution in response to natural or vaccine-induced infection have enhanced our understanding of their role in the pathogenesis of disease.

Major studies have been made over the past few years in the field of cellular immunology. Advances in lymphocyte cell separation techniques[12] have been extremely useful in differentiating lymphocyte populations into various functional groups. It is now possible to study the reactivity *in vitro* of lymphocytes to mitogens and specific antigens. Virus-infected target cells can be labelled with radioactive isotopes and the interaction of lymphocytes in the presence or absence of antibody or complement can be studied *in vitro*. Several chemical factors termed lymphokines, which are substances elaborated by lymphocytes in response to specific antigens and mitogens, have been defined and these, together with antigen–antibody complexes, have been implicated in immunopathological injury to the host[13]. Observations of hosts, immunodeficient either in their cellular or humoral response to viruses, have given us a broader understanding of the role of the immune response in the pathogenesis of viral and bacterial diseases. An immunodeficiency disorder such as agammaglobulinaemia may also play a part in the persistence of enteroviral infections in humans[14].

Successful transplantation of organs has been made possible with the use of immunosuppressive drugs to preclude graft versus host reactions. Such drugs along with cytotoxic chemicals, which are used in the treatment of neoplastic disease and which also can be immunosuppressive, have been shown to activate viruses which persist in the host in a latent state. These activated viral infections pose serious problems to patients and can be lethal[15,16].

While all these advances have served to enhance our understanding of persistent viral infections, one must bear in mind that not all persistent infections cause disease. Inapparent persistent infections are common and only in certain instances does the persistent infection manifest itself as a harmful infectious disease.

In this chapter we will review the role of the immune response in persistent recurrent viral infections. We will limit ourselves to human infections using animal models only when they seem appropriate.

13.2 DEFINITION OF PERSISTENT RECURRENT INFECTIONS

Most viral infections are self-limiting; in some individuals viruses produce clinical disease while in others the infection never progresses beyond the sub-clinical stage. Viruses of the herpes virus group have been shown to produce sub-clinical disease. Antibody surveys reveal that herpes antibody is present in the majority of persons 10 years of age and older. In spite of demonstrable antibody, recurrent herpes infections do occur in certain individuals. Herpes simplex virus is a classic example of a virus which can cause a persistent and recurrent infection.

Recovery from acute viral infections in most cases produces long-term immunity. Secondary attacks by the same virus are uncommon. Although antibody is detectable over long periods it is conceivable that virus may remain dormant at a site not available to antibody, yet continue to produce enough antigenic stimulus to maintain the level of antibody throughout the life of the host. When the equilibrium between virus and host defences is disrupted, for example by immunosuppression, ageing, etc., virus may be activated with the subsequent expression of clinical disease. Thus any virus which produces acute infections has the potential for persistence and given the proper set of circumstances apparent disease may recur.

13.3 PATTERNS OF DISEASES ASSOCIATED WITH PERSISTENT AND RECURRENT INFECTIONS

Acute clinical illness followed by persistent latent infection with demonstrable virus – Congenital rubella and cytomegalovirus (CMV) infections fall into this class. The virus can be recovered for long periods. Antibody of the IgM type is present indicating active infection.

Acute clinical illness followed by latent infection with one or more recurrence of acute disease during which infectious virus is demonstrable – Herpes simplex and varicella-zoster infections of man fall into this category. Antibody of the IgG type is always present.

Acute apparent infection with subsequent inapparent infection followed by subacute or chronic disease in which virus remains masked – Subacute sclerosing panencephalitis (SSPE) which may follow acute measles infection is representative of this group. High levels of measles antibody are detected in the serum and the CSF.

Protracted progressive infection followed by apparent disease ultimately ending in death with infectious virus demonstrable in early and late infection – Kuru and CJD infections in man, scrapie in sheep and goats and mink encephalopathy come under this category. No immune response is detectable in the host and no non-host protein is evident.

Protracted or life-long latent infection without apparent disease in which immunosuppressive therapy unmasks the latent virus – Virus infections of the papova group (JC and BK virus) of man as well as some herpes infections fall into this group. Antibody is present after initial infection, which generally occurs early in life, and persists indefinitely.

Acute apparent or inapparent infection followed by persistent infection in which virus-coded products (antigen) can be demonstrated for long periods of time – Hepatitis B infections come under this heading. Antibody to some antigens may be present in certain cases.

13.4 MECHANISMS OF VIRAL PERSISTENCE

Mims[17] has reviewed several factors which may contribute to the persistence of virus within the host. These include:

(a) Viruses with low pathogenicity in certain host cells; rubella, visna and cytomegalo viruses are cited as examples.

(b) Virus infections with ineffective antibody response (tolerance), e.g. neonatally-acquired lymphocytic choriomeningitis (LCM) infection of mice.

(c) Virus infections in which there may be ineffective cell-mediated immune response; SSPE may fall into this category.

(d) Persistent viral infections in which there may be a defective interferon response.

(e) Persistent infections in which no immune response of any kind is observed, e.g. kuru and CJD in man, scrapie in sheep and goats and mink encephalopathy.

(f) Viral infection of lymphocytes and macrophages may account for the persistence of EB virus, Aleutian mink disease and equine infectious anaemia.

That one or more of these mechanisms may contribute to the persistence of virus in a particular disease process is well within the realm of probability.

13.5 DNA VIRUSES WHICH CAUSE PERSISTENT RECURRENT INFECTIONS IN HUMANS

13.5.1 Hepatitis B

The discovery of Australia antigen, at present referred to as hepatitis B surface antigen or HBs-Ag by Blumberg[18], and the demonstration of its association with hepatitis B infection [19,20] has made it possible to answer previously unresolved questions regarding this disease. Epidemiological and serological evidence has shown that there are approximately 120 million carriers of HBs-Ag in the world. HBs antigenaemia occurs with high frequency in tropical and sub-tropical countries[21]. If the production of HBs-Ag is due to active multiplication of hepatitis B virus (HBV) this would represent one of the most common persistent viral infections known to man.

13.5.1.1 Replication of Hepatitis B virus

Intrahepatic distribution of HBV has been studied with immunochemical techniques both in man and experimentally infected chimpanzees. Following infection, the viral genome is transported to the nucleus of the hepatocytes. Replication of viral DNA coupled with virus-specific production of core protein leads to the assembly of core antigen (HBc-Ag) in the nucleus. Quite independently, viral coded HBs-Ag is synthesized in the cytoplasm of the hepatocyte. HBs-Ag has been shown to possess a group-specific 'a' determinant with subtype determinants of either 'd' or 'y'. Two other subtype determinants 'w' or 'r' have also been reported. A 46 nm particle termed the Dane particle[22] has been observed in the endoplasmic reticulum of the hepatocyte by electron microscopy and represents the completed virion of HBV. Assembly of the particle is completed within the cytoplasm and subsequently transported from the cell. Viral DNA and DNA polymerase have been shown to be associated with the core particle.

13.5.1.2 Disease pattern associated with HBV infection

HBV infection may be divided into three major categories:

(1) Acute hepatitis with transient antigenaemia (HBs-Ag), with the subsequent appearance of anti-HBc-Ag and anti-HBs-Ag antibodies. This comprises approximately 70% of the cases.

(2) Acute infection which is sub-clinical and occurs when HBs-Ag appears for only a short period of time if at all. This pattern is observed in 25% of HBV infections.

(3) A silent infection in which HBs-Ag persists with the appearance of anti-HBc-Ag antibody, but not anti-HBs-Ag antibody. This latter group, which comprises about 5% of HBV cases, represents the silent carriers which form the classical source of transfusion-associated hepatitis B infection. Some chronic HBs-Ag carriers also carry an 'e' antigen or HBe-Ag in their sera. These individuals seem prone to chronic active hepatitis and sera from these individuals are thought to be highly infectious.

13.5.1.3 Immune response in HBV infections

As indicated previously, the presence of anti-HBs-Ag in the serum indicates a past infection with HBV. The presence of HBs-Ag in the serum indicates a latent infection. Hepatitis caused by HBV is thought to be due to immune lymphocytes recognizing altered antigens on the surface of infected hepatocytes and also immune complex formation of HBs-Ag and anti-HBs-Ag antibody. Several extrahepatic manifestations of hepatitis B are thought to be due to HBV antigen and antibody complex formation. These manifestations include glomerulonephritis[23], polymyelgia rheumatica[24], infantile papular acrodermatitis (Gianotti's disease)[25], and essential mixed cryoglobulinaemia[26]. It is likely that the HBV antigen–antibody complexes cause the vascular damage observed in each of these pathological processes.

13.5.1.4 Humoral antibody responses in HBV infection

Antibody to HBs-Ag usually occurs during the HBs antigenemic phase, late in the incubation period and prior to or at the onset of hepatocellular injury. During this prehepatic phase maximum HBV-associated DNA polymerase activity is observed in the serum[27]. The onset of anti-HBs-Ag formation is indicated by the appearance of anticomplementary activity in the serum[28] and by the demonstration of antigen–antibody complexes in the particulate fraction of the serum using ultrastructural analysis[29]. Anti-HBs-Ag antibody can be detected over an extended period of time[30].

13.5.1.5 Cellular immune response

HBV-associated antigens can induce specific cellular immune responses in experimental animals[31]. Guinea-pigs immunized with HBs-Ag develop delayed cutaneous hypersensitivity to HBs-Ag but not to HBc-Ag; conversely, animals immunized with HBc-Ag develop delayed cutaneous hypersensitivity to HBc-Ag but not to HBs-Ag[32]. Studies with athymic nude mice have shown that the cellular immune response to HBs-Ag appears to depend upon thymus-derived T cells[33].

Lymphocyte stimulation and leukocyte-migration inhibition assays have also been used successfully to measure cell-mediated immunity to HBV antigens[34,35]. Dudley et al.[36], using leukocyte-migration inhibition, demonstrated cellular immunity to HBV-associated antigens in seven of eight patients with circulating HBs-Ag. Using purified HBs-Ag Laiwah et al.[37] demonstrated a reasonable correlation between antigen-induced lymphocyte stimulation and leukocyte-migration inhibition assays. The correlation was only demonstrable during the convalescent phase following the clearance of HBs-Ag.

Using the leukocyte-migration inhibition assay with purified HBs-Ag Desaules and his co-workers[38] studied cellular immune responses in asymptomatic HBs-Ag carriers and in patients who had cleared the antigen after acute infection. They found a reduction of migration inhibition activity in the majority of HBs-Ag carriers when compared to patients who had cleared the antigen after acute infection. Furthermore, they found the migration inhibition response of HBs-Ag carriers to purified protein derivative (PPD) to be normal, suggesting that the depressed immune response to HBs-Ag might be responsible for the chronic antigenaemia.

Edington and Chisari[39] discovered a defect in E-rosette formation of T lymphocytes from hepatitis patients. The defect was found to be due to a rosette-inhibiting factor detected in the sera of patients with hepatitis. Rosette-inhibiting factor was found during the first 4 weeks following maximum blood transaminase levels and appeared to persist for 12 weeks or more in patients who progressed to chronic hepatitis, most of whom eventually became negative for HBs-Ag. Rosette-inhibiting factor was found to be a discrete plasma protein which was different from any previously described immunoregulatory factors. Thus it was suggested that a T-lymphocyte abnormality may be of importance in the pathogenesis of acute and chronic hepatitis. The authors speculated further that hepatocellular injury and persistence of viral synthesis may be due to the hepatocyte surface expression of viral and cellular antigens as well as to the specificity and the character of the host immune response. Termination of HBV infection was viewed as a suppression of the viral genome rather than an eradication of infected cells.

13.5.1.6 *Other immunological factors*

Several workers have reported an association between certain histocompatibility antigens and viral hepatitis. Mackay and Morris[40] reported an increased incidence of HLA-A1 and HLA-B8 in patients with chronic active hepatitis. This finding was confirmed by Galbraith and his associates[41]. Page et al.[42] presented evidence that increased incidence of HLA-A1 is secondary to that of HLA-B8 because of a linkage disequilibrium.

Recent studies of HLA antigens by Hillis and his colleagues[43] showed an association between HBs antigenaemia and HLA-BW15, BW17 and BW35. These findings were disputed by another group[44], however, as they were only able to demonstrate an association between HLA-B8 and HBs antigenaemia.

13.5.1.7 *Occurrence of different specificity of HBs-Ag and anti-HBs-Ag in humans and experimental animals*

Recent studies by Koziol et al.[45] demonstrated that the antigenaemia which developed in a dentist with acute icteric hepatitis was due to restricted specificity. Anti-HBs-Ag antibody which was present in the serum of the patient prior to the infection was shown to react with only one subdeterminant, a_1, of the HBs-Ag. The anti-HBs-Ag/a_1 antibody coexisted with HBs-Ag of subtype ayw in the acute phase serum. This observation was further confirmed by Tabor et al.[46] who found three patients having both detectable HBs-Ag and anti-HBs-Ag antibody in their sera.

Further sub-typing revealed that in each case the anti-HBs-Ag antibody was directed at a different subtype from that of the circulating HBs-Ag, indicating that reinfection or simultaneous infection with a second subtype had occurred. Several other investigators have confirmed these findings[47–49].

13.5.1.8 Occurrence of defective Dane particles in sera of HBs-Ag carriers

Recent studies by Gerin[50] have shown defective and incomplete Dane particles in the sera of two chronic carriers of HBs-Ag. The significance of this observation to our understanding of the persistence of HBV remains open to conjecture.

13.5.1.9 Hepatitis A

The demonstration of hepatitis A virus (HAV) in stool specimens using immune electron microscopy[51], and the subsequent transmission of the virus to marmoset monkeys, have led workers to suggest that HAV may be the causative agent of hepatitis in man[52]. HAV has not yet been cultivated in cell culture. However, the livers of infected marmosets have been used as a source of virus for neutralization tests in primates[52]. Furthermore, inactivated virus from marmoset livers has been used as an antigen in complement-fixation[53] and immune adherence tests[54]. Serological surveys have shown that antibody to HAV is acquired early in life[55]. No persistent antigenaemia has been demonstrated in humans or experimentally infected animals. Based upon these observations it seems unlikely that HAV plays any role in persistent chronic hepatitis.

13.5.1.10 Non-A non-B hepatitis

Two recent reports have shown that non-A non-B hepatitis can be transmitted parentally to chimpanzees[56, 57]. In both studies the animals developed biochemical and histological evidence of hepatitis. They subsequently recovered, however, with no further biochemical or histological signs of infection. No clinical disease was observed in these experimentally infected primates. Since the inocula for transmission studies were derived from specimens from an acute as well as a chronic hepatitis case, this suggested the possibility that a chronic carrier state exists in non-A non-B hepatitis. Such animal transmission studies will be used further to study the nature of non-A non-B hepatitis agent or agents, its pathogenesis in man, and the development of serological tests for diagnostic and epidemiological purposes.

13.5.2 Herpes simplex virus type 1 and type 2 infections

Herpes simplex virus type 1 (HSV-1) and herpes simplex virus type 2 (HSV-2) are excellent examples of viruses which cause persistent recurrent infections. The association of HSV-2 with cervical cancer[58-60] and the susceptibility of HSV-1 infection to IUDR, one of the first drugs used in the chemotherapy of viral infections[61], have stimulated renewed interest in these two serotypes. Since HSV remains latent in the sensory ganglion and because it can be isolated and reactivated in culture from the ganglion, it has been postulated that the sensory ganglion represents the privileged site of latency for the virus. The virus is thought to travel via nerve pathways during reactivation[62-64].

In spite of these observations, the factors which contribute to recurrence are poorly understood. It is generally assumed that an immunological response may be involved in the reactivation of herpes simplex.

13.5.2.1 Humoral immune response

Herpes viruses possess the ability to spread from cell to contiguous cell in culture in the presence of anti-herpes antibody. Recurrent herpes infections are common even though affected individuals possess serum antibody to HSV. A prospective study by Douglas and Couch[65] of humans with a history of recurrent infections showed that virus can be recovered intermittently from oral secretion in the absence of disease. They were unable, however, to isolate virus from parotid gland secretions. Virus was also recovered from acute lesions, and the frequency of isolations declined significantly after the first week. Serum-neutralizing antibody levels were not found to be related to recurrence of the infection or to virus isolations, and the local IgA response did not appear to play a role in recurrence of herpes infection. They concluded that antibody is most probably not involved in recurrent infection. A study by Doerr et al.[66] showed that in nearly all cases of primary HSV infection, IgM antibody to HSV was detected, particularly in cases with CNS involvement (encephalitis/meningitis). In one case IgM antibody was detected for 11 weeks after the onset of illness and in another case it was detected in the CSF for 6 weeks. Serum IgM antibodies were rarely detected in localized herpes infections which were due primarily to reactivation.

13.5.2.2 Cell-mediated immunity

In addition to humoral responses various cellular immune assays in vitro have revealed a cell-mediated immune response less than 1–2 weeks after the primary infection[67]. Positive delayed hypersensitivity skin-test responses in individuals with antibody have been described[68]. It has been demonstrated that depletion of T cells or of macrophages leads to increased mortality in experimental animals infected with HSV[69, 70].

Individuals with hepatic recurrences display a wide variety of cell-mediated responses as measured by cellular immune assays in vitro. The information gathered so far suggests a correlation between an observed depression of certain lymphokines such as macrophage-migration inhibition factor and an increased predilection to herpes virus recurrences[71-73]. Two recent studies by Lopez and O'Reilly[74] and O'Reilly et al.[75] showed that individuals with recurrent disease were found to have higher neutralizing antibody titres to herpes virus than normal subjects. The neutralizing antibody titres of normal individuals were found to correlate well with their lymphocyte transformation response, whereas a similar correlation was not observed in patients with recurrent disease. Virus-specific lymphoproliferative responses were routinely detected in patients with recurrent infection, irrespective of the clinical stage of the disease. In contrast, a transient depression of herpes-specific leukocyte migration-inhibition factor and interferon production was routinely observed at the time of and immediately prior to virus-induced vesicular eruptions. During convalescence, however, production of these mediators was again observed in response to inactivated antigen.

Using antibody-dependent cellular cytotoxicity techniques Kohl et al.[76] showed that, in the presence of herpes antibody, adherent human peripheral blood mononuclear leukocytes, which possess monocyte-macrophage characteristics, and non-adherent peripheral blood mononuclear leukocytes were cytotoxic to herpes virus-infected target cells. They also showed that this reaction occurred irrespective of the immune status of the donor.

A similar study with the same assay was performed to determine the cellular immune status of neonates. Using HSV-1 and HSV-2 infected target cells, effector cell activity was detected in all 13 cord blood samples tested; cord blood mononuclear cells displayed moderately reduced cytotoxicity as compared to adult mononuclear cells. The antibody-dependent cytotoxic activity against HSV-infected cells was shown to be transported across the placenta, providing further evidence that IgG is involved in the reaction[77].

Conflicting reports have appeared recently regarding the type of mononuclear cells which takes part in the antibody-dependent cytotoxic reaction against herpes virus. Studies by Russell and Kaiser[78] show that a null cell and not the K cell or 'killer' cell is most probably involved in the reaction. Another study showed that non-phagocytic cells with low avidity Fc receptors are the effector cells. Some had surface immunoglobulins and others lacked both B and T receptors. Low levels of killing were observed without the addition of anti-herpes antibody to the test system and killing appeared to depend upon the same subpopulation as the antibody-dependent effector cells[79].

13.5.2.3   Role of Fc receptors in HSV infection

Herpes virus is known to produce Fc receptors on the surface of infected cells[80,81]. Costa and Rabson[82] speculated that the appearance of Fc receptors confers a biological advantage on the virus by binding immunoglobulin molecules or antigen–antibody complexes on the cell surface. This might favour the virus by blocking viral antigenic sites or by consuming antibody directed at viral surface antigen or by modifying the replication of the virus. The significance of these speculations to HSV persistence remains to be answered.

13.5.2.4 Herpes infection and histocompatibility antigens of the HLA system

Recurrent herpes labialis has been reported to be associated with the A1 and B8 loci antigens of the HLA system[83].

13.5.3 Epstein–Barr virus (EBV)

Epstein–Barr virus (EBV), a member of the herpes virus group, is the causal agent of infectious mononucleosis[84], and is also associated with two neoplasms of man, Burkitt's lymphoma and nasopharyngeal carcinoma[85]. Infectious mononucleosis (IM) is a benign self-limited lymphoproliferative disease marked by the appearance of atypical lymphocytes in the peripheral blood. EBV causes lymphoproliferation in vitro[86] and the virus is required for the successful establishment and propagation of lymphoid cell lines. It is now well established that EBV transforms bone-marrow-derived or B-cell lymphocytes and that these cells can be used to establish continuous lymphoblastoid cell lines[87,88]. Most of the atypical lymphocytes present in acute infectious mononucleosis possess characteristics similar to thymus-derived (T) cells[89]. Since T cells are known to play a major role in the defence against viral diseases[90], it has been postulated that these lymphocytes are involved in the elimination of EBV-transformed B lymphocytes[91–95].

13.5.3.1 Humoral immunity to EBV in infectious mononucleosis

Hampar et al.[96], using immunoferratin electron microscopy, demonstrated IgM in the sera of patients with infectious mononucleosis but not in the sera of healthy individuals with IgG antibody to EB viral capsid antigen (VCA). This finding was subsequently confirmed by others using an immuno-fluorescence test to detect IgM[97,98]. Characteristic humoral antibody responses to EBV in patients with infectious mononucleosis are as follows: by the third day of onset the patient's lymphocytes contain EB virus-associated complement-fixing antigen (EBNA) in a nuclear location. Heterophile antibody usually does not appear until the third day of symptoms with a maximum titre occurring by the 15th day. EBV-specific IgM antibody is demonstrable by the 8th day and increases in titre by the 15th day. VCA-specific antibody of the IgG class is undetectable on the 3rd day but is present on the 8th day, rising to maximum titres 2 weeks later. No correlation has been found between the levels of EBV–VCA-specific antibodies, heterophile antibodies, EBNA antibody and the severity of clinical symptoms and haematological changes[99-101]. EBV IgM antibody assays, if done properly, serve as an excellent tool for diagnosing IM[102,103].

13.5.3.2 *Cell-mediated immunity to EBV in infectious mononucleosis*

Denman and Pelton[104] showed that lymphocytes from IM patients had some cytotoxic activity *in vitro* against an EB virus-producing lymphoid cell line. Several workers have demonstrated with a ^{51}Cr-labelled lymphoblastoid cell line that the cytotoxic action is mediated by the T lymphocyte and that the cytotoxic activity is directed only against those cell lines which carry the EBV genome[105-107]. The hypothesis that T cells in acute infectious mononucleosis function by eliminating infected B cells has been further supported by studies of Klein *et al.*[108]. They showed a very small proportion of EBNA-positive cells among a non-sheep red blood cell binding cell fraction in the circulation of patients with acute infectious mononucleosis. They also isolated T cells from patients which were specifically cytotoxic to EBV-carrying target cells. The EBV-specific T-cell activity could be correlated with the presence of T lymphoblasts and the activity disappeared rapidly after the acute phase of the disease.

Products of the major histocompatibility complex are important as target structures in T-lymphocyte-mediated cytolysis. It is generally assumed that cytotoxic T cells do not recognize specific viral antigens but rather a modification of histocompatibility antigens induced by viral infection. This 'altered self' hypothesis led to the prediction that murine cells expressing viral antigens but lacking H-2 determinants would be resistant to T-cell-mediated cytolysis[109]. Indeed this fact was established by Zinkernagel and Oldstone[110] using murine F9 teratoma cells. Similar observations were made by Tursz *et al.*[111] who showed that EBV-genome-carrying Daudi cells lacking HLA markers were resistant to cytolysis by EBV-sensitized peripheral T lymphocytes from IM patients.

Recent studies by Jondal[112] showed that, in the sera of normal EBV-positive individuals, antibodies directed against EBV-determined membrane antigens had the capacity to induce antibody-dependent cellular cytotoxicity against EBV-superinfected lymphoid cell lines. Sera from normal EBV-negative individuals did not possess this activity. Sera from patients with acute IM who have been shown to possess EBV-specific killer T cells did not induce antibody-dependent cytotoxicity. The cytotoxic activity observed in cell lines carrying the EBV genome is presumed to be due to a lymphocyte-dependent membrane antigen.

13.5.3.3 *Immunodeficiency and EBV*

Purtilo *et al.*[113] reported that among males of certain families EBV infection causes fatal infectious mononucleosis, agammaglobulinaemia or malignant

B-cell lymphoma. This unusual susceptibility to EBV was shown to be inherited as an X-linked recessive trait.

13.5.3.4 *Endogenous reactivation of EBV infections*

Studies by Sumaya[114] have suggested that endogenous reactivation of EBV occurs in a certain proportion of people positive for antibody to EBV-specific VCA and early antigen. Sera containing antibody to early antigen were further tested for the presence of EBV-specific IgM antibody and antibodies to EBV-specific nuclear antigen (EBNA). Since none of the individuals had a history of infectious mononucleosis it was suggested that the appearance of anti-early antigen antibody was due to endogenous reactivation of latent EBV.

13.5.4 Cytomegalovirus

Cytomegalovirus, another member of the herpes virus group, causes intra-uterine infection in 0.7–18.0% of newborn babies. Several follow-up studies have shown a high frequency of at least mild developmental disorders of the central nervous system among congenitally infected infants[115,116]. Some congenital infections are symptomless and at birth only a few congenitally infected babies show typical severe cytomegalic inclusion disease, with hepatosplenomegaly, thrombocytopenia, seizures and chorioretinitis[117].

CMV infections are also common in the first months of life. This type of infection is termed perinatal[118]. CMV has been isolated from the uterine cervix most frequently towards the end of pregnancy and many authors have suggested that cervical virus may be responsible for perinatal infection. It has been shown that perinatal CMV infection is asymptomatic and like congenital CMV leads to virus excretion persisting for several months or years in spite of appreciable levels of circulating antibody[119,120]. CMV is excreted in maternal milk and this finding has led some workers to suggest that breast feeding constitutes a possible route of transmission of the virus from mother to child[121].

13.5.4.1 *Humoral immunity*

Antibody to CMV is produced following CMV infection and it appears to persist for life. The primary antibody response to CMV is highly specific. No cross-reactivity is seen between CMV and other members of the herpes virus group as determined by CF tests. CMV-specific IgM antibody is detected in neonates and elevated IgM in the cord blood also may be indicative of a possible CMV infection[122].

13.5.4.2 *Cell-mediated immunity*

Studies of murine cytomegalovirus infection in mice have suggested that T cells are critical for recovery from murine CMV infection. T-cell-deficient nude mice succumb to experimental CMV infection when inoculated with sublethal doses of CMV[123,124].

Wild mice depleted of T cells with antithymocytic antisera have an increased rate of mortality due to disseminated CMV[125]. Further studies by Booss and Wheelock[126] showed that there was a depression of T-cell function in CMV-infected mice, and that this depression was at least partially mediated by humoral mechanisms.

Rola-Pleszczynski et al.[127] studied cell-mediated immunity in mothers and infants with congenital infection due to CMV. Cell-mediated immunity was measured with a ^{51}Cr-release microassay. The data suggested that a specific impairment in cell-mediated immunity to CMV existed in mothers of infants with congenital CMV infection and in some individuals who persistently excrete CMV.

Diamond et al.[128] showed that peripheral blood leukocytes from 14 healthy non-immune human donors were capable of destroying CMV-infected fibroblasts but not uninfected fibroblasts. Antibody did not appear to mediate the response. Unlike adult leukocytes, cord blood leukocytes were ineffective in destroying CMV-infected target cells. Schauf et al.[129] showed that three infants with CMV infection had a significantly reduced percentage of T cells, compared to age-matched controls. They further showed that compensatory increases in the percentage of IgG-bearing null cells had occurred. Furthermore, two patients displayed decreased lymphocyte reactivity to PHA and PWM. They concluded that these abnormalities may have resulted from CMV infection of the lymphocytes and that the infection might be responsible for prolonged excretion of CMV in the urine.

13.5.4.3   Cytomegalovirus and Guillain–Barré syndrome

Recent studies suggest an association between CMV and Guillain-Barré syndrome. Schmitz and Enders[130] found IgM antibody to CMV in 10 of 94 patients with Guillain-Barré leading them to speculate that CMV may be the causative agent of Guillain-Barré. Dowling and his co-workers[131] measured complement-fixing antibody to CMV, adenovirus and measles virus in the sera of 92 patients with Guillain-Barré and 120 controls. Thirty patients had markedly elevated levels of CF antibody to CMV.

13.5.5   Varicella-zoster virus

Herpes zoster (shingles) is an acute infection of adults with varicella-zoster (V-Z) virus, which also causes chicken-pox in children. Patients with shingles usually can be shown to have suffered previously from chicken-pox and the disease is thought to be due to reactivation of V-Z virus in subjects previously exposed to this agent. Varicella or chicken-pox is a common infection of children which is self-limiting with occasional complications such as pneumonia and encephalitis. Herpes zoster is also common and is found more often in older age groups. Varicella-zoster virus is thought to persist in the sensory ganglion following varicella infection. When the host defence mechanisms deteriorate virus replicates in the sensory ganglion and is subsequently transported down the sensory nerve and released around the sensory nerves of the skin, producing the characteristic cluster of zoster vesicles[132]. While the characteristic pathology of affected ganglia has been known for some time, V-Z virus has recently been demonstrated in CNS tissue by electron microscopy and immunofluorescence[133, 134].

13.5.5.1 Humoral immune response

Varicella-CF antibody to V-Z is detectable following the primary attack but antibody levels are no longer detectable after a few months. CF antibody to varicella cross-reacts with HSV thus limiting the use of the CF test. Because V-Z virus remains cell-associated, neutralization tests are not usually practicable although some laboratories have reported the use of the test for V-Z antibody determinations[135]. Several other tests are available, such as the indirect immunofluorescence antibody test[136], indirect haemagglutination test[137] and platelet aggregation test[138]. The newly developed fluorescent technique for the detection of V-Z antibodies to membrane antigen of infected cells has been very useful and may correlate with susceptibility to the disease[139].

13.5.5.2 Herpes zoster

The humoral antibody response following herpes zoster infection appears to be secondary in nature. IgM-reactive antibody to V-Z virus was detected in one study[140] but not in another[141]. The latter study found two sub-classes of IgG: fast-migrating and slow-migrating. Varicella sera lacked specific neutralizing activity in the rapidly migrating fraction but neutralizing activity was demonstrated in both fractions of sera from patients with zoster.

13.5.5.3 Cell-mediated immunity

Russell et al.[142] found that lymphocytes obtained from patients in the acute phase of zoster, exhibited an impaired transformation response in vitro to V-Z antigens when compared to normal controls who presumably had had prior infection. Lymphocytes from patients with acute zoster, however, responded normally to phytohaemagglutinin (PHA) and PPD. Jordan and Merigan[143] demonstrated lymphocyte transformation to V-Z antigen with lymphocytes collected from zoster patients who were 2–11 weeks convalescent and from varicella-immune children. The hyporesponsiveness to V-Z antigen observed by Russell *et al.*[142] in the acute phase of the disease is probably transient in nature with normal lymphocyte reactivity reappearing during convalescence.

13.5.5.4 *Interferon production*

The production *in vitro* of interferon by lymphocytes from varicella-immune and non-immune individuals stimulated with V-Z antigen indicates that the reaction is apparently non-specific in nature. Vesicle interferon levels of zoster patients have also been examined. Patients who have disseminated lesions exhibit a delay in vesicle interferon production compared to those whose vesicles remain localized. Local interferon production and humoral antibodies may be important host responses in V-Z infection[143].

13.5.6 Adenoviruses

Rowe *et al.*[144] described a virus which caused spontaneous degeneration of cell cultures derived from surgically removed adenoids and tonsils. Similar viruses were isolated from military personnel suffering from acute respiratory disease[145]. The term adenovirus was adopted in 1956 to describe this group of agents. Adenoviruses have been shown to persist in human tissue at extremely low levels. In a series of studies it was found that human adenoviruses may persistently infect about one in 10^8 cells of the adenoids or tonsils[146] and the virus could be isolated from at least 50% of the surgically removed tonsils[147]. Adenovirus shedding into the gastrointestinal tract may occur for prolonged periods of time without an observable effect on the host.

Studies in our laboratory have shown that some chimpanzees excrete adenovirus in the urine for periods of a year or more. The agent designated Pan 11 was isolated from three chimpanzees. All animals had serum-neutralizing antibodies to the agent. Except for one animal which had chronic interstitial nephritis all were healthy. Three individuals who worked with the infected animals developed neutralizing antibody to the virus. Newborn hamsters inoculated with Pan 11 virus developed rhabdomyosarcoma which was transplantable[148]. IgG and IgA antibodies were detectable in the urine of animals excreting Pan 11 virus. Neutralizing antibody to Pan 11 virus was detected in the IgG fraction but not in the IgA fraction[149]

Roos *et al.*[150] reported the isolation of a virus from the brain of a patient dying from radiation-treated lymphosarcoma who also had a 3–4-week history of a neurological disease diagnosed as subacute encephalitis. The virus was shown to be closely related to adenovirus 32 by neutralization test and to adenovirus 27 by haemagglutination-inhibition test. The authors suggested that the reduced immunological defences of the patient. may account for the expression of this agent.

The latency of adenoviruses or their reactivation later in life is currently open to speculation. The virus–host interaction in persistence and/or reactivation of adenoviruses deserves further investigation.

13.5.7 Papovaviruses

Certain viruses of this group can cause latent infections in their natural host, e.g. polyoma in mice and SV-40 in rhesus monkeys. Some viruses within this group are commonly found in the urine either in natural infections or in experimentally infected animals. Serum antibody to these agents is readily demonstrable in natural hosts. SV-40 virus was discovered to be a contaminant of poliomyelitis virus vaccines but not before several million people had been vaccinated with these vaccines.

13.5.7.1 Papovaviruses and progressive multifocal leukoencephalopathy

Progressive multifocal leukoencephalopathy (PML) is a rare subacute demyelinating disease of man. The disease is generally seen as a complication of Hodgkin's disease, sarcoidosis or leukemia. It has also been reported in immunosuppressed patients following organ transplantation or in cases of systemic lupus erythematosus[151].

In 1971 Padgett et al.[152] recovered a virus (JC virus) from the brain of a PML case and this agent, though not identical to SV-40, shared some cross-reactivity. Weiner et al.[153] isolated agents from two patients with PML which were identical to SV-40. Another papovavirus (BK virus) was isolated by Gardner et al.[154] from the urine of a patient following renal transplantation. Since most of the patients with PML either have disorders of the reticuloendothelial system or are on immunosuppressive therapy, no serum antibody to these agents has been detected. Serological surveys have shown that low levels of antibody to SV-40 in human populations with no history of killed or live polio vaccine inoculations may have been due to infection with a different but antigenically related papovavirus[155]. More recent sero-epidemiological surveys have shown that antibody to JC and BK viruses is quite common in children and adults[156-158]. Brown et al.[159], in a sero-epidemiological survey to determine the distribution of antibody to papova-virus in primitive isolated populations, observed different patterns of antibody to JC, BK and SV-40 papovavirus. A few extremely isolated populations were without antibody to BK virus. In other areas, however, antibody prevalence increased with age. Antibody prevalence in families was found to be similar to that of the general population. Similar age patterns of antibody to JC virus was also noticed when sera were tested for antibody to JC virus; however, the experience with the two viruses showed that they occurred independently in several populations. Sera with no antibody to BK virus were examined for SV-40 virus antibody. Five per cent of the sera gave positive results suggesting that antibody to SV-40 may be due to BK or closely related papovaviruses in humans unexposed to contaminated vaccines or simian sources of SV-40 infection. It is noteworthy that the two cases of PML from which SV-40 was isolated[153] had no history of inoculations with killed or live polio vaccine. It thus appears that papovaviruses cause infections in man, and that PML is a rare manifestation in an immunologically compromised host. Since immunosuppression can be caused by multiple factors, the specific immunosuppressive mechanisms which precipitate PML are as yet unknown. The elucidation of such mechanisms is of immense importance to the understanding of the disease[160].

13.6   RNA VIRUSES WHICH CAUSE PERSISTENT RECURRENT INFECTIONS IN HUMANS

13.6.1   Subacute sclerosing panencephalitis (measles virus)

Subacute sclerosing panencephalitis (SSPE) is a slow, progressive inflammatory disorder of the CNS of children and young adults. Convincing evidence implicating measles virus as the aetiological agent of SSPE has accumulated over the years culminating in the successful isolation of measles virus from brain biopsies of SSPE patients[161,162]. Although it is now generally accepted that SSPE is a chronic virus infection of the brain caused by measles virus the pathogenesis of the disease still remains obscure. It is generally assumed that the immune system is somehow involved in the causation of the disorder[163].

13.6.1.1   *Humoral immunity in SSPE*

A heightened antibody response to measles virus is observed in nearly all patients with SSPE. Measles virus antibody was first demonstrated by Connolly et al.[164] in the serum and CSF of three patients with SSPE. High levels of complement-fixing (CF) and haemagglutination-inhibiting antibody were found in the serum of two patients and in one the titre increased 16-fold during the course of the illness indicating active infection. Numerous investigators subsequently confirmed their observations[165-170].

In a follow-up study Connolly[171] showed that the measles serum : CSF antibody ratio was considerably lower in three patients with SSPE than the poliomyelitis type 2 serum : CSF antibody ratio, suggesting endogenous measles antibody production within the CNS. Kolar[172] examined the CSF of a large number of SSPE patients and found a high frequency with elevated γ-globulin levels. Tourtellotte et al.[173] observed a similar rise in the level of γ-globulin within the CSF and calculated that approximately 95% of the brain IgG was synthesized within the CNS. Other investigators[174], using radioisotopically-labelled immunoglobulin G administered intravenously in patients with SSPE, supported this concept by demonstrating that CSF immunoglobulin G may arise from a non-vascular source.

Salmi et al.[175] identified different measles virus-specific antibodies in matched CSF and sera of eight SSPE patients using neutralization, haemolysis-inhibition (HLI), haemagglutination-inhibition (HI), CF and immunodiffusion tests. They found the relative content of antibodies against various measles virus products to differ among individuals. The major fraction of antibodies detected in CF and immunodiffusion tests reacted with measles nucleocapsid antigen. Comparison of antibodies against measles virus products and against group-specific vertex capsomere antigen of adenovirus in matched CSF and serum samples revealed the production of measles virus-specific antibody within the CNS of all eight SSPE cases tested.

Gel electrophoresis studies of CSF and serum of SSPE patients have revealed several homogeneous bands in the γ region with slightly different electrophoretic mobilities[176-178]. The evidence indicates that these bands represent homogeneous groups of measles virus-specific antibody and that each homogeneous IgG population possesses antibody activity to specific measles virus structural components[179]. Recent studies of CSF from six SSPE patients indicated that the mobility of oligoclonal IgG was different in all CSF samples[180]. Moreover, measles virus antibody to different measles virus components in these IgG fractions was shown to be evenly distributed in the slow- and fast-moving IgG fractions. Vandvik et al.[181] showed that the IgG isolated from the sera, CSF and brain extracts of SSPE patients was electrophoretically homogeneous and it differed from the heterogeneous IgG antibodies isolated from control individuals following natural measles infection. They found that in the CSF or brain of SSPE patients most or all of the oligoclonal IgG possessed measles antibody activity. The biological significance of the homogeneous antibody response in SSPE remains to be determined.

Although IgG has been shown to predominate in the sera of SSPE patients, IgM measles-specific antibody has been reported[182], and more recently IgD antibodies directed against measles virus components also have been demonstrated[183].

Immunofluorescent studies have detected the presence of measles virus–antibody–complement complexes on the ganglia and glial cells of SSPE patients suggesting that antibodies might somehow be involved in the pathogenesis of the disease[184,185]. That such complexes can cause disruption of measles virus-infected cells is well documented. Cytolysis of measles virus-infected cells in the presence of antibody and complement (C) was reported by Minogaiwa and Yamada[186], and was shown to be due to a reaction between measles antibody and viral antigen on the surface of infected cells. Using ^{51}Cr-release assay with measles virus-infected carrier cells Kibler et al.[187] found cytotoxic antibody to be present in the sera and

CSF of SSPE patients as well as in the sera of individuals recovering from acute measles virus infection. The range of cytotoxic antibody titres was only slightly higher in the SSPE sera than in early and atypical measles sera. Late measles sera and CSF from SSPE patients were less cytotoxic for carrier cultures. Oldstone *et al.*[188] showed that cultured cells from the brain of a patient with SSPE were lysed by the patient's own serum. Lysis was dependent on the presence of antibody to measles virus and complement and only occurred when viral antigen was present on the cell surface. The authors suggested that similar events may operate *in vivo* and play a major role in the pathogenesis of tissue injury in patients with SSPE.

Immunocytotoxicity of measles-infected HeLa cells have been shown by Joseph and his colleagues[189] to be mediated by the alternative complement pathway and measles antibody of the immunoglobulin G class. Cytolytic measles antibody in sera and CSF from patients with SSPE was found to be totally functional as was the alternative complement pathway. Joseph *et al.*[190] have shown in antibody-binding studies that cells acutely infected with measles virus can express 2–3 times more viral surface antigen than persistently infected cells. Moreover, cells persistently infected with measles virus were found to be more refractory to immune cytotoxic activity than acutely infected cells, and this may be due to the lower levels of viral surface antigen in persistently infected cells. The authors speculated that the relative lack of measles virus surface antigen on SSPE infected cells[163] might allow these cells to persist in SSPE patients despite the presence of cytolytic antibody.

Modulation of viral surface antigens has also been shown to occur following the addition of measles antibody in the absence of complement[191]. Measles antigen disappeared rapidly from the cell surface after treatment with antibody and the denuded cells were found to be less susceptible to the cytolytic activity of antibody and complement. It was conjectured that modulation of measles viral antigen in the presence of antibody without complement might also occur *in vivo* and if surface antigen on infected cells was absent then virus would be able to persist in the presence of cytolytic antibody.

Investigators, using radiolabelled [125]I C3, have reported the presence of immune complexes in the CSF and serum of patients with SSPE[188]. Immune complex deposits of measles virus–antimeasles antibody and complement have been demonstrated on the glomerular basement membrane of kidney and other tissues of SSPE patients[192,193]. The significance of these findings with respect to the pathogenesis of SSPE is uncertain.

13.6.1.2 Cellular immunity in SSPE

The role of the cellular immune system in the pathogenesis of SSPE is unknown. In 1968 Burnet[194] postulated T-lymphocyte unresponsiveness in patients with SSPE due to the persistence of measles antigen in the thymus. If so no cellular immune reaction to measles should be observed in SSPE patients. Since then a number of conflicting studies have appeared in the literature. Several workers have demonstrated cellular immune abnormalities in SSPE patients in support of Burnet's hypothesis. Gerson et al.[195] reported depressed cellular immune function in four patients with SSPE using six skin-test antigens including measles, dinitrochlorobenzene responsiveness and delayed allogenic skin reactions. Similar observations were made by Kolar[172]. Moulias et al.[196] demonstrated lymphocyte unresponsiveness to measles virus in leukocytes from SSPE patients using macrophage-migration inhibition and blast transformation as measures of cellular immunity. Cell-mediated immune function against antigens other than measles, however, appeared normal. Similar observations have been reported by others[197-199].

Conversely, numerous workers have reported no evidence of impairment of cell-mediated immune function to measles antigen in SSPE patients. Using purified measles antigen Saunders et al.[200] demonstrated increased lymphocyte transformation in an SSPE patient compared with a healthy matched control. Immunocompetent lymphocytes were also demonstrated by skin testing and macrophage-migration inhibition in another case of SSPE using concentrated measles virus[201]. HeLa cells persistently infected with SSPE measles virus were shown to stimulate lymphocytes from SSPE patients[202]. Using the macrophage-migration inhibition test, the mixed lymphocyte virus-infected cell culture test and the lymphocytotoxic assay Ahmed et al.[203] reported that leukocytes from four SSPE patients were extremely responsive to conventional measles and SSPE measles virus preparations. Kreth et al.[204,205] showed that lymphocytes from SSPE patients elicited a vigorous response to measles virus using a lymphocytotoxic assay against ^{51}Cr-labelled target cells persistently infected with measles virus. Steele et al.[206] and Perrin et al.[207] reported similar findings.

In the light of these more recent experimental findings it is now the general feeling that Burnet's hypothesis of cellular immune impairment can no longer explain the pathogenesis of SSPE. An alternative hypothesis is therefore needed to explain the mechanism(s) by which the virus escapes immune elimination in the presence of high titres of measles-specific antibody and competent cellular immunity. Sell et al.[208] suggested that a blocking factor may explain virus persistence. They showed that stimulation of lymphocytes from SSPE patients by SSPE virus-infected HeLa cells could be blocked by a heat-labile factor in the plasma or spinal fluid. Allen et al.[209] also described a heat-labile inhibitory factor of mitogen-induced lymphocyte transformation in the plasma of an SSPE patient.

Conversely, Swick et al.[210] reported the presence of a heat-stable blocking factor of lymphocyte transformation in the plasma of patients with SSPE. Ahmed et al.[203] demonstrated a blocking agent in the plasma and CSF of four patients with SSPE which blocked the response *in vitro* of their lymphocytes to SSPE measles virus. The blocking factor was specific for SSPE virus and did not block the response of lymphocytes to non-specific mitogens, bacterial antigens or other viral antigens. Preliminary experiments indicated that the blocking factor is IgM or antigen–antibody complexes. It was postulated that the blocking factor may be responsible for the inability of the immune system to eliminate measles virus from the CNS. Steele *et al.*[206] using a ^{51}Cr-cytotoxicity microassay demonstrated that serum and CSF from SSPE patients inhibited the cellular immune response to SSPE-infected cells but not to measles-infected cells. Preliminary characterization indicated that the blocking factor was IgM or antigen–antibody complexes.

In contrast, Kreth and ter Meulen[211] showed that pretreatment of SSPE peripheral lymphoid cells with SSPE serum or CSF neither blocked nor increased measles virus-specific cytotoxicity in virus-infected target cells when cells were subsequently tested in CSF-containing tissue culture medium. However, killing activity was found to be enhanced by the addition of SSPE serum or CSF to the cytotoxic assay. Non-SSPE measles antibody also caused enhancement. In view of these findings and in an effort to explain virus persistence in SSPE the authors speculated that virus-infected brain cells in SSPE patients were probably protected from an immune attack by antibody-induced antigenic modulation of viral determinants on the surface of infected cells.

Kreth and Wiegand[212], in a study of SSPE lymphocytes to determine if T or K cells were involved in the killing of ^{51}Cr-labelled measles virus-infected target cells, found the cytotoxicity to be mediated by K cells. Perrin *et al.*[207] corroborated their findings. Moreover, they were unable to demonstrate a blocking factor of cell-mediated cytotoxicity in the sera of SSPE patients. They were able, however, to demonstrate enhanced killing of measles virus-infected target cells in the presence of either serum or purified IgG-containing antibodies to measles virus.

Several animal models of SSPE now exist in which persistent infections of the CNS have been established with either conventional or SSPE strains of measles virus. Models include the hamster[213–215], ferret[216–218], monkey[219], and dog[217]. The humoral immune responses in these animals appear to parallel those of human SSPE patients with adequate to elevated levels of measles antibody. Definitive cellular immune studies, however, have yet to appear.

13.6.2 Chronic progressive panencephalitis (rubella)

Weil *et al.*[220] reported a case of chronic progressive panencephalitis in a 12-year-old boy with congenital rubella syndrome. The disease was characterized by late onset with prolonged progressive neurological deterioration.

It was of interest that although the disease resembled SSPE clinically and pathologically, rubella virus and not measles virus was isolated from the brain of the patient. Antibody to rubella virus was extremely high in the serum and CSF whereas serum antibody to measles was less than 1 : 8. Cellular immune studies with leukocytes from the patient revealed a normal migration-inhibition response to rubella antigen. Furthermore, heat-inactivated serum from the patient inhibited lymphocyte-mediated cyto-toxicity of ^{51}Cr-labelled rubella virus-infected target cells. CSF from the patient had no effect on the lymphocyte cytotoxic response. Townsend et al.[221] described three patients with congenital rubella syndrome who developed progressive neurological illness. Examination of the sera and CSF of these patients revealed high antibody titres to rubella virus in two patients and all had elevated CSF protein and γ-globulin levels. Attempts to isolate virus from the brains of these patients proved unsuccessful although patho-logical examination of the brains of two showed a widespread subacute panencephalitis. In view of these findings the authors stressed that viruses other than measles virus can produce a clinical picture similar to SSPE.

13.6.2.1 Congenital rubella

Prenatal infection of infants with rubella virus may produce chronic infection and congenital malformation. In infants with congenital rubella, virus frequently can be isolated at birth, particularly from infants infected during the first trimester of pregnancy. A virus-excretory phase usually follows during which the agent can be isolated from the urine, CSF, faeces, throat secretions and various tissues such as lung, thymus and circulating lympho-cytes[222–224] for as long as 16–18 months after birth[225–228]. Most infants, however, stop excreting virus by 6 months of age[228–230], although rubella virus has been isolated from the lens material of a 3-year-old congenitally infected child[223]. During viral shedding affected infants may show clinical signs of infection and most possess high titres of neutralizing antibody[222, 231,232]. Some children, however, exposed to rubella virus in utero may possess elevated antibody titres without clinical disease[233]. The mechan-ism(s) whereby the virus is allowed to persist, particularly in the presence of high titres of neutralizing antibody, is unknown. A defect in the immune system has been postulated as a possible mechanism to explain rubella virus persistence.

13.6.2.2 Humoral immunity in congenital rubella

Several groups of workers have reported IgM levels in the cord sera of some infants with congenital rubella[222,234–236] indicating an active immune response by the fetus. IgM levels were found to be elevated with greater frequency in the clinically more severe cases. Elevated levels of IgM in certain infants with rubella have also been observed during the early months of life[231,235-237]. Cessation of viral shedding has been shown to correlate well with concomitant drops in IgM levels[231,237,238]. Some affected infants also display elevated IgA levels[234,235]. Conversely, dysgammaglobulinaemia and antibody deficiency syndromes have also been described in a number of cases. The most frequent patterns have been elevated IgM levels with IgG and IgA deficiencies[231,239-241]. Although immunological abnormalities in the levels of different immunoglobulins do exist in some patients there is little evidence to indicate that these aberrations are in any way involved in establishing or maintaining persistence of the virus.'

Specific anti-rubella antibodies of both fetal and maternal origin have been demonstrated in infants with congenital rubella[229]. Most studies have shown that these infants possess neutralizing antibody, haemagglutinating antibody and CF antibody. Alford et al.[225] have shown that rubella antibody is present in the fetal serum between the 12th and 16th weeks of gestation. The antibody appeared to be maternal IgG as it was found in a lower concentration in the blood of the fetus than in the blood of the mother. Maternal IgG antibodies are lost during the first few months of life and then the infant begins to produce endogenous IgG[222,232,242]. Fetal IgM antibody was found by Alford et al.[225] to be produced about the 20th week of gestation. The production of IgM and IgG is strong evidence against the theory that immunological tolerance is involved in the pathogenesis of congenital rubella.

Michaels[237,243] demonstrated that in some infants with congenital rubella a defect in humoral immunity to antigens other than rubella virus exists during virus shedding. In two infants prenatally infected with rubella there was evidence of impairment of the antibody response to measles and poliomyelitis vaccine viruses, diphtheria toxoid and blood group substances. Several workers have also reported that infants with congenital rubella have a greater frequency of infections which tends to support the concept of immunological impairment[231,239]. Infants who stop shedding virus however no longer show a suppression of the immune response[237,243].

13.6.2.3   Cellular immunity in congenital rubella

A defect in cellular immune function also has been postulated to explain viral persistence in congenital rubella. Delayed hypersensitivity to *Candida albicans* has been found to be diminished in some patients with congenital rubella[229,244]. Olsen et al.[245] showed that lymphocytes of four patients with congenital rubella virus were unresponsive to PHA stimulation *in vitro*. In a subsequent study Montgomery[246] reported a similar effect in eight of 14 patients tested. Olsen et al.[247] showed that the depression lasted only for the duration of the infection. White and Leikin[244] have shown that lymphocyte reactivity *in vitro* to vaccinia virus in patients who were previously immunized with vaccinia and who were no longer shedding rubella virus was reduced significantly. However, they observed a normal blast-transformation response to PHA in the same patients. Simons and Fitzgerald[224] demonstrated depressed lymphocyte reactivity in three of seven patients, all of whom were viremic at the time of testing. Marshall et al.[248] found that lymphocyte responsiveness in vitro to PHA was normal in 20 patients with congenital rubella. Six of these patients were excreting virus at the time of the tests. Fuccillo et al.[249] studied cell-mediated immunity to rubella virus in children with documented congenital rubella syndrome. Using a ^{51}Cr-lymphocytotoxicity microassay they demonstrated cell-mediated immunity to rubella virus in only three of 11 children. None of the children, with the exception of a 5-month-old infant, were shedding virus at the time of the study. The authors suggested that the lack of cellular immunity in the majority of children tested might explain the persistence of the virus in the postpartum period. The mechanism(s) by which the virus is eventually eliminated is also open to conjecture. They suggested that temporary cell-mediated immunity might occur in these cases or that the virus infection is self-limiting and terminates with the death of the infected cells[250].

The studies to date indicate that not all patients with congenital rubella display depressed lymphocyte reactivity in vitro following exposure to non-specific mitogens and specific antigens. In some studies the impaired reactivity appears to be only transient in nature and is found only during the active phase of the disease. Others have shown the depression to last well beyond the termination of virus shedding. Additional studies are needed to determine if cessation of virus shedding coincides with the development of cellular immunity.

13.6.3 Foamy viruses

The oncornaviruses or RNA tumour viruses have long been known to produce tumours in animals under natural or experimental conditions. They have also been shown to transform cell cultures in vitro. Their involvement in human disease is unknown although man may be affected[251].

The foamy viruses persistently infect a wide variety of animals and share many physicochemical similarities with the oncornaviruses[252]. One major difference, however, is that foamy viruses do not produce tumours under natural or experimental conditions, nor do they cause cellular transformation in vitro. The foamy viruses nevertheless are receiving increasing attention because of recent human isolations.

It is of interest that of three human foamy virus isolations, all have been from patients afflicted with neoplasms. Simian foamy virus (SFV) type 1 was isolated from a patient with chronic myeloid leukaemia[253]. Foamy viruses have also been isolated from Africans with nasopharyngeal carcinoma[254] and Burkitt's lymphoma[255]. The nasopharyngeal isolate was shown to be closely related to SFV type $6^{256,257}$ and the Burkitt's isolate appears to be a variant of SFV type 3^{258}.

Persistent foamy virus infections occur in the presence of neutralizing antibody. These agents elicit a normal humoral antibody response in naturally infected hosts and laboratory animals. Hooks et al.[259] showed that foamy viruses in cell culture are able to spread from cell to contiguous cell in the presence of foamy virus antibody. Furthermore, the addition of antibody and complement to the infected cells failed to cause lysis. They concluded that these data, along with their observations that foamy viruses are poor inducers of interferon and relatively resistant to the antiviral action of interferon, may serve to explain, at least in part, the manner in which persistence is achieved. Hooks and Detrick-Hooks[260] also showed that the cellular immune response to PHA was depressed in rabbits persistently infected with SFV type 7. The humoral response, however, appeared normal. The authors suggested that the observed cellular immune depression might be of importance in initiating foamy virus persistence.

13.7 UNCONVENTIONAL VIRUSES WHICH CAUSE PERSISTENT INFECTIONS IN HUMANS

In this review we have considered the immune response of the host persistently infected with conventional viruses that are either DNA or RNA in nature. There is also, however, a group of transmissible virus-like agents which produce fatal infections of the brain that have been classified as the subacute spongiform virus encephalopathies[261]. Within this group are two diseases of man, kuru and Creutzfeldt–Jakob disease, and two diseases of animals, scrapie of sheep and goats and transmissible mink encephalopathy (TME). The most challenging outcome of the discovery that chronic progressive non-inflammatory degenerative CNS diseases (sporadic, as in most cases of Creutzfeldt–Jakob disease (CJD); epidemic, as in kuru; or familial, as in CJD and kuru) are slow infections caused by viruses with incubation periods measured in years or decades, during which virus replication is active and continuous in most tissues of the infected host, is the realization that the aetiological agents of these infections form a group of micro-organisms new to microbiology and to investigators in the field of infectious diseases. Although the agents manifest many of the properties of 'classic conventional' viruses, they possess a series of atypical biological and physical properties that clearly differentiate them from any other known group of micro-organisms affecting mammalian hosts.

A number of excellent review articles have been published on the clinical, histopathological, epidemiological, and viral characteristics of kuru[262-272], scrapie[262,267,273-277], and mink encephalopathy[267,278,279]. They are characterized as *subacute*, since they are not associated with a febrile response, a cerebrospinal pleocytosis or changes in clinical chemistry or haematological values; *spongiform*, since the histopathologic lesion induced is an *intracellular* vacuolation of neurons and astrocytes restricted to the grey matter of the brain; *virus*, in that they are filterable, serially transmissible and self-replicating; and *encephalopathies*, because they are not associated with an inflammatory reaction during any stage of disease.

In spite of the fact that kuru, CJD, scrapie and mink encephalopathy are clearly transmissible diseases caused by small (mol. wt. 150 000), highly stable viruses, which are widely distributed throughout host tissues for periods of from several months to several years before infection becomes apparent and a slowly progressive course takes place, the most disturbing feature has surely been the consistent failure to demonstrate antibody to the virus or an immunopathological process to explain the disease. Complement-fixation, precipitation, gel-diffusion, and direct and indirect immunofluorescence tests on various agent-containing targets or examination of infected brain, spleen, kidney, and lymph nodes for the presence of immune complexes have consistently produced negative results. Neutralization tests using conventional methods and numerous modifications of the classic virus neutralization tests also failed to demonstrate the presence of antiviral antibody. Passive protection types of tests, such as those required to demonstrate neutralization of hog cholera virus by inoculating serum from animals with naturally acquired infections, or serum from a wide variety of mammalian and avian hosts hyperimmunized with high concentration of virus, into test animals at various time periods before challenging them with minimum doses of virus, have been negative. Similar results were obtained using antiglobulin-potentiated neutralization tests. Mice that had been splenectomized and thymectomized at birth and animals immunosuppressed with antilymphocytic serum and cyclophosphamide, when exposed to high and low concentrations of scrapie, developed disease with incubation periods only slightly longer than non-treated control mice[280-288].

If the virus or viruses of kuru, CJD, scrapie and TME do not induce antibody in their infected hosts, this implies that the agent or agents do not produce antigens in the manner of all known viruses. And this may, indeed, be the case. Their small size, the lack of a virion recognizable by electron microscopy, and the intimate association of the virus with host membrane may well mitigate recognition by the host. Animals infected with kuru, CJD, scrapie and TME make a normal response to antigens such as sheep erythrocytes and bovine serum albumin. Endogenous and exogenous interferon does not affect the spongiform viruses, nor is the ability of the host to produce interferon altered. In spite of the negative nature of these immunological findings we do not accept the hypothesis that these agents are truly non-antigenic. More thoroughly purified preparations of the viruses and more sensitive tests for studying their antigenicity will ultimately result in the development of an antigen–antibody system which will provide a better understanding of the relationships between the agents and the diseases they produce.

13.8 SUMMARY AND CONCLUSIONS

The term 'immunity' means any form of resistance against a potentially pathogenic organism or toxin. Allison[289] points out that immunity against viruses has many components, including resistance of individual host cells to infection, local factors such as temperature or acidity, formation of interferon, resistance of macrophages and other leukocytes, and specific humoral and cell-mediated immune responses. In acute viral infections all these factors may exert an influence on the outcome of an infection. In cases of persistent and recurrent virus infections the situation is obviously more complex, for in such infections it appears that the host defence mechanisms are unable to control the infection adequately. Rapid progress in the fields of humoral and cellular immunology, molecular biology and, to a greater extent, genetics has contributed significantly to our understanding of the underlying mechanisms in persistent infections. In the case of the unconventional viruses it appears that immunological factors neither potentiate, complicate, nor control the disease. In more conventional virus infections, in which the virus is never eliminated and viraemia persists throughout the life of the host in the presence of high levels of neutralizing antibody in the serum, replication within macrophages and the possibility of immune complexes may be the underlying mechanisms. And, finally, in latent and recurrent infections it appears that the spread of viruses within the host is under the control of cell-mediated immune mechanisms.

References

1. Von Magnus, P. (1951). Propagation of PR-8 strain of influenza A virus in chick embryos. III. Properties of the incomplete virus produced in serial passages of the undiluted virus. *Acta Pathol. Microbiol. Scand.*, **29**, 157
2. Huang, A. S. and Baltimore, D. (1970). Defective viral particles and viral disease processes. *Nature (Lond.)*, **226**, 325
3. Holland, J. J. and Villarreal, L. P. (1974). Persistent noncytocidal vesicular stomatitis virus infections mediated by defective 'T' particles that suppress virion transcriptase. *Proc. Nat. Acad. Sci. USA*, **71**, 2956
4. Fields, B. N. (1972). Genetic manipulation of reovirus – a model for modification of disease. *N. Engl. J. Med.*, **237**, 1023
5. Youngner, J. S., Dubovi, E. J., Quagliana, D. O., Kelly, M. and Preble, O. T. (1976). Role of temperature-sensitive mutants in persistent infection initiated with vesicular stomatitis virus. *J. Virol.*, **19**, 90
6. Preble, O. T. and Youngner, J. S. (1972). Temperature-sensitive mutants isolated from L cells persistently infected with Newcastle disease virus. *J. Virol.*, **9**, 200
7. Stoller, V., Peleg, J. and Shenk, T. E. (1974). Temperature sensitivity of a Sindbis virus mutant isolated from persistently infected *Aedes aegypti* cell culture. *Intervirology*, **2**, 337

8. Baltimore, D. (1970). RNA-dependent DNA polymerase in virions of RNA tumour viruses. *Nature (Lond.)*, **226**, 1209

9. Temin, H. M. and Mitzutani, S. (1970). RNA-dependent DNA polymerase in virion of Rous sarcoma virus. *Nature (Lond.)*, **226**, 1211

10. Simpson, R. W. and Inuma, M. (1975). Recovery of infectious proviral DNA from mammalian cells infected with respiratory syncytial virus. *Proc. Nat. Acad. Sci. USA*, **72**, 3230

11. Zhdnov, V. M. (1975). Integration of viral genomes. *Nature (Lond.)*, **256**, 471

12. Boyum, A. (1968). Separation of leucocytes from blood and bone marrow. *Scand. J. Clin. Lab. Invest.*, **21** (Suppl.), 97, 51

13. Oldstone, M. B. A. and Dixon, F. J. (1975). Immune complex disease associated with viral infections. In: *Viral Immunology and Immunopathology* (A. L. Notkins, ed.), chap. 20, pp. 341–356 (New York: Academic Press)

14. Wilfert, C. M., Buckley, R., Rosen, F., Whisnat, J., Oxman, M. N., Griffith, J. F., Katz, S. L. and Moore, M. (1977). Persistent enterovirus infections in agammaglobulinemia. In: *Microbiology 1977* (D. Schlessinger, ed.), p. 488 (Washington, D.C.: American Society for Microbiology)

15. Ho, M., Dowling, J. N., Armstrong, J. A., Suwansirikul, S., Wu, B., Youngblood, L. A. and Saslow, A. (1976). Factors contributing to the risk of cytomegalovirus infection in patients receiving renal transplants. *Yale J. Biol. Med.*, **49**, 17

16. Dowling, J. N., Saslow, A. R., Armstrong, J. A. and Ho, M. (1976). The relationship of immunosuppression to cytomegalovirus infection. *Yale J. Biol. Med.*, **49**, 77

17. Mims, C. A. (1974). Factors in the mechanisms of persistence of viral infections. *Progr. Med. Virol.*, **18**, 1

18. Blumberg, B. S. (1964). Polymorphisms of serum proteins and the development of isoprecipitins in transfused patients. *Bull. N.Y. Acad. Med.*, **40**, 377

19. Blumberg, B. S., Sutnick, A. T. and London, W. T. (1968). Hepatitis and leukemia: Their relation to Australia antigen. *Bull. N.Y. Acad. Med.*, **44**, 1566

20. Prince, A. M. (1968). An antigen detected in the blood during the incubation period of serum-hepatitis. *Proc. Nat. Acad. Sci. USA*, **60**, 814

21. Szmuness, W. (1975). Recent advances in the study of the epidemiology of Hepatitis B. *Am. J. Pathol.*, **3**, 629

22. Dane, D. S., Cameron, C. H. and Briggs, M. (1970). Virus-like particles in serum of patients with Australia antigen-associated hepatitis. *Lancet*, **i**, 695

23. Combes, B., Sastny, P., Shorey, J., Barrera, A., Carter, W. W., Hull, A. and Eigenbrot, E. H. (1971). Glomerulonephritis with deposition of Australia antigen antibody complex in glomerular basement membrane. *Lancet*, **ii**, 234

24. Bacon, P. A., Doherty, S. M. and Zukerman, A. J. (1975). Hepatitis B antibody in polymyelgia rheumatica. *Lancet*, **ii**, 476

25. Gianotti, F. (1973). Papular acrodermatitis of childhood: An Australia antigen disease. *Arch. Dis. Child.*, **48**, 794

26. Levo, Y., Gorevic, P. D., Kasab, H. J., Franklin, Z. D. and Franklin, E. C. (1977). Association between hepatitis B virus and essential mixed cryoglobulinemia. *N. Engl. J. Med.*, **296**, 1501

27. Krugman, S., Hoofnagle, J. H., Gerety, R. J., Kaplan, P. M. and Gerin, J. (1974). Viral hepatitis B: DNA polymerase activity and antibody to hepatitis core antigen. *N. Engl. J. Med.*, **290**, 1331

28. Shulman, N. R. and Barker, L. M. (1969). Virus-like antigen, antibody and antigen–antibody complexes in hepatitis measured by complement fixation. *Science*, **165**, 304

29. Almeida, J. D. and Waterson, A. P. (1970). Immune complexes in hepatitis. *Lancet*, **ii**, 983

30. Barker, L. F., Peterson, M. R., Shulman, R. and Murray, R. (1973). Antibody responses in viral hepatitis type B. *J. Am. Med. Assoc.*, **223**, 1005

31. Irwin, G. R., Hierholzer, W. J. and McCollum, R. W. (1972). Delayed hypersensitivity to hepatitis-associated antigen in guinea-pigs. *J. Infect. Dis.*, **125**, 73

32. Gerety, R. J., Hoofnagle, J. H. and Barker, L. F. (1974). Humoral and cell-mediated immune responses to two hepatitis B virus antigens in guinea-pigs. *J. Immunol.*, **113**, 1223

33. Roberts, I. M., Bernard, C., Vyas, G. M. and Mackay, I. R. (1975). 'T' cell dependence of immune response to hepatitis B antigen in mice. *Nature (Lond.)*, **254**, 606

34. Laiwah, A. A. C. Y. (1971). Lymphocyte transformation by Australia antigen. *Lancet*, **ii**, 470

35. Ito, K., Nakagawa, J. and Okimoto, Y. (1972). Chronic hepatitis migration inhibition of leukocytes in the presence of Australia antigen. *N. Engl. J. Med.*, **286**, 1005

36. Dudley, F. J., Guistino, V. and Sherlock, S. (1972). Cell-mediated immunity in patients positive for hepatitis associated antigen. *Br. Med. J.*, **4**, 754

37. Laiwah, A. A. C. Y., Chandhuri, A. K. R. and Anderson, J. R. (1973). Lymphocyte transformation and leukocyte migration inhibition by Australia antigen. *Clin. Exp. Immunol.*, **15**, 27

38. Desaules, M., Frei, P. C., Libanska, J. and Wuilleret, B. (1976). Lack of leukocyte migration inhibition by hepatitis B antigen and normal non-specific immunoreactivity in asymptomatic carriers. *J. Infect. Dis.*, **134**, 505

39. Edington, T. and Chisari, F. C. (1975). Immunological aspects of hepatitis B infection. *Am. J. Med. Sci.*, **270**, 213

40. Mackay, L. R. and Morris, P. J. (1972). Association of autoimmune active chronic hepatitis with HL-A1, 8. *Lancet*, **ii**, 793

41. Galbraith, R. M., Edelleston, A. L. W. F., Smith, M. G. M., Williams, R., McSween, R. N. M., Watkinson, G., Dick, H., Kennedy, L. A. and Batchleov, J. R. (19—). Histocompatibility antigens in active chronic hepatitis and primary biliary cirrhosis. *Br. Med. J.*, **3**, 604

42. Page, A., Sharp, H. L., Greenberg, L. S. and Yunis, E. (1975). Genetic analysis of patients with chronic active hepatitis. *J. Clin. Invest.*, **56**, 530

43. Hillis, W. D., Hillis, A., Bias, W. B. and Walker, W. G. (1977). Association of hepatitis B surface antigenemia with HLA locus B specificities. *N. Engl. J. Med.*, **296**, 1310

44. Patterson, M. J., Hourani, M. R. and Mayor, G. H. (1977). HLA antigens and hepatitis B virus. *N. Engl. J. Med.*, **297**, 1124

45. Koziol, D. E., Alter, H. J., Kirchner, J. P. and Holland, P. V. (1976). The development of HBs-Ag-positive hepatitis despite the previous existence of antibody to HBs-Ag. *J. Immunol.*, **117**, 2260

46. Tabor, E., Gerety, R. J., Smallwood, L. A. and Barker, L. F. (1976). Induction of antibody to the 'y' determinant of HBs-Ag in a chimpanzee carrier of HBs-Ag sub-type 'adw'. *J. Immunol.*, **117**, 2038

47. Le Bouvier, G. L., Capper, R. A., Williams, A. E., Pelletier, M. and Katz, A. J. (1976). Concurrently circulating HBs-Ag and heterotypic anti-HBs antibody. *J. Immunol.*, **117**, 2262

48. Sasaki, T., Ohkubo, Y., Yamashita, Y., Imai, M., Miyakawa, Y. and Mayumi, M. (1976). Co-occurrence of hepatitis B surface antigen of a particular subtype and antibody to a heterologous subtype specificity in the same serum. *J. Immunol.*, **117**, 2258

49. Moraczewska, Z., Kazimierz, M. and Holland, P. (1978). Simultaneous presence in serum of HBs-Ag and anti-HBs-Ag of different specificities. *Intervirology*, **9**, 189

50. Gerin, J. (1978). Personal communication

51. Feinstone, S. M., Kapikian, A. Z. and Purcell, R. H. (1973). Hepatitis A: Detection by immune electron microscopy of a virus-like antigen associated with acute illness. *Science*, **182**, 1026

52. Provost, P. J., Ittensohn, O. L., Villarejos, V. M., Arguedas, J. and Hilleman, M. R.

(1973). Etiologic relationship of marmoset-propagated CR-326 hepatitis A virus to hepatitis in man. *Proc. Soc. Exp. Biol. Med.*, **142**, 1257

53. Provost, P. J., Ittensohn, O. L., Villarejos, V. M. and Hilleman, M. R. (1975). A specific complement fixation test for human hepatitis A employing CR-326 virus antigen: Diagnosis and epidemiology. *Proc. Soc. Exp. Biol. Med.*, **148**, 962

54. Krugman, S., Friedman, M. and Lattimer, C. (1975). Viral hepatitis type A: Identification by specific complement fixation and immune adherence tests. *N. Engl. J. Med.*, **292**, 1141

55. Szmuness, W., Dienstag, J. L., Purcell, R. H., Harley, E. J., Stevens, C. E. and Wong, D. C. (1976). Distribution of antibody to hepatitis A antigen in urban adult populations. *N. Engl. J. Med.*, **295**, 755

56. Alter, H. J., Purcell, R. H., Holland, P. V. and Popper, H. (1978). Transmissible agent in non-A and non-B hepatitis. *Lancet*, **i**, 459

57. Tabor, E., Gerety, R. J., Drucker, J. A., Seeff, L. B., Hoofnagle, J. H., Jackson, D. R., Milton, A., Barker, L. F. and Pineda-Tamondong, G. (1978). Transmission of non-A, non-B hepatitis from man to chimpanzees. *Lancet*, **i**, 463

58. Rawls, W. E., Tompkins, W. A. F. and Melnick, J. L. (1969). The association of herpes virus type 2 and carcinoma of the uterine cervix. *Am. J. Epidemiol.*, **89**, 547

59. Nahmias, A. J., Josey, W. E., Naib, Z. M., Luce, C. F. and Guest, B. A. (1970). Herpes virus hominis type 2 infection – association with cervical cancer. *Am. J. Epidemiol.*, **91**, 547

60. Aurelian, L., Royston, I. and Davis, H. J. (1970). Antibody to genital herpes simplex virus – association with cervical atypia and carcinoma *in situ. J. Nat. Cancer Inst.*, **45**, 455

61. Kaufman, H. E. (1963). Treatment of deep hepatic keralitis with IDU and corticosteroids. *Eye, Ear, Nose, Throat Digest*, **25**, 37

62. Stevens, J. G. and Cook, M. L. (1975). Maintenance of latent herpetic infection – an apparent role for anti-viral IgG. *J. Immunol.*, **113**, 1685

63. Stevens, J. G. (1977). Herpes simplex infections as models for latency. In: *Microbiology 1977* (D. Schlesinger, ed.), p. 509 (Washington, D.C.: American Society for Microbiology)

64. Walz, A. M., Price, R. W. and Notkins, A. C. (1975). Latent infection with herpes simplex virus type 1 and 2: viral reactivation *in vivo* after neurectomy. *Science*, **184**, 1185

65. Douglas, R. G. and Couch, R. B. (1970). A prospective study of chronic herpes virus infection and recurrent herpes labialis in humans. *J. Immunol.*, **104**, 289

66. Doerr, H. W., Gross, G., Schmitz, H. and Enders, G. (1976). Neutralizing serum IgM antibodies in infections with herpes simplex virus hominis. *Med. Microbiol. Immunol.*, **162**, 183

67. Nahmias, A. J., Shore, S. L., Kohl, S., Starr, S. E. and Ashman, R. B. (1976). Immunology of herpes simplex virus infection. *Cancer Res.*, **36**, 836

68. Yamamoto, Y. (1966). A re-evaluation of the skin test of herpes simplex virus. *J. Microbiol.*, **10**, 67

69. Nahmias, A. J., Hirsch, M. S., Kramer, J. H. and Murphy, F. (1969). Effect of antithymocyte serum on herpes virus hominis (type 1) infection in adult mice. *Proc. Soc. Exp. Biol. Med.*, **132**, 696

70. Zisman, B., Hirsch, M. S. and Allison, A. C. (1970). Selective effects of anti-macrophage serum, silica, and anti-lymphocyte serum on pathogenesis of herpes virus infection of young adult mice. *J. Immunol.*, **104**, 1155

71. O'Reilly, R. J. and Lopez, C. (1975). Cyclic deficiency of lymphokine production in patients with recurrent herpes labialis or progenitalis. *Fed. Proc.*, **34**, 947

72. Rasmussen, L. E., Jordan, G. W., Stevens, D. A. and Merrigan, T. C. (1974). Lymphocyte interferon production and transformation after herpes simplex infections in humans. *J. Immunol.*, **112**, 728

73. Wilton, J. M., Ivanyi, L. and Lehner, T. (1972). Cell-mediated immunity in herpes virus hominis infections. *Br. Med. J.*, **1**, 723

74. Lopez, C. and O'Reilly, R. J. (1977). Cell-mediated immune responses in recurrent herpes virus infections. I. Lymphocyte proliferation assay. *J. Immunol.*, **118**, 895

75. O'Reilly, R. J., Chibbaro, A., Anger, E. and Lopez, C. (1977). Infection associated deficiency of lymphokine production in patients with recurrent herpes labialis or herpes progenitalis. *J. Immunol.*, **118**, 1095

76. Kohl, S., Starr, S. E., Oleske, J. M., Shore, S. L., Ashman, R. B. and Nahmias, A. J. (1971). Human monocyte-macrophage mediated antibody-dependent cytotoxicity to herpes simplex virus-infected cells. *J. Immunol.*, **118**, 729

77. Shore, S. L., Milgrom, H., Wood, P. A. and Nahmias, A. J. (1977). Antibody-dependent cellular cytotoxicity to target cells infected with herpes simplex viruses: Functional adequacy in the neonate. *Pediatrics*, **59**, 22

78. Russel, A. S. and Kaiser, J. T. (1976). Cell-mediated immunity to herpes simplex virus in man. *J. Allergy Clin. Immunol.*, **58**, 539

79. Heron, I., Moller-Larsen, A. and Berg, K. (1977). Effector cell involved in cell-mediated cytotoxicity to cells infected with herpes simplex type 1 virus. *Infect. Immun.*, **16**, 48

80. Watkins, J. F. (1964). Adsorption of sensitized sheep erythrocytes to HeLa cells infected with herpes simplex virus. *Nature (Lond.)*, **202**, 1364

81. Yasuda, J. and Milmgrom, H. (1968). Hemadsorption of herpes simplex infected cell cultures. *Int. Arch. Allergy Appl. Immunol.*, **1**, 33

82. Costa, J. C. and Rabson, A. L. (1975). Role of Fc receptors in herpes simplex virus infection. *Lancet*, **i**, 77

83. Sasazuki, T., McDevitt, H. O. and Grumet, C. F. (1977). The association between genes in the major histocompatibility complex and disease susceptibility. In: *Annual Review of Medicine: Selected Topics in the Clinical Sciences* (W. Creger, ed.). (Palo Alto, California: Annual Reviews, Inc.)

84. Henle, W. and Henle, G. (1972). Epstein–Barr virus: The cause of infectious mononucleosis. In: *Oncogenesis and Herpesviruses* (I. M. Biggs, G. de The and L. N. Payne, eds.), p. 269 (Lyon, France: International Agency for Research on Cancer)

85. Klein, G. (1976). The Epstein–Barr virus and neoplasia. *N. Engl. J. Med.*, **293**, 1353

86. Miller, G. (1971). Human lymphoblastoid cell lines and Epstein–Barr virus: A review of their interrelationships and their relevance to the etiology of leukoproliferative states in man. *Yale J. Biol. Med.*, **43**, 358

87. Pattengale, P. K., Smith, R. W. and Gerber, P. (1974). B-cell characteristics of human peripheral and cord blood lymphocytes. *J. Nat. Cancer Inst.*, **52**, 1081

88. Schneider, U. and Zur-Hansen, H. (1975). Epstein–Barr induced transformation of human leukocytes after cell-fractionation. *Int. J. Cancer*, **15**, 29

89. Sheldon, P. J., Papamichail, M. and Hemsted, G. (1973). Thymic origin of atypical lymphoid cells in infectious mononucleosis. *Lancet*, **i**, 1153

90. Notkins, A. L. (1974). Immune mechanisms by which the spread of viral infections is stopped. *Cell. Immunol.*, **11**, 478

91. Roysten, I. (1973). Epstein–Barr virus and infectious mononucleosis. *Lancet*, **ii**, 1152

92. Pattengale, P. K., Smith, R. A. and Perlin, E. (1974). Atypical lymphocytes in acute infectious mononucleosis. *N. Engl. J. Med.*, **291**, 1145

93. Guiliano, V. J., Jasin, H. E. and Ziff, M. (1974). The nature of atypical lymphocytes in infectious mononucleosis. *Clin. Immunol. Immunopathol.*, **3**, 90

94. Pagano, J. S. (1974). Epstein–Barr viral genome and its interactions with human lymphoblastoid cells and chromosomes. In: *Viruses, Evolution and Cancer* (K. Maramorosch and E. Kurstak, eds.), pp. 79–116 (New York: Academic Press)

95. Carter, R. L. (1975). Infectious mononucleosis model for self-limiting lymphoproliferation. *Lancet*, **i**, 846

96. Hampar, B., Hsu, K. C., Martos, L. M. and Walker, J. L. (1971). Serologic evidence that

herpes type virus is the etiologic agent of heterophile-positive infectious mononucleosis. *Proc. Nat. Acad. Sci. (Wash.)*, **68**, 1407

97. Schmitz, H. and Scherer, M. (1972). IgM antibodies to Epstein–Barr virus in infectious mononucleosis. *Arch. Gesamte Virusforsch.*, **37**, 332

98. Banatuala, J. E., Best, J. M. and Walker, D. K. (1972). Epstein–Barr virus specific IgM in infectious mononucleosis, Burkitt's lymphoma and nasopharyngeal cancer. *Lancet*, **i**, 1205

99. Neiderman, J. C., McCollum, R. W., Henle, G. and Henle, W. (1968). Infectious mononucleosis – clinical manifestations in relation to EB virus antibodies. *J. Am. Med. Assoc.*, **203**, 205

100. Henle, W., Henle, G., Neiderman, J. C., Halita, K. and Klemola, E. (1971). Antibodies to early antigens induced by Epstein–Barr virus in infectious mononucleosis. *J. Infect. Dis.*, **124**, 58

101. Henle, G., Henle, W. and Horowitz, C. A. (1974). Antibodies to Epstein–Barr virus associated nuclear antigen in infectious mononucleosis. *J. Infect. Dis.*, **130**, 231

102. Evans, A. S., Neiderman, J. C., Cenabre, L. C., West, B. Z. and Richards, V. A. (1975). A prospective evaluation of heterophile and Epstein–Barr virus-specific IgM antibody test in clinical and subclinical infectious mononucleosis: specificity and sensitivity of the tests and persistence of antibody. *J. Infect. Dis.*, **132**, 546

103. Nikoskelainen, J., Leikola, J. and Klemola, E. (1974). IgM antibodies specific for Epstein–Barr virus in infectious mononucleosis without heterophile antibodies. *Br. Med. J.*, **4**, 72

104. Denman, A. M. and Pelton, B. K. (1974). Control mechanisms in infectious mononucleosis. *Clin. Exp. Immunol.*, **18**, 1

105. Svedmyr, E. and Jondal, M. (1975). Cytotoxic effector cells, specific for B-cell lines transformed by Epstein–Barr virus are present in patients with infectious mononucleosis. *Proc. Nat. Acad. Sci. (Wash.)*, **72**, 1622

106. Roysten, I., Sullivan, J. L., Periman, P. O. and Perlin, E. (1975). Cell-mediated immunity to Epstein–Barr virus transformed lymphoblastoid cells in acute infectious mononucleosis. *N. Engl. J. Med.*, **293**, 1159

107. Hutt, L. M., Huang, Y. T., Dascomb, H. E. and Pagano, J. (1975). Enhanced destruction of lymphoid cell lines by peripheral blood leukocytes taken from patients with acute infectious mononucleosis. *J. Immunol.*, **115**, 243

108. Klein, G., Svedmyr, E., Jondal, M. and Persson, P. O. (1976). EBV-determined nuclear antigen (EBNA) positive cells in the peripheral blood of infectious mononucleosis patients. *Int. J. Cancer*, **17**, 21

109. Doherty, P. C., Blanden, R. V. and Zinkernagel, R. M. (1976). Specificity of virus-immune effector T cells for H2K or H2D compatible interaction – implications for H-antigen diversity. *Transplant. Rev.*, **29**, 89

110. Zinkernagel, R. M. and Oldstone, M. B. A. (1976). Cells that express viral antigens but lack H-2 determinants are not lysed by immune thymus-derived lymphocytes but are lysed by other antiviral immune attack mechanisms. *Proc. Nat. Acad. Sci. (Wash.)*, **73**, 3666

111. Tursz, T., Fridman, W. H., Senik, A., Tsapis, A. and Fellous, M. (1977). Human virus-infected target cells lacking HLA antigens resist specific T-lymphocyte cytolysis. *Nature (Lond.)*, **269**, 806

112. Jondal, M. (1976). Antibody-dependent cellular cytotoxicity (ADCC) against Epstein–Barr virus-determined membrane antigens. I. Reactivity in sera from normal persons and from patients with infectious mononucleosis. *Clin. Exp. Immunol.*, **25**, 1

113. Purtilo, D. T., DeFlorio, D., Hutt, L. M., Bhawan, J., Yang, J. P. S., Otto, R. and Edwards, W. (1977). Variable phenotypic expression of an X-linked recessive lymphoproliferative syndrome. *N. Engl. J. Med.*, **297**, 1077

114. Sumaya, C. V. (1977). Endogenous reactivation of Epstein–Barr virus infections. *J. Infect. Dis.*, **155**, 374

115. Starr, J. G., Bart, R. D. Jr. and Gold, E. (1970). Inapparent congenital cytomegalovirus infection: clinical and epidemiological characteristics in early infancy. *N. Engl. J. Med.*, **282**, 1075

116. Melish, M. E. and Hanshaw, J. B. (1973). Congenital cytomegalovirus infection. Developmental progress of infants detected by routine screening. *Am. J. Dis. Child.*, **126**, 190

117. Hanshaw, J. (1971). Congenital cytomegalovirus infection: A fifteen-year prospective. *J. Infect. Dis.*, **123**, 555

118. Levinshon, E. M., Foy, H. M., Kenny, G. E., Wentworth, B. B. and Grayston, J. T. (1969). Isolation of cytomegalovirus from cohort of 100 infants throughout first years of life. *Proc. Soc. Exp. Biol. Med.*, **132**, 957

119. Reynolds, D. W., Stagno, S., Hosty, T. S., Tiller, M. and Alford, C. A. Jr. (1973). Maternal cytomegalovirus excretion and perinatal infection. *N. Engl. J. Med.*, **289**, 1

120. Numazaki, Y., Yano, N., Morizuka, T., Takai, S. and Ishida, N. (1970). Primary infection with human cytomegalovirus: virus isolation from healthy infants and pregnant women. *Am. J. Epidemiol.*, **91**, 410

121. Hays, K., Danks, D. M. and Gibas, H. (1972). Cytomegalovirus in human milk. *N. Engl. J. Med.*, **287**, 177

122. Reynolds, D. W., Stagno, S., Stubbs, K. G., Dahle, A. J., Livingston, M. M., Saxon, S. S. and Alford, C. A. Jr. (1974). Inapparent congenital cytomegalovirus infection with elevated cord IgM levels. *N. Engl. J. Med.*, **290**, 291

123. Olding, I. B., Jensen, F. C. and Oldstone, M. B. (1975). A pathogenesis of cytomegalovirus infection. I. Activation of virus from bone marrow derived lymphocytes by *in vitro* allogenic reaction. *J. Exp. Med.*, **141**, 561

124. Starr, S. E. (1976). Murine cytomegalovirus infection in nude mice. *Clin. Res.*, **24**, 69a

125. Gardner, M. B., Officer, J. E., Parker, J., Estes, J. D. and Rongey, R. W. (1974). Induction of disseminated virulent cytomegalovirus infection by immunosuppression of naturally chronically infected wild mice. *Infect. Immun.*, **10**, 966

126. Booss, J. and Wheelock, E. F. (1977). Progressive inhibition of T-cell function preceding clinical signs of cytomegalovirus infection in mice. *J. Infect. Dis.*, **135**, 478

127. Rola-Pleszczynski, M., Frenkel, L. D., Fucillo, D. A., Hensen, S. A., Vincent, M. M., Reynolds, D. W., Stagno, S. and Bellanti, J. A. (1977). Specific impairment of cell-mediated immunity in mothers of infants with congenital infection due to cytomegalovirus. *J. Infect. Dis.*, **135**, 386

128. Diamond, R. D., Keller, R., Lee, G. and Finkel, D. (1977). Lysis of cytomegalovirus-infected human fibroblasts and transformed human cells by peripheral blood lymphoid cells from normal human donors. *Proc. Soc. Exp. Biol. Med.*, **154**, 259

129. Schauf, V., Strelkauskas, A. J. and Deveikis, A. (1976). Alteration of lymphocyte subpopulation with cytomegalovirus infections in infancy. *Clin. Exp. Immunol.*, **26**, 478

130. Schmitz, H. and Enders, G. (1977). Cytomegalovirus as a frequent cause of Guillain-Barré syndrome. *J. Med. Virol.*, **1**, 21

131. Dowling, P. D., Menonna, J. and Cook, S. (1977). Cytomegalovirus complement fixation antibody in Guillain-Barré syndrome. *Neurology*, **27**, 1153

132. Hope-Simpson, R. E. (1965). The nature of herpes zoster: a long-term study and new hypothesis. *Proc. R. Soc. Med.*, **58**, 9

133. Esiri, M. M. and Tomilson, A. H. (1972). Herpes zoster: demonstration of virus in trigeminal nerve and ganglion by immunofluorescence and electron microscopy. *J. Neurol. Sci.*, **15**, 35

134. Ghatak, N. R. and Zimmerman, H. M. (1973). Spinal ganglion in herpes zoster: a light and electromicroscopic study. *Arch. Pathol.*, **95**, 411

135. Caunt, A. E. and Shaw, D. G. (1969). Neutralization tests with varicella-zoster virus. *J. Hyg.*, **67**, 343

136. Schmidt, N. J., Lennette, E. H., Woodie, J. D. and Ho, H. H. (1965). Immunofluorescent staining in the laboratory diagnosis of varicella-zoster virus infections. *J. Lab. Clin. Med.*, **66**, 403

137. Furukawa, T. and Plotkin, S. A. (1972). Indirect hemagglutination test for varicella-zoster infection. *Infect. Immun.*, **5**, 835

138. Palosuo, T. (1972). Varicella and herpes zoster: differences in antibody response revealed by the platelet aggregation technique. *Scand. J. Infect. Dis.*, **4**, 83

139. Williams, V., Gershon, A. A. and Brunell, P. A. (1974). Serologic response to varicella-zoster membrane antigens measured by indirect immunofluorescence. *J. Infect. Dis.*, **130**, 699

140. Ross, C. A. and McDaid, R. (1972). Specific IgM antibody in serum of patients with herpes zoster infection. *Br. Med. J.*, **4**, 522

141. Leonard, L. L., Schmidt, N. J. and Lennette, E. H. (1970). Demonstration of viral antibody activity in two immunoglobulin G subclasses in patients with varicella-zoster infection. *J. Immunol.*, **104**, 23

142. Russell, A. S., Maini, R. A., Bailey, M. and Dumondi, D. C. (1972). Cell-mediated immunity to varicella-zoster antigen in acute herpes zoster (shingles). *Clin. Exp. Immunol.*, **14**, 181

143. Jordon, G. W. and Merigan, T. C. (1974). Cell-mediated immunity to varicella-zoster virus: *in vitro* lymphocyte response. *J. Infect. Dis.*, **130**, 495

144. Rowe, W. P., Huebner, R. J., Gilmore, L. K., Parrot, R. M. and Ward, T. G. (1953). Isolation of a cytopathogenic agent from human adenoids undergoing spontaneous degeneration in tissue culture. *Proc. Soc. Exp. Biol. Med.*, **84**, 570

145. Hilleman, M. R. and Werner, J. H. (1954). Recovery of new agents from patients with acute respiratory illness. *Proc. Soc. Exp. Biol. Med.*, **85**, 183

146. Strohl, W. A. and Schleinger, R. W. (1965). Quantitive studies of natural and experimental adenovirus infection of human cells. II. Primary cultures and the possible role of asynchronous viral multiplication in the maintenance of infection. *Virology*, **26**, 208

147. Evans, A. S. (1958). Latent adenovirus infections of the human respiratory tract. *Am. J. Hyg.*, **67**, 256

148. Asher, D. M., Hooks, J. J., Amyx, H. L., Luber, N. P., Asher, L. V. S., Gibbs, C. J. Jr. and Gajdusek, D. C. (1978). Persistent shedding of adenovirus in the urine of chimpanzees. *Infect. Immun.*, **21**, 129

149. Asher, L. V. S., Asher, D. M., Shah, K. V., Amyx, H. L., Gibbs, C. J. Jr. and Gajdusek, D. C. (1978). Antibodies in urine of chimpanzees with chronic adenoviral viruria. *Infect. Immun.*, **21**, 458

150. Roos, R., Chou, S. M., Rogers, N. G., Basnight, M. and Gajdusek, D. C. (1972). Isolation of an adenovirus 32 strain from human brain in a case of subacute encephalitis. *Proc. Soc. Exp. Biol. Med.*, **139**, 636

151. Zu Rhein, G. and Varakis, J. (1974). Progressive multifocal leukoencephalopathy in a renal allograft regiment. *N. Engl. J. Med.*, **291**, 798

152. Padgett, B. L., Zu Rhein, G. M., Walker, D. L., Eckroade, R. J. and Dessel, B. H. (1971). Cultivation of papova-like virus from human brain with progressive multifocal leuko-encephalopathy. *Lancet*, **i** (7712), 1257

153. Weiner, L. P., Herndon, R. M., Narayan, O., Johnson, R. T., Shah, K., Rubinstein, L. J., Preziosi, T. J. and Conley, F. K. (1972). Isolation of virus related to SV-40 from patients with progressive multifocal leukoencephalopathy. *N. Engl. J. Med.*, **286**, 385

154. Gardner, S. D., Field, A., Coleman, D. and Hulme, B. (1971). New human papovavirus (BK) isolated from urine after renal transplantation. *Lancet*, **i** (7712), 1253

155. Shah, K. V., Ozer, H. L., Pond, H. S., Palma, L. D. and Murphy, G. P. (1971). SV-40

neutralizing antibodies in sera of US residents without history of polio immunization. *Nature (Lond.)*, **231**, 448

156. Gardner, S. D. (1973). Prevalence in England of antibody to human polyomavirus (BK). *Br. Med. J.*, **1**, 77

157. Shah, K. V., Daniel, R. W. and Warszawski, R. M. (1973). High prevalence of antibodies to BK virus, an SV-40 related papovavirus in residents of Maryland. *J. Infect. Dis.*, **128**, 784

158. Padgett, B. L. and Walker, D. L. (1973). Prevalence of antibodies in human sera against JC virus, an isolate from a case of progressive multifocal leukoencephalopathy. *J. Infect. Dis.*, **127**, 467

159. Brown, P., Tsai, T. and Gajdusek, D. C. (1975). Seroepidemiology of human papovaviruses. Discovery of virgin population and some unusual patterns of antibody prevalence among remote peoples of the world. *Am. J. Epidemiol.*, **102**, 331

160. Brody, J. A. and Gibbs, C. J. Jr. (1976). Chronic neurological diseases. In: *The Viral Infections of Human Epidemiology and Control* (A. S. Evans, ed.), pp. 519–537 (New York and London: Plenum Book Company)

161. Horta-Barbosa, L., Fuccillo, D. A. and Sever, J. L. (1969). Subacute sclerosing panencephalitis: isolation of measles virus from a brain biopsy. *Nature (Lond.)*, **221**, 974

162. Payne, F. E., Baublis, J. V. and Itabashi, H. H. (1969). Isolation of measles virus from cell cultures of brain from a patient with subacute sclerosing panencephalitis. *N. Engl. J. Med.*, **281**, 585

163. ter Meulen, V., Katz, M. and Muller, D. (1972). Subacute sclerosing panencephalitis: a review. *Curr. Top. Microbiol. Immunol.*, **57**, 1

164. Connolly, J. H., Allen, I. V., Hurwitz, L. J. and Millar, H. D. (1967). Measles virus antibody and antigen in subacute sclerosing panencephalitis. *Lancet*, **i**, 542

165. Legg, N. J. (1967). Virus antibodies in subacute sclerosing panencephalitis: a study of 22 patients. *Br. Med. J.*, **3**, 350

166. Griffith, J. F. and Katz, S. L. (1968). Subacute sclerosing panencephalitis, laboratory findings in six cases. *Neurology*, **18**, 95

167. Adels, B. R., Gajdusek, D. C., Gibbs, C. J. Jr., Albrecht, P. and Rogers, N. (1968). Attempts to transmit subacute sclerosing panencephalitis and isolate a measles-related agent, with a study of the immune response in patients and experimental animals. *Neurology*, **18**, 30

168. Kennedy, C. (1968). A ten-year experience with subacute sclerosing panencephalitis. *Neurology*, **18**, 58

169. Sever, J. L. and Zeman, W. (1968). Serological studies of measles and subacute sclerosing panencephalitis. *Neurology*, **18**, 95

170. Berman, P. H., Giles, J. P. and Krugman, S. (1968). Correlation of measles and subacute sclerosing panencephalitis. *Neurology*, **18**, 91

171. Connolly, J. H. (1968). Additional data on measles virus antibody and antigen in subacute sclerosing panencephalitis. *Neurology*, **18**, 87

172. Kolar, O. (1968). Immunopathologic observations in subacute sclerosing panencephalitis. *Neurology*, **18**, 107

173. Tourtellotte, W. W., Parker, J. A., Herdon, R. M. and Cuadros, C. V. (1968). Subacute sclerosing panencephalitis: brain immunoglobulin-G, measles antibody and albumin. *Neurology*, **18**, 117

174. Cutler, R. W. P., Merler, E. and Hammerstad, J. P. (1968). Production of antibody by the central nervous system in subacute sclerosing panencephalitis. *Neurology*, **18**, 129

175. Salmi, A. A., Norrby, E. and Panelius, M. (1972). Identification of different measles virus specific antibodies in the serum and cerebrospinal fluid from patients with subacute sclerosing panencephalitis and multiple sclerosis. *Infect. Immun.*, **6**, 248

176. Booij, J. (1959). Agar-agar electrophoresis as an aid in cerebrospinal fluid diagnostics. *Folia Psychiatr. Neurol. Jpn.*, **62**, 37

177. Lowenthal, A. (1964). Agar gel electrophoresis in neurology. In: *Neurology* (Amsterdam: Elsevier Press, Inc.), pp. 1–204

178. Link, H., Panelius, M. and Salmi, A. A. (1973). Immunoglobulins and measles antibodies in subacute sclerosing panencephalitis. *Arch. Neurol.*, **28**, 23

179. Vandvik, B. and Norrby, E. (1973). Oligoclonal IgG antibody response in the central nervous system to different measles virus antigens in subacute sclerosing panencephalitis. *Proc. Nat. Acad. Sci.*, **70**, 1060

180. Norrby, E. and Vandvik, B. (1975). Relationship between measles virus-specific antibody activities and oligoclonal IgG in the central nervous system of patients with subacute sclerosing panencephalitis and multiple sclerosis. *Med. Microbiol. Immunol.*, **162**, 63

181. Vandvik, T., Norrby, E., Nordal, H. J. and Degre, M. (1976). Oligoclonal measles virus-specific IgG antibodies isolated from cerebrospinal fluids, brain extracts and sera from patients with subacute sclerosing panencephalitis and multiple sclerosis. *Scand. J. Immunol.*, **5**, 979

182. Connolly, J. H., Haire, M. and Hadden, D. S. M. (1971). Measles immunoglobulins in subacute sclerosing panencephalitis. *Br. Med. J.*, **1**, 23

183. Luster, M. I., Armen, R. C., Hallum, J. V. and Leslie, G. A. (1976). Measles virus-specific IgD antibodies in patients with subacute sclerosing panencephalitis. *Proc. Nat. Acad. Sci.*, **73**, 1297

184. ter Meulen, V., Muller, D. and Joppich, G. (1969). Immunohistological, microscopical and neurochemical studies on encephalitides. *Acta Neuropathol.*, **12**, 244

185. Vandvik, B. (1973). Immunopathological aspects in the pathogenesis of subacute sclerosing panencephalitis, with special reference to the significance of the immune response in the central nervous system. *Ann. Clin. Res.*, **5**, 308

186. Minagawa, T. and Yamada, M. (1971). Studies on the persistent infection with measles virus in HeLa cells. III. Immunolysis of cells in carrier state by anti-measles sera. *Jpn. J. Microbiol.*, **15**, 341

187. Kibler, R., Deller, A. and ter Meulen, V. (1974). Cytotoxic antibody activity in measles and subacute sclerosing panencephalitis (SSPE) infection. *Med. Microbiol. Immunol.*, **160**, 179

188. Oldstone, M. B. A., Bokisch, V. A., Dixon, I. J., Barbosa, L. H., Fucillo, D. and Sever, J. L. (1975). Subacute sclerosing panencephalitis: destruction of human brain cells by antibody and complement in an autologous system. *Clin. Immunol. Immunopathol.*, **4**, 52

189. Joseph, B. S., Cooper, N. R. and Oldstone, M. B. A. (1975). Immunologic injury of cultured cells infected with measles virus. I. Role of IgG antibody and the alternative complement pathway. *J. Exp. Med.*, **141**, 761

190. Joseph, B. S., Perrin, L. H. and Oldstone, M. B. A. (1976). Measurement of virus antigens on the surfaces of HeLa cells persistently infected with wild type and vaccine strains of measles virus by radioimmune assay. *J. Gen. Virol.*, **30**, 329

191. Joseph, B. S. and Oldstone, M. B. A. (1975). Immunologic injury in measles virus infection. II. Suppression of immune injury through antigenic modulation. *J. Exp. Med.*, **142**, 864

192. Dayan, A. D. and Stokes, M. I. (1972). Immune complexes and viceral deposits of measles antigens in subacute sclerosing panencephalitis. *Br. Med. J.*, **2**, 374

193. Philips, P. E. (1972). Immune complexes in subacute sclerosing panencephalitis. *N. Engl. J. Med.*, **286**, 949

194. Burnet, F. M. (1968). Measles as an index of immunological function. *Lancet*, **ii**, 610

195. Gerson, K. L. and Haslam, R. H. A. (1971). Subtle immunologic abnormalities in four boys with subacute sclerosing panencephalitis. *N. Engl. J. Med.*, **285**, 78

196. Moulias, R. S., Reinert, P. and Goust, J. M. (1971). Immunologic abnormalities in SSPE. *N. Engl. J. Med.*, **285**, 1099

197. Vandvik, B. (1970). Immunologic studies in subacute sclerosing panencephalitis. *Acta Neurol. Scand. Suppl.*, **46** (Suppl. 43), 232

198. Lischner, H. W., Grover, W. D. and De Forest, A. (1971). Proliferative response of lymphocytes to measles antigen in tissue culture in subacute sclerosing panencephalitis (SSPE). In: *Proceedings of the Fourth Annual Leukocyte Culture Conference* (O. R. McIntyre, ed.), p. 565 (New York: Appleton-Century-Crofts)

199. Sharma, M. K, Grover, W. D. and Huff, D. S. (1971). Studies of immunologic competence in subacute sclerosing panencephalitis (SSPE). *Clin. Res.*, **19**, 730

200. Saunders, M., Knowles, M., Chambers, M. E. and Caspary, E. A. (1969). Cellular and humoral responses to measles in subacute sclerosing panencephalitis. *Lancet*, **i**, 72

201. Mizutani, H., Saito, S., Nihei, K. and Izuchi, T. (1971). Cellular hypersensitivity in subacute sclerosing panencephalitis. *J. Am. Med. Assoc.*, **216**, 1201

202. Thurman, G. B., Ahmed, A., Strong, D. M., Knudsen, R. C., Grace, W. R. and Sell, K. W. (1973). Lymphocyte activation in subacute sclerosing panencephalitis virus and cytomegalovirus infections: in vitro stimulation in response to viral-infected cell lines. *J. Exp. Med.*, **138**, 839

203. Ahmed, A., Strong, D. M., Sell, K. W., Thurman, G. B., Knudsen, R. C., Wistar, R. Jr. and Grace, W. R. (1974). Demonstration of a blocking factor in the plasma and spinal fluid of patients with subacute sclerosing panencephalitis. I. Partial characterization. *J. Exp. Med.*, **139**, 902

204. Kreth, H. W., Kaeckell, Y. M. and ter Meulen, V. (1974). Cellular immunity in SSPE patients. *Med. Microbiol. Immunol.*, **160**, 191

205. Kreth, W. H., Kaeckell, Y. M. and ter Meulen, V. (1975). Demonstration of in vitro lymphocyte-mediated cytotoxicity against measles virus in SSPE. *J. Immunol.*, **114**(3), 1042

206. Steele, R. W., Fuccillo, D. A., Hensen, S. A., Vincent, M. M. and Bellanti, J. A. (1976). Specific inhibitory factors of cellular immunity in children with subacute sclerosing panencephalitis. *J. Pediatr.*, **88**(1), 56

207. Perrin, L. H., Tishon, A. and Oldstone, M. B. A. (1977). Immunologic injury in measles virus infection. III. Presence and characterization of human cytotoxic lymphocytes. *J. Immunol.*, **118**(1), 282

208. Sell, K. W., Thurmond, G. B. and Ahmed, A. (1973). Plasma and spinal fluid blocking factor in SSPE. *N. Engl. J. Med.*, **228**, 215

209. Allen, J., Oppenheim, J. J., Brody, J. A. and Miller, J. (1973). Labile inhibitor of lymphocyte transformation in plasma from a patient with subacute sclerosing panencephalitis. *Infect. Immun.*, **8**, 80

210. Swick, H., Brooks, W. H., Roszman, T. L. and Caldwell, P. (1976). A heat-stable blocking factor in the plasma of patients with subacute sclerosing panencephalitis. *Neurology*, **26**, 84

211. Kreth, H. W. and ter Meulen, V. (1977a). Cell-mediated cytotoxicity against measles virus in SSPE. I. Enhancement by antibody. *J. Immunol.*, **118**(1), 291

212. Kreth, H. W. and Wiegand, G. (1977b). Cell-mediated cytotoxicity against measles virus in SSPE. II. Analysis of cytotoxic effector cells. *J. Immunol.*, **118**, 296

213. Wear, D. J. and Rapp, F. (1971). Latent measles infection of the hamster central nervous system. *J. Immunol.*, **107**, 1593

214. Byington, D. P. and Johnson, K. P. (1972). Experimental subacute sclerosing panencephalitis in the hamster: correlation of age with chronic inclusion-cell encephalitis. *J. Infect. Dis.*, **126**, 18

215. Johnson, K. P. and Norrby, E. (1974). Subacute sclerosing panencephalitis (SSPE) agent in hamsters. III. Induction of defective measles infection in hamster brain. *Exp. Mol. Pathol.*, **21**, 166

216. Katz, M., Rorke, L. B., Masland, W. S., Koprowski, H. and Tucker, S. H. (1968). Trans-

mission of an encephalitogenic agent from brains of patients with subacute sclerosing panencephalitis to ferrets. Preliminary report. *N. Engl. J. Med.*, **279**, 793

217. Notermans, S. L. H., Tijl, W. F. J., Willems, F. T. C. and Slooff, J. L. (1973). Experimentally induced subacute sclerosing panencephalitis in young dogs. *Neurology*, **23**, 543

218. Thormar, H., Jervis, G. A., Karl, S. C. and Brown, H. R. (1973). Passage in ferrets of encephalitogenic cell-associated measles virus isolated from brain of a patient with subacute sclerosing panencephalitis. *J. Infect. Dis.*, **127**, 678

219. Albrecht, P., Shabo, A. L., Burns, G. R. and Tauraso, N. M. (1972). Experimental measles encephalitis in normal and cyclophosphamide-treated rhesus monkeys. *J. Infect. Dis.*, **126**, 154

220. Weil, M. L., Itabashi, H. H. and Carnay, L. (1975). Chronic progressive panencephalitis due to rubella virus simulating subacute sclerosing panencephalitis. *N. Engl. J. Med.*, **292**, 994

221. Townsend, J. J., Barringer, J. R., Wolinsky, J. S., Malamud, N., Mednick, J. P., Panitch, H. S., Scott, R. A. T., Oskira, L. S. and Cremer, N. E. (1975). Progressive rubella panencephalitis. *N. Engl. J. Med.*, **292**, 990

222. Bellanti, J. A., Artenstein, M. S., Olson, L. C. and Buescher, E. L. (1965). Congenital rubella, clinicopathologic, virologic and immunologic studies. *Am. J. Dis. Child.*, **110**, 464

223. Menser, M. A., Harley, J. D., Hertzberg, R., Dorman, D. C. and Murphy, A. M. (1967). Persistence of virus in the lens for three years after prenatal rubella. *Lancet*, **ii**, 387

224. Simons, M. J. and Fitzgerald, M. G. (1968). Rubella virus and human lymphocytes in culture. *Lancet*, **ii**, 937

225. Alford, C. A. Jr., Neva, F. A. and Weller, T. H. (1964). Virologic and serologic studies on human products of conception after maternal rubella. *N. Engl. J. Med.*, **271**, 1275

226. Rawls, W. E. and Melnick, J. L. (1966). Rubella virus carrier cultures derived from congenitally infected infants. *J. Exp. Med.*, **123**, 795

227. Rawls, W. E., Phillips, C. A., Melnick, J. L. and Desmond, M. M. (1967). Persistent virus infection in congenital rubella. *Arch. Ophthal. (Chicago)*, **77**, 430

228. Lindquist, J. M., Plotkin, S. A., Shaw, L., Gilden, R. V. and Williams, M. L. (1965). Congenital rubella syndrome as a systemic infection. Studies of affected infants born in Philadelphia (USA). *Br. Med. J.*, **2**, 1401

229. Cooper, L. Z. and Krugman, S. (1967). Clinical manifestations of postnatal and congenital rubella. *Arch. Ophthal.*, **77**, 434

230. Plotkin, S. A., Cochran, W., Lindquist, J. M., Cochran, G. G., Shaffer, D. B., Scheie, H. G. and Furukawa, T. (1967). Congenital rubella syndrome in late infancy. *J. Am. Med. Assoc.*, **200**, 435

231. Soothill, J. F., Hayes, K. and Dudgeon, J. A. (1966). Immunoglobulin in congenital rubella. *Lancet*, **i**, 1385

232. Alford, C. A. Jr. (1965). Studies on antibody in congenital rubella infections. I. Physicochemical and immunologic investigations of rubella-neutralizing antibody. *Am. J. Dis. Child.*, **110**, 455

233. Butler, N. R., Dudgeon, J. A., Hayes, K., Peckham, C. S. and Wybar, K. (1965). Persistence of rubella antibody with and without embryopathy. *Br. Med. J.*, **2**, 1027

234. Stiehm, E. R., Amann, A. J. and Cherry, J. P. (1966). Elevated cord macroglobulins in the diagnosis of intrauterine infections. *N. Engl. J. Med.*, **275**, 971

235. Alford, C. A. Jr., Schaefer, J., Blankenship, W. J., Straumfjord, J. V. and Cassody, G. (1967). A correlative immunologic, microbiologic and clinical approach to the diagnosis of acute and chronic infections in newborn infants. *N. Engl. J. Med.*, **277**, 437

236. McCracken, G. H., Hardy, J. B., Chen, T. C., Hoffman, L. S., Sever, J. L. and Gilkson, M. R. (1969). Serum immunoglobulin levels in newborn infants. II. Survey of cord and follow-up sera from 123 infants with congenital rubella. *J. Pediatr.*, **74**(3), 383

237. Michaels, R. H. (1969). Immunologic aspects of congenital rubella. *Pediatrics*, **43**, 339

238. Singer, D. B., South, M. A., Montgomery, J. R. and Rawls, W. E. (1969). Congenital rubella syndrome. Lymphoid tissue and immunologic function. *Am. J. Dis. Child.*, **118**, 54

239. Hancock, M. P., Huntley, C. C. and Sever, J. L. (1968). Congenital rubella syndrome with immunoglobulin disorder. *J. Pediatr.*, **72**, 636

240. Schimke, R. N., Boland, C. and Kirkpatrick, C. H. (1969). Immunologic deficiency in the congenital rubella syndrome. *Am. J. Dis. Child.*, **118**, 626

241. Claman, H. N., Suratte, V., Githens, J. H. and Hathaway, W. E. (1970). Histocytic reaction in dysgammaglobulinemia and congenital rubella. *Pediatrics*, **46**, 89

242. Vesikari, T. (1972). Immune response in rubella infections. *Scand. J. Infect. Dis.*, **4** (Suppl.), 1

243. Michaels, R. H. (1972). Suppression of antibody response in congenital rubella. *J. Pediatr.*, **80**, 583

244. White, L. R. and Leikin, S. (1968). Immune competence in congenital rubella: lymphocyte transformation, delayed hypersensitivity and response to vaccination. *J. Pediatr.*, **73**, 229

245. Olson, G. B., South, M. A. and Good, R. A. (1967). Phytohaemagglutinin unresponsiveness of lymphocytes from babies with congenital rubella. *Nature (Lond.)*, **214**, 695

246. Montgomery, J. R., South, M. A., Rawls, W. E., Melnick, J. L., Olson, G. B., Dent, P. B. and Good, R. A. (1967). Viral inhibition of lymphocyte response to phytohaemagglutinin. *Science*, **157**, 1068

247. Olson, G. B., Dent, P. B., Rawls, W. E., South, M. A., Montgomery, J. R., Melnick, J. L. and Good, R. A. (1968). Abnormalities of *in vitro* lymphocyte responses during rubella virus infections. *J. Exp. Med.*, **128**, 47

248. Marshall, W. C., Cope, W. A., Soothill, J. F. and Dudgeon, J. A. (1970). *In vitro* lymphocyte response in some immunity deficiency diseases and in intrauterine virus infections. *Proc. R. Soc. Med.*, **63**, 351

249. Fuccillo, D. A., Steele, R. W., Hensen, S. A., Vincent, M. M., Hardy, J. B. and Bellanti, J. A. (1974). Impaired cellular immunity to rubella virus in congenital rubella. *Infect. Immun.*, **9**, 81

250. Rawls, W. E., Desmyter, J. and Melnick, J. L. (1968). Virus carrier cells and virus-free cells in fetal rubella. *Proc. Soc. Exp. Biol. Med.*, **129**, 477

251. McAllister, R. M., Nicolson, M., Gardner, M. B., Rongey, R. W., Rasheed, S., Sarma, D. S., Huebner, R. J., Hatanaka, M., Oroszlan, S., Gilden, R. V., Kabigting, A. and Vernon, L. (1972). C-type virus released from human cultured rhabdomyosarcoma cells. *Nature New Biol.*, **235**, 3

252. Hooks, J. J. and Gibbs, C. J. Jr. (1975). The foamy viruses. *Bacteriol. Rev.*, **39**, 169

253. Young, D., Samuels, J. and Clarke, J. K. (1973). A foamy virus of possible human origin isolated in BHK-21 cells. *Arch. Gesamte Virusforsch.*, **42**, 228

254. Achong, B. G., Mansell, P. W. A., Epstein, M. A. and Clifford, P. (1971). An unusual virus in cultures from a human nasopharyngeal carcinoma. *J. Nat. Cancer Inst.*, **46**, 299

255. Balayan, M. S. (1977). (Personal communication)

256. Nemo, G. J., Brown, P. W., Gibbs, C. J. Jr. and Gajdusek, D. C. (1978). Antigenic relationship of human foamy virus to the simian foamy viruses. *Infect. Immun.*, **20**, 69

257. Brown, P., Nemo, G. and Gajdusek, D. C. (1978). Human foamy virus: further characterization, seroepidemiology, and relationship to chimpanzee foamy viruses. *J. Infect. Dis.*, **137**, 421

258. Nemo, G. J., Oda, H., Balayan, M. S., Gibbs, C. J. Jr. and Gajdusek, D. C. (1978). Characterization of a foamy virus isolated from a Burkitt's lymphoma patient. *Proc. 78th Ann. Mtg. Am. Soc. Microbiol.*, p. 265

259. Hooks, J. J., Burns, W. H., Hayashi, K., Geis, S. and Notkins, A. L. (1976). Viral spread in the presence of neutralizing antibody: mechanisms of persistence in foamy virus infection. *Infect. Immun.*, **14**, 1172

260. Hooks, J. J. and Detrick-Hooks, B. (1977). Foamy virus induced immunosuppression. *J. Gen. Virol.* (In press)

261. Gibbs, C. J. Jr. and Gajdusek, D. C. (1969). Infection as the aetiology of spongiform encephalopathies (Creutzfeldt–Jakob disease). *Science*, **165**, 3897, 1023–1025
262. Gajdusek, D. C. (1977). Unconventional viruses and the origin and disappearance of kuru. In: *Les Prix Nobel en 1967*, pp. 161–216 (Stockholm: The Nobel Foundation, P. A. Norstedt and Soner)
263. Beck, E., Daniel, P. M., Asher, D. M., Gajdusek, D. C. and Gibbs, C. J. Jr. (1973). Experimental kuru in the chimpanzee: a neuropathological study. *Brain*, **96**, 441–462 (plus plates)
264. Beck, E., Bak, I. J., Christ, J. F., Gajdusek, D. C., Gibbs, C. J. Jr. and Hassler, R. (1975). Experimental kuru in the spider monkey. Histopathological and ultrastructural studies of the brain during early stages of incubation. *Brain*, **98**, 592–612 (plus plates)
265. Gajdusek, D. C. (1973). Kuru in the New Guinea highlands. In: *Tropical Neurology* (J. D. Spillane, ed.), pp. 376–383 and plates 29–31 (London: Oxford University Press)
266. Gajdusek, D. C. (1977). Unconventional viruses and the origin and disappearance of kuru. *Science*, **197**, 943
267. Gajdusek, D. C. and Gibbs, C. J. Jr. (1975). Familial and sporadic chronic neurological degenerative disorders transmitted from man to primates. In: *Primate Models of Neurological Disorders, Proceedings of the Symposium on Primate Models of Neurological Disorders, Institute of Psychiatry, London, August 28–30, 1974* (B. S. Meldrum and C. D. Marsden, eds.), *Advances in Neurology*, vol. 10, pp. 291–317 (New York: Raven Press)
268. Klatzo, I., Gajdusek, D. C. and Zigas, V. (1959). Pathology of kuru disease. *Lab. Invest.*, **8**, 799
269. Beck, E., Daniel, P. M., Matthews, W. B., Stevens, D. L., Alpers, M. P., Asher, D. M., Gajdusek, D. C. and Gibbs, C. J. Jr. (1969). Creutzfeldt–Jakob disease: the neuropathology of a transmission experiment. *Brain*, **92**, 699
270. Gibbs, C. J. Jr. and Gajdusek, D. C. (1976). Studies on the viruses of subacute spongiform encephalopathies using primates their only available indicator. In: *Proceedings of the First Inter-American Conference on Conservation and Utilization of American Nonhuman Primates in Biomedical Research, Lima, Peru, June 2–4, 1975*. Scientific Publication No. 317, pp. 83–109 (Washington, D.C.: Pan American Health Organization)
271. Lampert, P. W., Gajdusek, D. C. and Gibbs, C. J. Jr. (1972). Subacute spongiform virus encephalopathies. Scrapie, kuru and Creutzfeldt–Jakob disease. *Am. J. Pathol.*, **68**, 626
272. Traub, R., Gajdusek, D. C. and Gibbs, C. J. Jr. (1977). Transmissible virus dementias. The relation of transmissible spongiform encephalopathy to Creutzfeldt–Jakob disease. In: *Aging and Dementia* (M. Kinsbourne and L. Smith, eds.), pp. 91–172 (Flushing, New York: Spectrum Publications, Inc.)
273. Beck, E., Daniel, P. M. and Parry, H. B. (1964). Degeneration of the cerebellar and hypothalamo-neurohypophysical systems in sheep with scrapie; and its relationship to human system degenerations. *Brain*, **87**, 153
274. Dickinson, A. G. (1976). Scrapie in sheep and goats. In: *Slow Virus Diseases of Animals and Man* (R. H. Kimberlin, ed.), pp. 267–305 (Amsterdam: Elsevier)
275. Fraser, H. (1976). The pathology of natural and experimental scrapie. In: *Slow Virus Diseases of Animals and Man* (R. H. Kimberlin, ed.), pp. 267–305 (Amsterdam: Elsevier)
276. Hadlow, W. J. (1961). The pathology of experimental scrapie in the dairy goat. *Res. Vet. Sci.*, **2**, 289
277. Hourrigan, J. L. (1965). The scrapie eradication program. In: *Slow, Latent and Temperate Virus Infections* (D. C. Gajdusek, C. J. Gibbs, Jr. and M. Alpers, eds.), NINDB Monograph No. 2, pp. 263–272 (Washington, D.C.: U.S. Government Printing Office)
278. Hartsough, G. R. and Burger, D. J. (1965). Encephalopathy of mink. I. Epizootiologic and clinical observations. *J. Infect. Dis.*, **115**, 387

279. Marsh, R. F. (1974). Slow virus diseases of the central nervous system. *Adv. Vet. Sci. Comp. Med.*, **18**, 155

280. Gibbs, C. J. Jr. and Gajdusek, D. C. (1978). Atypical viruses as the cause of sporadic, epidemic, and familial chronic diseases in man. In: *Perspectives in Virology* (M. Pollard, ed.), vol. 10, pp. 161–198 (New York: Raven Press)

281. Gibbs, C. J. Jr. (1967). Search for infectious etiology in chronic and subacute degenerative diseases of the central nervous system. *Curr. Top. Microbiol. Immunol.*, **40**, 44

282. Hotchin, J. and Buckley, R. (1977). Latent form of scrapie virus: A new factor in slow-virus disease. *Science*, **196**, 668

283. McFarlin, D. E., Raff, M. C., Simpson, E. and Nehlsen, S. H. (1971). Scrapie in immunologically deficient mice. *Nature (Lond.)*, **223**, 336

284. Marsh, R. F., Pan, I. C. and Hanson, R. P. (1970). Failure to demonstrate specific antibody in transmissible mink encephalopathy. *Infect. Immun.*, **2**, 727

285. Pattison, I. H., Millson, G. C. and Smith, K. (1964). An examination of the action of whole blood, blood cells, or serum on the goat scrapie agent. *Res. Vet. Sci.*, **5**, 116

286. Porter, D. D., Porter, H. G. and Cox, N. A. (1973). Failure to demonstrate immune response to scrapie infection in mice. *J. Immunol.*, **111**, 1407

287. Asher, D. M., Gibbs, C. J. Jr. and Gajdusek, D. C. (1976). Pathogenesis of subacute spongiform encephalopathies. *Ann. Clin. Lab. Sci.*, **6**, 84

288. Moulton, J. E. and Palmer, A. C. (1959). Attempts to demonstrate the transmissible agent of scrapie in experimentally infected goats by means of fluorescent antibody. *Cornell Vet.*, **49**, 349

289. Allison, A. C. (1972). Immune responses in persistent virus infections. *J. Clin. Pathol.*, **6**, 121

14
Immunology of Slow Infections

J. M. ADAMS

14.1   INTRODUCTION   497

14.2   SLOW INFECTIONS IN ANIMALS AND MAN   498

14.3   VISNA AND MAEDI IN SHEEP   501

14.4   LYMPHOCYTIC CHORIOMENINGITIS   501

14.5   HERPES GROUP OF VIRUSES   502
          14.5.1   *Herpes simplex viruses*   502
                    14.5.2   *Cytomegaloviruses*   503
                    14.5.3   *Epstein–Barr virus*   503
                    14.5.4   *Varicella zoster virus*   504

14.6   RUBELLA VIRUS   504

14.7   MEASLES VIRUS   504

14.8   THE IMMUNE SYSTEM   506

14.9   VIRUS ISOLATION   507

14.10 SUMMARY   509

14.1   INTRODUCTION

Both the immune system and slow infections are concepts of recent origin. It has only been in the past 10–15 years that immunology has emerged as the study of a system, recognized by the medical community in the same way as the cardiovascular, respiratory, and central nervous systems. The concept of slow infection was originated by the late Björn Sigurdsson in 1954. Veterinary research on the viral aetiology of chronic neurologic diseases such as scrapie in sheep and encephalopathy of mink later became experimental models for subacute and chronic degenerative demyelinating diseases of the nervous system of man. About this time Societ virologists claimed that they found transmissable agents of amyotrophic lateral sclerosis and multiple sclerosis. In 1958, G. W. A. Dick et al.[1] published a study entitled, *Virus of Acute Encephalomyelitis of Man and Multiple Sclerosis*. These investigators were successful in obtaining the virus of a vaccine which had been studied in Russia for the treatment of multiple sclerosis and for which some success had been claimed. Dick and his associates found that the vaccine appeared to have been derived from the rabies virus and they failed to demonstrate any neutralization of the virus from which the vaccine had been prepared with sera from patients with multiple sclerosis.

In more recent years it has become apparent that slow infections may be triggered by 'slow viruses'. Kuru and Creutzfeldt–Jakob disease in man, scrapie in sheep and transmissable mink encephalopathy (TME), are 'slow infections' which implies that the agent persists in body cells and multiplies without causing the death of the cell. The infecting agent is recognized by the body's immune system whose reaction may be responsible for the damage and, evidence is accumulating that, in addition to these so-called 'slow virus' infections, certain common human degenerative diseases such as rheumatoid arthritis, multiple sclerosis and leukaemia might also be the result of slow and inapparent viral infections.

14.2 SLOW INFECTIONS IN ANIMALS AND MAN

The original criteria for slow infections were defined by Sigurdsson as *first*, a long initial period of latency lasting several months or years; *second*, a protracted clinical course usually ending in serious disease and death; *third*, the infection is limited to a single species and a single organ or tissue system.

Slow infection refers to the incubation period and a prolonged clinical illness, but does not necessarily indicate that the infecting agent is limited as far as the relative significance of host and virus factors in the pathogenesis of disease is concerned. Slow infections can then best be considered as clinical entities sharing in common a long incubation period followed by disease which is frequently limited to single-organ systems and may be species specific.

Recently, observations implicating an infectious aetiology of certain chronic degenerative brain diseases of man have introduced a new concept of causation of human disease. It appears that man can sometimes incubate an infectious agent for many months or years without any evidence of disease.

It may then become symptomatic and ultimately death may result with a pathological process which shows few or none of the classic features of inflammation and none of the usual signs classically associated with infection. Host immunity may remain unaltered.

Degenerative diseases originally defined and described by veterinarians may represent mechanisms which augment our understanding of a number of diseases in man such as multiple sclerosis (MS) and subacute sclerosing panencephalitis (SSPE). These illnesses frequently have prolonged incubation periods implicating infection which began during childhood or even in infancy.

Table 14.1   Comparison of conventional and unconventional agents*

Conventional agents	*Unconventional agents*
1. Virions of standard viral structure demonstrable by electron microscopy inside and outside of cells. Demonstrable in the nuclear or cytoplasmic sites characteristic of their virus family.	No virions recognizable inside or outside of cells. Infectivity appears to be associated with membranes. Cytopathology demonstrable by electron microscopy is of membranes.
2. Have nucleic acid genomes. Multiplication inhibited by inhibitors of nucleic acid synthesis, virions inactivated by u.v. irradiation, etc., as with other viruses.	No evidence of nucleic acid genomes.
3. Antigenic in the manner of other viruses although some may modify the host's immune response.	Appear not to be antigenic. No immune response demonstrated, so far, in the host.
4. Physical stability characteristic of their virus family.	Unusual stability to heat, ultraviolet irradiation and chemicals.
5. Induce familiar inflammatory as well as degenerative changes in host tissues (providing the host has cells capable of inflammatory response).	Only degenerative changes in host tissues.
6. Capable of disease production in several organs and tissues.	Only CNS disease demonstrated, so far.

* By permission of the author, Robert Hanson and Ross Laboratories

A number of infections in man and animals have prolonged incubation periods and lead to progressive central nervous system deterioration and ultimately death. In these slow infections the agent may persist without appreciable or significant damage to tissue cells. Robert Hanson of the University of Wisconsin has composed a classification which divides agents belonging to *conventional* virus groups and those as yet undefined as viruses and hence distinctly *unconventional*. *Conventional* and *unconventional* agents are compared with each other (see Table 14.1) for further clarification of this complex problem.

Slow infections are associated with two classes of agents. First, the *conventional* viruses which meet the usual morphological and biochemical criteria and second, agents which lack the characteristic features usually exhibited by viruses.

The *unconventional* agents are known to cause scrapie of sheep, transmissable mink encephalopathy (TME), Kuru, and Creutzfeldt–Jakob disease in man. They are classified as slow infections because of long incubation periods and a slow but relentless course and the symptoms and signs are limited to the central nervous system where they produce damage without evidence of inflammation.

Table 14.2 Slow diseases in man of possible virus aetiology

Disease	Tissue involved
Multiple sclerosis	CNS
Schilder's disease	CNS
Devic's disease	CNS
Amyotrophic lateral sclerosis*	CNS
Progressive muscular atrophy*	CNS
Chronic bulbar paralysis*	CNS
Parkinsonian dementia	CNS
Paralysis agitans (Parkinson's disease)	CNS
Alzheimer's disease	CNS
Pick's disease	CNS
Chronic polymyositis	Muscle

* From Neuron Disease
From: *Slow Viruses* by David H. Adams and Thomas M. Bell (1976), Addison-Wesley Publishing Co., Reading, Mass., London, Amsterdam, Sydney, Tokyo

Investigators have failed to characterize the properties of non-conventional agents, but from filtration studies it appears that their size is somewhere between 7 and 50 nm and they should, therefore, be readily visualized with modern electron microscopes, but nothing resembling a virion or a specific structure has been identified. There is an apparent lack of nucleic acid in the infectious unit of these agents which weighs strongly against their being viruses of recognized types. No antibodies have been found against the agents. Almost all that is known about them is that they replicate, cause disease and pass through filters which retain bacteria. These strange agents have characteristics which are not usually associated with typical viruses, thus they are resistant to inactivation by ultraviolet radiation and are highly resistant to heat and formalin. Scrapie, TME, Creutzfeldt–Jakob disease and kuru have each been transmitted to primates. The disease processes appear to be limited to the central nervous system in animals and man, e.g. Creutzfeldt–Jakob disease, is a progressively fatal degenerative brain disorder highlighted by dementia, ataxia and tremor. There is no sign of active infection, in the blood or cerebrospinal fluid (CSF) in this disease and immunologically there is no evidence of antibodies or immunoglobulins which would serve to identify a specific infecting agent. Pathologically there is evidence of glial proliferation or scaring which occurs without the usual signs of inflammation. These changes are similar to those seen in kuru and in scrapie of sheep and goats. Practically all the degenerative diseases of unknown aetiology, especially those involving the CNS, may be considered as candidates to be classified as slow diseases. (See Table 14.2.)

We can list the *conventional viruses* related to these slow infections of the central nervous system; visna of sheep, subacute sclerosing panencephalitis (SSPE), rabies and lymphocytic choriomeningitis (LCM) of mice. The viruses produce disease in several organs and stimulate the production of demonstrable antibody.

14.3 VISNA AND MAEDI IN SHEEP

Visna represents an infection with a conventional RNA virus giving rise to slow infection of the brain of sheep. Slowness is dramatized by the fact that some sheep fail to develop the disease for periods up to 4 years following inoculation of the virus. The infection causes extensive pathological changes in the brain with widespread proliferation of glial and mononuclear cells accompanied by demyelination in the white matter. Ill sheep show certain features in common with human demyelinating diseases, postinfectious encephalomyelitis and multiple sclerosis. In a recent study[2] it was reported that in addition to brain lesions, many lambs developed pneumonia with lymphocytes and plasma cells in germinal centres in the lung and that visna virus was isolated from the lung. The data showed that visna virus can produce persistent infection in the lungs as well as in the brain of sheep. In infection of American lambs, virus was recovered by cultivation of cells from their brains. It is concluded[2] that sheep provide a possible model for the study of virus-induced demyelinating disease. Although a possible model for human disease, no disease in man has been found to be caused by the visna virus.

Visna virus in tissue culture causes multinucleated giant cells like those induced by measles virus. Visna antisera with a neutralizing titre 1:256 failed to neutralize measles virus and no relationship with measles was detected by several tests such as indirect fluorescent antibody studies and haemagglutination-inhibition (HI)[3].

Maedi is similar to visna and has a close antigenic relationship. In tissue culture maedi virus produces a characteristic cytopathic effect with complete cell destruction.

14.4 LYMPHOCYTIC CHORIOMENINGITIS

Hotchin[4] who studied lymphocytic choriomeningitis (LCM) virus infection experimentally induced in mice showed that the animals inoculated at birth had long continuing infection with high levels of virus for about 10 months at which time the mortality rose sharply and reached nearly 90% by 20 months after inoculation. This slow virus infection in mice called *persistent tolerant infection* (PTI) by Hotchin is continuously active at a high level during the life-span of the infected animal. This is in contrast to *latent infections* in which the level of virus in the infected animals is low; furthermore in PTI unlike in latency, there is little evidence of antibody.

Hotchin summarized his studies as follows: (1) the viruses actively multiply for long periods of time without apparent disease, (2) the agents are not recognized as foreign by the host, and (3) an immune reaction to these agents is either very delayed or does not occur at all. Finally, the disease produced may be an autoimmune response caused by the end of tolerance, but the final disease may be a gradual process of erosion of the affected cells by the virus. PTI appears to be a fundamental prerequisite of some slow infections. (Recently Hotchin[5] found hospital personnel becoming infected by the virus of lymphocytic choriomeningitis as a result of contact with Syrian hamsters and these infected individuals developed severe illness.) Hotchin has concluded that LCM virus in mice represents a model for the study of slow infections in human beings and Hotchin and Buckley[6] suggested comparable human diseases could appear in later life as a result of perinatal infection.

Oldstone and Dixon[7] have suggested that antigen–antiviral antibody complexes cause chronic infections. They point out that generalized infections may provide the environment necessary for forming complexes with the host antiviral antibody and complement and conclude that the disease described by Hotchin is neither viral nor autoimmune; they prefer to call it immune-complex disease.

14.5   HERPES GROUP OF VIRUSES

14.5.1   Herpes simplex viruses

The herpes viruses include herpes simplex (HSV), varicella zoster (VZ), cytomegalovirus (CMV), and Epstein–Barr virus. All of the herpes viruses of man have the potential to remain latent in the host after apparent recovery from the primary infection.

Herpes simplex virus (HSV) type 1, infects most of the population of the United States, usually between 6 months and 5 years of age. The initial infection may be mild or serious, or quite inapparent. The type 2 herpes virus is usually responsible for genital herpes, skin lesions below the waist, neonatal herpes, and meningitis. Roizman[8] states that 75% of those who contract primary infection as evidenced by antibodies against the virus are affected sometime during their lives with recurrent herpetic eruptions. Antibodies almost invariably are present in patients who have recurrent herpes infections. Physical or emotional provocations may initiate the typical herpes lesions, possibly because of a selective defect in cell-mediated immunity in certain individuals, and the virus may produce progressive disease in immunologically compromised individuals. (See Chapter 10.)

Leider and associates[9] suggest that herpes simplex encephalitis is caused by a reactivation of latent infection. They found that of 52 patients with signs of CNS disease associated with HSV, 18 had a history of recurrent herpes labialis before onset of encephalitis, suggesting that the disease may have been a manifestation or reactivation of herpes simplex infection. A mechanism for persistence is of great importance. Virus may spread by direct extension from cell to cell, and thus avoid contact with antibody. Infectious episodes may be terminated by interferon or by other non-specific responses and Roizman observed that cells resistant to HSV produce interferon following infection. It has been postulated by some virologists that the HSV persists in sensory ganglia, since HSV has been repeatedly recovered under special conditions from human trigeminal ganglia. On the other hand, the virus may remain silent in deep cells of the affected areas of the skin.

Stimuli associated with physical and emotional provocations of the host may be manifested in the form of typical herpetic lesions. Where does the virus persist in the host in the interval between recurrences? How does infection become arrested? Is it possible that virus spreads by direct extension from cell to cell and thus avoids contact with antibodies?

In considering the persistence of HSV in relation to cancer, Sabin[10] concluded that there is at present no acceptable epidemiological or other evidence that these viruses alone or in conjunction with some unknown factors are involved in any human cancer. He adds that the potentially oncogenic human cytomegaloviruses should be in an even more suspect category because they may be isolated from the cervix, uterus and other organs much more frequently than herpes simplex viruses.

14.5.2 Cytomegaloviruses

Cytomegaloviruses are a major cause of mental retardation and also cause auditory loss. Infection by these agents occurs in about 1% of newborn infants, but rapidly rises to 10–20% during the 3rd and 4th month of life. This suggests that infection is acquired soon after birth or that infection acquired at birth may become evident very slowly.

14.5.3 Epstein–Barr virus

Another herpes virus, the Epstein–Barr virus (EBV), which is associated with Burkitt's lymphoma, raises the possibility that an extremely common virus may produce malignancy as well as a benign infection due to differences in host resistance. The EBV is worldwide in distribution and it has been shown that about 80% of the low-income population in Philadelphia had antibodies to EBV in their sera associated with infectious mononucleosis[11].

14.5.4 Varicella zoster virus

Chicken-pox and herpes zoster are different clinical manifestations to infection with the same virus. Chicken-pox represents a primary infection with the VZ virus, whereas recurrent infection with the same agent produces localized herpes zoster eruption in the immunocompetent host. The most likely explanation is that the virus is incompletely eliminated following previous infections remaining inactive or latent for long periods within the host cell before being reactivated to produce disease.

14.6 RUBELLA VIRUS

Congenital rubella is a chronic, generalized slow infection causing eye defects such as chorioretinitis, cataracts, and glaucoma. Microcephaly, and mental retardation are common. The frequency of defects is related directly to infection of the mother early in pregnancy. The characteristic findings include thrombocytopenia, enlarged liver, and evidence of bleeding, with petechiae commonly present. Virus persists in congenital rubella despite serum antibodies. Virus may be isolated readily from the urine, faeces, throat secretions and cerebrospinal fluid, as well as from the peripheral blood, bone marrow, lungs, tissue and middle ear fluid. Virus persistence may end spontaneously when the child reaches 12–18 months of age. Virus may be isolated postmortem from essentially every organ and gland, including the brain. The virus-infected cells are morphologically indistinguishable from non-infected cells but their growth rate and ultimate doubling potential is greatly reduced. Rubella antiserum, when added to cell cultures infected with the virus does not rid the culture of virus. Infection early in embryonic life results in slower growth rate, and thus smaller organs and a smaller baby. A significant correlation was found between failure to thrive and virus persistence.

14.7 MEASLES VIRUS

Of the slow infections caused by viruses, none is more definitive than subacute sclerosing panencephalitis (SSPE). Most of the cases occur between the ages of 5 and 10 years, but may rarely appear during adolescence or adult life.

The onset of illness reveals subtle changes in personality, or unexplained deterioration of school performance, followed by myoclonic seizures, and neurological signs, including paresis, blindness, memory impairment, stupor, and coma. A fatal outcome is the rule, although there are rare case reports of recovery or significant improvement of neurological function. Pathologically, the classic changes of encephalitis including necrosis, gliosis, and perivascular mononuclear infiltration and intranuclear inclusion bodies are clearly identified by fluorescent antibody and electron microscopy as representing the nucleocapsids of measles virus. High levels of measles antibody can be demonstrated in the serum and cerebrospinal fluid. Following a primary measles illness, the patient is seemingly well for months or years. High antibody levels in the cerebrospinal fluid are produced locally in the brain.

The virus which has been isolated from patients with SSPE behaves immunologically like measles virus, in that it is neutralized by measles antibody, shows specific fluorescence when stained by labelled antimeasles antibody, and produces a similar cytopathology when inoculated into cell cultures. Normal measles virus infections may severely affect the nervous system as manifest by acute encephalitis which appears within a few days of the infection, and ends in one way or another in days or weeks. The condition may persist and progress for months or even years.

Measles encephalitis in many instances may be classed as an acute demyelinating, subacute, or chronic-progressive disease. Post-mortem studies show characteristic multinucleated giant cells, viral inclusion bodies in both the cytoplasm and the nucleus, all of which are the characteristic hallmark of the measles virus in the CNS[12]. Studies provide evidence for persistence of virus months and years following the initial measles illness[3].

These changes have been observed in other viral diseases such as canine distemper and rinderpest (a disease of cattle), both of which have symptomological and immunological similarities to measles. A disease of mature dogs, known as old dog encephalitis has been shown to have immunological and pathological similarities to distemper and measles, and consequently is of importance as a possible animal model for the study of severe demyelinating diseases of animals and man[13].

The fundamental observations of Charcot established neurology on the basis of pathological changes. Pierre Marie, an eminent student of Charcot, expounded his teachings and correlated typical symptom complexes with neuropathological findings. In lectures to the New Sydenham Society, Pierre Marie stated: 'Eruptive fevers must be mentioned, namely measles, scarlatina, and above all – smallpox. Cases are numerous in which insular sclerosis has been known to occur during convalescence after the affection: tremor of the limbs, with more or less paresis, disorder of speech, which becomes slow and scanning, nystagmus, and in short, all of the characteristic symptoms of insular sclerosis may exist. At times these symptoms cease and entirely disappear, but they may also continue and confirmed insular sclerosis occurs'[3].

Multiple sclerosis (MS) strikes most commonly in the years between 20 and 40, although it is known to occur occasionally in children. There is clear evidence that measles virus can produce slow infection; for example, SSPE develops many years after childhood measles. Furthermore, Enders-Ruckle[14] has reported persistent measles virus isolated from lymph tissues in the monkey and in two adult humans, all possessing naturally acquired measles antibodies, but this has not been confirmed in other laboratories. A genetic defect in cellular immunity to measles and related viruses has been postulated to explain the aetiology of MS.

The defect may be in immunodeficiency of the T cells, making it difficult for the patient to eradicate the infectious agent. The defect may be associated with the presence of LD-7a determinant. Multiple sclerosis may occur in persons with a genetically determined defect in cellular immunity to measles or to related viruses. However, we must know much more about the possible relationship between the virus and CNS pathology before reaching definite conclusions. Demyelination might result directly from viral damage to cells, but it might instead be due to the kind of antigen–antiviral antibody complex postulated in some other demyelinating diseases.

14.8   THE IMMUNE SYSTEM

Viruses such as measles, vaccinia, varicella zoster and those of the herpes group, and many others, are known to cause slow infections and induce a normal response in the normal host.

Notkins[15] proposes that viruses induce immunopathological lesions as follows: *first*, the virus is a foreign antigen; *second*, it is self-replicating, and so can produce a continuous supply of antigen over a long period of time. Certain viruses induce new antigens on the surface of infected cells. Then they may produce disease by infecting cells in the immune system and so produce immunological derangement. His studies show that herpes simplex, vaccinia, influenza and Newcastle virus all induce new antigens on the surface of infected cells. The interaction of specific antiviral antibody and complement with these new antigens results in cell damage or injury. As a consequence, a long interval may exist between initial exposure and the eventual expression of the disease.

Slow viral infections are a virus–host relationship in which the virus fails to cause acute disease and the host fails to kill the virus. Ultimately, either viral infection itself or host response to the virus result in the evolution of pathological changes and clinical disease. Slow infections are not latent infections and should be differentiated from acute infections followed by chronic sequelae. The causative agents in slow infections belong to two groups of agents previously referred to but transmissible and failing to evoke an immune response, finally causing degenerative changes limited to the central nervous system of the host. Classic viruses which cause slow infections are capable of causing acute infections. They represent DNA and RNA large and small viruses. The measles virus which causes subacute sclerosing panencephalitis causes progressive disease in face of an accentuated humoral antibody response. Mechanisms for slow infections include chronic dysfunction, inefficient cytopathic infection with unneutralized virus and persistent infection in which only the host's immune response causes disease. No single mechanism of pathogenesis applies to all slow infections. It has been suggested that all viral infections may represent a complex and dynamic interaction of virus and host usually resolved by clearance of virus, death of the host or establishment of a symbiotic equilibrium. Incompetence of either virus or host can result in prolonged unresolved interaction leading to slow and persistent disease.

Levy et al.[16] reported the increased capacity of lymphocytes from patients with multiple sclerosis to adhere to human epithelial cells infected with measles virus. When lymphocytes from affected patients were mixed with measles-infected human epithelial cells the lymphocytes formed rosettes around about 70% of the measles-infected cells. Lymphocytes from controls, either healthy or with other neurological and non-neurologic diseases formed rosettes around only 30% of measles-infected cells. It seems unlikely that so large a percentage of peripheral lymphocytes would be directed to measles specific determinants. Is it possible that measles infection alters normal cell surface structures and provides a general recognition site for a T cell or measles-associated determinants cross-reactive with such recognition structures? Levy et al.[16] suggest that multiple sclerosis is not a disease confined to the central nervous system but patients have one lymphocyte subpopulation or circulating substance that adhers to lymphocytes and augments their measles-inherent lymphocyte activity.

14.9 VIRUS ISOLATION

Enders-Ruckle[14], as already indicated, investigated the maintenance of immunity following measles. Her study demonstrated latent persistence of infectious virus or its subunits in the immune host which was considered responsible for permanent immunity to measles. In contrast, it is possible that intracellular virus is freed and immediately neutralized by circulating antibodies. A further consideration concerns the fact that the virus may be present in a non-infectious incomplete form. Studies demonstrated lifelong persistence of both kinds of complement-fixing antibodies in measles-immune persons. Significantly, her research detected persisting infectious virus in lymphoid tissues of measles-immune humans and monkeys.

The problem of identification or isolation of causative agents of severe demyelinating disease and of slow infections continues to be one of the most challenging unsolved problems to concern virologists, immunologists, oncologists and many other investigators.

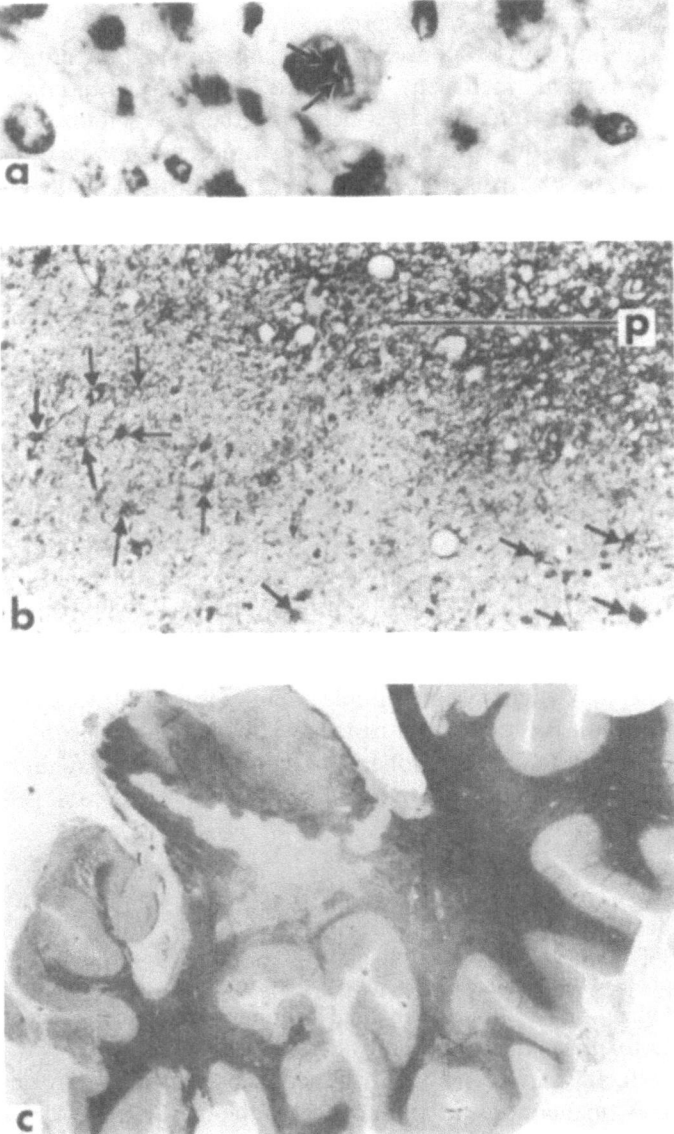

Figure 14.1 Neuropathology. (a) Nerve cell of the pons with pathological changes of the cytoplasm and two intranuclear inclusion bodies (arrows). (Haematoxylin & Eosin × 720); (b) Dense fibre gliosis within a *plaque* (P) of the frontal white matter and numerous astrocytes (arrows) in the surrounding tissue. (Holzer stain × 100); (c) Multiple small and large confluent demyelinated *plaques* within the subcortical white and grey matter. (Heidenhain–Woelcke stain). (From ter Meulen *et al.*[17] with permission of the authors and The Lancet Ltd)

In a 40-year-old man who developed encephalitis 3 days after the onset of acute measles and died 6 weeks later, ter Meulen[17] isolated measles virus by means of co-cultivation of cells derived from the patient's brain when cultured with a continuous line of African green monkey kidney cells. They established a cytopathic effect which was characterized by the formation of multinucleated giant cells with cytoplasmic and intranuclear inclusion bodies. Only co-cultivation of the brain cells with green monkey tissue cells yielded infectious virus. Photomicrographs of the brain tissue showed large and small multiple confluent demyelinated *plaques* within white and grey matter. They showed gliosis within a plaque. Pathological changes revealed cytoplasmic and intranuclear inclusion bodies. (See Figure 14.1.)

Pathak and Webb[18] reported viral inclusion bodies in post-mortem material 'similar to paramyxoviruses with a close resemblance to measles virus' from a 36-year-old female who died after severe multiple sclerosis and had high measles antibody titres in her serum and cerebrospinal fluid.

A recent report by Kiessling and associates[19] found a measles-virus-specific IgM response in SSPE. All their patients with SSPE had high titres of measles antibodies in both serum and CSF; both IgM and IgG were present, but IgM was more pronounced in CSF than in serum. The investigators postulated that virus-specific IgM in CSF indicates persistence of virus; and thus in other chronic diseases of the central nervous system such as multiple sclerosis, sensitive tests such as indirect radioimmunoassay might be employed to identify IgM and presumably persistent viral infection.

Other viruses aetiologically related to slow infections have been isolated by the cell-fusion technique. Parainfluenza type 1 has been isolated from brain cells of patients with multiple sclerosis[20], and Prineas[21] found virus-like tubules in electron micrographs of brain cells from patients with multiple sclerosis. He suggested that multiple sclerosis brain lesions may be initiated by periodic seeding of virus-bearing lymphocytes at selective sites in the white matter of the brain.

14.10 SUMMARY

Evidence for slow infections with rubella and cytomegaloviruses is established. The herpes group of viruses is recognized as causing possible recurrent latent and slow infections. The same characteristics are evident in infectious hepatitis type A and serum hepatitis type B[22, 23]. It is clear that measles virus can cause slow infection; this is supported by immunological and pathological findings in experimental studies as well as in humans[24]. Several clinics have reported measles antibodies in the sera and cerebrospinal fluid of patients with subacute sclerosing panencephalitis and multiple sclerosis. Measles virus has been isolated from patients with subacute sclerosing panencephalitis occurring years following childhood measles[25-28]. Current interest in slow virus infections is concerned with aetiology and pathogenesis of multiple sclerosis. Measles virus has been associated with the presence of plaques, gliosis and viral inclusion structures. Viral aetiology is implicated; it is premature to assume that all cases are caused by one kind of virus.

Using the more sensitive radioimmunoassay technique, Johnson and associates[29] report 18 of 25 multiple sclerosis patients have elevated measles antibodies in their cerebrospinal fluid, confirming the pathogenic role of measles virus in multiple sclerosis.

References

1. Dick, G. W. A., McKeown, F. and Wilson, D. C. (1958). Virus of acute encephalomyelitis of man and multiple sclerosis. *Br. Med. J.*, **1**, 7
2. Narayan, O., Silverstein, A. M., Price, D. *et al.* (1974). Visna virus infection of American lambs. *Science*, **183**, 1202
3. Adams, J. M. (1975). Persistent or slow viral infections and related diseases (Medical Progress). *West. J. Med.*, **122**, 380
4. Hotchin, J. (1967). Immune and autoimmune reactions in the pathogenesis of slow virus disease. *Curr. Top. Microbiol. Immunol.*, **40**, 33
5. Hotchin, J., Sikora, E., Kinch, W. *et al.* (1974). Lymphocyte choriomeningitis in a hamster colony causes infection of hospital personnel. *Science*, **185**, 1173
6. Hotchin, J. and Buckley, R. (1977). Latent form of scrapie virus: a new factor in slow-virus disease. *Science*, **196**, 668
7. Oldstone, M. B. A. and Dixon, F. J. (1971). Virus-antiviral antibody complexes. In: *Progress in Immunology – First International Congress of Immunology*, p. 763 (New York and London: Academic Press)
8. Roizman, B. (1965). An inquiry into the mechanisms of recurrent herpes infections of man. In: *Perspectives in Virology*, **Vol. IV**, p. 283 (New York: Harper and Row)
9. Leider, W., Magoffin, R. L., Lennette, E. H. *et al.* (1965). Herpes-simplex-virus encephalitis – its possible association with reactivated latent infection. *N. Engl. J. Med.*, **273**, 341
10. Sabin, A. B. (1975). Misery of recurrent herpes: What to do? *N. Engl. J. Med.*, **293**, 986
11. Henle, G. and Henle, W. (1970). EB virus in the aetiology of infectious mononucleosis. *Hosp. Pract.*, **33** (July)
12. Adams, J. M. and Brown, W. J. (1969). Studies on inclusion bodies in early and late demyelinating diseases. *Int. Arch. Allergy Appl. Immunol.*, **36**, 83 Pathogenesis and Etiology of Demyelinating Diseases (Basel: S. Karger)
13. Adams, J. M. *et al.* (1975). Old dog encephalitis and demyelinating diseases in man. *Vet. Pathol.*, **12**, 220
14. Enders-Ruckle, G. (1965). Methods of determining immunity resulting from measles. *Arch. Virus-forsch.*, **16**, 182
15. Notkins, A. L. (1971). Immunological injury of virus-infected cells by antiviral antibody and complement. In: *Progress in Immunology – First International Congress of Immunology*, p. 780 (New York and London: Academic Press)
16. Levy, N. L., Auerbach, P. S. and Hayes, E. C. (1976). A blood test for multiple sclerosis based on the adherence of lymphocytes to measles-infected cells. *N. Engl. J. Med.*, **294**, 1423
17. ter Meulen, V., Muller, D., Kackell, Y., Katz, M. and Meyermann, R. (1972). Isolation of infectious measles virus in measles encephalitis. *Lancet*, **ii**, 1172
18. Pathak, S. and Webb, H. E. (1976). Paramyxovirus-like inclusions in brain of patient with severe multiple sclerosis. *Lancet*, **i**, 311

19. Kiessling, W. R., Hall, W. W., Yung, L. L. and ter Meulen, V. (1977). Measles-virus specific immunoglobulin-M response in subacute sclerosing panencephalitis. *Lancet*, i, 324

20. ter Meulen, V., Koprowski, H., Iwasaki, Y. and Kackell, Y. M. and Muller, D. (1972). Fusion of cultured multiple-sclerosis brain cells with indicator cells: Presence of nucleocapsids and virions and isolation of parainfluenza-type virus. *Lancet*, ii, 1

21. Prineas, J. (1972). Paramyxovirus-like particles associated with acute demyelination in chronic relapsing multiple sclerosis. *Science*, **178**, 760

22. Greenberg, H. B., Pollard, R. B., Lutwick, L. T., Gregory, P. B., Robinson, W. S. and Merigan, T. C. (1976). Effect of human leukocyte interferon on hepatitis virus infections in patients with chronic active hepatitis. *N. Engl. J. Med.*, **295**, 517

23. Ho, M. (1976). Interferon and hepatitis B virus. *N. Engl. J. Med.*, **295**, 562

24. Brown, W. J. and Adams, J. M. (1973). Measles virus and multiple sclerosis. Presented at the *International Symposium on the Aetiology and Pathogenesis of the Demyelinating Diseases*, September 2–4, 1973, Kyoto, Japan

25. Connolly, J. H. *et al.* (1967). Measles-virus antibody and antigen in subacute sclerosing panencephalitis. *Lancet*, i, 542

26. Lennette, E. H., Magoffin, R. L. and Freeman, J. M. (1968). Immunologic evidence of measles virus as an etiologic agent in subacute sclerosing panencephalitis. *Neurology*, **18**, 95

27. Horta-Barbosa, L., Fuccillo, D. A., Sever, J. L., Seman, W. (1969). Subacute sclerosing panencephalitis: isolation of measles virus from a brain biopsy. *Nature (Lond.)*, **221**, 975

28. Payne, F. E., Baublis, J. V. and Itabashi, H. H. (1969). Isolation of measles virus from cell cultures of brain from a patient with subacute sclerosing panencephalitis. *N. Engl. J. Med.*, **281**, 585

29. Johnson, K. P. *et al.* (1978). *J. Clin. Microbiol.*

Index

ablastin, 80
Absidia spp., 54
Acanthamoeba
  castellani, 256
  polyphaga, 256
Acremonium spp., 61
actin binding deficiency, 182, 183, 185
Actinomyces spp., 248
Actinomycetes, 39
adenosine deaminase (ADA) deficiency, 174,
  175, 176, 177, 179
adenoviruses, 470, 471
adjuvants, 9, 12, 394, 398, 410
adrenalin, 226, 227, 302
adrenalitis, 394
agammaglobulinaemia, 119, 122, 130, 174,
  359, 456, 466
  measles, 246
  Swiss type, 130, 174
albinism, partial occulocutaneous, 128
Aleutian mink virus, 318, 458
alexin, 118
alimentary tract parasites, 94–9
alkylating agents, 144
allergens, 258
allergic reaction, types, 215, 216, 218;
    see also type
allergy, 215–58
  association of types, 230, 231
  bacterial, 222, 231, 252–6
  contact dermatitis, 224
  cytotoxic, 222
  'delayed' reaction, 223, 224
  drug products, 222, 254
  eczema, 253, 254
  erythema, 254, 255
  food, 99
  fungal antigens, 246–51
  helminth allergens, 251, 252, 258
  IgA deficiency, 164, 165
  infection, 224, 231
  inhaled particles and antigens, 256–8
  M. leprae, 238, 239
  M. tuberculosis, 231–8
  papular skin reactions, 254, 255
  respiratory, 24, 26, 29, 34

streptococcal infection, 222; *see also*
    autoimmunity
Streptococcus pneumoniae, 239–44
syphilis, 244
vasculitis, 223, 240, 241, 252, 253, 306, 325,
    413, 424, 449
viral antigens, 244–6; *see also* auto-
    immunity, immune complexes
Alzheimer's disease, 500
amoebiasis, invasive, 95, 96, 97, 101
amoebic dysentery, 95, 96
amyotrophic lateral sclerosis, 498, 500
anaemia
  aplastic, 55, 124, 182
  autohaemolytic in infectious mono-
    nucleosis, 413
  haemolytic, 7, 36, 124, 166, 246, 412
  nutritional, 7
  pernicious, 165, 166
anaesthesia, 118, 142, 143
anaphylatoxin activity, 301
anaphylaxis, 218, 219, 400
anergic serum, 135, 137, 138
anergy
  clinical conditions, 271–7
  delayed hypersensitivity, 270–88
  fungal infections, 39, 40, 43, 46, 287
  infectious disease, 269–88
  'positive', 270, 288
  recall antigens, 134–7
angioneurotic oedema, 188
angio-oedema, 240
anion polymers, 349
ankylosing spondylitis, 413
antibiotics, 144, 169
  in chronic infections, 423, 425
antibody deficiency, 158–69
  classification, 159, 160
  genetically determined 'acquired', 161
  treatment, 167–9
  see also immunodeficiency, hypogamma-
    globulinaemia
antibody formation in histoplasmosis, 43, 44
anticomplementary activity, 205, 210
antigenaemia, detection, 33
antigenic competition, 287

antigenic structure of bacteria, 397, 398
antigenic variation, 78, 79, 80, 81, 84, 103,
    423, 424
anti-idiotypic antibody, 305
anti-IgA antibody, 165, 195
antinuclear factor, 432
α_1-antitrypsin, 9
aphthous stomatitis, 242
arenavirus, 245
armadillo, 434
arthritis
    chronic infections, 424, 433, 439, 449
    hepatitis B antigen, 245, 413
    IgA deficiency, 165
    reduced immune response, 36
    sex-linked infantile hypogamma-
        globulinaemia, 124
    swine erysipelas, 412
    yersinia infection, 412
Arthus reaction, 222, 223, 224, 233, 253, 254,
    255, 306, 322, 330, 401, 433
Ascaris lumbricoides, 219, 251
aspergilloma, 26, 60
aspergillosis, 26, 31, 32, 33, 34
    allergic bronchopulmonary (ABA), 61, 62,
        223, 249, 251
    invasive, 60
Aspergillus
    clavatus, 256
    fumigatus, 30, 46, 60, 61, 62, 219, 223, 231,
        236, 240, 247, 249, 250, 251, 256
    spp., 26, 54, 61, 186, 193, 271, 352, 360,
        361, 362, 363, 364, 365
    terreus, 46
asplenia, 12, 13, 191
asthma, 26, 34, 55, 60–2, 164, 191, 219, 249,
    250, 255
ataxia–telangiectasia, 131, 132, 187
Aureobasidium
    pullulans, 256
    spp., 61
Australia antigen, 458
auto-allergic disease, 222
auto-antibodies, 101, 102, 241, 244, 320
autoimmune disease
    complement, 129, 130
    IgA deficiency, 165
autoimmunity
    infectious disease, 389–413
    intracellular antigens, 402
    leprosy, 432
    mechanisms, 391, 392
    streptococci, 397, 402–10; *see also* allergy
    syphilis, 402
    tissue injury, 400, 401
    virus infections, 393, 395, 396, 413;
        see also allergy, immune complexes
azetidine, 394, 395

azothiaprine, 143

Babesia
    microti, 84, 102
    spp., 79, 83
Bacillus subtilis, 220, 257
bacterial endotoxins, 9–11
bacterial killing, 128, 129, 183, 185, 186, 208,
    209, 360
bactericidal disorders, 117, 119, 126, 127, 128
Bacteroides spp., 372
Balantidium coli, 95
Bark Stripper's disease, 62
bartonellosis, 7
basophils, 303
B-cell
    absence, 124
    chronic infections, 425
    deficiency, 122
    EB virus, 465, 467
    function, 154, 155, 156, 390, 391
    IgA deficiency, 125
    immune complexes, 304
    malignancies, 356
    malnutrition, 203, 204
    protozoal infections, 102
    receptors, 304
    suppressor, 283
    tolerance, 391, 392
BCG
    disseminated, 174
    vaccination, 190, 228, 233, 237, 238
beryllium, 235
biological detergents, 220, 257
Bird Fancier's disease, 26, 62, 63, 64, 219, 224
BK virus, 458, 471
Blastomyces
    dermatidis, 48, 49, 50, 248
    spp., 30, 43, 46
blastomycosis, 25, 26, 32, 447, 448
    African, 49
    immune response, 48–50
    North American, 48
    South American, 50
blocking factors, 59, 305, 425
blood transfusion, hazards, 165, 195
bone marrow
    grafting, 177–9
    transplants in candidiasis, 59
Bordetella pertussis, 235, 394
Botrytis spp., 61
Brucella spp., 348, 356
brucellosis, 257
Burkitt's lymphoma, 318, 320, 465, 479
burns, altered host defence, 118, 121, 141,
    142, 349, 360

Camplyobacter (Vibrio) foetus, 100

cancer
  B-cell lymphoma, 467
  cervical, 463, 503
  chemotherapy, 144, 456
  cryptococcosis, 52
  foamy viruses, 479, 480
  herpes simplex virus type 2, 463
  IgA deficiency, 124, 125
  immunodeficiency, 133
  immunosuppression, 144
  invasive aspergillosis, 60
  leprosy, 276, 431
  lymphoreticular, 128
  nasopharyngeal, 318, 320, 465, 479
  rhabdomyosarcoma, 470
  solid tumours, 145, 359
  sporotrichosis, 40
  uterus, 503
Candida
  albicans, 2, 8, 28, 29, 33, 35, 41, 55, 57,
    59, 60, 134, 180, 208, 219, 221, 222,
    224, 231, 236, 247, 251, 252, 253, 256,
    271, 355, 364
    allergy, 248, 249, 250, 353
    chronic infection, 448, 449
    compromised host, 366, 367
  guilliermondii, 55
  krusei, 55
  parapsilosis, 55
  spp., 10, 26, 32, 35, 38, 54, 101, 127, 130,
    162, 172, 174, 193, 271, 273, 352, 356,
    360, 361, 362, 363, 366, 367, 368, 371,
    373
  tropicalis, 55
candidiasis, 26, 31, 33, 34, 35, 55–60
  chronic mucocutaneous, 35, 125, 126, 173,
    181, 232, 448, 449
carbohydrate
  determinants, 398
  metabolism in leukaemia, 145
cardiolipins, 244, 402
carrageenan, 235
carriers, 391, 392
cartilage hair hypoplasia, 171
cell-mediated immunity, 348, 349, 356
cell-mediated studies of fungal infections, 30,
    31
cell wall structure, β-haemolytic
    streptococcus, 397, 398
cerebrospinal fluid
  coccidioidomycosis, 48
  cryptococcosis, 52, 53, 54
ceruloplasmin, 9
Chaetonium spp., 61
Chaga's disease; *see* trypanosomiasis, South
    American
Chediak–Higaski syndrome, 5, 119, 128, 184
chemotactic factor inactivator (CFI), 278, 279

chemotactic factors, 401
chemotaxis, 347, 348
  complement, 301, 401
  defects, 117, 128, 129, 137, 138, 139, 140,
    141, 184, 360
  malnutrition, 208
chemotherapy, chronic infections, 423, 425
chicken-pox, 504
chloramphenicol, 144
chorea, 406
chorioretinitis, 467
choroid plexus, immune complexes, 299
chromium, 5
chromomycosis, 25, 32, 39
chronic bulbar paralysis, 500
chronic granulomatous disease (CGD), 119,
    120, 122, 127, 128, 183, 185–7
chronic polymyositis, 500
ciliate parasite, 95
Cladosporium spp., 61
Clostridium tetani, 120
cobalt, 5
cobra venom, 307
Coccidia, 85, 89–94
  classification, 89
Coccidioides
  immitis, 30, 41, 46, 248, 274
  spp., 43, 46, 47, 356, 360, 361
coccidioidomycosis, 25, 26, 30, 31, 32, 34
  geographical distribution, 46
  immune response in, 45–8
coeliac disease, 99
collagen, 395, 398
colonization resistance, 346
complement
  cryptococcosis, 53, 54
  deficiencies, 36, 122, 129, 130, 358
  disorders, 118, 187–9
  fungal infections, 29
  haemolytic activity, 205, 206
  malnutrition, 205
  protozoan infection, 84, 92
  see also immune complexes
concanavalin A, 247
congenital toxoplasmosis, 90, 91
conjunctivitis, 34, 61
consumptive opsinopathy, 141
conventional viruses, 499, 500, 501
copper, 5, 8, 9
corticosteroids, 351, 374, 448
Corynebacterium
  diphtheriae, 241, 255
  parvum, 84, 282
Coxackie B virus, 318
C-reactive protein (CRP), 9, 11, 240, 247, 278
Creutzfeld–Jakob disease (CJD), 455, 458,
    480–2, 499, 500
'crisis' forms, 83, 84

Crohn's disease, 165, 190
cross-reacting antigens
    parasite and host, 391, 396–402
    streptococci, 404–9
cryoglobulinaemia, 319
cryoglobulins, 310, 321, 323, 432, 433
cryptococcosis, 25, 26, 31, 32
    immune response in, 52–4
Cryptococcus
    neoformans, 29, 33, 52, 53, 54, 274, 363,
        364, 368
    spp., 271, 356, 361, 371
Cryptostroma corticale, 256
C-substance, 240, 247
cyclophosphamide, 35, 443
cystic fibrosis, 62
cystitis, chemical, 367
cytomegalovirus, 271, 318, 356, 363, 365, 370,
    457, 467, 468, 503
cytotoxic drug therapy, 357, 358, 359, 367

D-amino acids, 394
Dane particles, 459, 462
decontamination
    systems, 120, 121, 154
    techniques, 375, 376, 377
degenerative diseases, 499, 500, 501
demyelinating diseases, 501
Dengue haemorrhagic fever virus, 245, 318,
    319, 320
dermatomyositis, 125, 165, 166, 187, 396
Dermatophagoides
    antigens, 164
    spp., 219, 220
dermatophytosis, 22, 25, 31, 37–9
determinants of infection, 117, 120–2
Devic's disease, 500
diabetes, 52, 55, 133, 144, 351
diagnosis and immune response to fungi, 28,
    29, 30–3
Dientamoeba fragilis, 95
Di George's syndrome, 36, 125, 126, 158,
    169, 170, 171, 179
dimorphism, 24, 49
DI particles, 455
Dirofilaria immitis, 251
distemper, canine, 505
DNA viruses, 458–72, 506
drugs, immune suppressive effects, 120, 143,
    144, 189
Duncan's disease, 191
dye-test for *Toxoplasma*, 91
dwarfism, immunodeficiency, 132

Echinococcus granulosus, 251
ECHO virus, 167
Ectromelia, 10

eczema
    bacterial allergens, 253, 255
    candidiasis, 55
    host-defence, 129, 131, 132
    Wiskott–Aldrich syndrome, 180
ekiri, 244
'Elisa' assays, 33, 221, 311
emperipolesis, 402
encephalitis, 167, 245, 394, 503, 505, 509;
    see also panencephalitis
encephalomyelitis, 501
encephalopathy
    progressive multiple leuko- (PML), 471
    subacute spongiform, 480
    transmissible mink (TME), 458, 480, 481,
        498, 499, 500
    see also panencephalitis
endocarditis, 321, 322, 331
enhancement, 393, 394, 424, 425
Entamoeba
    gingivalis, 95
    histolytica, 93, 95–7, 101, 104
        sensu stricta, 95
enzymatic changes, malnutrition, 209, 210
enzyme deficiencies, 128, 131, 145, 170, 173,
    175, 176, 185, 186
eosinophil chemotactic reactor (ECF-A), 218
eosinophils, 302, 303
epidermal desquamation, 254, 255
Epidermophyton spp., 37
Epstein–Barr virus (EBV), 191, 272, 318, 320,
    458, 465–7, 503
equine infectious anaemia virus, 318, 458
Erysipelothrix rhusiopathiae, 412, 413
erythema
    generalized, 254, 255
    nodosum, 246
        leprosum (ENL), 276, 322, 432, 433, 449
Escherichia coli, 5, 10, 13, 208, 209, 242,
    243, 244, 278, 347, 356, 362, 363, 364,
    411
    allergens, 243, 244
espundia, 440, 441, 442
extracts of fungi, 29, 37
exocytosis, 301, 302
extrinsic allergic alveolitis, 26, 29, 34, 62–4,
    219, 256, 257

Farmer's lung, 26, 62–4
Fernandez reaction, 430
α-fetoprotein, 180, 279
fetal liver grafts, 179
fever, 353, 370
fibrinogen, 9
foamy viruses, 479, 480
folic acid antagonists, 144
Freund's adjuvant, 394
fungal allergens, 246–51

fungal cell, 23, 24
fungal infections
  clinical spectrum, 447, 448
  defective resistance, 360, 361, 363, 365
  immunotherapy, 38
  non-specific tissue reactions, 26, 27
  normal immune response to, 21–64
  types, 25
  types of immune response, 27–30
fungal spores, 24, 25, 34, 41, 45, 46, 61, 62
Fusarium spp., 54, 61

gallium, 5
gastroenteritis, haemorrhagic in pigs, 243
genetic susceptibility, chronic infection, 427
genito-urinary tract infection, 99
Geotrichum spp., 31
Gianotti's disease, 460
Giardia
  intestinalis, 95, 97–9, 101
  lamblia, 98, 193, 361
  muris, 98, 99
glomerulonephritis
  acute experimental serum sickness, 306, 307
  chemotaxis and opsonization, 360
  chronic infections, 424
  experimental, 242
  post streptococcal infection, 222, 241, 320,
    321, 331, 397, 403, 409, 410
  schistosomiasis, 447
  subacute bacterial endocarditis, 321, 322,
    331
  yersinial infection, 412
  with HBs antigen, 319, 460
  viral allergens, 245
glucose-6-phosphate dehydrogenase
  deficiency, 126, 128, 185
glutathione reductase deficiency, 185, 186
glycoproteins, 345
goitre, 401
gonorrhoea, 100, 103
Goodpasture's syndrome, 410
graft-versus-host disease, 172, 174, 177, 178
  179, 195, 359
Gram-negative organisms, cell wall structure,
  398
Gram-positive organisms, cell wall structure,
  397
granulocyte
  function, 8, 10, 11, 347, 348
  transfusions, 354, 355, 374, 375
granulocytopaenia, 352, 355, 357, 359, 362,
  365, 366, 372
granulomatous response, 224, 234, 235, 273,
  279, 285, 287, 429
Graphium spp., 256
Guillain–Barré syndrome, 468

haemodialysis, 351
haemolytic anaemia; *see* anaemia
Haemophilus
  influenzae, 13, 130, 222, 243, 254, 255,
    347, 369, 377
  spp., 369
hair, 171, 184
hapten-carrier model, 82
haptens, 391, 392, 404
haptoglobin, 9
heat test, 227
HeLa cells, 93, 298, 318
helminth infections, 329, 330, 446, 447;
    see also schistosomiasis
Henhoch–Schonlein purpura, 187
hepatitis, 125, 165, 245, 272, 413
  A virus, 462
  B antigens, 245, 276, 319, 458, 459
  B virus, 272, 318, 356, 363, 368, 458–62
  non-A non-A agent, 462
hepatosplenomegaly, 467
herpes
  simplex, 356, 361, 363, 366, 395, 457,
    462–5, 502, 503
  viruses, 271, 349, 457, 458, 502
  zoster, 356, 361, 363, 368, 457, 468–70, 504
hexose monophosphate shunt (HMP), 127,
  185, 186
histamine, 218, 219, 220, 221, 224, 226
histocompatibility locus, 413
histiocytosis X, 176
Histoplasma capsulatum, 30, 41, 43, 44, 45,
  52, 248, 250, 273
Histoplasma
  cells, 27
  spp., 46, 271, 356, 361
histoplasmin, 41, 42, 43, 44
histoplasmosis, 25, 26, 28, 30, 31, 32, 277, 447
  disseminated, 273
  immune response in, 41–3
HLA antigens
  Farmer's Lung disease, 64
  leprosy, 427
  streptococcal antigens, 399, 400
  virus infections, 461, 465
  yersinial arthritis, 412
Hodgkin's disease, 36, 144, 271, 279, 357,
  361, 448, 471
Hoeppli phenomenon, 447
hog cholera virus, 318
host defence
  colonization resistance, 346
  defects, 117–46
  disturbances, 349–55
  in chronic infections, 422, 424
  mechanisms, 120–2, 344–9
  reinforcement, 377
hyaluronic acid, 392, 397, 399

hyperferraemia, 6, 7
hypersensitivity
    chronic infections, 422, 423
    delayed, 28; *see also* anergy, Type IV
        reaction
    pneumonitis, 62
    reactions, 218–30, 400, 401
    respiratory, 26
hyperthyroidism, 401
hypervitaminosis A, 3
hypocalcaemia, 125, 126
hypoferraemia, 6, 7
hypogammaglobulinaemia, 36, 145, 158, 191,
        352, 359
    congenital in girls, 161
    sex-linked infantile, 123, 124
    total, 132
    transient, 124, 162, 163
    variable, 161, 165–7
    with IgM, 161, 162
    X-linked pan-, 157, 159, 160, 161, 162,
        163, 166, 168, 192
hypoparathyroidism, 126

idiotype, 155
'Id' reactions, 38, 39, 55
IgA deficiency, 124, 125, 160, 163, 164, 361
IgE
    demonstration, 220, 221, 222
    elevated, 129, 164, 184, 204, 360
    fungal allergens, 249, 250
IgG
    chronic infections, 425
    deficiency, 125, 160, 166, 167
    replacement, 167, 168
    subclass properties and activities, 166, 219
IgM
    deficiency, 125, 160, 165
    hyper with immunodeficiency, 124, 161,
        162, 204
immune
    complexes, 295–331
        bacterial infections, 320–3, 404
        biological activities, 299–305
        cell interactions, 301–6
        chronic infections, 423, 424, 425, 439
        complement, 297, 300, 301, 307
        detection, 307–17
        fate, 298, 299
        fungal infections, 34
        glomerulonephritis, 410, 439, 460
        nature, 297
        parasitic disease, 323–30
        rheumatic fever, 404, 408
        site of formation, 297, 298, 299
        tissue injury, 306, 307
        virus infections, 298, 317–20, 460;
            see also allergy, autoimmunity

    facilitation, 425
    response
        fungal infections, 21–64
        intracellular protozoal, 94
        modification, 35, 36
immunity, defined, 154, 155, 390, 391
immunization, hazards, 195
immunoconglutinins, 297
immunodeficiency, 151–95; *see also*
        anergy, hypogammaglobulinaemia,
        immunosuppression
    acquired, 117, 120, 132–46, 161
    antibody mediated, 117, 123–5
    cell-mediated, 117, 125, 126, 169–73
    classification, 157
    combined cellular and humoral, 118, 130–2,
        173–82
    diagnosis, 191–4
    fungal infections, 35, 36
    giardiasis, 98, 103
    primary, 117, 119, 122–32
    secondary, 189–91
    severe combined (SCID), 130, 158, 159,
        174, 175, 176, 177, 178, 179, 192
    sex-linked with hyper IgM, 124, 160
    special hazards, 195
    variable, 159, 161, 181
immunodepression
    antigenic competition, 287
    parasitic infections, 104, 426
immunoglobulins
    cellular basis, 155, 156
    loss, 189, 190
    malnutrition, 203, 204
    mycotic infections, 29
    non-specific, 101, 102
    secretory, 204
    Type I reactions, 219
    Type III reactions, 222, 223
immunological derangement, 506
immunological spectra, chronic infections,
        426
immunological surveillance, 431
immunosuppression
    activation of viruses, 456
    associated disease states, 118, 144, 145
    congenital rubella, 478
    Entamoeba histolytica, 96
    fungal infections, 33, 35, 59
    haptenic determinants, 392
    pharmacological agents, 118, 143, 144
    toxoplasmosis, 91
    Treponema pallidum, 436, 438
    see also immunodeficiency
immunosuppressive serum factors, 277–9
immunotherapy, fungal infections, 34, 38
impetigo, 410
infantile papular acrodermatitis, 460

infection
  chronic, 421–49
  compromised host, 343–77
    diagnosis, 370–4
    treatment, 371–7
  intercurrent, 426, 443
  patterns of, 355
  persistent recurrent viral, 453–82
  persistent tolerant (PTI), 502
  predisposing factors, 355
  prevention, 353, 354
  super infections, 351, 371, 373
  type and defective resistance, 360, 361
infectious mononucleosis, 299, 318, 320, 465, 466
inflammatory response
  autoimmunity, 393
  compromised host, 352, 363, 364
  fungal disease, 26, 27
  host defence, 122, 347
  Trichomonas vaginalis, 99
influenza virus, 272, 273, 455, 506
interferon, 155, 232, 272, 345, 347, 349, 354, 458, 464, 470, 480, 503
iodine, 5
iridocyclitis, 433, 439
iron, 5, 6–8, 11, 155, 202
irradiation, viral infections, 361
isolation, 375, 376
Isospora
  belli, 90
  bigemina, 89
  hominis, 90
  natalensis, 90
isotype, 155

Jarisch–Herxheimer reaction, 423
JC virus, 458, 471
Job's syndrome, 119, 184

Kahler's disease, 352
kala-azar, 326, 327, 328, 329, 440, 441, 442
Kartagner's syndrome, 154
killer (K) cells, 304, 464
Kimura's disease, 249
Klebsiella
  pneumoniae, 362, 364
  spp., 10, 354, 362, 363, 372
Koch phenomenon, 231
kuru, 455, 458, 480–2, 498, 499, 500

lactic dehydrogenase virus, 318, 319
lactoferrin, 345, 347
Lamblia
  intestinalis, 98
  spp., 373
laminar air-flow isolator, 376
latent state, paracoccidioidomycosis, 50

lazy-leukocyte syndrome, 127, 128, 184
legionnaire's disease, 370
Leishmania
  braziliensis, 85, 440, 441, 442
    guyanaensis, 89
    panamensis, 89
  classification, 85, 103, 440
  donovani, 85, 88, 89, 102, 440, 441, 443
    chagasi, 89
  enriettii, 274, 442
  mexicana, 85, 441
    amazonesis, 89
    mexicano, 89
    pifanoi, 89
  peruviana, 85, 441
    uta, 89
  pifanoi, 441, 442
  spp., 85, 424, 440, 443
  tropica, 85–8, 102, 104, 440, 441, 442
    braziliensis, 85
leishmaniasis, 85–9, 440–4
  histological spectrum, 443, 444
  immune complexes, 329
  New World, 85, 89
  Old World, 85, 89
lepromin test, 239, 275, 411, 429
leprosy
  allergy, 238, 239, 244
  anergy, in lepromatous, 237, 424
  autoimmunity, 411
  cell mediated immunity, 286, 429, 430, 431
  clinical spectrum, 427, 428, 429
  delayed type hypersensitivity, 273, 275
  genetic susceptibility, 427
  granuloma formation, 429
  immune complexes, 322, 323, 331
  protozoal infections, compared with, 103
  reaction states, 432, 433
  serum factors, 277, 279, 431, 432
Leuconostoc mesenteroides, 392
leukaemia, 55, 60, 145, 351, 357, 358, 359, 471, 479, 498
  clinical picture of infections, 362–8, 369
leukocyte
  function, 5, 127, 128
  loss, 190
  mobility defects, 183, 184
leukocytic endogenous mediator, 9
leukokinin; see tuftsin
leukopenia, 177
levamisole, 228, 354
'life-island', 376
lipopolysaccharide (LPS), 10
Listeria
  monocytogenes, 2, 233, 271, 286, 363, 368
  spp., 348, 356, 357, 369, 370
lithium therapy, 354, 377

liver
    abscesses, 95, 96, 97, 186, 370
    chronic disease, 412
long-acting thyroid stimulator (LATS), 401
low density lipoprotein (LDL), 278
LTS antibody, 219
lupus erythematosus; see systemic lupus
    erythematosus
Ly antigens, 285
lymphocyte
    circulation, 279–83
    trapping, 282
lymphocytic choriomeningitis virus (LCM),
    245, 318, 319, 458, 501, 502
lymphocytotoxin, 132, 182
lymphoid atrophy, 206
lymphoid tissue hyperplasia, 166
lymphokines, 232, 235, 348, 456, 463
lymphoma
    American Burkitt's, 191
    IgM deficiency, 165
    immunosuppression, 145
    mycoses, 55
    transfer factor, 173
    Wiskott–Aldrich syndrome, 181
lymphopenia, episodic, 132
lymphoproliferative disorders, reduced
    resistance, 357, 358, 359, 365, 368, 370
β-lysine, 345, 347
lysis, 301
lysozyme, 145, 155, 345, 347

macrophage
    and T cells, 271, 390
    as suppressor, 283
    factors, 232
    function, 156, 190, 347, 348, 390
    immune complexes, 303
    lepromatous leprosy, 275, 279
    malnutrition, 208, 209, 210
    protozoal infections, 83, 84, 92, 102
    syphilis, 244
    tuberculin patch test, 229, 234, 235
    Type IV reactions, 401
    Wiskott–Aldrich syndrome, 131
maedi, 501
malabsorption, 124, 164, 166, 169
malaria, 7, 78, 82, 103, 323, 324, 331, 361,
    426; see also plasmodia
malnutrition
    cell-mediated response, 206–10
    fungal infections, 36
    immune status, 118, 133, 145, 146, 190,
        201–10, 426
    intestinal atrophy, 163
malignant disease; see cancer
Malt Worker's Lung, 63
manganese, 5

mast-cell, 219, 221, 301, 302, 303
measles virus, 190, 191, 206, 246, 272, 298,
    318, 320, 426, 455, 456, 457, 472–6,
    504–6, 507
mechanical factors, 154, 155
mercaptopurine, 143
metastasis, Leishmania, 85, 89
methotrexate, 144
microbial products, 2, 9–12
Micrococcus
    cararrhalis, 255
    tetragenus, 255
Microsporum spp., 37
Micropolyspora faeni, 63, 64, 256
migration inhibition factor (MIF), 234
    in candidiasis, 58
Mimea polymorphea, 192
minerals, 2, 5–9
mitogen, in protozoal infections, 102
Mitsuda reaction, 238, 429
monocytopaenia, 351, 357
mononuclear phagocytes, 303
M proteins, 397, 399, 409
Mucor spp., 26, 54, 360, 361, 362, 363, 364,
    365
mucous membranes, in host defence, 346, 350
multiple myeloma, 359, 369
multiple sclerosis, 498, 499, 500, 501, 505,
    506, 507, 509
mumps, 246, 271, 272
murein, 397
Mushroom Worker's Lung, 62
myasthenia gravis, 182
mycetoma, 25, 32, 35
    immune response in, 39
Mycobacterium
    avium, 237
    johnei, 229
    kansasii, 431
    leprae, 238, 239, 273, 274, 275, 286, 287,
        323, 427, 429–34, 438, 439
    lepraemurium, 274, 281, 283, 284, 285
    smegmatis, 12, 431
    spp., 356
    tuberculosis, 2, 4, 224, 225, 228, 229,
        231–8, 252, 257, 271, 273, 274, 349,
        352, 357, 370, 410, 430
    ulcerans, 237
Mycoplasma pneumoniae, 246
mycoses
    opportunist, 26, 54–60
    respiratory, 25, 26, 30
    subcutaneous, 23
myeloperoxidase, 328
    deficiency, 119, 127, 128, 129, 145, 185
myocardial antigens, 405, 406, 407, 408, 409

nasopharyngeal carcinoma, 318, 320, 465, 479

NADH oxidase deficiency, 127
NADPH oxidase deficiency, 127
NBT test, 193
Necator americanus, 446
Neisseria
    gonorrhoeae, 347
    meningitidis, 13
    spp., 193
nematode infections, 101
nephritis
    nephrotoxic serum, 240
    post streptococcal; *see* glomerulonephritis
neutropenia, 183
neutrophil disorders, 117, 119, 126, 127, 128, 137
neutrophils, 302
Newcastle disease virus, 2, 10, 506
Nezelof's syndrome, 36, 130, 174
Nocardia
    asteroides, 46, 363, 368
    brasiliensis, 248
    spp., 362
non-specific immunity, primary defects, 182–9
non-specific defence mechanism, blood parasites, 83, 84
non-specific resistance, infection, 1–14
non-specific tissue reactions, in fungal disease, 26, 27
nucleoside phosphorylase deficiency, 170
nude mice, 158
null cell, malignancies, 356
nursery workers, 41

O antigens, 398
occupation, sporotrichosis, 40, 41
oesophagitis, 366
old tuberculin (OT), 224
Onchocerca volvulus, 330, 446
onchocerciasis, 330, 424, 446
oncornavirus, 318, 479, 480
opsonin deficiency, 126, 141
opsonization, 348
opsonizing defects, 189, 355, 359, 360
orchitis, 394, 433
organ transplantation, 351, 356, 359, 369, 370, 471
Oriental sore, 440, 441
osteomyelitis, 186

Pan 11, 470
panencephalitis
    chronic progressive (rubella), 476–9
    subacute sclerosing (SSPE, measles), 318, 320, 457, 458, 472–6, 499, 501, 507
Papova viruses, 458, 471, 472
papular skin reactions, 254, 255
Paracoccidioides brasiliensis, 49, 50, 51, 52, 274

Paracoccidiomyces brasiliensis, 448
paracoccidioidomycosis, 25, 26, 31, 32
    immune response in, 50–2
parainfluenza virus, 509
paralysis agitans, 500
paramyxoviruses, 509
parasites
    ciliate, 95
    alimentary tract, 94–9
    blood stream (protozoal), 78–84
    intracellular (protozoal), 84–94
    luminal, 103
    mucous surfaces, 94–101
    urogenital tract, 94, 99–101
parathyroid hypoplasia; *see* Di George's syndrome
parenteral nutrition, 351
parkinsonian dementia, 500
Parkinson's disease, 500
'passive immune kill', 400
Pasteurella
    pseudo-tuberculosis, 410
    tularensis, 356
Penicillium
    casei, 256
    frequentans, 256
    spp., 30, 61
Pentatrichomonas hominis, 95
phagocytic disorders, 117, 126, 128, 183, 185
phagocytosis, 347, 348
    acquired disturbance, 358
phenytoin, 163
Phlebotomus spp., 440
phycomycoses, 26, 27, 33
Pick's disease, 500
piedra, 25
pigeon faeces, 52
pipecolic acid, 394
pityriasis versicolor, 25
plasmalogen, 407, 408
Plasmodia, 10
Plasmodium
    berghei, 3, 82
        yoelli, 286
    falciparum, 78, 81, 82, 324, 426
    knowlesi, 81
    malariae, 78, 81, 324
    ovale, 78
    spp., 81, 82, 101, 103
    vivax, 78
    yoelli, 83
platelets, 302
platinum, 220
Pneumocystis carinii, 130, 174, 193, 271, 352, 361, 363, 368, 369
    diagnosis and treatment in compromised host, 365

pneumonia
  diagnosis in compromised host, 364, 365
  streptococcal, 239, 240
pokeweed mitogen (PWM), 156, 287
poliomyelitis, 193
poliovirus, 272
polyarteritis nodosa, 245, 306, 319, 396
polyarthritis, 411
polyclonal antibody synthesis, 297
polymorphonuclear leukocyte (PMN),
    malnutrition, 208, 209, 210
polynucleotides, 349
polyoma virus, 471
polysaccharide antigens, 236, 258
pox viruses, 172
'predator' host, 90, 93
pregnancy, and *Entamoeba histolytica*, 96
'prey' host, 90
prick test, 220
progressive muscular atrophy, 500
proline, 394
proprionobacterium acnes, 345
prostaglandins, 218, 302
protective immunity in histoplasmosis, 44
Proteus mirabilis, 242
protozoa
  blood parasites, 78–84
  intracellular parasites, 84–94
protozoal infections, 77–104, 323, 324
  defective resistance, 361
Pseudomonas
  aeruginosa, 2, 362, 364, 377
  spp., 10, 354, 362, 363, 372, 373
purified protein derivative (PPD), 224
pyruvate kinase deficiency, 185, 186

rabies virus, 498, 501
radio-allergosorbent (RAST) tests, 62, 221,
    249
Raji cell radioassay, 314, 315
reference antigens, of fungi, 30, 55, 56
renal transplant recipients, 133
respiratory hypersensitivity, 60–64
respiratory syncytial virus, 246, 456
reticular dysgenesis, 174, 177
reverse transcriptase, 455, 456
'revivescence', 228
rheumatic fever, 240, 306, 397, 403, 404, 412
rheumatoid arthritis, 125, 165, 166, 187, 306,
    358, 360, 498
rheumatoid factor, 297, 393, 413, 432
Rh factors, 124
rhinitis, 34, 61
Rhizopus spp., 54
rinderpest (cattle), 505
ringworm infections; *see* dermatophytosis
RNA
  immune, 354

viruses, 472–80, 507
rosette-inhibiting factor, 461
rubella, 191, 272, 455, 457, 458, 476–9, 504

Salmonella
  gallinarum, 243
  infections, 7, 412
  spp., 10, 193, 348, 349, 352, 355, 356, 357,
    363, 368, 373
  typhi, 426
Sarcocystis
  fusiformis, 90, 93
  life cycle, 90, 93
  lindermanni, 90
  miescheriana, 90
  nomenclature, 89, 90
  spp., 89, 103 ·
sarcoid, 52
sarcoidosis, 270, 271, 275, 471
sarcoma, IgA deficiency, 124
scarlatina, 505
Schilder's disease, 500
Schistosoma
  japonicum, 329, 447
  mansoni, 329, 330
schistosomiasis, 251, 329, 330, 331, 446, 447
Schizotrypanum spp., 79
Schwachman's syndrome, 184
Schwartzman reaction, 244
scrapie, 458, 480, 481, 498, 499, 500
sepsis, 120, 121, 129, 133, 134, 135, 362, 363
septicaemia, 367, 368, 412
serodiagnosis
  fungi and actinomycetes, 28, 29, 30, 31–3,
    367
  plasmodia, 81
  toxoplasmosis, 91
  Trichomonas vaginalis, 100
  trypanosomes, 80
Serratia
  marcensus, 127
  marsescens, 185, 192
  spp., 362
serum sickness, 253, 302, 303, 304, 306, 307,
    321, 322, 324, 325, 404
  -like disease, 245, 423
  syndrome, 319, 330
Shigella
  flexneri, 244
  infections, 412
shock, altered host defence, 143
sickle cell disease, 7
siderophores, 6
simian foamy virus (SFV), 479
skin
  in host defence mechanisms, 120, 121, 344,
    345, 349, 350
  grafts, burns, 141

skin (*continued*)
  -reactive factor, 233
  tests
    diagnosis of infection, 30, 31, 135, 136, 137
    fungal antigens, 247, 248
    streptococcal antigens, 242
    techniques, 220
    Type I reaction, 218, 219, 220
    Type III reaction, 222, 223, 224
sleeping sickness, 78
slow-reacting substance (SRS-A), 218
slow viruses, 455, 458, 480–2, 497–510
smallpox, 133, 505
spleen, 12, 13, 283–5, 286, 359
  Leishmania, 85
  leprosy, 279, 280
splenectomy, 191, 358, 359, 360, 369
splenomegaly, 165
Sporobolomyces spp., 61
Sporothrix
  spp., 31, 54
  schenckii, 40, 41, 248
sporotrichosis, 25, 31, 32
  immune response in, 40, 41
Sporotrichum spp., 238
standardization of reactions, in fungal infections, 29, 30
Staphylococcus
  albus, 8, 255
  aureus, 4, 13, 120, 127, 134, 185, 193, 208, 221, 231, 242, 243, 252, 253, 254, 255, 256, 321, 353, 356, 362, 364, 365, 366, 367, 369, 372
  epidermis, 127, 134, 321
  faecalis, 255
  spp., 10
steroids, 143, 144
Stevens–Johnson syndrome, 246
Stormont test, 229
streptococcal
  antigens, 240, 241, 242
  impetigo, 410
  infection and immune complexes, 320, 321
Streptococci
  antigenic structure, 397
  β-haemolytic, 396, 397, 403
  nephritogenic, 410
Streptococcus
  group A, 13, 240, 241, 242, 252, 321, 347
  group D, 252
  haemolyticus, 255
  pneumoniae, 4, 10, 13, 221, 231, 239, 240, 254, 347, 364, 369, 377
  pyogenes, 4, 120, 347, 398
  spp., 275, 362
  viridans, 255
streptolysins, 240, 241

Strongyloides
  stercoralis, 99
  spp., 361
short-term sensitizing (STS) antibody, 219
suppressor cells, 283–5, 286, 287, 288
suppressor effects, 270
surgery, altered host defence, 118, 120, 133, 142, 143, 349
SV-40 virus, 471
syphilis, 103, 244, 277, 402, 424, 426, 436–9
systemic lupus erythematosus (SLE), 52, 125, 165, 285, 306, 325, 358, 360, 395, 396, 433, 471
  SLE-like syndrome, 186, 187
systemic reactions, 257, 258

T-cell
  chronic infections, 425
  dysfunction, 54, 125, 126, 130
  EB virus, 466
  function, 154, 155, 156, 390, 391
  fungal infections, 36, 59, 60
  help, 391
  immune complexes, 305
  immunodeficiency, 122, 130, 131
  lepromatous leprosy, 431
  malignancies, 356
  measles virus, 507
  protozoal infections, 103
  receptors, 305
  subpopulations, 285, 287, 401
  surface receptors, 287
  tolerance, 391, 425
  treatment of defects, 172, 173
  Type IV reactions, 228, 401
teeth, 367
tetany, congenital, 126
Thermoactinomyces
  sacchari, 256
  vulgaris, 63, 256
thrombocytopenia, 131, 162, 180, 412, 467
thymic aplasia, 36, 130, 271
thymic deficiency, congenital, 448
thymic dysplasia, 36
thymic hormones, 288
thymic hypoplasia; *see* Di George's syndrome
thymoma, 125, 159, 161, 182
thymopoietin, 173
thymosin, 131, 173
thymus
  extracts, 173
  foetal transplant, 126, 171, 172, 173, 179
  Plasmodium berghei, 82
  malnutrition, 206
thyroiditis, 165, 394, 412
tick-bone encephalitis, 456
tinea, 25

tolerance, 43, 286, 390, 391, 392, 393, 424, 425
Toxoplasma
  gondi, 89, 90, 91, 92, 102, 104, 271, 352, 356, 361, 363, 365, 369
  spp., 89, 90
transcobalamin II deficiency, 151, 162, 163
transfer factor (TF), 45, 48, 51, 59, 173, 182, 183, 228, 232, 288, 348, 354
transferin, 155, 228, 345, 347
trauma, altered host defence, 118, 120, 133, 138, 139, 140, 141, 143, 349
Treponema pallidum, 244, 274, 402, 424, 436, 438, 439
Trichinella spiralis, 251, 286
trichomoniasis, 103
Trichophyton
  gypseum, 271
  mentagrophytes, 31, 38, 39, 254
  spp., 37, 248
  rubrum, 31, 39
  verrucosum, 34
Trichomonas
  tenax, 95
  vaginalis, 95, 99–101, 102
Tritrichomonas foetus, 99
Trypanosoma
  brucei, 102, 103, 286
    brucei, 78, 79, 80, 81, 325
    gambiense, 78
    rhodesiense, 78, 103
  congolense, 78, 274
  gambiense, 273
  lewisi, 78, 80
  musculi, 3, 78, 80
  cruzi, 79, 82–4, 104, 444, 445
  rhodesiense, 325
  spp., 10
  vivax, 78
trypanosomiasis, 82, 83, 84, 273, 325–9, 426
  African, 79, 80, 81, 83, 84, 101, 102, 103, 325–6
  South American, 79, 83, 84, 102, 103, 444, 445; see Chaga's disease
temperature sensitive (TS) mutants, 455
tuberculin
  allergy; see allergy, Type IV
  depot, 227, 228, 238
  sensitivity, 238
  skin reaction, 225–30
tuberculosis, 228, 434–6
tuftsin, 13, 347
  deficiency, 128
Type I reaction, 218–22, 231, 236, 248, 400

Type II reaction, 222, 400
Type III reaction, 222–4, 231, 236, 248, 257, 400, 401
Type IV reaction, 224–30, 231, 236, 248, 401
Type V reaction, 401

ulcers, amoebic, 95, 96, 97
ulcerative colitis, 411
unconventional agents, 499, 500
urinary tract infections, in leukaemia, 367
urogenital tract parasites, 94, 99–101
urticaria, 240

vaccination
  BCG, 190, 228, 233, 237, 238
  blastomycosis, 50
  malaria, 82
  inactivated vaccine, 246
  Toxoplasma, 91
vaccines
  anti-fungal, 34
  anti-protozoal, 104
  bacterial, 256
vaccinia, 506
  disseminated, 193, 195
varicella, 132, 193, 271, 272, 361
varicella-zoster virus; see herpes zoster
vasculitis; see allergy
vesicular stomatitis virus, 395
viral allergens, 244, 245, 246
viral infections, 453–82
  defective resistance, 361
virulence, 120
visna, 501
vitamin
  A, 2, 3, 5, 202
  B$_{12}$, 163
  C, 3–5
  combinations, 5
  E, 5

Waldenström's disease, 352, 359, 369
Wasserman reaction, 402
Whipple's disease, 165
Wiskott–Aldrich syndrome, 36, 131, 173, 180, 181

yeasts, 24, 33
yersinia, 411, 412
Yersinia enterocolitica, 411

zinc, 235
zirconium, 235